Plumer's

Principles & Practice of
Intravenous Therapy

Plumer's

Principles & Practice of Intravenous Therapy

Sharon M. Weinstein, RN, CRNI, MS

Director, Office of International Affairs
Premier Hospitals Alliance, Inc.
Westchester, Illinois

Infusion Therapy Consultant
Former Faculty, Department of Surgery
University of Health Sciences/The Chicago Medical School
North Chicago, Illinois

Former Vice-Chair, Intravenous Nurses Certification Corporation

Past President, The Intravenous Nurses Society, Inc.

Leader, Intravenous Therapy Delegations to People's Republic of China,
    Commonwealth of Independent States, and Germany

Fifth Edition

J. B. Lippincott Company
Philadelphia

Acquisitions Editor: Margaret Belcher
Sponsoring Editor: Ellen Campbell
Project Editor: Barbara Ryalls
Indexer: Alexandra Nickerson
Design Coordinator: Doug Smock
Cover Designer: Mark James
Production Manager: Helen Ewan
Production Coordinator: Kathryn Rule
Compositor: Circle Graphics
Printer/Binder: R.R. Donnelley and Sons Company
Cover Printer: R.R. Donnelley and Sons Company

5th Edition

6   5   4   3   2   1

Library of Congress Cataloging-in-Publication Data
Weinstein, Sharon.
    Plumer's Principles & practice of intravenous therapy / Sharon
M. Weinstein.—5th ed.
        p.   cm.
    Rev. ed. of: Principles and practice of intravenous therapy /
revised by Ada Lawrence Plumer, Faye Consentino. 4th ed. c1987.
    Includes bibliographical references and index.
    ISBN 0-397-55009-X
    1. Intravenous therapy.   I. Plumer, Ada Lawrence. Principles and
practice of intravenous therapy.   II. Title.   III. Title: Principles
and practice of intravenous therapy.
    [DNLM: 1. Infusions, Parenteral. WB 354 W424p]
RM170.P57 1993
615.8'55—dc20
DNLM/DLC
for Library of Congress   92-48916
                                                                            CIP

Any procedure or practice described in this book should be applied by the healthcare practitioner under appropriate supervision in accordance with professional standards of care used with regard to the unique circumstances that apply in each practice situation. Care has been taken to confirm the accuracy of information presented and to describe generally accepted practices. However, the authors, editors, and publisher cannot accept any responsibility for errors or omissions or for any consequences from application of the information in this book and make no warranty express or implied, with respect to the contents of the book.

Every effort has been made to ensure drug selections and dosages are in accordance with current recommendations and practice. Because of ongoing research, changes in government regulations and the constant flow of information on drug therapy, reactions and interactions, the reader is cautioned to check the package insert for each drug for indications, dosages, warnings and precautions, particularly if the drug is new or infrequently used.

Contributors

Anne Marie Frey, RN, BSN, CRNI
 IV Nurse Clinician
 St. Christopher's Hospital for Children
 Philadelphia, Pennsylvania

Margaret M. McCluskey, RN, OCN, CRNI, MPH
 Oncology Nurse Consultant
 Health Educator
 Evanston Hospital Corporation
 Evanston, Illinois

Susan Y. Pauley, RN, CRNI
 IV Supervisor
 Massachusetts General Hospital
 Boston, Massachusetts

Christine Shaw Regan, RN, BSN
 Nutrition Support Coordinator
 Midwestern Regional Medical Center
 Zion, Illinois

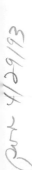

Preface

This fifth edition of **PLUMER'S PRINCIPLES & PRACTICE OF INTRAVENOUS THERAPY,** like its predecessor, provides the most current base of knowledge available for nurses and other health care professionals who share the responsibility of ensuring high-quality infusion care to patients in diverse settings. It meets the vital demand for clinically relevant and current information that the professional must have to provide competent care.

The level of nursing expertise required to deliver infusion care and the manner in which it is delivered have changed rapidly with technologic advances and the expanded range of delivery setting options. The evolution of emerging technology has mandated an unprecedented high level of expertise for delivering infusion therapy. Some technologic advances such as today's vascular access devices not only have ensured the availability of complex therapeutic modalities, but also have altered the face of care delivery settings to embrace high-tech care in the home and infusion centers, and enabled patients to participate in their own care.

Because the nursing professional is held accountable for providing multidimensional high-quality infusion care to the patient in such diverse settings, the nursing student and professional must have a reliable and comprehensive source of information on all aspects of current infusion therapy. **PLUMER'S PRINCIPLES & PRACTICE OF INTRAVENOUS THERAPY, FIFTH EDITION** has been completely updated and reorganized to create the resource that truly meets these needs.

While the structure of the fifth edition retains the six-section organization of the previous edition, the reader will immediately note the change in flow of information and the emphasis on an integrated approach to content. Part I reviews the history, legal implications and organization of the intravenous department. Risk management has been rewritten to encompass quality improvement, consistent with the approach of many health care organizations to a continuous quality improvement program. Staff nurse responsibilities for infusion therapy are included in Part I, plus a new section detailing the role and responsibility of the IV team nurse, since IV teams nationwide are experiencing new growth and visibility in a highly competitive health care market. The clearly defined IV team role adds a new focus to the text.

Part II has been reorganized to follow a natural progression of applicable anatomy and physiology, potential local and systemic complications, sources of contamination and principles of prevention, and relevant laboratory tests. The laboratory values have been updated and now address examples of conversion to Système Internationale (SI) units. The techniques chapter has been expanded to include therapeutic phlebotomy.

Part III, now titled Principles of Equipment Selection and Application, has also been completely updated. The equipment chapter expands to address both new developments in this rapidly changing field and the vast array of equipment now available to the practicing nurse. A comprehensive discussion of intravenous filtration, the concept of "bubble point," and the impact of filtration on IV patient outcome is included. Rate of administration and intra-arterial therapy have also been added to Part III, as have the chapters on central venous catheterization and advanced vascular access (formerly central venous catheters), in an effort to include all equipment and applications in one content area.

Part IV now addresses Applications of Infusion Therapy for Homeostasis, including principles and rationales of fluid and electrolyte balance and principles of parenteral fluid administration. The chapter on total parenteral nutrition has been updated by Christine Shaw Regan, RN, BSN, an experienced metabolic support nurse and former member of the American Society for Parenteral and Enteral Nutrition (ASPEN) Nurses' Committee, to reflect the latest trends in nutrition support nursing. Patient assessment and methods of determining nutritional status have been rewritten. Two appendices detail the role of the nutrition support nurse and guidelines for home total parenteral nutrition consistent with ASPEN Standards. The chapter on transfusion therapy, by Susan Y. Pauley, RN, CRNI, IV Supervisor at Massachusetts General Hospital and a nationally recognized leader in the field of infusion/transfusion therapy, has also been completely rewritten, with greater emphasis on the transmission of blood-borne diseases and the ramifications for practicing clinicians, and includes materials from the American Association of Blood Banks (AABB).

Part V is now titled Pharmacologic Applications of Intravenous Therapy and includes principles of drug administration in a rewritten, updated, and more comprehensive chapter. New tables address the subject of therapeutic drug monitoring and drug clearance times, a source of valuable information for the nurse responsible for the delivery of infusion therapy. A new chapter on pain management is also included in Part V, which discusses all aspects of subcutaneous, intravenous, intrathecal, and epidural pain relief. Nursing interventions are delineated to facilitate delivery of high-quality care to the patient with intractable pain. The chapter on cancer chemotherapy has been renamed Antineoplastic Therapy (consistent with the Standards of Practice of the Intravenous Nurses Society [INS] terminology) and completely rewritten and updated by Margaret M. McCluskey, RN, OCN, CRNI, MPH, an experienced oncology nurse educator and a member of the Oncology Nursing Society's (ONS) education committee.

Part VI, Special Applications of Intravenous Therapy, includes a chapter on Pediatric Intravenous Therapy, which has been rewritten and revised by Anne Marie Frey, RN, BSN, CRNI, a nationally recognized pediatric infusion specialist, to reflect the current state of the art and practice of pediatric infusion. The chapter on Home Infusion Therapy has also been revised to address the intricacies of the home care environment and the needs of patients for whom care is delivered outside the inpatient setting. Third-party payments, billing, and accreditation of home infusion programs are discussed, and new tables and figures provide a ready resource to nurses practicing in this clinical arena.

The fifth edition also addresses practice Standards of INS throughout. In short, this edition has been revised and rewritten with the intent of meeting the total resource needs of the nurse—student, new practitioner, or experienced clinician—responsible for delivering high-quality infusion care, regardless of the clinical setting in which care is provided. Comprehensive and current, **PLUMER'S PRINCIPLES & PRACTICE OF INTRAVENOUS THERAPY, FIFTH EDITION** is an essential tool in any setting in which IV therapy is provided.

Sharon M. Weinstein, RN, CRNI, MS

Special Acknowledgments

As professional nurses practicing infusion therapy, we know what it is that we do, but at times it is difficult to sum up the complexities of our practice. When I chose the infusion therapy specialty, I sought out the only reference available at that time: **PRINCIPLES & PRACTICE OF INTRAVENOUS THERAPY** by Ada Lawrence Plumer. From the original text, I taught myself all there was to know about intravenous therapy. I used it to develop policies and procedures for my first hospital-based IV team. I used it as the basis for my class content and to develop patient teaching tools. Plumer was my roadmap, my guidebook, my Bible. Now, many years later, Ada Plumer's book is my book. As an IV nursing professional, educator, author, and clinician, I am personally and professionally honored to follow Ada Lawrence Plumer as the author of **PLUMER'S PRINCIPLES & PRACTICE OF INTRAVENOUS THERAPY, FIFTH EDITION**. A leader, pacesetter, and cofounder of the professional society, Plumer set the tone for our professional practice, served as a mentor to many nurses and encouraged excellence in the delivery of intravenous nursing care. To Ada, and to Faye Cosentino, co-author of the fourth edition, I express my thanks . . . and the gratitude of countless other nursing professionals in whom you have instilled a passion for intravenous nursing practice.

Acknowledgments

PLUMER'S PRINCIPLES & PRACTICE OF INTRAVENOUS THERAPY, FIFTH EDITION, is the result of the collaborative efforts of its original authors, Ada Lawrence Plumer and Faye Cosentino; the outstanding contributing authors to this edition: Anne Marie Frey, RN, BSN, CRNI, Margaret M. McCluskey, RN, OCN, CRNI, MPH, Susan Y. Pauley, RN, CRNI, and Christine Shaw Regan, RN, BSN; and myself. I am most grateful to them. I would also like to thank the manufacturers of infusion products and equipment for their information and assistance, as well as the authors and publishers who permitted use of their copyright materials in this text.

A special thank you to Ellen Campbell, Margaret Belcher, and Diana Intenzo in the Nursing Division and to Barbara Ryalls in Production at J. B. Lippincott Company for their encouragement, support, and technical assistance in developing a fine manuscript—one that is worthy of supporting the Plumer name.

Thanks are extended to William Eudailey, PharmD, and to the late David Blaess, RPh, who taught me to apply the principles gleaned from Plumer's book to everyday practice.

And finally, thanks to my family, for understanding and acknowledging my passion for sharing my infusion therapy practice via the written word.

SMW

Contents

PART II
Principles of Venipuncture

CHAPTER 9

Potential Complications: Local and Systemic 83

CHAPTER 10

Sources of Contamination and Principles of Prevention 94

CHAPTER 11

Laboratory Tests 113

PART III
Principles of Equipment Selection and Application

PART IV
Applications of Intravenous Therapy for Homeostasis

PART V
Pharmacologic Applications of Intravenous Therapy

Plumer's

Principles & Practice of Intravenous Therapy

PART I

Practice of Intravenous Therapy

CHAPTER 1

History of Intravenous Therapy

EARLY HISTORY

The idea of injecting various substances, including blood, into the circulatory system is not new; it has been in the human mind for centuries. In 1628, William Harvey's discovery of the circulation of the blood stimulated increased experimentation. In 1656, Sir Christopher Wren, with a quill and bladder, injected opium intravenously into dogs, and 6 years later, J. D. Major made the first successful injection in man.[4]

In 1665, an animal near death from loss of blood was restored by infusion of blood from another animal. In 1667, a 15-year-old Parisian boy was the first human to receive a transfusion successfully; lamb's blood was administered directly into the circulation by Jean Baptiste Denis, physician to Louis XIV.[4] The enthusiasm aroused by this success led to promiscuous transfusions of blood from animals to man with fatal results, and in 1687, by an edict of church and parliament, animal-to-man transfusions were prohibited in Europe.

About 150 years passed before serious attempts were again made to inject blood into humans. James Blundell, an English obstetrician, revived the idea. In 1834, saving the lives of many women threatened by hemorrhage during childbirth, he proved that animal blood was unfit to inject into man and that only human blood was safe. Nevertheless, complications persisted; infections developed in donor and recipient. With the discovery of the principles of antisepsis by Pasteur and Lister, another obstacle was overcome, yet reactions and deaths continued.

The first attempt, recorded in 1821, to prevent coagulation during transfusion was by Jean Louis Prévost, a French physician, who, with Jean B. A. Dumas, used defibrinated blood in animal transfusions.[4]

TWENTIETH-CENTURY ADVANCES

In 1900, Karl Landsteiner proved that not all human blood is alike; classifications were made.[4] In 1914, a chemical, sodium citrate, was found to prevent blood from clotting.[4] Since then, rapid advances have been made.

Hugh Leslie Marriot and Alan Kekwick, English physicians, introduced the continuous slow-drip method of blood transfusion; their findings were published in 1935.[4]

Administration of parenteral fluids by the intravenous (IV) route has become widely used only during the past 40 years. The difficulty in accepting this procedure was the

Sharon M. Weinstein: PLUMER'S PRINCIPLES & PRACTICE OF INTRAVENOUS THERAPY, FIFTH EDITION, © 1993 J. B. Lippincott Company

result of lack of safe solutions. The solutions used contained substances called pyrogens, proteins that are foreign to the body and not destroyed by sterilization. These caused chills and fever when injected into the circulation. About 1923, with the discovery and elimination of these pyrogens, the IV administration of parenteral fluids became safer and more frequent.

Until 1925, the most frequently used parenteral solution was normal saline solution. Because of its hypotonicity, water could not be administered IV and had to be made isotonic; sodium chloride achieved this effect.[2] After 1925, dextrose was used extensively to make isotonic solutions and to provide a source of calories.[2]

In the early 1930s, administration of an IV injection was a major procedure reserved for the critically ill patient. The physician performed the venipuncture, assisted by a nurse. The success of IV therapy and the great increase in its use led to the establishment of a department of specially trained personnel for infusion therapy. In 1940, the Massachusetts General Hospital became one of the first hospitals to assign a nurse as an IV specialist. The services of the IV nurse consisted of administering IV solutions and transfusions, cleaning infusion sets, and cleaning and sharpening needles. Emphasis was placed on the technical responsibility of maintaining the infusion and keeping the needle patent. The sole requisite of the IV nurse was the ability to perform a venipuncture skillfully.

As knowledge of electrolyte and fluid therapy grew, more solutions became available, and further knowledge was needed to monitor the fluid and electrolyte status of the patient. Normal saline was no longer the only electrolyte solution. Today more than 200 commercially prepared IV fluids are available to meet every need of the patient.

In the middle 1940s, disposable plastic sets became available and eventually replaced the reusable rubber tubings.

A whole new approach to IV therapy and a respite to the starving patient evolved in 1965 when members of the Harrison Department of Surgical Research at the University of Pennsylvania showed that sufficient nutrients could be given to juvenile beagle dogs to support normal growth and development.[1] This led to what is known today as total parenteral nutrition.

In the middle 1960s, Dr. Stanley Dudrick developed the first formula for parenteral nutrition, a method by which sufficient nutrients are administered into the central vein to support life and maintain one's growth and development.

Glass containers were first used for IV solutions. Plastic bags were introduced in the 1970s; since air venting is not required, the risk of air embolism and airborne contamination was reduced. Today, plastic is the primary container for IV solutions. Glass containers are used when stability of the infusate in plastic is a concern.

The 1970s brought tremendous scientific, technologic, and medical advances, and IV therapy gained recognition as a highly specialized field. Nurses performed many of the functions formerly reserved for the medical staff—intra-arterial therapy, neonatal therapy, and antineoplastic therapy. Professional organizations were established to provide a forum for the exchange of ideas, information, experiences, and knowledge, with the ultimate goal of raising standards and increasing the level of patient care.

On October 1, 1980, the United States House of Representatives recognized the profession and declared an official day of honor for IV nurses: "Resolved, that IV Nurse Day be nationally celebrated in honor of the National Intravenous Therapy Association, Inc. on January 25 of each year." The proclamation was presented by the Honorable

Edward J. Mackey from the Fifth Congressional District of the Commonwealth of Massachusetts.[3]

RECENT INNOVATIONS

The Intravenous Nurses Society, Inc. (INS), formerly National Intravenous Therapy Association (NITA), has experienced tremendous growth nationwide. Educational offerings have been expanded to include advanced studies in an effort to meet the needs of the advanced practitioner. The Intravenous Nurses Certification Corporation (INCC) likewise expanded to include the National Board of IV Nurse Examiners, the LP/VN Board of Nurse Examiners, and an Executive Committee.

Professional IV nurses are encouraged to prepare for the credentialing process through videotapes, a core curriculum, educational programs, the society's professional journal, and published Standards of Practice.

Intravenous therapy delivery has permeated all clinical settings; the growth of high-tech infusion therapies followed. The growth of this specialty practice has resulted in expanded roles for IV nurses nationally and internationally.

Manufacturers have continued to keep pace with demands for technologically advanced products that ensure patient safety and reliability in the delivery of infusion therapy.

REFERENCES

1. Dudrick, S. J. (1971). Rational intravenous therapy. *American Journal of Hospital Pharmacy 28*, 83.
2. Elman, R. (1949). Fluid balance from the nurse's point of view. *American Journal of Nursing 49*, 222.
3. Gardner, C. (1982). United States House of Representatives honors the National Intravenous Therapy Association, Inc. *Journal of the National Intravenous Therapy Association 14*(1), 5(1), 14.
4. Schmidt, J. E. (1959) *Medical discoveries who and when* (p. 59). Springfield, IL: C. Thomas.

CHAPTER 2

Legal Implications of Intravenous Therapy

Because of the law and its interpretation, doubts and questions exist regarding the legal rights of nurses to administer IV therapy. As the scope of IV therapy has become more complex and specialized, nurses have become more involved in administration procedures formerly performed solely by physicians and considered medical acts. Since violation of the Medical Practice Act is considered a criminal offense, IV nurses should be well versed in such procedures.

PROFESSIONAL AND GOVERNMENTAL REGULATIONS

To alleviate the nurse's fears regarding possible liability for claimed violation of the Medical Practice Act, the medical profession has issued joint policy statements with nursing associations on a number of procedures, including IV therapy.

Joint statements are written when questions arise regarding the nurse's professional responsibility or obligation to perform specific therapeutic measures and these questions are not answered in existing statutes (ie, nursing practice acts and medical practice acts). This is considered the most useful way to deal with procedures performed by members of both professions.

Sponsors of joint statements are the state nurses' association, which is concerned with the area of nursing practice; the state medical society, which is concerned with therapeutic measures that were formerly considered solely the practice of medicine and which legally must be prescribed by the physician; and the state hospital association, which is concerned with institutional liability for therapeutic measures performed in member health care facilities.

Other ways of dealing with procedures are through rulings made by attorney generals, by state boards of nursing, and by the interpretation of the Nurse Practice Act. In some states, the nurse practice acts relating to the definition of nursing are global and do not refer to specific procedures because it is believed that with frequent changes in professional practice, it would not be feasible to have state legislators review such changes before implementation in a practice setting.

State boards of nursing have sought the input of IV nursing professionals and the professional societies to ensure high levels of care.

Sharon M. Weinstein: PLUMER'S PRINCIPLES & PRACTICE OF INTRAVENOUS THERAPY, FIFTH EDITION, © 1993 J. B. Lippincott Company

Professional nursing societies are taking an expanded role in decision-making as it pertains to the specialty practice. Standards of practice have been developed that provide a criterion for judgment and ensure maximal safety for the patient as well as protection for the physician, nurse, and health care organization.

To answer the question "Can I legally administer IV therapy?" each nurse must ask the following questions:

1. Does the state law delegate this function to the nurse?
2. Does the particular institution's or agency's policy, with the approval of the medical staff, permit the nurse to perform this function?
3. Is the nurse limited in the types of fluids and medications he or she may administer by a list delineated by the hospital?
4. Is the order written by a licensed physician for a specific patient?
5. Is the nurse qualified by education and experience to administer IV therapy?

Nurses may properly refuse to perform IV therapy if in their professional judgment they are not qualified and competent. It has been established by law that in a question of negligence, individuals are not protected because they have "carried out the physician's orders." They are held liable in relation to their knowledge, skill, and judgment.

In hospitals and states in which no written opinion relevant to IV therapy exists, what is the registered nurse's responsibility when ordered by a licensed staff physician to administer IV therapy? "A nurse is legally required to carry out any nursing or medical procedure she is directed to carry out by a duly licensed physician unless she has reason to believe harm will result to the patient from doing so."[1] To meet their legal responsibilities to patients, nurses must be qualified by knowledge and experience to execute the procedure, otherwise they may properly refuse to perform it. "Where there is no medical reason to question a physician's order, the nurse's failure to carry out such an order will subject her to liability for any consequent harm to the patient."[1]

States are recommending that schools of professional nursing include in their curriculum a course that will offer the student nurse clinical instruction and experience in IV therapy. IV nursing specialists have been instrumental in developing the content for such programs.

The Private Duty Nurse

A private duty nurse, who works under the direction, supervision, and control of a hospital and private physician, is subject to the rules and regulations of the hospital concerning all matters relating to nursing care. If the hospital policy-making committee has rules regarding who may and may not give IV therapy, the private duty nurse is subject to the same rules that apply to the staff nurse. To prevent any misunderstanding on the part of the private duty nurse, a specific sentence may be added to the hospital's joint policy statement noting that the private duty nurse who has complied with the criteria applicable to the administration of IV therapy may give an IV infusion.

The Agency Nurse

Temporary staffing agencies continue to proliferate nationwide, providing valuable assistance during times when a shortage of licensed professional personnel occurs. When given responsibility for the administration of intravascular therapies, agency personnel must be oriented to the facility's policies and procedures and the functions performed by a specialized department. Every effort should be made to ensure patient safety, public protection, and viability of the IV program.

LEGAL GUIDELINES

The IV nurse's fear of involvement in malpractice suits is increasing with the growth in complexity of therapy and numbers of IV specialists. Many of the functions performed by the nurse have important legal consequences. An understanding of the legal principles and guidelines involved is necessary if daily professional actions are not to result in unwanted malpractice suits. It will be easier to have a clearer understanding of these guidelines if a few of the legal terms are first defined.

Definitions

Criminal law relates to an offense against the general public because of its harmful effect on the welfare of society as a whole. Criminal actions are prosecuted by a government authority, and punishment includes imprisonment or fine, or both. The administration of IV therapy, if performed in an unlawful manner, can involve the nurse in criminal conduct. Violation of the Nursing Practice Act or the Medical Practice Act by an unlicensed person is considered a criminal offense.

Civil law deals with conduct that affects the legal rights of the private person or corporation. When harm occurs, the guilty party may be required to pay damages to the injured person.

A *tort* is a private wrong, by act or omission, which can result in a civil action by the harmed person. Common torts relevant to professional nursing practice include negligence, assault, battery, false imprisonment, slander, libel, and invasion of privacy. There are some defenses in civil actions, such as contributory negligence on the part of the plaintiff.

Coercion of a rational adult patient in order to insert a cannula constitutes *assault* (the threat to do harm) *and battery* (actually hitting or forcing). If the patient refuses treatment, and explanation and encouragement fail, the physician should be notified.

Malpractice is the negligent conduct of professional persons. Negligent conduct is not acting in a reasonable and prudent manner, with resultant damage to a person or that individual's property. It is not synonymous with carelessness, although a person who is careless is negligent.

If a nurse with no previous training administers an IV infusion, performs an arterial puncture, or adds medications to IV fluids, and does it as carefully as possible but harm results, a civil court may rule such conduct as negligent; that nurse should not have performed the act without previous training and experience. Such a negligent action is considered an act of malpractice because it involves a professional person. However, if the act of malpractice does not create harm, legal action cannot be initiated.

The *rule of personal liability* is "every person is liable for his own tortious conduct" (his own wrongdoing).[1] No physician can protect the nurse from an act of negligence by bypassing this rule with verbal assurance. The nurse involved cannot avoid legal liability even though another person may be sued and held liable. The physician who orders placement of a peripherally inserted central catheter (PICC) cannot assume responsibility for the nurse who is negligent in implementing the procedure. If harm occurs as a result of the action, the nurse is liable for this wrongdoing.

The rule of personal liability is relevant in medication errors. Medication errors are a common cause of malpractice claims against nurses.[2] Negligence results from the administration of a drug to the wrong patient, at the wrong time, in an incorrect dosage, or in an improperly prescribed manner. If the physician writes an incomplete or partially illegible order and the nurse fails to clarify it before administration and harm results, the nurse is liable for negligence. The same applies to the administration of IV fluids. Nurses have a legal and professional responsibility to know the purpose and effect of the IV fluids and medications they administer. They must take care to ensure that patients receive the prescribed volume of fluid at the prescribed rate of flow. Fluid administered in an amount above or below that ordered constitutes an error that can result in fluid and electrolyte imbalances and lead to serious consequences for the patient and litigation for the nurse.

Nursing Role

The act of *observation* is the legal and professional responsibility of the nurse. Frequent observation is imperative for the early detection and prevention of complications. Undetected complications that are allowed to increase in severity because of failure to observe the patient constitute an act of negligence on the part of the nurse.

The rule of personal liability applies to supervisors and nurses under their supervision. Supervisors usually will not be held liable for the negligence of nurses under their supervision because every person is liable for his or her own wrongdoing. However, a supervisor is expected to know if the nurse is competent to perform assigned duties without supervision. Supervisors who are negligent in the assignment of an inexperienced nurse or a nurse who requires supervision may be held liable for the acts of the nurse.[1] Nurses themselves are always held liable.

Nurse–patient relationships play a significant role in influencing patients to initiate legal liability against nurses. Intravenous nurses must be particularly aware of and attentive to the emotional needs of their patients. Inserting cannulas can cause pain and apprehension in patients. Specialists must develop appropriate interpersonal relationships. Nurses who are impersonal, aloof, and so busy with the technical process of starting an IV infusion that they have no time for establishing kindly relationships with patients are the suit-prone nurses whose personalities may initiate resentment and later malpractice suits. Patients most likely to sue are those who are resentful, frequently hostile, uncooperative, and dissatisfied with the nursing care. By demonstrating respect, care, and concern for all patients, as well as rendering skilled, efficient nursing care, nurses may avoid malpractice claims.

Policies and procedures should be detailed, and all nurses practicing infusion therapy should be required to know and review them periodically. Policies and procedures should follow national guidelines established by the Centers for Disease Control and Prevention (CDC) and Standards of Practice established by the Intravenous Nurses Society (INS). These guidelines provide a model for IV nurses and foster optimal care for the patient receiving IV therapy.

Credentialing

Credentialing of IV nurses nationwide began with the first certification examination in 1985. The credentialing process consists of three components: (1) licensure, (2) accreditation, and (3) certification. *Licensure* represents the entry into practice level afforded to all professional nurses who successfully complete the registered nurse examination.

Accreditation reflects a program or service meeting established guidelines. Accreditation is offered to facilities, agencies, and other health care providers by groups like the Joint Commission on Accreditation of Healthcare Organizations (JCAHO) and the Community Health Accreditation Program (CHAP), administered by the National League for Nursing (NLN).

Certification is the highest level attainable by the professional IV nurse. It is the process by which a society attests to the professional and clinical competence of the individual who successfully completes the process.

Evaluation of Adequate Performance

A standard must be carefully defined for the health care institution or the nurse to evaluate adequate performance. Tools useful in this process include the following:[2]

1. INS Standards of Practice
2. State Board of Nursing regulations for registered nurses and licensed practical/vocational nurses
3. American Nurses' Association Standards of Nursing Practice
4. Policies and procedures of the employing health care institution or agency

PLACEMENT OF THE PERIPHERALLY INSERTED CENTRAL CATHETER

The placement of a PICC requires special training and demonstrated competency on the part of the professional registered nurse. Each state sets its own practice guidelines, and not all states consider the placement of PICC catheters to be within the scope of professional nursing practice. It is incumbent on the institution or facility to contact the respective State Board of Nursing to determine policy. Each health care facility must establish criteria for qualification within its own legal guidelines. Such a program should include:

- Indications
- Advantages
- Placement technique
- Complications
- Care and maintenance
- Legal issues
- Product education

Minimal standards for successful completion of an educational program include the following:

- Satisfactory performance during initial probationary/review period
- Successful completion of in-house IV certification course
- Clinical competency evidenced by actual practice
- Successful completion of in-house requirements for PICC insertion

REFERENCES

1. Bernzweig, E. P. (1981). *Nurse's liability for malpractice* (3rd ed, p. 68). New York: McGraw-Hill.

2. Guarriello, D. L. (1983). Intravenous therapy and the law. *Journal of the National Intravenous Therapy Association, 6,* 278.

BIBLIOGRAPHY

Revised intravenous nursing standards of practice. (1990). *Journal of Intravenous Nursing,* (Suppl.), S17.

REVIEW QUESTIONS

1. Which of the following rules indicates that "every person is liable for his own tortious conduct"?
   a. negligent action
   b. personal liability
   c. tortious conduct
   d. Wrongdoing act

2. Coercion of a rational adult patient in order to insert a cannula is which of the following?
   a. assault
   b. battery
   c. a only
   d. a and b

3. The credentialing process consists of which of the following components?
   a. licensure
   b. accreditation
   c. certification
   d. all of the above

4. Tools used to evaluate adequate performance include which of the following?
   a. INS Standards of Practice
   b. State Board regulations
   c. Institutional policies/procedures
   d. all of the above

5. A PICC training program should include which of the following?
   a. practicum
   b. technique
   c. a and b
   d. b only

Organization of an Intravenous Department

INTRAVENOUS NURSING TEAMS _____

It is now well established that an IV nursing team enhances the level of care that an institution or facility may provide. The quality of patient care is improved because specialized nurses, freed from other responsibilities, are able to focus their attention on developing high standards of performance. Such nurses, cognizant of the potential dangers of infusion therapy, are vigilant and meticulous in performing and maintaining IV therapy. Their high standards of performance contribute to atraumatic venipunctures, conservation of veins for future use, and reduction of routine complications. The knowledge, skills, and abilities of these specialized nurses ensure patient safety. Intravenous nursing teams continue to proliferate nationwide as more health care institutions recognize their value.

With the increasing complexity of IV therapies and the potential dangers associated with this practice, hospitals have recognized the value of IV therapy teams. Parenteral departments have been established in a great many hospitals and home care programs nationwide.

LEADERSHIP _____

Because the functions performed by the IV department are not generally classified as nursing procedures, the responsibility for this department is often allocated to the head of another department directly involved in the functions of IV therapy, such as the director of the blood bank, the pharmacy, or the anesthesia department. The IV department fulfills an important function of the blood bank, administering bloods and blood components; is in close alliance with the pharmacy, administering infusions of which 50% to 80% contain drugs; and executes many of the functions performed by the anesthesiologist. IV departments may also function as self-contained cost centers within the institution's infrastructure.

PHILOSOPHY AND OBJECTIVES _____

In organizing a department, the first consideration should be to establish a philosophy and the objectives necessary to support such a philosophy. An example follows:

Sharon M. Weinstein: PLUMER'S PRINCIPLES &
PRACTICE OF INTRAVENOUS THERAPY, FIFTH
EDITION, © 1993 J. B. Lippincott Company

Philosophy

To administer safe and successful IV therapy in the best interests of the patient, the hospital, and the nursing profession.

Objectives

The objectives of an IV department are:

1. To develop skills and impart knowledge that will provide a high level of safety in the practice of IV therapy (embodies administration of solutions and drugs, administration of blood and blood components, placement of IV cannulas, and withdrawal of blood samples)
2. To encourage further education and knowledge in the field of IV therapy
3. To assist in keeping the nursing staff educated in the maintenance of IV therapy and other nursing needs relevant to IV therapy
4. To collaborate with orientation personnel in the development and implementation of continuing education in IV therapy
5. To develop nursing judgment in IV therapy
6. To keep abreast of the latest scientific and medical advances and their implications in the practice of IV therapy

FUNCTIONS OF THE DEPARTMENT

In organizing an IV department, the functions to be performed must be delineated. They may include:

1. Administration of parenteral fluids
2. Preparation and administration of drugs in solution
3. Administration of blood and blood components
4. Routine inspection and daily change of all infusion tubings and dressings
5. Therapeutic phlebotomy
6. Collection of venous blood samples for all laboratories: chemistry, bacteriology, hematology, blood bank, and so on. This includes:
   a. Collection of blood samples from central lines
   b. Knowledge of the requirements of the various laboratory tests, including the proper collection and handling of blood samples
7. Total parenteral nutrition
8. Antineoplastic therapy
9. Intra-arterial therapy
10. Pediatric IV therapy
11. Home infusion therapy
12. Outpatient procedures
13. Pain management

Policies and Procedures

Policies and procedures play a vital role in the functioning of a department, serving as a guide to its operations, providing the nurse with adequate instruction, and ensuring the patient of a high level of nursing care. They may also provide legal protection in determining whether or not an individual involved in negligent conduct has had adequate instruction in performing the act.

Policies and procedures should comply with state and federal laws, and national guidelines should be followed. The Joint Commission on Accreditation of Healthcare Organizations (JCAHO) publishes a manual for both hospital and home care accreditation. The American Association of Blood Banks (AABB) provides a technical manual with standards for care and administration of blood and component therapy. The Centers for Disease Control and Prevention (CDC) and Intravenous Nurses Society (INS) provide guidelines as well as Standards of Practice.[1]

Policies describing the responsibilities of the IV nurse vary significantly among hospitals and should be outlined to prevent confusion or misunderstanding. Examples of a few such policies follow.

Administration of Parenteral Fluids

1. IV nurses will, on written order, initiate all infusions, with the exception of those not approved for administration by the nurse.
2. No more than two attempts at venipuncture will be allowed.
3. Venipunctures should be avoided in the lower extremities except when the patient's condition may necessitate this use and this location has specifically been ordered by the physician.

Preparation and Administration of Intravenous Drugs

1. Nurses will, on written order, prepare and administer only those solutions, medications, and combinations of drugs approved in writing by the pharmacy and the therapeutics committee.
2. Nurses must check the patient's clinical record and question the patient regarding sensitivity to drugs that may cause anaphylaxis. They must observe the patient following initial administration of such drugs.

Use of Force in Performing Venipuncture

No coercion will ever be used on a rational adult patient. A patient may refuse treatment.

Patency Flushing

Flushing with heparinized saline solution to ensure and maintain patency of an intermittent IV cannula shall be accomplished at established intervals.[2] The concentration of heparinized saline used should not alter the patient's clotting factors.

Incompatibility Flushing

Flushing with 0.9% sodium chloride shall be done prior to and following administration of medications and solutions that are incompatible.

Product Integrity

All IV therapy products are to be checked for integrity before use.

Nursing Care Plan
A nursing care plan should be established within 24 hours of date/time of admission.

Peripheral Cannula Selection
The cannula selected should be of the smallest gauge and shortest length to accommodate the prescribed therapy. Only radiopaque catheters may be used.

Personnel Qualifications

The IV nurse is usually a registered nurse who is specially hired and trained, since IV therapy involves the administration of drugs, blood, and fluids requiring specialized judgment and skill. Because of the highly specialized therapy and the responsibility involved, the success of the department depends on the selection of its personnel. Not all nurses are successful as IV nurses.

The nurse, who will be drawing blood samples and giving transfusions where carelessness can mean a patient's life, must be conscientious. The importance of the job, the importance of being accurate, and the importance of careful patient identification must be realized by the nurse. Duties include mixing and administering drugs which, given IV, act rapidly. There is no margin for error.

Cooperation and teamwork are essential to the success of the department. No one individual's job is finished until the entire department has completed its work. If one nurse becomes involved in a time-consuming emergency, the others must be ready and willing to assist and accomplish the remaining work.

Mental and emotional stability are important in the nurse's success as an IV specialist. Manual dexterity, necessary in administering an IV infusion, is greatly affected by the mental and emotional attitude of the nurse. The performance of few procedures is so easily affected by stress as is the execution of a difficult venipuncture.

An understanding and pleasant personality are other assets necessary to the success of the individual and the department. The nurse has unpleasant functions to perform, which are better tolerated by the patient if the nurse is empathetic.

Tact is important. The nurse works in close conjunction with the hospital nursing staff, ancillary departments, and the patient. An inappropriate attitude and uncooperative personality can do much to impair harmony and disrupt care.

The nurse in charge of the IV department, who must assume responsibility for the teaching, training, and successful functioning of this department, should have a voice in selecting its personnel.

Once the functions of this department are classified, the work load should start at a reasonable level. It may be desirable to start by performing only a few designated functions, such as the administration of blood and fluids. After this program has been successfully organized, other functions may be added. By so doing, the problems that may arise when initiating such a program could be met and remedied, and the success of the department may be guaranteed from the outset.

Before this department can be operational, the hospital nursing staff must first be apprised of its functions.

Call System

A system for receiving calls must be organized, with special emphasis on emergency calls. Some systems work better than others under various conditions. The size of the hospital, number of patients, size and location of the department, and the functions to be performed must be taken into consideration in deciding which system would be most adaptable.

Requisitions

Requests for parenteral administrations and other functions may be filled out on requisitions and sent to the department. This system has the drawbacks of added paperwork, lost time involved, and the necessity of the IV nurse having to return to the department to pick up the requisitions. It may prove successful in a smaller hospital, where calls are not as numerous as in a large hospital and where the nurses are stationed in the blood bank or pharmacy.

Page System

The page operator lists the floor extensions as they are received. The IV nurse calls in every half hour to pick up calls. Any emergency call may be put through by means of voice page or by means of a radio pager.

Routine Rounds

Routine rounds may be made twice a day by the IV nurse. The requests for services are listed on a clipboard with the patient's name and room number. When orders have been filled, they are checked off by the IV nurse. Emergencies are handled by pager.

This system involves less expenditure of time by the nursing staff. It eliminates the necessity for placing calls or sending out requisitions. The IV department is freed from unnecessary phone calls. The charge nurse, with a glance at the board, immediately knows what procedures have been performed.

Preparation of Equipment

Setting up the necessary equipment for procedures to be performed must be allotted to either the IV department or the nursing staff.

Preparation of Equipment by the Intravenous Department

When preparation of equipment becomes the responsibility of the IV department, an equipment cart must be provided on each floor. This cart carries all necessary equipment for parenteral administration as follows:

IV solutions	Alcohol, povidone prep pads
Venous access devices	Syringes
Armboards	Sterile sponges
Administration sets	Antiseptic swabs and ointment
Filters	Transparent dressings
Tourniquet	IV start kits
Tape	

The professional IV nurse ascertains the accuracy of the physician's order and assembles supplies from the cart maintained on each nursing unit or from alternative means.

Other Systems
Regardless of the method of securing equipment for venipuncture, the IV nurse has a crucial role in determining accuracy of the order, assembling the appropriate equipment consistent with the therapy that has been ordered, and using the equipment in a safe manner.

Interdepartmental Communications

Patients with infusions in progress may visit ancillary hospital departments during their hospital stay, including medical imaging, nuclear medicine, surgery, and others. To ensure the success and viability of an IV therapy department/team, other departments within the institution must be oriented to the team's functions. If orders are written early in the day, it will be easier to meet all requests and to ensure timely delivery of therapy to each patient under the team's care.

DIDACTIC PROGRAM

An adequate teaching program and criteria for the evaluation of the IV nurse must be established. The criteria depend on the role of the IV nurse as dictated by hospital policies. The competency of the nurse must be evaluated and maintained. The IV nurse receives on-the-job training. The length of time involved in teaching depends on the individual and may range from 6 to 8 weeks. The following is a suggested outline for teaching IV, drug, and transfusion therapy.

Suggested Teaching Outline

    I. Legal implications of IV therapy
      A. State policy
        1. Review state rulings, joint policies related to IV therapy.
      B. Hospital policy
        1. Review health institution's or agency's policy, which has been approved by the medical staff.
        2. Responsibilities of nurse in administering IV therapy
        3. List of fluids and drugs delineated by the hospital for administration by the nurse
      C. National standards
        1. CDC
        2. INS
      D. Legal requirements
        1. Qualification by education and experience
        2. Adherence to hospital policy
        3. Thorough knowledge of fluids and drugs: their effects, limitations, and dosages
        4. Order by licensed physician for specific patient
        5. Skilled judgment
      E. Review of policy and procedure books
        1. Policy statements do not provide immunity if the nurse is negligent.
        2. The nurse is legally responsible for his or her own actions.

II. Equipment
  A. Review all types of equipment, their characteristics and usage.
  B. Review procedures for the proper handling of equipment, changing of administration sets, use of products.
  C. Adhere to established infection control procedures and guidelines in the use of equipment.
    1. Aseptic technique in manipulation of equipment
    2. Inspection of parenteral fluids and containers
    3. Scheduled change of administration sets

III. Anatomy and physiology as applied to IV therapy
  A. Review names and locations of peripheral veins of the upper extremity.
  B. Differentiate between arteries and veins. Recognize an inadvertent arterial puncture.
  C. Recognize dangers associated with the use of veins of the lower extremities.
  D. Understand factors that influence the size and condition of the vein.
    1. Trauma
    2. Temperature
    3. Diagnosis of the patient
    4. Psychological outlook of the patient
  E. Choose veins suitable for venipuncture
    1. To infuse various fluids and medications, with preservation of veins in mind
    2. To draw blood samples
    3. To administer blood

IV. IV therapy
  A. Methods of infusion
    1. Continuous
    2. Intermittent
    3. Electronic infusion device
  B. Manner and approach to the patient
    1. Explain the vasovagal reaction (an undesirable autonomic nervous system response).
    2. Alleviate fears.
      a. Make patient comfortable.
      b. Explain procedure.
      c. Reassure patient.
      d. Appear confident.
  C. Methods of venous distention
    1. Apply a broad tourniquet above selected site.
    2. Apply a blood pressure cuff inflated to 50 to 60 mm Hg or to just below diastolic pressure.
    3. Have patient clench fist periodically.
    4. Allow arm to hang dependent over the side of the bed.
    5. Tap lightly slightly distal to the proposed venipuncture site.
    6. Apply moist heat to entire extremity.
  D. Antiseptic and aseptic technique. Skin flora have been implicated as an important source of organisms responsible for catheter-associated

infection. Stress importance of handwashing. Adherence to aseptic technique is imperative, especially during preparation of the venipuncture site.

E. Choice of cannula (steel needle, catheter)
1. Purpose of the infusion
2. Condition and availability of the vein
3. Gauge and length of cannula depend on:
   a. Location of the vein
   b. Fluid used
   c. Purpose of the infusion
   d. Available venous access

F. Techniques of venipuncture
1. Steel needle
2. Syringe and needle
3. Vacuum tube and needle holder (commercially supplied)
4. Catheters (over-the-needle, through-the-needle). Complications associated with catheters include mechanical and chemical thrombophlebitis, infection, and catheter embolism.

G. Hazards and complications. Observing the patient, reporting reactions, and taking measures to prevent complications are the nurse's legal and professional responsibilities.
1. Systemic complications
   a. Infections (septicemia, fungemia)
      Preventive measures:
      (1) Use aseptic technique.
      (2) Inspect all fluids and containers before use.
      (3) Use fluids within 24 hours.
      (4) Change administration sets consistent with published standards.
      (5) Do not irrigate plugged cannulas.
      (6) Remove nonfunctioning sets and needles.
   b. Pulmonary embolism (occurs when a substance, usually a clot, becomes free floating and is propelled by the venous circulation to the right side of the heart and into the pulmonary artery)
      Preventive measures:
      (1) Use clot filters for infusing blood and blood components.
      (2) Use special blood filters of micropore size for infusing several units of stored bank blood.
      (3) Avoid using veins of the lower extremities.
      (4) Avoid irrigating plugged cannulas.
   c. Air embolism (may be fatal when small bubbles accumulate dangerously and form tenacious bubbles that block the pulmonary capillaries)
      Preventive measures:
      (1) Vigilance in preventing fluid containers from emptying. Infusions through a central venous catheter carry greater risk of running dry because a negative venous pressure is more likely.
      (2) Vented Y-type infusions or piggyback infusions allowing solutions to run simultaneously may introduce air into line if con-

tainer empties. Check valves, safety valves, and micropore filters (wet) reduce this risk.

   d. Circulatory overload (a real hazard in patients with impaired renal and cardiac functions)

   Preventive measures:

   (1) Maintain infusion at prescribed flow rate. Do not play "catch-up" if infusion is behind schedule.

   (2) Never apply positive pressure when infusing fluids and blood.

   (3) Do not administer fluids in excess of quantity ordered to maintain a keep-open infusion.

   (4) Be alert to signs of circulatory overload.

   e. Speed shock (systemic reaction occurring when a substance foreign to the body is rapidly introduced into the circulation)

   Preventive measures:

   (1) Slow injection of drugs

   (2) Use of controlled-volume chambers

   (3) Use of microbore drip sets

   (4) Use of double clamps—an extra clamp ensures greater safety should the initial clamp let go.

   (5) Ensure that IV fluid is flowing freely before regulating flow.

   f. Fluid and medication error

   Preventive measures:

   (1) Be familiar with IV fluids.

   (2) Know drug, dosage, and rate of administration.

   (3) Clarify orders.

   (4) Verify identity of the patient and the admixture.

  2. Local complications

   a. Phlebitis (mechanical, chemical, and septic)

   Preventive measures:

   (1) Do not use veins located over an area of joint flexion.

   (2) Anchor cannulas well to prevent motion and reduce the risk of introducing microorganisms into puncture wound.

   (3) Adequately dilute medications.

   (4) Use a cannula relatively smaller than the vein.

   (5) Use aseptic and antiseptic technique.

   (6) Remove cannula within 48 hours.

   (7) Remove cannula for:

     (a) Erythema

     (b) Induration

     (c) Tenderness by palpation of venous cord

     (d) Nonfunctioning needle

   b. Infiltration (recognize extravasation)

   (1) Check questionable extremity against normal extremity.

   (2) Apply a tourniquet tightly enough to restrict venous flow proximal to the injection site. If infusion continues regardless of this venous obstruction, extravasation is evident.

H. Intra-arterial therapy

  1. Arterial puncture

        a. Syringe and needle
        b. Indwelling catheter
    2. Constant arterial pressure monitoring
        a. Set-up procedure
    3. Arterial blood gases (ABG)
        a. Collection
        b. Interpretation
    4. Swan-Ganz catheter
        a. Basic knowledge
        b. Insertion
        c. Complications
V. Rationale of fluid and electrolyte therapy
  A. Fundamentals of fluid and electrolyte metabolism
    1. Body fluid compartments
    2. Electrolyte composition
    3. Acid–base balance
  B. Principles of fluid therapy
    1. Deficit
    2. Maintenance
    3. Replacement
  C. IV fluids
    1. Classification and effect
        a. Isotonic
        b. Hypotonic
        c. Hypertonic
    2. Parenteral fluids
VI. Drug therapy
  A. Hazards
    1. Incompatibilities
        a. Therapeutic (undesirable reaction from overlapping effect of two drugs)
        b. Physical (interaction that leads to a visible change such as color, precipitate, or gas bubbles)
        c. Chemical (invisible interaction, with degradation of drug and loss of therapeutic activity)
    2. Vascular trauma
    3. Speed shock
    4. Bacterial and fungal contamination
    5. Particulate contamination
    6. Medication errors
  B. Knowledge of the drug
    1. Dose and effect
    2. Recommended rate of infusion
    3. Reactions
    4. Contraindications
  C. Factors controlling stability and compatibility of admixtures
    1. Pharmaceutical agents in drug formation (buffers, preservatives, and stabilizers)

   2. Brand of drug (formulation varies)
   3. pH of drug, pH of IV fluid
   4. Concentration (degree of dilution)
   5. Order of mixing
   6. Diluent
   7. Period of time solution stands
   8. Light
   9. Temperature
  D. Preparation of admixture
     1. Procedure for transcribing orders on medication label
     2. Frequency with which medication order should be renewed
     3. Reconstitution of drug using aseptic and antiseptic technique
        a. Correct diluent
        b. Correct volume
        c. Absence of particulate matter
     4. Procedure for adding drug to fluid container
     5. Stability of the admixture
     6. Labeling
  E. Administration of drugs
     1. Verify identity of patient and admixture.
     2. Check for sensitivities of patient to any drug that may cause an-
        aphylaxis.
     3. Observe patient for untoward reactions when administering an initial
        dose of an antibiotic.
     4. Patients known to be sensitive to a drug require the presence of a
        physician.
     5. Inspect admixture each time before administration.
     6. Record drug, dosage, and amount of fluid on fluid intake chart and
        medication sheet.
VII. Transfusion therapy
  A. Principles of immunohematology
     1. Factors governing red blood cell destruction
     2. ABO compatibility
     3. Rh compatibility
     4. Handling and storage of blood
  B. Blood and blood components
     1. Uses
     2. Methods of administration
     3. Reactions and protocol to follow
  C. Administration of blood and blood components
     1. Order for the transfusion must be written on the day the transfusion is
        scheduled.
     2. Substantiate identity of patient and blood.
     3. Inspect blood before administration.
     4. Follow proper technique in administration.
     5. Observe patient.
     6. Document in patient's record.

REFERENCES

1. Centers for Disease Control. (1982). Guidelines for prevention of intravascular infection. *Journal of the National Intravenous Therapy Association, 5*(1), 39.

2. *Revised intravenous nursing standards of practice.* (1990). *Journal of Intravenous Nursing,* (Suppl.), S7.

REVIEW QUESTIONS

1. Parenteral infusion teams are a part of the program in which of the following?
   a. home care companies
   b. acute care hospitals
   c. clinics
   d. all of the above

2. Leadership of the IV department may be:
   a. self-directed
   b. pharmacy
   c. administration
   d. any of the above

3. Policies and procedures should comply with which of the following?
   a. state and federal laws
   b. local ordinances
   c. county rules and regulations
   d. local law

4. Concentration of heparinized saline used should:
   a. not alter patient's clotting factors
   b. alter patient's clotting factors
   c. minimally alter patient's bleeding time
   d. not alter patient's bleeding time

5. A cannula selected for peripheral infusion therapy should be:
   a. largest gauge and longest length
   b. smallest gauge and shortest length
   c. largest gauge and shortest length
   d. smallest gauge and longest length

CHAPTER 4

Risk Management and Quality Improvement

RISK MANAGEMENT

Given the growth of infusion therapy practice and the movement of such practice to alternative care settings, the potential for associated risks is more intense than ever. The institution in which IV care is administered must assume responsibility for providing as safe an environment as possible to ensure patient safety and positive patient outcomes. The institution is also responsible for the quality of care provided by its agents.

MALPRACTICE CLAIMS

The hospital or involved professional person (or both) may be charged with malpractice if an injury occurs AND (1) a standard of care or duty can be established, (2) the standard of care or duty was not met, (3) the patient was harmed or injured because the standard was not met, and (4) it was possible to foresee that injury or harm would result from not meeting the standards (depending on state law).

Several systems are used to identify, investigate, and control unfavorable situations, thus the term *risk management*.

Incident Reports

An incident report is required for any accident or error resulting in actual or potential injury or harm. The report should contain only factual statements regarding the incident. Each report must be immediately followed by a full investigation into all possible causes, and corrective action must be taken immediately to prevent its recurrence. Reporting all unexpected incidences, accidents, and errors can help identify problem patterns.

Patient Safety

Establishment and monitoring of safety and security surveillance programs can be effective in preventing unsafe or insecure environments that can result in injuries.

Sharon M. Weinstein: PLUMER'S PRINCIPLES & PRACTICE OF INTRAVENOUS THERAPY, FIFTH EDITION, © 1993 J. B. Lippincott Company

QUALITY ASSURANCE

The Joint Commission on Accreditation of Healthcare Organizations (JCAHO) mandates an ongoing program for monitoring quality. Ideally, the program must objectively and systematically monitor and evaluate the appropriateness and quality of patient care. Although the JCAHO, at the time of survey, does not always examine the IV team functions from a departmental standpoint, the organization does examine very carefully outcome parameters, standards of practice, policies and procedures within various hospital departments, including, but not limited to, pharmacy, nursing, emergency, and critical care. JCAHO also surveys home infusion programs and carefully scrutinizes such programs before awarding the JCAHO accreditation standing.[5]

Opportunities to improve the quality of infusion care and to ensure positive patient outcomes should be pursued. The process focuses on (1) problem identification, (2) problem evaluation, (3) data collection and analysis, (4) implementation of corrective action, (5) problem reevaluation, and (6) problem resolution.

The quality assurance process should be reviewed quarterly, and reports should be given to the institution's risk management department. The purpose of the risk management program is to provide preventive functions and activities in the health care organization. The quality assurance process is only one facet of the organization's risk management program.

PROBLEM IDENTIFICATION

Problems may be identified by many sources. These include incident reports, patient complaints, employee complaints, questionnaires, surveys, interviews, review of statistical data, and suggestions from patients, visitors, or other department members.

To determine if a problem warrants further investigation, the following questions need to be answered:

1. Is the problem related to quality of patient care?
2. Does the problem arise frequently enough to require correction?
3. Can the problem be solved?
4. Are the benefits to patient care from solving the problem worth the cost of investigation and solution?

Some problems are serious and require immediate solutions. Many will cross departmental lines and require cooperation from other department members. Priority-based decisions must be hospital specific.

PROBLEM EVALUATION

Methods used for problem evaluation may include criterion-based studies, interviews with patients and staff members, surveys, and observations. Experimental designs can be an excellent method for problem evaluation. However, such designs can be complex and costly.

Criteria

Criteria act as a yardstick and refer to the standards on which the judgments will be based. They can be divided into three main categories: structure, process, and outcome. *Structure* refers to resources available, such as staffing capabilities, management, equipment, information systems, and facilities or building. *Process* refers to how the care should be delivered. Assumptions are made that some aspects of care should be provided in certain ways. *Outcome* is based on the principle that care is delivered to bring about certain results. For many studies, structure, process, and outcome criteria may be combined.

Policy and procedure manuals are the hospital standards or criteria on which procedure monitoring may be judged. Criteria may also be based on standards developed and tested by another hospital or listed in professional literature. To ensure an acceptable level of patient care, all manuals must be revised periodically and kept in accordance with national standards.

References to be used for IV practice standards include: (1) Intravenous Nurses Society (INS), *Standards of Practice*; (2) Centers for Disease Control and Prevention (CDC), *Guidelines for the Prevention and Control of Nosocomial Infections*; (3) American Association of Blood Banks (AABB), *Safe Transfusion*; (4) JCAHO, *Accreditation Manual for Hospitals or Home Care*.[1,2,4,5]

When evaluating studies, people tend to find what they are looking for. To minimize this effect of self-fulfilling prophecy, the criteria must be objective and measurable. To avoid subjectivity, care should be taken to use clear, concise terms that can be answered by yes or no, or by numbers. This objectivity must also be kept in mind when preparing a survey or an interview or performing an observation.

Regardless of what method of problem evaluation is used, to achieve meaningful results, standardization, reliability, and validity of the test are of utmost importance when selecting and designing any quality assurance study.

Standardization

Performing the study with standard directions under standard conditions to a sample group for whom the study is intended results in a standardized test. Using random sampling ensures that every patient or event has an equal chance of being selected.

Random sampling may be achieved by selecting all patients whose hospital identification band ends in an odd number or every other occurrence.

Reliability

The best method of estimating the reliability of a study is to perform that study with the same group on two different occasions. Correlating the results of the test–retest method considers different patient samples and errors caused by different conditions. If the study cannot be repeated without significant result variance, it cannot be considered reliable.

Validity

Validity of the study refers to whether or not it contains a fair sample of the multiple situations it is supposed to represent. For example, if the sample number is too small or if the proportion of critically ill patients varies, the test cannot be considered valid for a hospital-wide study.

DATA ANALYSIS AND INTERPRETATION

Once the study methodology and criteria have been established, data collection begins. Data are the results obtained from the study. Raw data are the individual results before these results have been compiled into a form that can be analyzed and interpreted.

Data are usually collected in a form that can be analyzed by statistics. This allows mathematical methods for analyzing, interpreting, and reporting these separate elements in summary form. The two main kinds of statistics are descriptive and inferential.

Compliance

Compliance refers to those situations in which the criteria are met. Noncompliance refers to the situations in which the criteria are not met. Both compliance and noncompliance are usually expressed in percentages. The expected compliance rate should be reasonable and achievable.

If the compliance rate appears high, one must carefully examine the conditions required for a standardized, reliable, and valid study of the identified problem. If all these conditions are being met, one must examine the criteria to be sure that the identified problem is being addressed. Continuing with a study showing a high rate of compliance will not give the necessary information to solve an identified problem.

Descriptive Statistics

Descriptive statistics allow for meaningful reporting of findings in a small amount of space, even though a large amount of raw data may vary a great deal.

In summarizing study results, descriptive statistics are used to calculate: (1) the average result, (2) the difference between individual results and the average, and (3) the relationship between the average result on one part of the study and the average result on another part.[3]

Comparing average results tells a good deal about the relationship between the two parts.

Arithmetic Mean
In statistical analysis, the average result is called the mean. To find the mean, simply total all results and divide the answer by the total number in the study.

This is especially helpful when comparing performances of team members.

Median
Median is the result that falls exactly in the middle of all the score results. The same number of people scored above it as scored below it.

Mode
In any test or study situation, several people can achieve the same score or test result. The score or result that is seen most frequently is called the mode.

Standard Deviation
The difference between individual results and the mean indicates the extent to which figures in a given set vary from the mean. This tells how much variation is present between the group and the individual.

To calculate the standard deviation:

1. Calculate the mean for each score.
2. Subtract the mean from each score and square the answer.
3. Add all the squares together.
4. Divide the sum by the total number of scores.
5. Take the square root of that value.

In most quality assurance studies, it is not necessary to actually perform the mathematical calculations. It is sufficient to know that normally 68% of the scores will fall, plus or minus, within a given range from the mean. Calculating the difference between each score and the mean will identify those with abnormal deviations.

If the study design allows for measurement of two different factors, comparing data that pertain to each factor can provide additional information.

Only from a well-designed experimental study can one expect to find that one thing causes another to occur. All other methods allow one to say only that there appears to be a correlation between two things.

Correlation

Correlation refers to an association between occurrences. A *high positive correlation* indicates that A has a high frequency of occurrence when it is associated with B. A *high negative correlation* indicates that A occurs rarely when it is associated with B.

Reporting studies to a central quality assurance committee enhances communications within the hospital. Such a committee encourages use of all information as efficiently as possible. It can also help a new participant by providing suggestions or assistance with all steps of a study.

Most quality assurance programs use standard hospital-wide forms for reporting the study. This form should be a short summary of all the steps taken, study results, and what corrective action is planned. All raw data must be retained by the person performing the study.

Personal confidentiality of all participants in the study must be maintained. Copies of any study should be limited strictly to those demonstrating a need to know.

IMPLEMENTATION OF CORRECTIVE ACTION

Factors to consider when choosing a corrective action include: (1) areas for change that the environment can best accommodate, (2) areas of potential barriers or constraints, (3) areas of potential support, and (4) the needed resources.

Each strategy must be analyzed for expected costs, advantages and disadvantages, anticipated benefits, and the feasibility of implementation.

Before developing the plan the following questions must be answered.

WHY is it being implemented?

WHAT must be done to make the plan operational?

WHO will be involved with and responsible for accomplishing it?

WHERE will implementation take place?

WHEN will it be completed?

The best method of corrective action will depend on each particular problem and individual situation. Methods may include policy or procedure revision, equipment change, a new information system, continuous monitoring, or in-service education.

PROBLEM REEVALUATION

After corrective action has been implemented, a reevaluation is necessary to determine if the applied corrective action results in minimization or solution of the problem. Without follow-up, the success of the entire evaluation process cannot be ensured.

This evaluation should tell if the anticipated change did in fact occur. If so, is the change sufficient to solve the problem? One also must decide if any needs still remain and if so, how they will be met. If change did not occur, one must find the reasons and decide if a new strategy is required.

Frequently, reevaluation is performed by repeating the first evaluation and comparing preaction data with postaction data.

Any evaluation method may be used provided it contains the necessary elements to obtain standardized, reliable, valid results.

PROBLEM RESOLUTION

The final step in the process is the development of a plan to ensure the maintenance of the quality of care achieved with the corrective action. Periodic or continuous screening may be required. An IV team quality audit process may be involved. Surveys, patient satisfaction questionnaires, or personal interviews may be used. An IV checklist incorporated into daily care may provide an excellent source for quick identification of potential problems. Given the expanding role of IV nurses to encompass alternative site care within an institution or facility, checklists addressing patient teaching of self-administration, use of electronic infusion devices, discharge medications, and other facets of care may be developed.

POTENTIAL STUDY AREAS

Potential study areas for quality assurance within IV practice are diverse and interface with multiple hospital departments. Suggested areas to be studied include (1) hazardous materials and handling of hazardous waste, (2) infection control, (3) handwashing, and (4) product integrity.

QUALITY IMPROVEMENT

The greatest impact on the quality assurance process within health care organizations has been the influence of Deming and others who have introduced the concept of Total Quality Improvement (TQI) or Continuous Quality Improvement (CQI). Such processes provide a mechanism for examining the process, rather than the individual involved, and encourage participation across interdepartmental lines to improve the process itself. Quality improvement teams within an organization are appointed and study areas are identified; process improvement is the direct result of the CQI program.

REFERENCES

1. American Association of Blood Banks. (1981). *Safe transfusion*. Washington, DC.
2. Centers for Disease Control. (1983). *Guidelines for the prevention and control of nosocomial infections*. Atlanta.
3. Colton, T. (1974). *Statistics in medicine*. Boston: Little, Brown.
4. *Revised intravenous nursing standards of practice.* (1990). *Journal of Intravenous Nursing*, (Suppl.), S3–S11.
5. Joint Commission on Accreditation of Healthcare Organizations. (1992). *Accreditation manual for hospitals or home care*. Chicago.

BIBLIOGRAPHY

Cobb, M. D. Evaluating medication errors. (1986). *Journal of Nursing Administration 16*(4), 41–44.
Gardner, C. (1987). Risk management of medication errors. *Journal of the National Intravenous Therapy Association 10*(4), 266–278.
Gardner, C. (1987). Risk management of medication errors. *Journal of the National Intravenous Therapy Association 10*(3), 186–196.

REVIEW QUESTIONS

1. An incident report should contain what type of information?
   a. factual
   b. anecdotal
   c. editorialized
   d. subjective

2. The quality assurance process focuses on which of the following components?
   a. problem identification
   b. problem evaluation
   c. data collection and analysis
   d. all of the above

3. Which of the following organizations mandates an ongoing program for monitoring quality?
   a. Centers for Disease Control and Prevention
   b. Joint Commission on Accreditation of Healthcare Organizations
   c. American Society for Healthcare Risk Management
   d. American Association of Blood Banks

4. The quality assurance process should be reviewed how frequently?
   a. monthly
   b. quarterly
   c. semiannually
   d. annually

5. Researchers who have influenced the quality assurance process include:
   a. Deming
   b. Evanson
   c. Riding
   d. Colton

CHAPTER 5

The Staff Nurse's Responsibility in Infusion Therapy

Administration of safe, high-quality infusion therapy in the health care organization depends on the contributions of many members of the health care team. The staff nurse plays a primary role in maintaining the infusion and in protecting the patient from the hazards and complications associated with routine IV therapy. Policies regarding the responsibilities of the staff nurse vary significantly among health care institutions and are often influenced by the presence or absence of a full-service IV team.

National standards of practice and guidelines have been established to protect the patient. Each nurse within an organization must be cognizant of the policies and procedures relevant to infusion therapy and be familiar with nursing responsibilities to provide a safe level of care for the patient.

The role of an IV team and possible delineation of responsibilities must be part of the orientation program and ongoing education for all nurses to provide a team approach to safe IV care.

STANDARDS OF PRACTICE

The Intravenous Nurses Society's (INS) Standards of Practice is an authoritative document that outlines the nurse's scope of practice and educational requirements and defines autonomy, accountability, and responsibility for the specialty practice of infusion therapy. Institutional policies and procedures should be developed and implemented based on these standards and interpretations, regardless of the clinical setting in which care is delivered.

NURSING CARE PLAN

A nursing care plan should be established within 24 hours of completion of the initial nursing assessment. The care plan should:

- Reflect nursing diagnosis
- Evaluate progress and effectiveness of care

Sharon M. Weinstein: PLUMER'S PRINCIPLES & PRACTICE OF INTRAVENOUS THERAPY, FIFTH EDITION, © 1993 J. B. Lippincott Company

- Include time frames for goal achievement
- Be modified consistent with the patient's clinical progress

MONITORING

Ongoing monitoring provides information regarding a patient's response to the pre-scribed therapies. Patients receiving IV therapies should be monitored at frequent, established intervals based on practice setting, prescribed therapy, condition, and age. Monitoring should:

- Be established in policies and procedures
- Minimize risk of potential complications of routine IV therapy
- Include cannula site, flow rate, clinical data, patient response

INTRAVENOUS ADMINISTRATION SET CHANGE

Routine changing of administration sets is an infection control measure. Administration sets are changed consistent with the type of set used and the specific therapy ordered for the patient.[2]

Primary Continuous
1. Change every 48 hours and immediately on suspected contamination or when the integrity of the product has been compromised.
2. Avoid touch contamination.
3. Use aseptic technique.

Secondary
1. Change every 48 hours and immediately on suspected contamination or when the integrity of the product has been compromised.
2. Avoid touch contamination.
3. Use aseptic technique.

Primary Intermittent
1. Change every 24 hours and immediately on suspected contamination or when the integrity of the product has been compromised.
2. Remove attached needles after each use, and aseptically attach a new, sterile needle.
3. Maintain asepsis.
4. Avoid touch contamination.
5. Change of add-on devices should coincide with changing of the administration set.

Total Parenteral Nutrition
1. Change every 24 hours and immediately on suspected contamination or when the integrity of the product has been compromised.

2. Use aseptic technique.

3. Sets specific for electronic infusion devices should be changed every 24 hours unless physical properties or visual inspection requires more frequent set change.

Lipid Emulsion

1. Discard after each use unless additional units are added consecutively.

2. If consecutive administration is used, change every 24 hours.

3. Change immediately on suspected contamination or when the integrity of the product has been compromised.

Blood/Blood Components

1. Change after each unit given.

2. Change immediately on suspected contamination or when the integrity of the product has been compromised.

3. Use aseptic technique.

4. Do not use for more than 4 hours.

5. Change add-on filters consistent with set change.

6. Use each set for only one unit to identify the unit responsible for a possible reaction.

Hemodynamic and Arterial Pressure Monitoring

1. Change set, dome, and pressure tubing every 48 hours and immediately on suspected contamination or if the integrity of the product has been compromised.

2. Use aseptic technique.

3. Change of add-on devices should coincide with set change.

INTRAVENOUS CONTAINERS

The risk of infection is great if aseptic technique is not observed.

1. Wash hands before parenteral fluids are opened and administered.

2. Inspect fluid containers before use for cracks, leaks, damaged caps, and expiration date.

3. Inspect fluid for discoloration, turbidity, and evidence of particulate matter.

4. Check label to ensure evidence of time and date opened, any additives, and appropriateness of infusate for the patient for whom ordered.

DRESSING CHANGES

A sterile, occlusive dressing is an appropriate infection control measure.

1. Gauze dressings should be applied aseptically and securely taped.

2. Change every 48 hours and immediately if the integrity of the dressing has been compromised.

3. When a transparent semipermeable membrane (TSM) is used over gauze, it is considered a gauze dressing and should be changed every 48 hours.

4. Do not cover site dressings with roller bandages.

5. TSM dressings should be changed at established intervals using aseptic technique or when the integrity of the dressing has been compromised.

AMBULATING THE PATIENT

Special precautions must be taken when ambulating patients with infusions. The fluid container must be kept sufficiently high at all times to maintain a constant flow. Any cessation in the rate must be detected immediately and remedied before a clot is allowed to plug the needle.

FREQUENT OBSERVATION

Fluid maintenance requires frequent observation of patients receiving infusions. The attending nurse should visit the patient frequently, checking the rate of flow, the amount of solution remaining, and the site of infusion, as described in the following sections.

Rate of Flow

Because the rate of flow, once established, is often difficult to maintain, the staff nurse should check and readjust the flow whenever necessary. Flow control devices may be used to assist in regulating a prescribed administration rate. Electronic infusion devices may be used when warranted by the patient's age, condition, and prescribed therapy.

When Infusion Stops

When an infusion stops, the cause must be immediately investigated and remedied. The following procedure is to be used:

1. Check for infiltration.
2. Check the fluid level in the bottle.
3. Check for kinking of the tubing.
4. Open the clamp.
5. Check air vent. Has it been inserted if required and is it patent?
6. Check the cannula for patency by kinking the tubing a few inches from the cannula while pinching and releasing the tubing between the cannula and the kinked tubing. Resistance, if encountered, should be treated with caution because a clot may have plugged the cannula. If the patient complains of pain, a sclerosed vein may be the cause of the cessation of flow. In either case, the cannula must be removed.
7. Is the cannula in line with the vein or up against the wall of the vein? A slight adjustment, by moving the cannula, may remedy the problem.
8. If the IV solution is cold, as in the case of blood, venous spasm may result. Heat

placed directly on the vein will relieve the spasm and increase the flow of the infusion.

9. If the infusion is blood, check the filter; heavy sediment may be slowing the flow. Replace the filter if necessary.

10. Increase the height of the bottle to increase gravity.

11. If unable to restart the flow after these procedures have been followed, restart the infusion.

Amount of Solution in the Container

Air embolism and *blood embolism* are significant hazards of infusion therapy and may be associated with delay in changing solution containers. Subsequent solutions should be added before the level of fluid falls in the drip chamber. Failure to do this results in the following problems:

Plugged Cannula

Intravenous solutions flow into the vein by means of gravity. Once the fluid level has dropped in the tubing to about the level of the patient's chest, the blood will be forced back into the cannula, occluding the lumen of the cannula. Occluded cannulas should be removed, not irrigated. Fibrinous material injected into the vein can propagate a thrombus, possibly resulting in an infarction. Irrigation may embolize small infected cannula thrombi, which could result in septicemia. Aspiration aimed at dislodging the fibrin may cause the vein to collapse around the cannula point, traumatizing the vessel wall.

Trapped Air

If the bottle (in an air-venting system) is changed after the level of fluid drops in the tubing and before the cannula plugs, the air is trapped in the tubing and forced into the patient by pressure of the fresh solution. Fatal air embolism can result. The use of plastic bags, containers that contain no air, and administration sets that have no junctions through which air can leak have reduced the risk of introducing air into the patient's veins. Air can be introduced at the beginning of an infusion by not completely clearing the set of air or when changing containers. Infusions through a central venous catheter carry an even greater risk of air embolism than do those through a peripheral vein. Air embolism can occur during tubing changes involving the central venous catheter. It has been suggested, through animal experimentation, that a normal adult should tolerate air embolism of as much as 200 mL, but for persons in poor health smaller amounts may be fatal; less than 10 mL might be fatal in a gravely ill person.[1]

Before the flow ceases and the bottle empties, replace the empty bottle with fresh solution using the following procedure:

1. Vent fresh bottle if vent is required.

2. Kink tubing to prevent air from being introduced into the flowing solution.

3. Change container. Hang solution bottle before unkinking tubing.

4. Readjust rate if necessary.

Nonfunctioning (leaking or plugged) sets should be removed.

The 0.2-μm Air-Eliminating Filter

A 0.2-μm air-eliminating filter protects the patient from air embolism, bacteria, and particulate matter. INS advocates the use of the 0.2-μm air-eliminating filters for routine administration of IV fluids.[2]

Recommendations for the Use of 0.2-μm Air-Eliminating Filters[2]

1. The filter should be placed at the terminal end of the administration set, that is, as close to the cannula as possible.

2. The filter should be changed at the time of administration set change.

3. Lipid emulsions, blood, and blood products should not be administered through the filter.

4. Consideration must be made to the administration of some drugs since their dosage may be affected by the filter; follow the manufacturer's recommendations.

5. The psi of the filter must be compatible with the electronic infusion device in use.

Infiltration or Inflammation at Injection Site

Failure to recognize an infiltration before the swelling has increased to a sizable degree may:

1. Cause damage to the tissues.

2. Prevent the patient from receiving necessary and urgent medication.

3. Limit veins available for future therapy.

If the question of infiltration exists, compare the questionable extremity with the normal extremity. An infusion has infiltrated if:

1. Swelling occurs about the site of the cannula.

2. A tourniquet applied above the cannula does not stop the flow of fluid.

Checking for an infiltration by a backflow of blood into the adapter is not a reliable method because:

1. In small veins, the cannula may approach the size of the vein, occluding the lumen and obstructing the flow of blood; the solution flows undiluted so that no backflow of blood is obtained.

2. The cannula may have punctured the vein, causing an infiltration, and at the same time be within the lumen of the vein, or the bevel may be only partially within the lumen of the vein, causing a swelling and still producing a backflow of blood on test.

Inspect the injection site for erythema, induration, or tenderness by palpating the venous cord. If any of these signs occur, remove the cannula. When replacing it, sterile equipment should be used and the site changed, preferably to the opposite arm. Should infection be noted, the cannula and the infusate should be cultured and lot numbers of sets and infusions recorded.

DISCONTINUATION OF THERAPY

To discontinue an infusion, use the following procedure:

1. Stop flow by clamping off tubing.
2. Remove all tape from cannula. Do not use scissors.
3. With a dry sterile sponge held over the injection site, remove cannula. The cannula must be removed nearly flush with the skin. This prevents the point from damaging the posterior wall of the vein, thus encouraging the process of thrombosis. Visually ascertain that the length of the cannula removed corresponds with length inserted. Information should be noted on the dressing.
4. Apply pressure instantly and firmly. Do not rub. Hematomas occur from cannulas carelessly removed and render veins useless for future use.

Small adhesive bandages, such as Band-Aids®, should not be used unless specifically ordered. It must be emphasized that such a bandage is not used to stop bleeding and does not take the place of pressure. If ordered, it should be applied only after pressure has been applied and the bleeding stopped.

REFERENCES

1. Fireitag, J., & Miller L. (Eds.). (1980). *Manual of medical therapeutics* (23rd ed., p. 293). Boston: Little, Brown.

2. *Revised intravenous nursing standards of practice.* (1990). *Journal of Intravenous Nursing,* (Suppl.), S57.

BIBLIOGRAPHY

Alfaro, R. (1986). *Application of nursing process: A step-by-step guide* (p. 108). Philadelphia: J. B. Lippincott.

Hogan, G. F. (1986). Signature requirements for drug orders in medical records. *American Journal of Hospital Pharmacy, 43*(5), 1152.

REVIEW QUESTIONS

1. The INS Standards document defines:
   a. scope of practice
   b. educational requirements
   c. a only
   d. a and b

2. Ongoing monitoring provides information regarding:
   a. care plan
   b. set change
   c. patient's response to therapy
   d. family's feelings about therapy

3. To minimize the risk of phlebitis, routine IV tubing should be changed at what frequency?
   a. 24 hours
   b. 36 hours
   c. 48 hours
   d. 72 hours

4. Tubing used to administer total parenteral nutrition should be changed at what frequency?
   a. 24 hours
   b. 36 hours
   c. 48 hours
   d. 72 hours

5. Which of the following is an appropriate occlusive dressing?
   a. adhesive strip
   b. gauze and tape
   c. transparent semipermeable membrane
   d. elastoplast

6. The 0.2-μm filter protects the patient from which of the following?
   a. air
   b. bacteria
   c. particulate matter
   d. all of the above

7. Which of the following is NOT true of failure to recognize an infiltration?
   a. damage to the tissues occurs
   b. patient prevented from receiving medication
   c. limited access available
   d. patient's care will not be compromised

8. Which of the following is NOT a sign of infusion phlebitis?
   a. redness
   b. swelling
   c. tenderness
   d. pus

9. An IV nursing care plan should reflect which of the following?
   a. nursing diagnosis
   b. time frames for goal achievement
   c. evaluation of process and effectiveness of care
   d. all of the above

10. Monitoring of infusion therapy:
   a. minimizes risk
   b. eliminates risk
   c. maximizes risk
   d. produces risk

CHAPTER 6

The Intravenous Team Nurse

Specialized teams of IV nurses provide clinical expertise and cost-effective care and decrease the risk of complications related to infusion therapy. Ideally, registered nurses with clinical and theoretical expertise should be responsible for administering IV therapy.

It is estimated that 70% to 80% of all hospitalized patients receive IV therapy and that the home infusion market will continue to escalate beyond expectations. An IV nursing team can best provide positive patient outcomes for infusion therapy regardless of the clinical setting in which care is delivered.

In the hospital environment, such a team should function 7 days a week and should consist of registered nurses with a minimum of 2 years of medical/surgical nursing experience. The number of nurses involved should be consistent with the institution's needs and patient census. The team should be supervised by a registered nurse educated in the specialty practice. Team functions should be defined in policies and procedures and should be based on published Standards of Practice.[1]

Cost effectiveness may be established through high productivity levels, minimal patient complications, and optimal use of all equipment. The team should be a budgeted item and established as an independent department. The team should interact with the following hospital departments: pharmacy and therapeutics, new products, infection control, nutritional support, transfusion therapy, quality improvement, and risk management.

ASSESSMENT

Assessment of the patient receiving infusion therapy is an ongoing process that aims to achieve desired patient outcomes. Assessment is based on knowledge, experience, and observation skills and includes the patient's appropriateness and available venous access for the type of therapy prescribed. Assessments should be documented in the clinical record and may require immediate interventions.

INITIATION

Intravenous therapy is initiated for therapeutic or diagnostic purposes on a physician's written and signed order. The physician's written order should include solution and/or medication, dosage, volume, rate, frequency, and route of administration. Appropriate-

Sharon M. Weinstein: PLUMER'S PRINCIPLES & PRACTICE OF INTRAVENOUS THERAPY, FIFTH EDITION, © 1993 J. B. Lippincott Company

ness of the therapy should be determined using the principles of the nursing process: assessment, planning, implementation, and evaluation. The patient has the right to refuse treatment.

SITE SELECTION

Site selection is aimed at minimizing the potential risk of complications related to routine IV therapy and preserving veins for future use.

Peripheral

1. Assess patient's condition; age, diagnosis, size, and availability of veins.
2. Vein should accommodate gauge and length of the cannula.
3. Consider purpose and duration of therapy.
4. Subsequent cannulations should be made proximal to the previously cannulated site.

Arterial

1. Assess patient's condition; age, diagnosis, size, condition and location of arteries.
2. Consider purpose and duration of therapy.
3. Determine presence of a pulse and distal circulation.
4. Perform Allen's test when selecting the brachial or radial artery.
5. Frequency of site rotation should be established in institutional policies.

Peripherally Inserted Central (PICC)

1. Assess patient's age and condition; vein condition, size and location.
2. Consider type and duration of therapy.
3. Vein should accommodate gauge of catheter.
4. Perform anatomic measurements before catheter insertion.
5. Area of antecubital fossa is usual site.

Central

1. Site selection, other than peripherally inserted central catheters, is a medical act.
2. Most appropriate veins are internal jugular and subclavian.
3. Distal tip should be located in superior vena cava.

CANNULA SELECTION

Selection of an appropriate cannula will minimize potential complications of routine IV therapy.

Peripheral

1. Select smallest gauge and shortest length to accommodate the prescribed therapy.
2. Catheters should be radiopaque.
3. Stainless steel needles should be limited to short-term or single-dose administration.

Arterial

1. Select smallest gauge and length that will accommodate prescribed therapy.
2. Stainless steel needles should not be used for indwelling arterial access.
3. Radiopaque catheters should be used.

Peripherally Inserted Central

1. Radiopaque catheters should be used.
2. Length of catheter should be such that tip resides in the superior vena cava.
3. Knowledge of the use and placement of these catheters is required.
4. Only products designed for PICC placement should be used.

Central

1. Select based on patient's condition and prescribed therapies.
2. Radiopaque catheters should be used.
3. Consideration should be given to catheters placed entirely under the skin (implanted) or that partially exit the skin (tunneled).
4. Consideration should be given to patient preference, length of therapy, life-style, and ease of maintenance.
5. Consideration should be given to the use of multiple lumens.

HAIR REMOVAL

Excess hair may be removed to enhance site preparation and to facilitate catheter insertion, taping, and dressing adherence. The method used is clipping with a scissors. Shaving is not recommended because potential microabrasions caused by the razor may increase the risk of infection. The use of depilatories may potentiate an allergic reaction.

SITE PREPARATION

Peripheral

Cleansing the insertion site before initiation of therapy reduces the potential for infection. An appropriate antimicrobial solution should be used, such as tincture of iodine 1% to 2%, iodophors, 70% isopropyl alcohol, or chlorhexidine. Extremely dirty skin should be cleaned with soap and water before the antimicrobial solution is applied. Hair removal should be consistent with published standards.

The skin cleansing solution should be applied in a concentric circle, from the center to the periphery of the intended site, and allowed to air dry. If the patient has a known allergy to iodine, the solution of choice is 70% isopropyl alcohol applied with friction for a minimum of 30 seconds or until the applicator is clean.

Peripherally Inserted Central

The site should be cleansed as with any peripheral line placement since a sterile field is required. The catheter that is not enclosed in a sterile protective cover requires surgical scrub and garb for the nurse and surgical preparation and sterile draping of the patient.

Central

Aseptic cleansing with an appropriate antimicrobial solution is required. Central catheters requiring medical placement may be placed percutaneously or surgically. Percutaneous placement requires the use of mask, sterile gloves, gown, and a surgical scrub.

CANNULA PLACEMENT

Peripheral

Placement should be established in written policies and procedures. When aseptic placement has been compromised, as in an emergency, the catheter should be replaced when the patient has been stabilized. Before use, all products should be inspected for integrity. Manufacturer's guidelines for placement should be followed. Radiopaque, over-the-needle catheters are the state-of-the-art and the preferred choice for routine therapy.

Peripherally Inserted Central

Such catheters should be placed for a definite therapeutic indication. The length should allow for appropriate placement without alteration of tip integrity. Aseptic technique should be used. Radiographic confirmation of catheter tip location should be obtained before initiation of prescribed therapy, consistent with manufacturer's guidelines for the use of a particular product and published standards.

Central

Placement of central catheters is a medical act. The nursing role in assisting in catheter placement should be defined in written policies and procedures. The Valsalva maneuver should be used to reduce the risk of air embolism.

CANNULA STABILIZATION

All cannulas should be stabilized in a manner that does not interfere with assessment and monitoring of the IV site or impede delivery of the infusate. Products available for stabilization include tape, transparent semipermeable membrane dressings, steri-strips, and sutures.

JUNCTION SECUREMENT

The securement of junction points of IV tubing and add-on devices minimizes the risk of complications of routine IV therapy. Junction securement devices include tape, clasping devices, Luer lock and slip connections, and others.

DRESSINGS

Sterile dressings are infection control measures and should be applied in an aseptic manner. Dressings include tape and gauze and transparent semipermeable membrane materials. Intravenous nursing responsibilities are the same as those for the staff nurse.

NEEDLE/STYLET DISPOSAL

The recapping of needles/stylets increases the potential risk to the clinician. Needles and stylets should be disposed of in nonpermeable, rigid, tamper-proof containers. Needles and stylets should not be recapped, broken, cut, or bent. Standards established by the Occupational Safety and Health Administration (OSHA) and the Joint Commission on Accreditation of Healthcare Organizations (JCAHO) should be followed.

MONITORING

All patients receiving infusion therapy should be monitored at prescribed intervals consistent with established policy, their clinical condition, and the type of therapy being administered. Monitoring includes:

- Cannula site
- Flow rate
- Clinical status
- Patient response to therapy

SITE CARE

Periodic site care enables the professional to observe and evaluate the skin–cannula junction and surrounding tissue and is a valid infection control measure. Site care includes aseptically cleaning the skin–cannula junction with an appropriate antiseptic solution, applying an antimicrobial or antibiotic ointment consistent with institutional policy, and applying an occlusive, sterile dressing.

DOCUMENTATION

Documentation of care delivered provides a mechanism for recording and retrieving information. Documentation in the clinical record should include information to identify IV procedures, prescribed treatments, complications, and nursing interventions.

Labeling provides easily identified information relevant to the cannula, type of dressing, solution, medication, administration set, and the identification of the professional responsible for cannula placement.

Documentation also provides a statistical base for retrieval of pertinent information to be reviewed at established intervals. Analysis of such information contributes to objective data concerning quality, cost effectiveness of care, and patient's clinical outcomes.

CANNULA REMOVAL

Cannula removal should be established in institutional policies and procedures and is directed at minimizing complications of routine IV therapy.

Peripheral

1. Remove every 48 hours or immediately on suspected complication/contamination.
2. Schedule removal to coincide with administration set change.
3. When cannula-related infection is suspected, remove cannula immediately.
4. Cannula may be cultured if necessary.
5. Pressure should be applied to the site and a dry, sterile dressing should be applied.

Arterial

1. Change cannula every 96 hours or immediately on suspected complication/contamination.[2]
2. The integrity of the cannula should be documented.

Peripherally Inserted Central

1. Remove immediately on suspected complication or contamination.
2. Consider a central catheter when the tip is located in the superior vena cava or subclavian vein.
3. Use caution in the removal of peripherally inserted central catheters, especially if the catheter has been in place for some time.
4. On removal, apply pressure, an antiseptic ointment, and a sterile gauze dressing to site.
5. Application of ointment may occlude skin tract and prevent air embolism.
6. Change dressing and assess site every 24 hours until site has epithelialized.

Central

1. Optimal time for removal is unknown.
2. Precautions should be taken to minimize air embolism.
3. If resistance is encountered, physician should be notified.
4. On removal, apply pressure, an antiseptic ointment, and a sterile gauze dressing.
5. Application of ointment may occlude skin tract and prevent air embolism.
6. Change dressing and assess site every 24 hours until site has epithelialized.

Tunneled/Implanted

1. Removal of these devices is a medical act.
2. Optimal time for removal is unknown.
3. Assess site at predetermined intervals following removal.

REFERENCE

1. Revised *intravenous nursing standards of practice.* (1990). *Journal of Intravenous Nursing,* (Suppl.), S3.

2. *Revised intravenous nursing standards of practice.* (1990). *Journal of Intravenous Nursing,* (Suppl.), S31.

BIBLIOGRAPHY

Hadaway, L. (1988). Nursing diagnosis applied to I.V. nursing practice. *Journal of Intravenous Nursing, 11*(2), 109–111.

Ryan, K. A. (1989). Standardized care plans for I.V. therapy. *Journal of Intravenous Nursing, 12*(2), 94–98.

REVIEW QUESTIONS

1. Which of the following represents the percentage of hospitalized patients receiving infusion therapy?
   a. 40–50
   b. 60–65
   c. 70–80
   d. 85–95

2. The IV team should be directly supervised by which of the following:
   a. RN educated in the specialty practice
   b. RN educated in another specialty practice
   c. RPh
   d. EdD

3. Which of the following statements is true?
   a. The patient has a right to refuse treatment.
   b. The hospitalized patient gives up his rights to refuse treatment.
   c. The rights of the hospitalized patient differ from those of the outpatient.
   d. The rights of the outpatient are greater.

4. Which of the following statements is NOT true of peripheral cannula selection?
   a. Select smallest gauge and shortest length to accommodate the prescribed therapy.
   b. Catheters should be radiopaque.
   c. Stainless steel needles should be limited to short-term or single-dose use.
   d. Stainless steel needles are appropriate for long-term peripheral therapy.

5. Which of the following statements is NOT true of peripherally inserted central catheters?
   a. Radiopaque catheters should be used.
   b. Length of catheter should be such that tip does not reside in superior vena cava.
   c. Knowledge of use and placement of these lines is required.
   d. Only products designed for PICC placement should be used.

6. The appropriate method to remove excess hair is:
   a. shave with safety razor
   b. clip with scissors
   c. shave with straight razor
   d. use depilatory

7. Appropriate antimicrobial solutions for skin prep include which of the following?
   a. tincture of iodine 1%–2%
   b. chlorhexidine
   c. 70% isopropyl alcohol
   d. iodophors

8. Percutaneous placement of a central catheter requires use of:
   a. mask
   b. sterile gloves
   c. gown
   d. surgical scrub

9. Placement of central catheters is:
   a. a nursing act
   b. a medical act
   c. defined in policy
   d. defined in procedure

10. Needles and stylets should NOT be:
   a. recapped
   b. clipped
   c. broken
   d. bent

PART II

Principles of Venipuncture

CHAPTER 7

Anatomy and Physiology Applied to Intravascular Therapy

ANATOMY AND PHYSIOLOGY

Intravascular therapy consists of the introduction of fluids, blood, and drugs directly into the vascular system, that is, into arteries, into bone marrow, and into veins. The *arteries* are used as a route to introduce radiopaque material for diagnostic purposes, such as arteriograms for cerebral disorders, as well as for monitoring blood pressure, determining arterial blood gases, and administering chemotherapy. The dangers of arterial spasm and subsequent gangrene present problems that make this type of therapy hazardous for therapeutic use. The *bone marrow*, because of its venous plexus, is used for intravascular therapy, by the intraosseous route. The *veins*, because of their abundance and location, present the most readily accessible route.

Applied to intravascular therapy, knowledge of the anatomy and physiology of veins and arteries is essential to the proficiency of the clinician and to ensure positive patient outcome. Through a study of the superficial veins, the nurse acquires a sense of discrimination in the choice of veins for IV use. Many factors must be considered in selecting a vein; the anatomic characteristics offer a basis for good judgment. The size, location, and resilience of the vein affect its desirability for infusion purposes.

Familiarity with the principles underlying venous physiology is also of prime value to the nurse. An understanding of the reaction of veins to the nervous stimulation of the vasoconstrictors and vasodilators enables the clinician to (1) increase the size and visibility of a vein before attempting venipuncture and (2) relieve venous spasm and thus assist in infusion maintenance. The primary goal of therapy is to provide a positive outcome for the patient. Painless and effective therapy is desirable, promoting the patient's comfort, well-being, and often complete recovery from disease or trauma. An integral part of this goal is the recognition and prevention of complications. Through their knowledge of anatomy and physiology, clinicians can minimize this risk.

Phlebitis and *thrombosis* are by far the most common complications resulting from parenteral therapy. Although seemingly mild, they do present serious consequences: (1) they cause moderate to severe discomfort, often taking many days or weeks to subside, and (2) they limit the veins available for further therapy. Injury to the endothelial lining of the vein contributes to these local complications. A thorough understanding of the peripheral veins alerts the clinician to observe precautions in performing venipunctures.

Sharon M. Weinstein: PLUMER'S PRINCIPLES & PRACTICE OF INTRAVENOUS THERAPY, FIFTH EDITION, © 1993 J. B. Lippincott Company

Proper technique minimizes the trauma to the vessel wall and provides an entry as painless and safe as possible. Examination of the superficial veins of the lower extremities alerts the nurse to the dangers resulting from their use. By avoiding venipunctures in veins susceptible to varicosities and sluggish circulation, the likelihood of phlebitis and thrombosis is decreased and the secondary risk of *pulmonary embolism* is reduced.

Awareness of the characteristics that differentiate veins from arteries assists the clinician in reducing the risk of *necrosis* and *gangrene*; these serious complications occur when a medication is inadvertently injected into an artery.

An understanding of the anatomy and physiology of the veins and arteries enables the clinician to recognize the existence of an *arteriovenous anastomosis*; failure to recognize this condition results in repeated and unsuccessful venipunctures performed in an attempt to initiate the infusion. These repeated punctures compound the trauma to the inner lining of the vein and increase the risk of the local complications already described, any one of which limits the number of available veins, interrupts the course of therapy, and causes unnecessary pain and even dire consequences for the patient.

THE VASCULAR SYSTEM

The circulatory system is divided into two main systems, the pulmonary and the systemic, each with its own set of vessels. The *pulmonary system* consists of the blood flow from the right ventricle of the heart to the lungs, where it is oxygenated and returned to the left atrium. The *systemic system*, the larger of the two, is the one that concerns the IV nurse. It consists of the aorta, arteries, arterioles, capillaries, venules, and veins through which the blood must flow. The blood leaves the left ventricle, flows to all parts of the body, and returns to the right atrium of the heart via the vena cava. The *systemic veins* are divided into three classes: (1) superficial, (2) deep, and (3) venous sinuses.[2]

Superficial Veins

The superficial or cutaneous veins are those used in venipuncture. They are located just beneath the skin in the superficial fascia. These veins and the deep veins sometimes unite; in the lower extremities they unite freely.[1] For example, the small saphenous vein, a superficial vein, drains the dorsum of the foot and the posterior section of the leg; it ascends the back of the leg and empties directly into the deep popliteal vein. Before the small saphenous vein terminates in the deep popliteal, it sends out a branch that, after joining the great saphenous vein, also terminates in a deep vein, the femoral vein. Because of these deep connections, great concern arises when it becomes necessary to use the veins in the lower extremities. Thrombosis may occur, which could easily extend to the deep veins and cause pulmonary embolism. Understanding this, the nurse should refrain from using these veins.

Varicosities occurring in the lower extremities, although readily available to venipuncture, are not a satisfactory route for parenteral administration. The relatively stagnant blood in such veins is likely to clot, resulting in a superficial phlebitis. Medication injected below a varicosity may result in another potential danger, a collection of the infused drug in the varicosity. This is caused by the stagnant blood flow. This "pocket" of infused medication may delay the effect of the drug when immediate action is desired; another concern is the danger of untoward reactions to the drug, which may occur when this accumulation reaches the general circulation.

Arteriovenous Anastomosis

Deep veins are usually enclosed in the same sheath with the arteries. Occasionally an arteriovenous anastomosis may occur congenitally or as the result of past penetrating injury of the vein and adjacent artery. When such trauma occurs, the blood flows directly from the artery into the vein; as a result, the veins draining an arteriovenous fistula are overburdened with high-pressure arterial blood. These veins appear large and tortuous. In these unusual circumstances, the nurse's quick recognition of an arteriovenous fistula may prevent pain, complications, and loss of time resulting from repeated unsuccessful attempts to start the infusion.

Arteries and Veins

Knowledge of the characteristics differentiating veins from arteries and the position of each is important so that the nurse may avoid the complications of an inadvertent arterial puncture. Arteries and veins are similar in structure; both are composed of three layers of tissue. A close examination of these layers reveals their differing characteristics.

Tunica Intima or the Inner Layer

The first layer consists of an inner elastic endothelial lining, which also forms the valves in veins. These valves are absent in arteries. The endothelial lining is identical in the arteries and the veins, consisting of a smooth layer of flat cells. This smooth surface allows the cells and platelets to flow through the blood vessels without interruption under normal conditions. Care must be taken to avoid roughening this surface when performing a venipuncture or removing a needle from a vein. Any trauma that roughens the endo-thelial lining encourages the process of thrombosis, whereby cells and platelets adhere to the vessel wall.

Many veins contain valves, which are semilunar folds of the endothelium. These valves are found in the larger veins of the extremities; their function is to keep the blood flowing toward the heart. Where muscular pressure would cause a backing up of the blood supply, these valves play an important role. They occur at points of branching and often cause a noticeable bulge in the veins. Applying a tourniquet to the extremity impedes the venous flow. When suction is applied, as occurs in the process of drawing blood, the valves compress and close the lumen of the vein, preventing the backward flow of blood. Thus, these valves interfere with the process of withdrawing blood. Recognizing the presence of a valve, the nurse may resolve the difficulty by slightly readjusting the needle.

These valves are absent in many of the small veins, which can therefore be used when, because of obstruction from a thrombus in the ascending vein, they would otherwise prove useless. The cannula may be inserted below the thrombosis, with its direction toward the distal end of the extremity; this results in a rerouting of the fluid and avoidance of the thrombosed portion.

Tunica Media or the Middle Layer

The second layer consists of muscular and elastic tissue. The nerve fibers, both vaso-constrictors and vasodilators, are located in this middle layer. These fibers, constantly receiving impulses from the vasoconstrictor center in the medulla, keep the vessels in a state of tonus. They also stimulate both arteries and veins to contract or relax. The middle layer is not as strong and stiff in the veins as in the arteries, and therefore the veins tend to collapse or distend as the pressure within falls or rises. Arteries do not collapse.

Stimulation by a change in temperature or by mechanical or chemical irritation may produce spasms in the vein or artery. For instance, interrupting a continuous infusion to administer a pint of cold blood may produce vasoconstriction; this results in spasm, impedes the flow of blood, and causes pain. Application of heat to the vein promotes vasodilation, which will relieve the spasm, improve the flow of blood, and relieve the pain. The same results are obtained by heat when an irritating drug has caused vasoconstriction. In this situation, heat relieves the spasm and increases the blood flow and protects the vessel wall from inflammation caused by the medication—with heat dilating the vein and increasing the flow of blood, the drug becomes more diluted and less irritating. The use of heat to achieve vasodilation is also an aid when it becomes necessary to use veins that are small and poorly filled.

Spasms produced by a chemical irritation in an artery may have dire consequences. A single artery supplies circulation to a particular area. If this artery is damaged, the related area will suffer from impaired circulation and possibly from necrosis and gangrene. If a chemical agent is introduced into the artery, a spasm may result—a contraction that could shut off the blood supply completely. This problem is not as serious when veins are used because many veins supply a particular area; if one is injured, others will maintain the circulation.

Tunica Adventitia or the Outer Layer

The third layer consists of areolar connective tissue; it surrounds and supports the vessel. In arteries this layer is thicker than in veins because it is subjected to greater pressure from the force of blood within.

Arteries need more protection than veins and are so placed that injury is less likely to occur. Whereas veins are superficially located, most arteries lie deep in the tissues and are protected by muscle. Occasionally an artery is located superficially in an unusual place; this artery is then called an *aberrant artery*. An aberrant artery must not be mistaken for a vein. If a chemical that causes spasm is introduced into an aberrant artery, permanent damage may result.

Arteries pulsate and veins do not, a helpful differentiating characteristic.

Superficial Veins of the Upper Extremities

The superficial veins of the upper extremities are shown in Figures 7-1 and 7-2. They consist of the following: digital, metacarpal, cephalic, basilic, and median veins.

The Digital Veins

The dorsal digital veins flow along the lateral portions of the fingers and are joined to each other by communicating branches.[2] At times, these veins are available as a last resort for fluid administration. In some patients, they are prominent enough to accommodate a small-gauge needle. With adequate taping the fingers can be completely immobilized, thereby preventing the needle from puncturing the posterior wall of the vein and causing extravasation of fluid.

The Metacarpal Veins

The three metacarpal veins are formed by the union of the digital veins.[2] The position of these veins makes them well adapted for IV use; in most cases, the needle and adapter lie

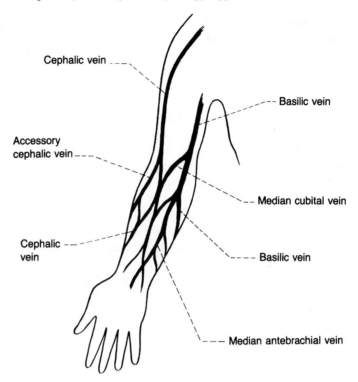

Cephalic vein

Accessory
cephalic vein

Cephalic
vein

Basilic vein

Median cubital vein

Basilic vein

Median antebrachial vein

FIGURE 7-1   Superficial veins of the forearm.

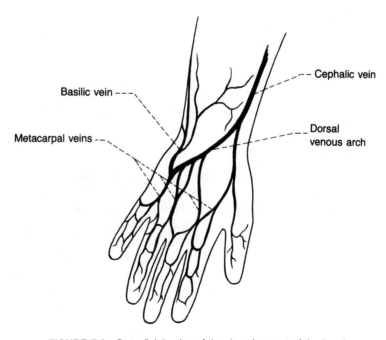

Basilic vein

Metacarpal veins

Cephalic vein

Dorsal
venous arch

FIGURE 7-2   Superficial veins of the dorsal aspect of the hand.

flat between the joints and the metacarpal bones of the hand, the bones themselves providing a natural splint. The early use of the metacarpal veins is important in a course of parenteral therapy. Irritating fluid passing through a vein traumatized by previous puncture causes inflammation and pain. Therefore, performing venipunctures for fluid administration at the distal end of the extremity, early in the course of therapy, is beneficial; it enables the nurse to initiate each successive venipuncture above the previous puncture site. Unnecessary inflammation and pain are avoided and opportunity for multiple venipunctures is provided.

Occasionally the use of the metacarpal veins in the elderly is contraindicated. Because of inadequate tissue and thin skin in this area, extravasation of blood on venipuncture may readily occur.

The Cephalic Vein

The cephalic vein has its source in the radial part of the dorsal venous network formed by the metacarpal veins. Receiving tributaries from both surfaces of the forearm, it flows upward along the radial border of the forearm.[2] Because of its size and position, this vein provides an excellent route for transfusion administration. It readily accommodates a large cannula and, by virtue of its position in the forearm, a natural splint is provided for the cannula and adapter.

The *accessory cephalic vein* originates from either one of two sources—a plexus on the back of the forearm or the dorsal venous network. Ascending the arm, it joins the cephalic vein below the elbow. Occasionally it arises from that portion of the cephalic vein just above the wrist and flows back into the main cephalic vein at some higher point.[2] The accessory cephalic vein readily receives a large cannula and is a very good choice for use in blood administration.

The Basilic Vein

The basilic vein has its origin in the ulnar part of the dorsal venous network and ascends along the ulnar portion of the forearm. It diverges toward the anterior surface of the arm just below the elbow, where it meets the median cubital vein. During a course of IV therapy, this large vein is often overlooked because of its inconspicuous position on the ulnar border of the hand and forearm; when other veins have been exhausted, this vein may still be available. By flexing the elbow and bending the arm up, the basilic vein is brought into view.

The Median Veins

The *median antebrachial vein* arises from the venous plexus on the palm of the hand and extends upward along the ulnar side of the front of the forearm; it empties into the basilic vein or the median cubital vein. This vein, when prominent, affords a route for parenteral fluid administration. However, there are frequent variations of the superficial veins of the forearm, and this vein is not always present as a well-defined vessel.

The *median cephalic* and *median basilic veins* in the antecubital fossa are the veins most generally used for withdrawal of blood. Because of their size and superficial location, they are readily accessible for venipuncture. They accommodate a large cannula, and because of the muscular and connective tissue supporting them, they have little tendency to roll.

The median cephalic vein crosses in front of the brachial artery; therefore, care must be taken during venipuncture to avoid puncturing the artery. Accidental intra-arterial injection of a drug could result in permanent damage.

The basilic vein, outside the antecubital fossa on the ulnar curve of the arm, is the least desirable for venipuncture. When the cannula is removed, a hematoma may readily occur if the patient flexes his or her elbow to stop the bleeding rather than elevating the arm in the preferred manner.

THE SKIN

The skin is made up of two layers, the epidermis and the dermis. The *epidermis* is the uppermost layer, which forms a protective covering for the dermis. Its degree of thickness varies in different parts of the body. It is thickest on the palms of the hands and the soles of the feet and thinnest on the inner surface of the limbs. Its degree of thickness also varies with age. In an elderly patient, the skin on the dorsum of the hand may be so thin that it does not adequately support the vein for venipuncture when parenteral infusions are required.

The *dermis*, or underlayer, is highly sensitive and vascular. It contains many capillaries and thousands of nerve fibers. These nerve fibers are of different types and include those that react to temperature, touch, pressure, and pain. The number of nerve fibers varies in different areas of the body. Some areas of the body skin are highly sensitive; other areas are only mildly sensitive. The insertion of a needle in one area may cause a great deal of pain, yet another area may be virtually painless. In my experience, the inner aspect of the wrist is a highly sensitive area. Venipunctures are performed here only when other veins have been exhausted.

SUPERFICIAL FASCIA

The superficial fascia, or subcutaneous areolar connective tissue, lies below the two layers of skin and is, in itself, another covering. It is in this fascia that the superficial veins are located. It varies in thickness. When a cannula is inserted into this fascia, there is free movement of the skin above. Great care in aseptic technique must be observed because an infection in this loose tissue spreads easily. Such an infection is called *cellulitis*.[1]

REFERENCES

1. Kimber, D. C., Gray, C. E., & Stackpoles, C. E. (1966). *Textbook of anatomy and physiology* (15th ed., pp. 69, 398, 423–431). New York: Macmillan.

2. Warwick, R., & Williams, P. L. (Eds.). (1973). *Gray's anatomy of the human body* (28th ed., pp. 700–703). Philadelphia: Lea & Febiger.

REVIEW QUESTIONS

1. Layers of the skin include:
   a. dermis
   b. epidermis
   c. fascia
   d. tunica intima

2. Which veins are most useful for venous sampling?
   a. median cephalic
   b. cutaneous
   c. median basilic
   d. accessory cephalic

3. An infection involving connective tissue is known as:
   a. cellulitis
   b. phlebitis
   c. thrombophlebitis
   d. phlebothrombosis

4. Superficial veins of the upper extremity include which of the following:
   a. digital
   b. metacarpal
   c. cephalic
   d. median basilic

5. An artery located superficially in an unusual location is known as:
   a. aberrant
   b. arteriovenous
   c. residual
   d. superficial

6. The basilic vein originates in which part of the dorsal venous network?
   a. radial
   b. ulnar
   c. metacarpal
   d. dorsal digital

7. The systemic system contains:
   a. aorta
   b. arteries
   c. ligaments
   d. veins

8. The pulmonary system contains:
   a. blood flow from right ventricle to lungs
   b. blood flow from left ventricle to lungs
   c. blood flow to the body
   d. blood flow from the body

9. A medication inadvertently injected into an artery may result in:
   a. necrosis
   b. gangrene
   c. cellulitis
   d. pustule formation

10. The bone marrow, because of its venous plexus, may be used for intravascular therapy via which route of administration?
    a. intravenous
    b. intramuscular
    c. subcutaneous
    d. intraosseous

_____

CHAPTER 8

Techniques of Intravenous Therapy

APPROACH TO THE PATIENT _____

The nurse's approach to the patient may have a direct bearing on that patient's response to IV therapy. Because an undesirable response can affect the patient's ability to accept treatment, the nurse's manner and approach are significant factors.

Although routine for the nurse, IV therapy may be a new and frightening experience to the patient unfamiliar with the procedure. Patients may have heard rumors of fatalities associated with infusions or may misinterpret the treatment. By explaining the procedure, the nurse will alleviate fears and help the patient to accept therapy.

The critically ill patient is particularly susceptible to fears, which can at times become exaggerated, triggering an undesirable autonomic nervous system response usually known as a *vasovagal reaction*. Such a reaction may manifest itself in the form of syncope and can be prevented if the nurse appears confident and reassures the patient. Sympathetic reaction may follow syncope and result in vasoconstriction. Peripheral collapse then limits available veins, complicating the venipuncture. Repeated attempts at venipuncture can result in an experience so traumatic as to affect the further course of fluid therapy. Only a skilled clinician should perform a venipuncture on an anxious patient with limited and difficult veins. (See Chapter 25 for special considerations in the pediatric patient.)

Reactions to exaggerated fear may not only make therapy difficult but may constitute a real threat to the patient with severe cardiac disease. Fear incites stimulation of the adrenal medulla to secrete the vasopressors, which help maintain blood pressure and increase the work of the heart. Increased adrenal cortical secretions result in sodium and chloride retention, which causes water retention, and loss of cellular potassium, which draws water with it into the intravascular system. Increased antidiuretic hormone secretions cause a decreased urinary output, which results in retention of fluids and an increase in blood volume.[6] Such an increase may be sufficient to send a patient with an overburdened vascular system into pulmonary edema.

SELECTING THE VEIN _____

The selection of the vein may be a deciding factor in the success of the infusion and in the preservation of veins for future therapy. The most prominent vein is not necessarily the most suitable for venipuncture; prominence may be from a sclerosed condition, which

Sharon M. Weinstein: PLUMER'S PRINCIPLES & PRACTICE OF INTRAVENOUS THERAPY, FIFTH EDITION, © 1993 J. B. Lippincott Company

occludes the lumen and interferes with the flow of solution, or the prominent vein may be located in an area impractical for infusion purposes. Scrutiny of the veins in both arms is desirable before a choice is made. The prime factors to be considered in selecting a vein are suitable location, condition of the vein, purpose of the infusion, and duration of therapy.

Location

Most superficial veins are accessible for venipuncture (Figure 8-1), but some of these veins, because of their location, are not practical. The antecubital veins are such veins, located over an area of joint flexion where any motion could dislodge the cannula and cause infiltration or result in mechanical phlebitis. If these large veins are impaired or damaged, phlebothrombosis may occur, which can limit the many available hand veins. The antecubital veins offer excellent sources for withdrawing blood and may be used numerous times without damage to the vein, provided good technique and sharp needles are used. But one infusion of long duration may traumatize the vein, limiting these vessels that most readily provide ample quantities of blood when needed.

Because of the close proximity of the arteries to the veins in the antecubital fossa,

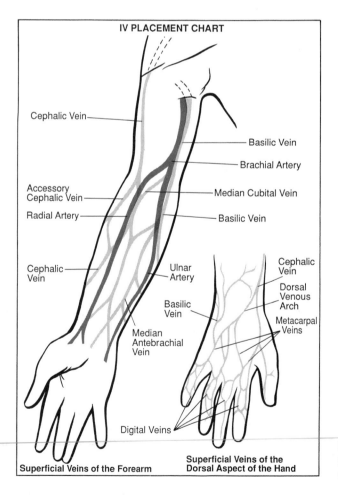

IV PLACEMENT CHART

Cephalic Vein

Basilic Vein

Brachial Artery

Accessory Cephalic Vein

Median Cubital Vein

Radial Artery

Basilic Vein

Cephalic Vein

Ulnar Artery

Cephalic Vein

Dorsal Venous Arch

Basilic Vein

Metacarpal Veins

Median Antebrachial Vein

Digital Veins

Superficial Veins of the Forearm

Superficial Veins of the Dorsal Aspect of the Hand

FIGURE 8-1 IV placement chart. (Courtesy: Becton Dickinson Vascular Access, Sandy, UT)

special care must be taken to prevent intra-arterial injection when medications are introduced. An artery can generally be detected by the thicker and tougher wall, the brighter red blood, and usually the presence of a pulse. Aberrant arteries in the antecubital area have been found to exist in one person out of ten. When a patient complains of severe pain in the hand or arm on infusion, an arteriospasm due to an intra-arterial injection is to be suspected, and the infusion must be stopped immediately.

Surgery often dictates which extremity is to be used. Veins should be avoided in the affected arm of an axillary dissection, such as a radical mastectomy; the circulation may be impaired, affecting the flow of the infusion and increasing the edema. When the patient is turned sideways during the operation, the upper arm is used for the IV infusion; increased venous pressure in the lower arm may interfere with the free flow of the solution.

The use of the veins in the lower extremities is frequently challenged. These objections arise from the danger of pulmonary embolism caused by a thrombus extending into the deep veins. Complications may also arise from the stagnant blood in varicosities; pooling of infused medications can cause untoward reactions when a toxic concentration reaches the circulating blood. Because of the stagnant blood, varicosities are susceptible to trauma. Phlebitis interferes with ambulation of the patient.

The Centers for Disease Control and Prevention (CDC) guidelines strongly recommend that "in adults, the upper extremity (or if necessary, subclavian and jugular sites) should be used in preference to lower extremity sites for IV cannulation. All cannulas inserted into a lower extremity should be changed as soon as a satisfactory site can be established elsewhere."[3]

Condition of the Vein

Frequently, the dorsal metacarpal veins provide points of entry that should be used first to preserve the proximal veins for further therapy. The use of these veins depends on their condition. In some elderly patients, the dorsal metacarpal veins may be a poor choice; blood extravasation occurs more readily in small thin veins, and difficulty may be encountered in adequately securing the cannula because of thin skin and lack of supportive tissue. At times these veins do not dilate sufficiently to allow for successful venipuncture; when hypovolemia occurs the peripheral veins collapse more quickly than do the large ones.

Palpation of the vein is an important step in determining the condition of the vein and in differentiating it from a pulsating artery. A thrombosed vein may be detected by its lack of resilience, by its hard, cordlike feeling, and by the ease with which it rolls. Use of such traumatized veins can result only in repeated venipunctures, pain, and undue stress.

Occasionally, when thrombosis from multiple infusions interferes with the flow of solution and limits available veins, the venipuncture may be performed with the cannula inserted in the direction of the distal end; lack of valves in these small peripheral veins permits rerouting of the solution and bypassing of the involved vein.

Often, large veins may be detected by palpation and offer advantages over the smaller but more readily discernible veins. Because of the small blood volume, the more superficial veins may not be easily palpated and may not make a satisfactory choice for venipuncture.

Continual use by the nurse of the same fingers for palpation will increase their sensitivity. The thumb should never be used because it is not as sensitive as the fingers;

also a pulse may be detected in the nurse's thumb, and this may be confused with an aberrant artery.

Although not apparent, edema may conceal an available vein; application of finger pressure for a few seconds often helps to disperse the fluid and define the vein.

Purpose of the Infusion

The purpose of the infusion dictates the rate of flow and the solution to be infused—two factors that inherently affect the selection of the vein. When large quantities of fluid are to be rapidly infused, or when positive pressure is indicated, a large vein must be used. When fluids with a high viscosity such as packed cells are required, a vein with an adequate blood volume is necessary to ensure flow of the solution.

Large veins are used when hypertonic solutions or solutions containing irritating drugs are to be infused. Such solutions traumatize small veins; the supply of blood in these veins is not sufficient to dilute the infused fluid.

Duration of Therapy

A prolonged course of therapy requires multiple infusions, which makes preservation of the veins essential. Performing the venipuncture distally with each subsequent puncture proximal to the previous one and alternating arms will contribute to this preservation.

The patient's comfort should also be considered when infusions are required over an extended period of time; avoiding areas over joint flexion and performing venipunctures on veins located on the dorsal surface of the extremities will provide more freedom and comfort to the patient.

SELECTING THE CANNULA

Infusions may be administered through a cannula or steel needle (Figures 8-2 and 8-3). Typical cannulas include:

1. Over-the-needle catheter (ONC). Once the venipuncture is made, the catheter is slipped off the needle into the vein and the steel needle removed. The intravenous Nurses Society (INS) does not recommend the use of obturators, which are inserted into the catheter to maintain patency for intermittent infusion.

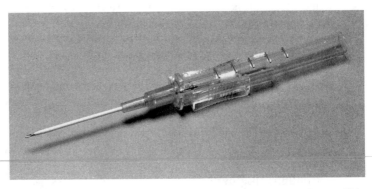

FIGURE 8-2 Protectiv™ IV cannula. (Courtesy: Critikon, Inc., Tampa, FL)

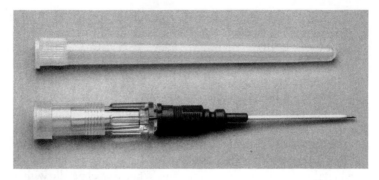

FIGURE 8-3 Over-the-needle IV catheter. (Courtesy: Abbott Laboratories, North Chicago, IL)

2. Inside-the-needle catheter (INC). The venipuncture is performed and the catheter is then pushed through the needle until the desired length is within the lumen of the vein; the cutting edge is then protected by a shield to prevent the catheter from being severed.

The choice of catheter depends on the purpose of the infusion and the condition and availability of the veins.

The ONCs are used routinely today to ensure a ready route for the administration of blood and fluid.

The INCs are used when a longer catheter is desired. They afford less risk of infiltration than does the steel cannula, often being used for administering drugs or hypertonic solutions that may cause necrosis if extravasation occurs.

The cutdown catheter is used when veins become exhausted from prolonged therapy, obesity obscures the veins, and peripheral veins have collapsed from shock.

Catheters are made of a diversity of materials; for many years polyvinylchloride was used almost exclusively. Ideally, to reduce the risk of thrombi formation on the catheter, the catheter should be of a hemorepellant material. Silicone catheters are thought to be helpful in this respect. Catheters should be radiopaque for detection by x-ray in the event the catheter is severed and lost in the circulation.

Steel needles are of two types, the steel cannula (not recommended for infusion purposes) and the winged infusion device or small-vein needle. The gauge refers to both the inside and the outside diameters of the lumen—the smaller the gauge, the larger the lumen. Steel needles are often thin walled. Because the wall of the needle is thinner than that of the standard needle, a larger lumen is obtained for the same external diameter, offering the advantage of enhanced flow rates. Today, the steel needle is most commonly used for venous sampling purposes.

The winged infusion device or small-vein needle is similar to the steel cannula, with the hub replaced with two flexible wings. Originally designed for pediatric and geriatric use, it has been used in prolonged therapy for all ages. Two types of small-vein needles are available, one with a short length of plastic tubing and a permanently attached resealable injection site, the other with a variable length of plastic tubing permanently attached to a female Luer adapter that accommodates an administration set. The small-vein needle with the resealable injection site offers a method for the intermittent administration of medications or fluids. A dilute solution of heparin maintains patency of the needle when it is not in use.

The small-vein needle is approximately ¹/₂ inch long and ranges in size from a 27-gauge bore to a 16-gauge bore. It has definite advantages: the short bevel reduces the risk of infiltration from puncture to the wall of the vein, and the plastic wings provide a firm grip for inserting the needle and better control in performing the venipuncture. The wings fold flat against the skin, affording better anchoring power than the straight steel needle with a bulky hub.

The factors to be considered in selecting a steel needle are length of bevel, gauge, and length of the needle.

A short *bevel* reduces the risk of (1) trauma to the endothelial wall, (2) infiltration from a puncture to the posterior wall, and (3) hematoma or extravasation occurring when the steel needle enters the vein. When a steel needle with a long bevel is inserted into the vessel, blood may leak into the tissues before the entire bevel is within the lumen of the vein.

Whenever possible, the *gauge* of the needle should be appreciably smaller than the lumen of the vein to be entered; when the gauge of the needle approaches the size of the vein, trauma may occur. When a large needle occludes the flow of blood, irritating solutions flowing through the vein with no dilution of blood may cause chemical phlebitis. Mechanical phlebitis may result from motion and pressure exerted by the needle on the endothelial wall of the vein.

When large amounts of fluid are required, a needle of adequate size must be used; a small lumen interferes with the flow of solution. As Adriani stated,

> The flow of blood varies inversely as the fourth power of the radius of the lumen of the needle. Thus, a needle with an internal radius of 1 mm. delivering 1 cc. of blood with a fixed pressure on the plunger or in the infusion bottle delivers only ¹/₁₆ of a cc. when the radius is reduced to ¹/₂ mm.[1]

A large needle is also required with fluids of high viscosity. The rate of flow of the solution decreases in proportion to the viscosity of the fluid.

The flow of the solution varies inversely with the *length of the needle shaft*. If the length of the needle is increased, other conditions being equal, the volume flowing will be reduced.[1] Use of a short needle for infusions reduces the risk of infiltration. Because a short needle affords more play than a long needle, more motion is needed to puncture the vessel wall.

SECURING APPROPRIATE ENVIRONMENT

The importance of proper lighting should not be overlooked. A few extra seconds spent in obtaining adequate light may actually save time and free the patient from unnecessary venipunctures. The ideal light is either an ample amount of daylight or a spotlight that does not shine directly on the vein but leaves enough shadow for clearly defining the vessel.

VENOUS DISTENTION

Special care must be taken to distend the vein adequately. To achieve this, a soft rubber tourniquet is applied with enough pressure to impede the venous flow while the arterial flow is maintained; if the radial pulse cannot be felt, the tourniquet is too tight. To fill the veins to capacity, pressure is applied until radial pulsation ceases and then released until pulsation begins. A blood pressure cuff may be used; inflate the cuff and then release it until the pressure drops to just below the diastolic pressure.

The tourniquet is applied to the midforearm if the selected vein is in the dorsum of the hand. If the selected vein is in the forearm, the tourniquet is applied to the upper arm.

Very little pressure is applied when performing venipunctures on patients with sclerosed veins. If the pressure is too great or the tourniquet is left on for an extended length of time, the vein will become hard and tortuous, causing added difficulty when the cannula is introduced. For some sclerosed veins, a tourniquet is unnecessary and only makes the phlebotomy more difficult.

If pressure exerted by the tourniquet does not fill the veins sufficiently, the patient may be asked to open and close his or her fist. The action of the muscles will force the blood into the veins, causing them to distend considerably more. A light tapping will often help fill the vein. It may be helpful, before applying the tourniquet, to lower the extremity below the heart level to increase the blood supply to the veins. Occasionally, these methods are inadequate to fill the vein sufficiently. In such cases, application of heat is helpful. To be effective the heat must be applied to the entire extremity for 10 to 20 minutes and retained until the venipuncture is performed.

PREPARATION FOR VENIPUNCTURE

Check Solution and Container

Careful inspection must be made to ensure that the fluid is clear and free of particulate matter and that the container is intact—there are no cracks in the glass bottle or holes in the plastic bag. The label must be checked to verify that the correct solution is being used and that the container is not outdated. Indicate the time and the date the bottle is opened; after 24 hours the fluid is outdated and should not be used.

Attach Administration Set to Fluid Container

The set is attached to the container by closing the roller clamp to equalize pressure, squeezing the drip chamber, and entering the bottle with a thrust, not a twisting motion. The chamber is released, causing immediate function of the air vent and filling of the drip chamber on the suspension of the bottle. This prevents leakage of fluid through the air vent and expedites clearing the infusion set of air, thus preventing bubbles from entering the tubing. In systems that do not require air venting—plastic bags and semirigid bottles—squeezing the drip chamber before insertion avoids the introduction of air into the container.

Height of the Fluid Container

The fluid container is suspended at approximately 3 feet above the injection site. At this height, adequate pressure is provided to achieve a maximum flow rate. The greater the height of the container, the greater the force with which the fluid will flow into the vein should the adjusting clamp release, and the greater the risk of speed shock.

Preparing the Patient and Providing Privacy

Visitors should be asked to leave the room during the procedure; curtains should be pulled if a roommate is present. The patient should be in a comfortable position with the arm on a flat surface. If necessary, a strip of tape is used to secure the arm to an armboard to prevent an uncooperative or disoriented patient from jerking the arm while the cannula is being inserted.

If the area selected for venipuncture is hairy, clipping the hair will permit better cleansing of the skin and make removal of the cannula less painful when the infusion is terminated. Shaving is not recommended, consistent with INS Standards. Products such as Skin-Prep decrease bacterial flora and should be considered for use before venipuncture.

TECHNIQUES IN VENIPUNCTURE

Direct Method or One-Step Entry

This method is performed with a thrust of the cannula through the skin and into the vein with one quick motion. The cannula enters the skin directly over the vein. This technique is excellent as long as large veins are available. However, because often one must resort to the use of small veins, this is not the preferred technique. Such an attempt at entry into the small veins will result in hematomas.

Indirect Method

This method consists of two complete motions:

1. Insertion of the cannula through the skin. The cannula enters the skin below the point where the vein is visible; entering the skin above the vein tends to depress the vein, obscuring its position.
2. Relocation of the vein and entry into the vein.

Recommended Skin Preparation[3]

The injection site should be scrubbed with an antiseptic and allowed to remain in contact for at least 30 seconds before venipuncture.

1. Tincture of iodine 1% to 2%, iodophor, or chlorhexidine may be used.
2. Isopropyl 70% alcohol is recommended if the patient is sensitive to iodine.

BASIC VENIPUNCTURE

The basic venipuncture is performed as follows:

1. Put on gloves.
2. Apply tourniquet and select vein.
3. Prepare skin according to recommendations.
4. After establishing a minimum rate of flow by adjusting the clamp, kink the infusion tubing between the third and little fingers of the right hand. When the kinked tubing is released, the minimum rate of flow will prevent a rapid infusion

of fluid and drugs with the potential danger of speed shock. Obstructing the flow of solution manually expedites the procedure and leaves the hands free for anchoring the steel cannula and caring for any collected blood samples.

5. Hold the patient's hand or arm with the left hand, using the thumb to keep the skin taut and to anchor the vein to prevent rolling.

6. Place the steel cannula in line with the vein, about 1/2 inch below the proposed site of entry (Figure 8-4). The bevel-up position of the cannula facilitates venipuncture and produces less trauma to the skin and the vein on puncture.

   To prevent extravasation in small veins, it is often necessary to enter the vein with the bevel down; any readjustment of the cannula should be made before releasing the tourniquet to prevent puncturing the vein and producing a hematoma.

7. Insert the cannula through skin and tissue at a 45° angle.

8. Relocate the vein and decrease the cannula angle slightly.

9. Slowly, with downward motion followed at once by raising point, pick up vein, leveling cannula until almost flush with skin.

10. On entering the vein there may be a flashback of blood, which indicates successful entry (Figure 8-5). With experience, the fingers will become sensitive to the cannula's entering the vein—the resistance encountered as the cannula meets the wall of the vein and the snap felt at the loss of resistance as the cannula enters the lumen. This is more difficult to discern on thin-walled veins with small blood volume. To prevent a through puncture, advance the cannula slowly, checking at each movement for a flashback of blood.

11. Release the tourniquet and remove the introducer (Figure 8-6).

12. Release the pressure exerted by the little finger, connect administration set to hub, and allow the solution to flow (Figure 8-7).

13. Check carefully for any signs of swelling.

If the vein has sustained a through puncture (evidenced by a developing hematoma) and the venipuncture is unsuccessful, the cannula should be immediately removed and

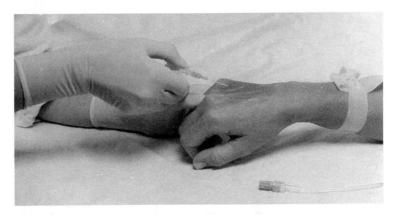

FIGURE 8-4   Venipuncture with over-the needle catheter. (Courtesy: Critikon, Inc., Tampa, FL)

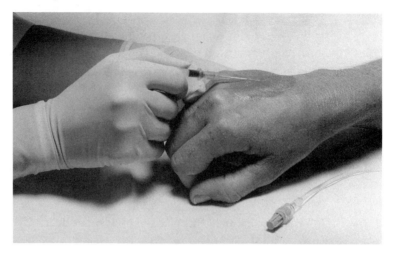

FIGURE 8-5   Evidence of flashback. (Courtesy: Critikon, Inc., Tampa, FL)

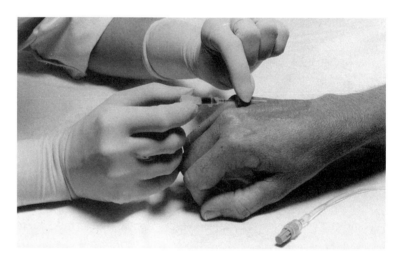

FIGURE 8-6   Catheter is advanced and the introducer is removed. (Courtesy: Critikon, Inc., Tampa, FL)

pressure applied to the site. Never reapply a tourniquet to the extremity immediately after a venipuncture; a hematoma will occur, limiting veins and providing an excellent culture medium for bacteria.

ANCHORING THE VASCULAR ACCESS DEVICE

The Cannula

1. Use ¹/₂-inch wide tape over the hub. Tape the cannula flush with the skin; no elevation of the hub is necessary, and it would only increase the risk of a through puncture from the point of the cannula.

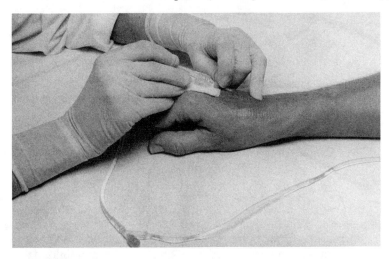

FIGURE 8-7 Primed administration set is connected to the catheter hub. (Courtesy: Critikon, Inc., Tampa, FL)

2. Place a ¹/₂-inch strip of tape—adhesive up—under the hub of the cannula. Place one end tightly and diagonally over the cannula. Repeat with the other end, crossing the first. This secures the cannula firmly and prevents any sideward movement. Avoid placing tape directly over the actual injection site.

3. Loop the tubing and secure it with tape independently of the cannula. This eliminates dislodging the cannula by an accidental pull on the tubing.

4. Apply an occlusive dressing over the cannula entrance site to allow for routine, standardized inspection.

5. Indicate type, gauge, insertion date, and initials near the dressing and in the clinical record. Variations in taping are shown in Figures 8-8 and 8-9.

The Armboard

The use of an armboard is helpful for immobilizing the extremity when undue motion can result in infiltration or phlebitis. It is a valuable aid in restraining the arm when infusions are initiated on uncooperative, disoriented, or elderly patients or children, or when the

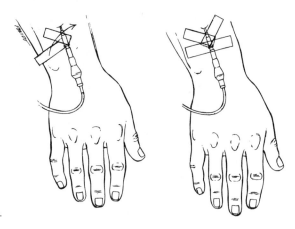

FIGURE 8-8 Chevron taping technique.

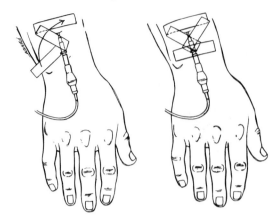

FIGURE 8-9 Variations in taping of over-the-needle cannula.

cannula is inserted on the dorsum of the hand or in an area of joint flexion. When the metacarpal veins are used, the fingers should be immobilized to prevent any movement of the cannula that could result in phlebitis.

The function of the hand may be endangered and even permanently impaired by the widespread hospital practice of flattening the hand on an armboard during IV therapy. This complication results from failure to recognize that the hand has both transverse and longitudinal arches and that if the knuckle joints (metacarpophalangeal) are immobilized in a straight position, they will develop contracture that will prevent motion. Patients on long-term therapy with edema or muscular weakness are particularly vulnerable. Intensive physical therapy, splinting, and even surgery may be required to restore mobility.

To preserve maximal function, the hand should be immobilized in a functional position on the armboard.

If a plastic armboard is used, cover it with absorbent paper or bandage to prevent the arm from perspiring and sticking to the board. Make certain that any tape placed on the cannula is independent of the board so that a motion of the arm on the board will not cause a pull on the cannula. If restraint of the arm is necessary, the restraint is secured to the board, not to the patient's arm above the puncture area; such restraint might act as a tourniquet, causing a backflow of blood into the cannula, resulting in clotting and obstruction of the flow.

Armboards have changed dramatically, and many manufacturers now provide sophisticated devices aimed at ensuring patient comfort (Figure 8-10).

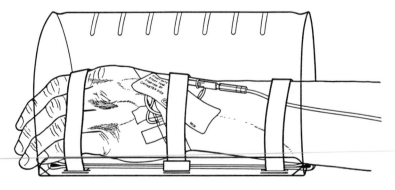

FIGURE 8-10 Genny Denny IV shield. (Courtesy: TADCO Inc., Farmington, NM)

APPLICATION OF AN OCCLUSIVE DRESSING

Consistent with INS Standards of Practice, an occlusive dressing should be applied over the infusion site. The occlusive dressing may be either gauze and tape or a transparent semipermeable membrane (TSM) dressing.

The following procedure is applicable to the Tegaderm pouch dressings manufactured by 3M (Figure 8-11). The professional is encouraged to follow the manufacturer's recommendations for the use of a specific product.

Infusion sites should be labeled with type of cannula (Figure 8-12), length and size, date, time, and initials of individual who initiated the infusion. Many labels are available to facilitate this practice (Figure 8-13).

THE INSIDE-THE-NEEDLE CATHETER

Because this type of catheter is associated with a higher incidence of serious complications, it is seldom used. The inherent danger of infection from bacteria invading the vein through the cutaneous opening and being carried along the plastic cannula makes thorough skin preparation necessary. Trauma caused by the insertion of a large catheter is increased when performed by an inexperienced clinician.

A catheter severed by the cutting edge of the needle can result in a serious complication when lost in the bloodstream. A catheter introduced into a vein over a joint flexion increases the risk of complication if the extremity is not immobilized.

An INC facilitates prolonged therapy but increases the risk of thrombophlebitis. Limiting the length of time the catheter is in use reduces the incidence of phlebitis; a time limit is sometimes difficult to enforce, however, because veins may be exhausted in a critically ill patient whose life depends on infusion therapy.

Insertion of the Inside-the-Needle Catheter

1. Put on gloves.
2. Apply a tourniquet and select the vein.
3. Prepare the injection site area according to recommendations.
4. Make the venipuncture.
5. Gently thread the catheter through the lumen of the needle into the vein until the desired length has been introduced.
6. Apply digital pressure on the vein to hold the catheter in place; withdraw the needle.
7. Apply pressure with a sterile sponge for 30 seconds to minimize bleeding through the puncture site.
8. Attach the needle to the infusion set, and regulate the flow rate. NEVER WITHDRAW THE CATHETER BACK THROUGH THE NEEDLE. If the venipuncture is unsuccessful, the needle and catheter must be removed together; to pull the catheter back through the needle may sever the catheter and result in its loss in the circulation.
9. Slip the shield from the base of the needle over the bevel and tape; the shield must be kept in place to protect the cutting edge of the needle and prevent its

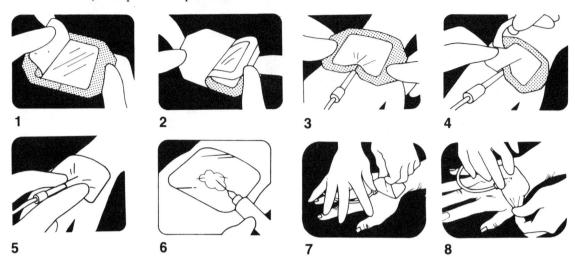

INSTRUCTIONS FOR USE*

1. Remove sterile dressing from package. Remove and discard the center cut-out "window." Part 1.

   Tegaderm pouch dressings do not have a cut-out "window."

2. Peel the paper liner from the dressing, exposing the adhesive surface. Part 2.

3. Position the dressing over the catheter site or wound. If using the peripheral IV dressing with the frame opening, place the opening over the catheter hub. Firmly rub the dressing from the center out toward the edges. Part 3.

4. Remove the paper frame from the dressing while smoothing down the dressing edges. Part 4. If on IV site, seal securely around catheter hub. Part 5. Again, firmly smooth dressing from the center toward the edges.

5. You may observe the site or wound without removing the dressing. It is normal for wound fluid to accumulate under a Tegaderm dressing. If exudate threatens to compromise adhesion of the dressing, aspirate the fluid with a small gauge needle using sterile technique. Part 6. Patch the puncture site with a small piece of Tegadrem dressing.

   For cosmetic purposes, Tegaderm dressing may be covered with a layer of gauze. Tape the gauze to skin around the dressing.

6. To remove the dressing, grasp one edge of the dressing and slowly pull from the skin in the direction of hair growth. Part 7. Or, grasp one edge of the dressing and pull the dressing straight out to stretch it and release adhesion. Part 8. IV catheters should always be stabilized with one hand during dressing removal.

APPLICATION HINTS

1. Choose the size dressing appropriate for the application. Especially for wounds where exudate is likely, choose a dressing size that will provide at least a two-inch margin of dressing adhered to healthy, dry skin. When using Tegaderm pouch dressing, the wound margins should be under the pouch area of the dressing.

2. Adhesive products do not adhere to wet or oily surfaces. Soaps, detergents, ointments, and skin lotions can lower adhesion. Clean and dry skin thoroughly before dressing application.

3. Firm rubbing of the dressing improves the adhesion. Always rub the dressing from the center out to the edges after application.

4. Protective skin barriers and skin tackifiers are not necessary under Tegaderm dressings but, if they are used, **allow them to dry completely** before dressing application. Alcohol trapped under a dressing can be a skin irritant.

5. Do not stretch a Tegaderm dressing during application. Applying an adhesive product with tension can cause mechanical trauma to the skin. **Stretching can also cause adhesion failure.**

FIGURE 8-11   Application of Tegaderm pouch dressing. (Courtesy: 3M Healthcare, St. Paul, MN. Reprinted with permission of 3M Company.)

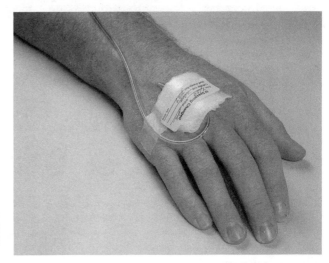

FIGURE 8-12 Labeling of the venipuncture site consistent with INS Standards. (Courtesy: United Ad Label Co., Inc., Brea, CA)

severing the catheter. A tongue depressor is frequently used to secure the needle and catheter to further guard against kinking and breaking of the catheter at the junction of the needle.

10. Tape the catheter to prevent motion.

11. Ascertain the patency and position of the catheter in the vein.

12. Topical antibiotic or antiseptic ointment should be applied to the injection site.

13. Apply a sterile gauze or TSM dressing; the puncture made by the needle is larger than the inlying catheter, and seepage of fluid and infection can occur.

14. Indicate length, gauge, and type of catheter, initials of nurse, and date of insertion on tape near dressing and in medical record.

15. Use an armboard if the catheter lies over a point of flexion—motion contributes to phlebitis. The arm must not be fastened tightly to the armboard; vascular occlusion results in a plugged catheter, and stasis edema may occur.

16. Remove gloves. Wash hands.

THE OVER-THE-NEEDLE CATHETER

Venipuncture and Insertion

1. Put on gloves.

2. Apply a tourniquet and select the vein.

3. Prepare the injection site according to recommendations. If palpation of the vein is necessary, prepare the fingertip in the same manner. Do not touch the proposed insertion site.

4. Perform the venipuncture in the usual manner. When the needle has punctured the venous wall, introduce it 1/2 inch farther to ensure entry of the catheter into the lumen of the vein.

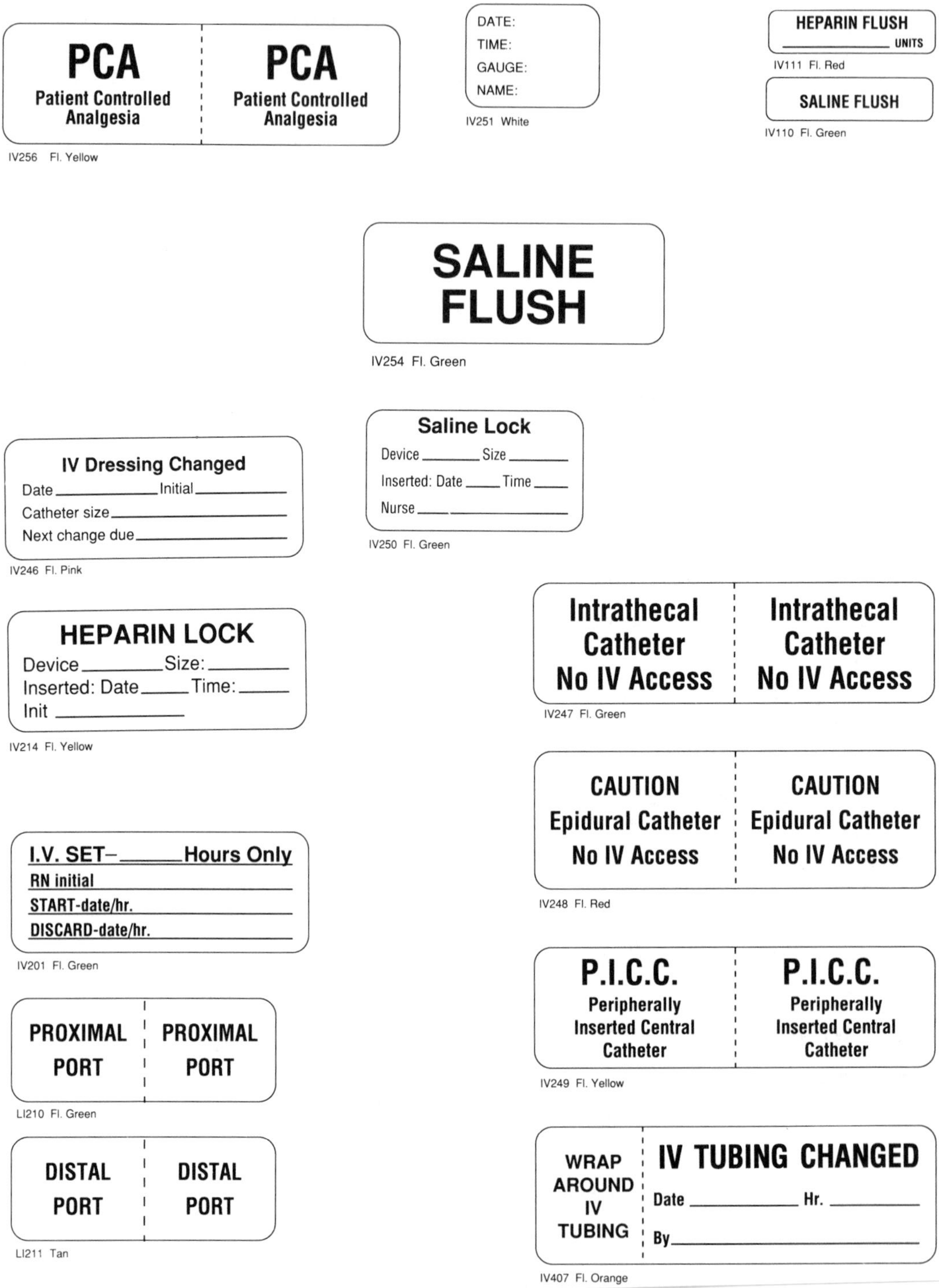

PCA
Patient Controlled
Analgesia

PCA
Patient Controlled
Analgesia

IV256 Fl. Yellow

DATE:
TIME:
GAUGE:
NAME:

IV251 White

HEPARIN FLUSH
_____ UNITS

IV111 Fl. Red

SALINE FLUSH

IV110 Fl. Green

SALINE FLUSH

IV254 Fl. Green

IV Dressing Changed
Date _____ Initial _____
Catheter size _____
Next change due _____

IV246 Fl. Pink

Saline Lock
Device _____ Size _____
Inserted: Date _____ Time _____
Nurse ___ _____

IV250 Fl. Green

HEPARIN LOCK
Device _____ Size: _____
Inserted: Date _____ Time: _____
Init _____

IV214 Fl. Yellow

**Intrathecal
Catheter
No IV Access**

**Intrathecal
Catheter
No IV Access**

IV247 Fl. Green

I.V. SET–_____ Hours Only
RN initial _____
START-date/hr. _____
DISCARD-date/hr. _____

IV201 Fl. Green

CAUTION
Epidural Catheter
No IV Access

CAUTION
Epidural Catheter
No IV Access

IV248 Fl. Red

**PROXIMAL
PORT**

**PROXIMAL
PORT**

LI210 Fl. Green

P.I.C.C.
Peripherally
Inserted Central
Catheter

P.I.C.C.
Peripherally
Inserted Central
Catheter

IV249 Fl. Yellow

**DISTAL
PORT**

**DISTAL
PORT**

LI211 Tan

**WRAP
AROUND
IV
TUBING**

IV TUBING CHANGED
Date _____ Hr. _____
By _____

IV407 Fl. Orange

FIGURE 8-13   Variety of site, tubing, and chart labels available. (Courtesy: United Ad Label Co., Inc., Brea, CA)

5. Hold the needle in place and slowly slide the catheter hub until the desired length is in the vein. IF THE VENIPUNCTURE IS UNSUCCESSFUL, DO NOT REINSERT THE NEEDLE INTO THE CATHETER. To do so can sever the catheter.

6. Remove the needle by holding the catheter hub in place. To minimize leakage of blood while removing the needle and connecting the infusion set, apply pressure on the vein beyond the catheter with the little finger.

7. Attach the administration set, which has been previously cleared of air, and regulate the rate of flow.

8. Topical antiseptic iodophor ointment should be considered or a broad-spectrum antiseptic ointment for patients sensitive to iodine.

9. Tape catheter securely to prevent motion that could contribute to phlebitis. Avoid taping over injection site; cover site with sterile sponge or TSM dressing.

10. Loop the tubing and tape independent of the catheter to prevent an accidental pull from withdrawing the catheter.

11. Indicate the length, gauge, and type of catheter, the date of insertion, and the initials of the nurse on the tape, close to the dressing, and again in the clinical record.

12. Remove gloves and wash hands.

MIDLINE CATHETER INSERTION

Landmark and Aquavene are registered trademarks of Menlo Care, Inc. The Landmark midline catheter (Figure 8-14) has been designed for peripheral infusion of general IV solutions and medications and venous sampling. Indications for midline IV therapy include antibiotics, hydration, pain medication, and peripheral nutrition solutions of

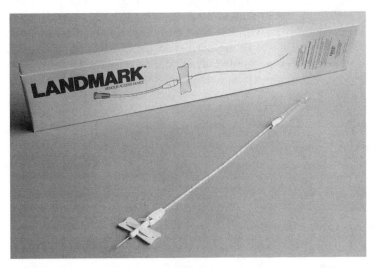

FIGURE 8-14 Landmark® Midline Catheter. (Courtesy: Menlo Care, Inc., Menlo Park, CA)

12.5% or less final glucose concentration, and selected antineoplastic agents (excluding vesicants, which the Oncology Nursing Society generally recommends be infused through a central line).

The procedure should be performed only by trained clinical staff and following careful consideration of the possible risks, including thrombosis, phlebitis, air embolism, infection, vascular perforation, bleeding, and catheter transection.

Vein Assessment

As with any venipuncture, adequate assessment of the patient and the venous status is essential to ensure success. The basilic vein is the vein of choice for longer line IV insertions because of its larger size, straighter course, and adequate hemodilution capability.

Procedure for Insertion

Before insertion, the clinician should carefully select the vessel site and aseptically prepare it consistent with institutional policy and recommended INS Standards of Practice, then establish a sterile field and apply gloves. The procedure for insertion is outlined in Figure 8-15.

HYPODERMOCLYSIS

Though seldom used, the IV nursing professional should be familiar with the terminology *hypodermoclysis* and its clinical applications. When performing a hypodermoclysis, the subcutaneous route is used as a vehicle for absorption of IV isotonic hydration fluids, usually lactated Ringer's solution. One-half ampule of Wydase is added to each 500 mL of IV solution to enhance absorption of the solution within the subcutaneous tissue.

A clysis needle, resembling the standard winged infusion needle, is entered into the lateral aspect of the patient's thigh and the infusion is initiated. Standard skin preparation consistent with INS Standards of Practice should be followed before the procedure and for removal of the needles at the completion of the clysis.[5] Some manufacturers provide therapy-specific clysis administration sets. In lieu of such a set, a standardized 78-inch administration set may be used.

PHLEBOTOMY

Phlebotomy is performed in many institutions by the professional IV nurse. The phlebotomy, a bleeding of between 400 and 500 mL blood, is performed for transfusion purposes, as well as therapeutically for acute pulmonary congestion, polycythemia vera, hemochromatosis, and porphyria cutanea tarda.

Blood for Transfusion Purposes

Routine Blood Bank Blood
When the bleeding is performed for routine bank blood, donor selection is based on the medical history and the physical examination (weight, temperature, pulse, blood pressure, and hemoglobin). The technique is according to the standards of the American Association of Blood Banks (AABB).[2]

Autotransfusion

Autotransfusion is used to return the patient's own blood to the circulation. The phlebotomy may be either:

1. *Blood bank procedure.* When the phlebotomy is performed in the blood bank, the usual blood bank procedure is followed. The blood can be stored at 4°C or the red cells can be frozen.

2. *Non–blood bank procedure.* When the bleeding is performed outside the confines of the blood bank, the same technique (according to the standards of the AABB) is used. However, the donor criteria can be modified; for example, a person with a history of cancer cannot make a routine donation but may donate for himself. Blood, which is suitable only for the donor, must be labeled with his name, hospital number, or social security number, and segregated from other donor bloods. The ABO type is confirmed just before transfusion.

An important fact to bear in mind is the possibility of sepsis; clinically undetected bacteremia may exist in the patient with a catheter, a tracheostomy, or a disease process.

Blood for Therapeutic Purposes

The therapeutic phlebotomy is a valuable means by which a quantity of blood is removed to promote the health of the donor. It requires a written order by the physician specifying the date, the amount of blood to be drawn, the frequency of bleeding, and the hemoglobin or hematocrit at which the patient should be bled. If the recipient's physician approves and if the label conspicuously indicates the diagnosis and a therapeutic bleeding, the blood may be used for transfusion.

Acute Pulmonary Congestion (Inpatient)

The phlebotomy is performed to reduce venous pressure and to relieve the work load on the heart of a patient suffering from acute pulmonary edema of cardiac failure or overtransfusion. Overtransfusion is much less likely to occur today because central venous pressure monitoring provides a valuable guide for fluid administration; also, drugs are available to increase cardiac output and lower the central venous pressure. Because the patient with acute pulmonary congestion is critically ill, the phlebotomy should probably be done by, or in the presence of, the patient's physician.

Polycythemia Vera (Inpatient or Outpatient)

The therapeutic phlebotomy is most frequently performed on the hospital patient for the production of remissions in the treatment of polycythemia vera, a disease characterized by a striking increase in the number of circulating red blood corpuscles. It is used to reduce the red cell mass, either alone or in combination with radioactive phosphorus (^{32}P), lowering the blood volume, reducing blood viscosity, and improving circulatory efficiency. The number of and interval between phlebotomies should be specified by the physician and the hematocrit value determined after the blood donation.

Hemochromatosis (Usually Outpatient)

Hemochromatosis is characterized by excessive body stores of iron. The phlebotomy is performed to reduce the total body iron concentration. Because these patients usually

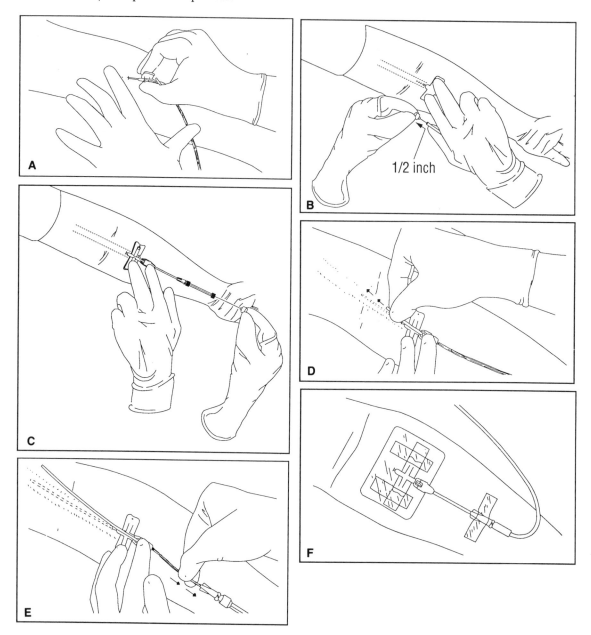

FIGURE 8-15   Procedure for insertion of Landmark® catheter. (**A**) Step 1: Insertion. *Squeeze butterfly wings upright (pebble side against fingers). Perform venipuncture. Check for flashback. Advance to butterfly hub.* (**B** and **C**) Step 2: Removal of stylet. *Release butterfly wings and hold flat. Release tourniquet. While holding needle safety tube, withdraw stylet fully until needle tip is enclosed in safety tube.* (**D**) Step 3: Advancement. *Hold butterfly wings flat. Pull sheath tab slowly forward to advance catheter to desired initial length.* (**E**) Step 4: Lock Catheter and Remove Sheath. *Continue to hold butterfly wings. Lock catheter in place by firmly pulling back on remaining extension tubing. Cut sheath.* (**F**) Step 5: Completion. *Remove needle safety tube and attach IV tubing or heparin lock to luer lock. Secure and dress site per institution policy. Immobilize arm for 30 minutes.* (Courtesy of Menlo Care, Inc., Menlo Park, CA)

Nursing Care Tips*

1. Landmark® package should be opened on a firm, flat surface. While holding the bottom layer with one hand, use your dominant hand to peel the top layer back in a horizontal motion (do not pull upward).

2. Landmark should not be flushed or placed in a saline/water bath prior to insertion as this will initiate hydration and softening of the Aquavene® catheter.

3. Blood pressure cuffs or tourniquets should not be placed on the arm where Landmark is indwelling.

4. Hemostats or any clamp with teeth/sharp edges should not be used on the catheter.

5. Method of blood sampling is at the discretion of the practitioner; however, a syringe is recommended to avoid collapsing a soft catheter lumen.

6. The internal volume of the hydrated Landmark catheter is approximately 0.3 mL (important to know when performing flushing or declotting procedures).

7. Needles used to inject through the heparin lock should be one (1) inch or less. Needles longer than this may puncture the catheter.

8. When changing tubing or the injection cap, maintain the exit site (hub) *at* or *below* the level of the patient's heart to prevent a possible air embolism.

9. The sterile dressing should be changed according to institution policy. It should remain dry and occlusive at all times.

10. Patients who are crutch walking should be carefully instructed to avoid any pressure on the inner surface area or axilla of the cannulated arm.

11. Upon removal of the Landmark catheter, the shape of the catheter may appear irregular or "vessel like." This is the normal conforming of the catheter to the anatomical shape of the patient's skin and vein.

12. Catheter removal should be performed using a slow and gentle method to prevent vasoconstriction and venospasm.

FIGURE 8-15   *(Continued)*

have a hematocrit value in the normal range, periodic checks on the hematocrit value are desirable.

Porphyria Cutanea Tarda (Usually Outpatient)
The mechanism of relief of these skin lesions by phlebotomy is not clear. Because these patients have a normal hematocrit reading, they are most likely to be bled too much; periodic hematocrit checks are desirable.

Procedure for Bleeding

To allay apprehension and to avoid a vasovagal reaction, the procedure should be explained and the patient reassured and put at ease.

Identification
1. Identify donor with the record and the order for the phlebotomy.
2. Make sure that identically numbered labels to donor record are attached to the blood collection container and to test tubes for donor blood samples.
3. Make sure that the processing tubes are correctly numbered and kept with the container during the collection of blood.

Donor Arm Preparation
Adequate preparation of the skin is vital in providing an aseptic site for venipuncture to protect both the donor and the recipient. In preparing the area, always start at the venipuncture site and move outward in concentric spirals for at least 1½ inches; use sterile materials and instruments.

1. Put on gloves

2. Using a 15% aqueous (not alcoholic) soap or detergent solution, scrub vigorously for at least 30 seconds with gauze or 60 seconds with cotton balls.

3. Apply 10% acetone in 70% isopropyl alcohol to remove the soap; let dry.

4. Apply tincture of iodine (3% in 70% ethyl alcohol) and allow to dry.

5. Use 10% acetone in 70% isopropyl alcohol to remove the iodine; allow to dry.

6. Place a dry sterile gauze over the site until ready to perform the venipuncture.

Alternative procedure:

1. Put on gloves

2. Use 0.7% aqueous scrub solution of iodophor compound (povidone–iodine or poloxamer–iodine complex), scrubbing the area for 30 seconds. Remove the foam; it is not necessary to dry the arm.

3. Prepare with iodophor complex solution (*eg*, 10% povidone–iodine); allow to stand 30 seconds. The solution need not be removed.

4. Place a dry sterile gauze sponge over the site until ready to perform the venipuncture. Do not repalpate vein.

Collection of Blood

The following procedure for the collection of blood using the plastic bag is reproduced from the AABB's *Technical Methods and Procedures*.[2] This procedure may be modified when the blood is to be discarded.

1. Inspect bag for any defects. Apply pressure to check for leaks. The anticoagulant solution must be clear.

2. Position bag carefully, being sure it is below the level of the donor's arm.
   a. If balance system is used, be sure counterbalance is level and adjusted for the amount of blood to be drawn. Unless metal clips and a hand sealer are used, make a very loose overhand knot in tubing. Hang the bag and route tubing through the pinch clamp.
   b. If balance system is not used, be sure there is some way to monitor the volume of blood drawn.
   c. If a vacuum-assist device is used, the manufacturer's instructions should be followed.

3. Reapply tourniquet or blood pressure cuff. Have donor open and close hand until previously selected vein is again prominent.

4. Uncover sterile needle and do venipuncture immediately. A clean, skillful venipuncture is essential for collection of a full, clot-free unit. Tape the tubing to hold needle in place and cover site with sterile gauze.

5. Open the temporary closure between the interior of the bag and the tubing, if present.

6. Have donor open and close hand, squeezing a rubber ball or other resilient object slowly every 10 to 12 seconds during collection. Keep the donor under observation throughout phlebotomy. The donor should never be left unattended during or immediately after donation.

7. Mix the blood and anticoagulant gently and periodically (approximately every

30 seconds) during collection. Mixing may be done by hand, by placing bag on a mechanical agitator, or by using a rocking vacuum-assist device.

8. Be sure blood flow remains fairly brisk, so that coagulation activity is not triggered. Rigid time limits are not warranted if there is continuous agitation, although units requiring more than 8 minutes to draw may not be suitable for preparation of platelet concentrates, fresh frozen plasma, or cryoprecipitate.

9. Monitor volume of blood being drawn. If a balance or vacuum-assist device is used, blood flow will stop after the proper amount has been collected. One mL of blood weighs 1.053 g, the minimum allowable specific gravity for female donors. A convenient figure to use is 1.06 g; a unit containing 405 to 495 mL should weigh 425 to 520 g plus the weight of the container with its anti-coagulant.

10. Clamp tubing temporarily using a hemostat, metal clip, or other temporary clamp. Next, collect blood-processing sample by a method that precludes contamination of the donor unit. This may be accomplished in several ways.

    a. If the blood collection bag contains an in-line needle (sid connector), make an additional seal with a hemostat, metal clip, hand sealer, or a tight knot made from previously prepared loose knot just distal to the in-line needle. Open the connector by separating the needles. Insert the proximal needle into a processing test tube, remove the hemostat, allow the tube to fill, and reclamp tubing. Carefully reattach sid connector. Donor needle is now ready for removal.

    b. If the blood collection bag contains an in-line processing tube, be certain that the processing tube, or pouch, is full when the collection is complete and the original clamp is placed near the donor needle. Entire assembly may now be removed from donor.

    c. If a straight-tubing assembly set is used, there are two alternative procedures. In the first method, remove the needle from the donor's arm as soon as the tubing is clamped. Take bag and assembly to sealer area or collect processing tube at the donor chair by placing a hemostat close to where donor tubing enters the bag, leaving the tubing full of blood. Remove the clamp next to donor needle, empty contents of donor tubing into the processing test tube, reapply clamp or permanently seal next to donor needle, remove hemostat next to donor bag, and allow the donor tubing to refill with blood, well mixed, from donor bag.

       In the second method, place two hemostats or temporary seals on the tubing. Cut tubing between the seals, put cut end of the tubing into the processing test tube, remove the proximal hemostat, allow tube to fill, and reclamp tubing.

11. Deflate and remove tourniquet. Remove needle from arm. Apply pressure over gauze and have donor raise arm (elbow straight) and hold gauze firmly over phlebotomy site with the other hand.

12. Discard needle assembly into rigid container designed to prevent accidental injury to and contamination of personnel.

13. Strip donor tubing as completely as possible into the bag, starting at seal. Work quickly, to avoid allowing the blood to clot in the tubing. Invert bag several times to mix thoroughly, then allow tubing to refill with anticoagulated blood from the bag. Repeat this procedure a second time.

14. Seal the tubing left attached to the bags into segments on which the segment number is clearly and completely readable. Knots, metal clips, or a dielectric sealer may be used to make segments suitable for crossmatching. It must be possible to separate segments from the container without breaking sterility of the container.
15. Reinspect container for defects.
16. Recheck numbers on container, processing tubes, and donation record. Be sure the expiration date of the unit is on the container label.
17. Place blood at appropriate temperature. Unless platelets are to be removed, whole blood should be placed at 1°C to 6°C immediately after collection. If platelets are to be harvested, blood should not be chilled but should be maintained at room temperature (about 20°C–24°C) until platelets are separated. Platelets should be separated within 6 hours after collection of the unit of whole blood.

Treatment of Adverse Donor Reactions
Stop the phlebotomy at the first sign of reaction and call the physician.

1. *Fainting*
   a. Elevate the donor's feet above head level.
   b. Loosen tight clothing.
   c. Ascertain that the donor has adequate airway.
   d. Apply cold compresses to forehead and back of neck.
   e. Check and record blood pressure, pulse, and respiration periodically.
2. *Nausea and vomiting*
   a. Instruct the donor to breathe slowly.
3. *Muscular twitching* or tetanic spasms of hands or face
   a. Instruct donor to rebreathe into a paper bag. DO NOT GIVE OXYGEN.
4. *Convulsions* (rare)
   a. Call for assistance.
   b. Prevent the donor from injuring himself or herself by turning the patient on the left side.
5. *For more serious reactions* or if donor does not respond
   a. Call for medical assistance.

Record the nature and treatment of all reactions on the donor's record; include opinion as to the future use of the donor for blood donations.

Suggested Procedure for Therapeutic Phlebotomy

The blood must be discarded. This procedure is not adequate for recipient protection.

Equipment
Phlebotomy pack (obtained from blood bank); if only double pack is available, ignore the satellite pack.
Counterbalance stand (obtained from blood bank) or small spring scale
Blood pressure cuff or tourniquet

Tincture of iodine (3% in 70% ethyl alcohol) or iodophor complex solution (10% povidone–iodine)

10% acetone in 70% isopropyl alcohol for use with tincture of iodine

Sterile sponges

Technique

Preparation

1. Put on gloves
2. Select the most suitable vein. Apply a tourniquet or a blood pressure cuff inflated to 50 to 60 mm Hg. Opening and closing the fist will make the vein more prominent. Remove the tourniquet.
3. Prepare the venipuncture site. Always start at the puncture site and move out in concentric spirals for 1½ inches.
   a. Apply tincture of iodine; allow to dry. *Question patient before applying; some patients may be allergic to iodine.*
   b. Apply 10% acetone in 70% isopropyl alcohol to remove iodine. Allow to dry. Iodophor complex (10% povidone–iodine) may be substituted for iodine. It does not cause skin reactions even in iodine-sensitive individuals. Do not wash off iodophor complex. Cover the site with dry sterile gauze to prevent contamination until the phlebotomy is begun.

Collection of Blood

1. Suspend bag from donor scale as far below donor's arm as possible.
2. If counterbalance scales are used, adjust the balance for amount of blood to be drawn.
3. Make loose overhand knot in donor tube near needle.
4. Apply tourniquet (do not impair arterial circulation).
5. *Do not touch or repalpate vein.*
6. Perform phlebotomy.
7. Tape needle in place and cover with sterile sponge.
8. Pinch bead into bag from junction of donor tube and bag to open lumen and allow blood to flow.
9. Instruct patient to open and close fist slowly.
10. Collect blood until bag falls on scale. If spring scales are used, collect until prescribed amount has been withdrawn.
11. Pull knot tight.
12. Release tourniquet, withdraw needle, and apply pressure with gauze pad until bleeding has stopped. *Do not flex arm.* The arm may be elevated while applying pressure.
13. Dispose of blood and equipment as directed by hospital procedure.
14. Record procedure in clinical record.

REFERENCES

1. Adriani, J. (1962). Venipuncture. *American Journal of Nursing, 62,* 66.
2. American Association of Blood Banks. (1985). *Technical manual* (9th ed., pp. 11–15). Washington, DC.
3. Centers for Disease Control. (1982). Guidelines for prevention of intravascular infection. *Journal of the National Intravenous Therapy Association, 5*(1), 39–50.
4. Dudley, H. A. (1960). Modified technique for intravenous cannulation. *Surgery, Gynecology and Obstetrics, 111,* 513.
5. *Revised intravenous nursing standards of practice.* (1990). *Journal of Intravenous Nursing,* (Suppl.), S41.
6. Metheny, N. M. (1992). *Fluid and electrolyte balance* (2nd ed., pp 8, 10). Philadelphia: J.B. Lippincott.

BIBLIOGRAPHY

Jemison-Smith, P., & Thrupp, L. D. (1982). Phlebitis, infections and filtration. *Journal of the National Intravenous Therapy Association, 5*(5), 329–335.
Turco, S. J. (1987). Infusion phlebitis: A review of literature. *Parenterals, 5*(3), 1–8.
Zenowich, D. (1981). Physics of maintaining I.V. flow. *Journal of the National Intravenous Therapy Association, 4*(3), 212–214.

REVIEW QUESTIONS

1. The term "vasovagal reaction" refers to an autonomic nervous system response to:
   a. stress
   b. fluid resuscitation
   c. sudden hydration
   d. circulatory overload

2. Veins used initially to preserve future venous access include which of the following?:
   a. cephalic
   b. metacarpal
   c. basilic
   d. digital

3. Prime factors to be considered in selecting a vein for infusion include which of the following?
   a. location
   b. condition
   c. purpose
   d. duration

4. Application of digital pressure applied to disperse fluid denotes presence of:
   a. hypertension
   b. edema
   c. circulatory collapse
   d. hypotension

5. The catheter most frequently used today is:
   a. through the needle
   b. cutdown
   c. over the needle
   d. subclavian

6. A needle commonly used for venous sampling is:
   a. steel
   b. aluminum
   c. silastic
   d. polyethylene

7. Trauma to the endothelial wall is minimized by use of:
   a. long bevel
   b. short bevel
   c. thin wall
   d. large needle

8. The basilic vein is the vein of choice for longer line IV insertions because of its:
   a. larger size
   b. straighter course
   c. adequate hemodilution
   d. density

9. Indications for midline therapy include which of the following?
   a. hydration
   b. antibiotics
   c. pain medication
   d. peripheral nutrition

10. Therapeutic phlebotomy may be performed for which of the following reasons?
    a. polycythemia vera
    b. hemochromatosis
    c. acute pulmonary congestion
    d. thrombocytopenia

Potential Complications: Local and Systemic

Intravenous therapy subjects the patient to numerous potential hazards, many of which can be avoided if the nurse understands the risks involved and uses all available measures to prevent their occurrence. Local complications occur frequently but are rarely serious. Systemic complications, though rarer, are serious and frequently life-threatening, requiring immediate recognition and medical attention.

LOCAL COMPLICATIONS _____

Occasionally local complications are not recognized until considerable damage is done. Early recognition may prevent (1) extensive edema depriving the patient of urgently needed fluid and medications, (2) necrosis, and (3) thrombophlebitis with the subsequent danger of embolism. The local complications occur as the result of trauma to the wall of the vein.

Thrombosis

Any injury that roughens the endothelial cells of the venous wall allows platelets to adhere and a thrombus to form. Because the point of the cannula traumatizes the wall of the vein where it touches, thrombi form on the vein and at the tip of the cannula. Thrombosis occurs when a local thrombus obstructs the circulation of blood. It must be remembered that thrombi form an excellent trap for bacteria, whether carried by the bloodstream from an infection in a remote part of the body or introduced through the subcutaneous orifice.[3]

Thrombophlebitis

Thrombophlebitis is the term used to denote a twofold injury—thrombosis plus inflammation. The development of thrombophlebitis is easily recognized. A painful inflammation develops along the length of the vein. If the infusion is allowed to continue, the vein progressively thromboses, becoming hard, tortuous, tender, and painful.[7] Early detection may prevent an obstructive thrombophlebitis, which causes the infusion to slow and finally stop. This condition is most painful, persisting indefinitely, incapacitating the patient, and limiting valuable veins for future therapy.

Sharon M. Weinstein: PLUMER'S PRINCIPLES & PRACTICE OF INTRAVENOUS THERAPY, FIFTH EDITION, © 1993 J. B. Lippincott Company

Usually a sterile inflammation develops from a chemical or mechanical irritation. When the inflammation is the result of sepsis, it is much more serious and carries with it the potential danger of septicemia and acute bacterial endocarditis.

There is always the inherent danger of embolism when thrombosis occurs. The more pronounced the inflammation and the more intense the pain, the more organized the thrombus is likely to become. It has been frequently stated that embolism is less likely to occur from the well-attached clot of thrombophlebitis than from phlebothrombosis.[6]

Phlebothrombosis

Phlebothrombosis denotes thrombosis and usually indicates that the inflammation is relatively inconspicuous. It is thought to give rise to embolism because the thrombus is poorly attached to the wall of the vein.[6] Both thrombophlebitis and phlebothrombosis have a degree of inflammation and are associated with potential embolism.

Contributing Factors
Any irritation involving the wall of the vein predisposes the patient to thrombophlebitis. Inflammation to the vein will occur from any foreign body and is mediated by the following: (1) duration of the infusion, (2) composition of the solution, (3) site of the infusion, (4) technique, and (5) method used.

Duration of the infusion is a significant factor in the development of thrombophlebitis. As the duration of time is lengthened, the incidence and degree of inflammation increase.

The *composition of the solution* may play a role. Venous irritation and inflammation may result from the infusion of hypertonic glucose solutions, certain drug additives, or solutions with a pH significantly different from that of the plasma. Solutions of dextrose are known to be irritating to the vein.[4,5] The United States Pharmacopeia specifications for pH of dextrose solutions range from 3.5 to 6.5; acidity is necessary to prevent "caramelization" of the dextrose during autoclaving and to preserve the stability of the solution during storage. Studies have shown a significant reduction in thrombophlebitis when buffered glucose solutions have been infused.[4] Neut, a sodium bicarbonate 1% solution, may be added to increase the pH of acid IV solutions. This additive, however, poses a problem of incompatibility when added to solutions containing drugs. The largest number of incompatibilities may be produced by changes in pH.[8] As an example, tetracycline hydrochloride, with a pH of 2.5 to 3.0, is unstable in an alkaline environment.

The *site of infusion* can be a factor contributing to thrombophlebitis. The veins in areas over joint flexion undergo injury when motion of the cannula irritates the venous wall. The veins in the lower extremities are especially susceptible to trauma, enhanced by the stagnant blood in varicosities and the stasis in the peripheral venous circulation.

Small veins are subject to inflammation when used to infuse an irritating solution. The infusion cannula may occlude the entire lumen of the vein, obstructing the flow of circulating blood; the solution then flows undiluted, irritating the wall of the vein.

Technique can mean the difference between a successful infusion and the complication of thrombophlebitis. Only minimal trauma results from a skillfully executed venipuncture, whereas a carelessly performed venipuncture may seriously traumatize the venous wall.

Phlebitis associated with sepsis may be related to the technique of the operator.

Infection is always a risk if sterile technique is not zealously observed. Thorough cleansing of the skin is important in preventing infections. Maintenance of asepsis is essential during long-term therapy, particularly in the use of the through-the-needle cannula.[2]

Methods used to infuse parenteral solutions may foster septic thrombophlebitis. This complication is most often associated with the through-the-needle cannula. The cannula threaded through the needle remains sterile, does not come in contact with the skin, but provides a large subcutaneous orifice facilitating entry of bacteria around the catheter and seepage of fluid.

The over-the-needle cannula is not without fault since it comes in direct contact with the skin before being introduced into the vein. However, the tight fit through the skin may bar further bacterial entry.

Preventive Measures

In performing venipunctures, the nurse should exercise every caution to avoid injuring the wall of the vein needlessly. Multiple punctures, through-and-through punctures, and damage to the posterior wall of the vein with the point of the cannula can cause thrombosis. The risk of phlebitis may be minimized if the nurse:

1. Refrains from using veins in the lower extremities.
2. Selects veins with ample blood volume when infusing irritating substances.
3. Avoids veins in areas over joint flexion; uses an armboard if the vein must be located in an area of flexion.
4. Anchors cannulas securely to prevent motion.

To prevent septic phlebitis, thorough preparation of the skin, together with aseptic technique and maintenance of asepsis during infusion, is imperative.

Periodic inspection of the injection site will detect developing complications before serious damage occurs. Complaints of a painful infusion make it necessary to differentiate between early phlebitis and venospasm from an irritating solution. If the latter is present, slowing the solution and applying heat to the vein will dilate the vessel and increase the blood flow, diluting the solution and relieving the pain. Following hypertonic solutions with isotonic fluids will flush the vein of irritating substances.

If inflammation accompanies the pain, a change in the injection site should be considered. To continue the infusion will only bring progressive trauma and limit available veins. Adherence to time limits for removal of the cannula reduces the incidence of phlebitis.[4]

Phlebitis is often graded using a set scale:

- 1+ = pain at site; erythema and/or edema; no streak; no palpable cord
- 2+ = pain at site; erythema and/or edema; streak formation; no palpable cord
- 3+ = pain at site; erythema and/or edema; streak formation; palpable cord[4]

During removal of the infusion cannula, care must be taken to prevent injury to the wall of the vein; the cannula should be removed at an angle nearly flush with the skin. Pressure should be applied for a reasonable length of time to prevent extravasation of blood.

Infiltration

Dislodgment of the cannula with consequent infiltration of fluid is not uncommon and too frequently is considered of minor significance. With the increasing numbers of irritating solutions and the frequency with which potent drugs are infused in IV solutions, serious problems may occur when the fluid invades the surrounding tissues. Hypertonic, acid, and alkaline solutions are contraindicated for hypodermoclysis and are not intended for other than venous infusions. If they are allowed to infiltrate, necrosis may occur.

If necrosis is avoided, edema may nevertheless:

1. Deprive the patient of fluid and drug absorption at the rate essential for successful therapy.
2. Limit veins available for venipuncture, complicating therapy.
3. Predispose the patient to infection.

Extravasation

Extravasation can easily be recognized by the increasing edema at the site of the infusion. A comparison of the infusion area with the identical area in the opposite extremity assists in determining whether there is a swelling.

Frequently the edema is allowed to increase to great proportions because of a misconception that a backflow of blood into the adapter is significant proof that the infusion is entering the vein. This is not a reliable method for checking a possible infiltration. The point of the cannula may puncture the posterior wall of the vein, leaving the greater portion of the bevel within the lumen of the vein. Blood return will be obtained on negative pressure, but if the infusion is allowed to continue fluid will seep into the tissues at the point of the cannula, increasing the edema.

Occasionally, a blood return is not obtained on negative pressure. This may occur when the needle occludes the lumen of a small vein, obstructing the flow of blood.

To confirm an infiltration, apply a tourniquet proximal to the injection site tightly enough to restrict the venous flow. If the infusion continues regardless of this venous obstruction, extravasation is evident.

Once an infiltration has occurred, the cannula should be removed immediately.

Drugs that contribute to extravasation necrosis are most often osmotically active, ischemia-inducing, or cause direct cellular toxicity. Mechanical compression within the infiltrated tissue can increase the extent of damage, as can infection of the resulting wound. If only superficial tissue loss occurs and remains free of infection, débridement will yield a clean bed capable of granulating. If deep structures are involved, spontaneous wound healing may be averted, resulting in the need for wide excision, débridement, grafting, or amputation to restore tissue integrity.

SYSTEMIC COMPLICATIONS

Septicemia

Septicemia is caused by invasion of the bloodstream by microorganisms or their byproducts, including bacteria, fungi, mycobacteria, and rarely viruses. Certain predisposing factors put the infusion therapy patient at risk, including age less than 1 year or greater than 60 years, the presence of granulocytopenia, an immunocompromised state, loss of skin integrity, and presence of a distant infection that might contribute to hematogenous seeding. Cannula factors can also contribute to development of septicemia, including the size of the cannula, the number of lumens, the function and use of the cannula, catheter material and bacterial adherence, and thrombogenicity.

Clinical manifestations of septicemia include chills, fever, general malaise, and headache. Supportive therapy for the patient with septicemia includes fluid replacement, blood pressure maintenance, oxygenation, cardiac output maintenance, nutritional support, and preservation of acid–base balance. Ancillary treatments involve administration of steroids, naloxone, and endotoxin vaccination.

Prevention programs support the use of 0.2-μm air-eliminating, bacterial-retentive filters. Intravascular systems should be considered potential portals for infection. Good handwashing techniques, line care protocols, adherence to Intravenous Nurses Society (INS) Standards of Practice for monitoring, maintenance of infusion, tubing changes, and catheter care all contribute to an environment that will not readily support development of septicemia in the patient receiving infusion therapies.

Sterile Solutions

All IV solutions should be inspected for abnormal cloudiness or for the presence of extraneous particulate matter.

Methods of sterilization of parenteral fluids vary with manufacturing companies. If the method used produces a vacuum in solution bottles, presence of a vacuum should be noted; lack of vacuum indicates possible loss of sterility and contamination.

Use of Freshly Opened Solutions
Protein solutions must be used as soon as the seal is broken. Refrigerating these opened solutions for future use can result in serious consequences.

Other solutions should be used within 24 hours. The wise practice of indicating on the container the time and date that the seal is broken safeguards patients from possible contaminated infusions, especially patients on keep-open infusions for intermittent drug therapy.

Protection of Solution from Contamination
In the drug-additive program, sterile technique is essential to prevent organisms from being introduced into the solution. All drugs must be reconstituted with a sterile diluent. Once opened, any unused diluent should be discarded.

Keep-open solutions, terminated temporarily for blood infusion or drug therapy, must be protected from contamination. Sterile caps are available for some containers.

Pulmonary Embolism

Pulmonary embolism occurs when a substance, usually a blood clot, becomes free floating and is propelled by the venous circulation to the right side of the heart and into the pulmonary artery.[6] Emboli may obstruct the main pulmonary artery or the arteries to the lobes, occluding arterial apertures at major bifurcations.[6] Obstruction of the main artery results in circulatory and cardiac disturbances. Recurrent small emboli may eventually result in pulmonary hypertension and right heart failure.[10]

Preventive Measures

Certain precautions must be taken to prevent this serious complication.

1. Blood or plasma must be infused through an adequate filter to remove any particulate matter that could result in small emboli.

2. Veins on the lower extremities should be avoided when venipunctures are performed. These veins are particularly susceptible to trauma, predisposing the patient to thrombophlebitis. Although superficial veins rarely seem to be the source of emboli consequence,[6] a thrombus may extend into the deep veins, resulting in a potentially viable clot; superficial and deep veins unite freely in the lower extremities.

3. Positive pressure should not be used to relieve clot formation. To check for patency of the lumen of the cannula, kink the infusion tubing about 8 inches from the cannula. Then kink and release the tubing between the cannula and the pinched tubing—if the tubing becomes hard and meets with resistance, obstruction is evident, necessitating removal and reinstatement of the infusion.

4. Special precautions should be observed in the drug-additive program. Reconstituted drugs must be completely dissolved before being added to parenteral solutions; it is the inherent nature of red cells to adhere to particles, adding to the danger of clot formation.

5. Solutions should be examined to detect any particulate matter.

Air Embolism

Although air embolism is a significant possible complication with air-dependent containers, it is much more frequently associated with central venous lines. There is a potential risk for air embolism on the insertion of a central venous catheter, on inadequate sealing of the tract subsequent to disconnection of a central venous catheter, with disconnection of central lines, and with bypassing the "pump housing" of an electronic volumetric pump with an IV piggyback connection. Fatal embolism may occur when small bubbles accumulate dangerously and form tenacious bubbles that block the pulmonary capillaries.[1] Recognition of the circumstances that contribute to this hazard and measures taken to prevent their occurrence are imperative for safe fluid therapy.

Gravity Infusions

If a vented container is allowed to run dry, air enters the tubing and the fluid level drops to the proximity of the patient's chest. The pressure exerted by the blood on the walls of the veins controls the level to which the air drops in the tubing. A negative pressure in the vein may allow air to enter the bloodstream. A negative pressure occurs when the extremity receiving the infusion is elevated above the heart.[8] Infusions flowing through a central venous catheter carry an even greater risk of air embolism when the container empties than those flowing through a peripheral vein; because the central venous pressure is less than the peripheral venous pressure, there is more apt to be a negative pressure that could suck air into the circulation. The nurse should take precautions while changing the administration set of a central venous infusion. The patient should be lying flat in bed and should be instructed to perform the Valsalva maneuver (forced expiration with the mouth closed) immediately before and during the time that the catheter is open to the air.

If the fluid container on a continuous infusion should empty, fresh solution will force the trapped air into the circulation. To remove the air from the administration set:

1. Place a hemostat close to the infusion cannula.
2. Hang the fresh solution.
3. With an antiseptic, clean the rubber section of the tubing proximal to the hemostat and below the air level in the tubing.
4. Insert a sterile needle to allow the air to escape.
5. Remove clamp and readjust flow.

The Y-type infusion set used with vented containers (Figure 9-1) is a less obvious source but one by which great quantities of air can be drawn into the bloodstream. Running solutions simultaneously is the contributing factor. If one vented container empties, it becomes the source of air for the flowing solution. This is explained by the fact that the atmospheric pressure is greater in the open tubing to the empty container than below the partially restricted clamp on the infusion side. Recurrent small air bubbles are constantly aspirated into the flowing solution and on into the venous system. The introduction of air may be prevented by running one solution at a time. Vigilance is

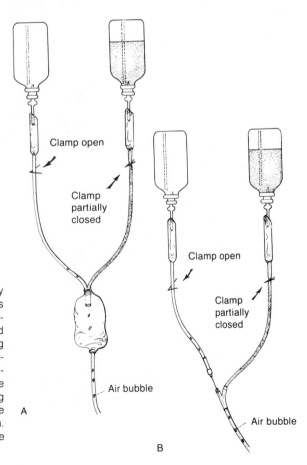

FIGURE 9-1 (**A**) The container runs dry during simultaneous infusion of fluids through a Y-type administration set. Pressure below the partially constricted clamp is less than atmospheric, allowing air from the empty container (atmospheric) to enter infusion. (**B**) A secondary infusion "piggybacked" through the injection site of a primary IV set. Lacking an automatic shut-off valve, air from the empty container will enter the circulation. The same principle is involved as in the Y-type set.

imperative if vented solutions are ordered to run simultaneously. The tubing must be clamped off completely before the solution container is allowed to empty.[9]

This same principle is involved in the piggyback setup for secondary infusions. The potential danger of air embolism exists whenever solutions from two vented sets run simultaneously through a common cannula. Advanced technologies have minimized the use of piggyback setups.

All connections of an infusion set must be tight. Any faulty opening or defective hole in the set allows air to be emitted into the flowing solution. If a stopcock is used, the outlets not in use must be completely shut off.

The regulating clamp on the infusion set should be located no higher than the chest level of the patient. Since the pressure exerted by the blood on the venous wall will normally raise a column of water from 4 to 11 cm above the heart, a restricting clamp placed above this point will result in a negative pressure in the tubing.[8] If great enough, the pressure can suck air into the flowing solution should a loose connection or a faulty opening exist between the clamp and the cannula.[8] The lower the clamp, the greater is the chance of any defects occurring above the clamp, where positive pressure can force the solution to leak out.[9]

An infusion set long enough to drop below the extremity gives added protection against air being drawn into the vein should the infusion bottle empty. Inlying pressure chambers on administration sets should be kept filled at all times. Manual compression of an empty chamber will force air into the bloodstream.

Occurrence of an Air Embolism
The nurse should be familiar with the symptoms associated with air embolism that arise from sudden vascular collapse: cyanosis, drop in blood pressure, weak rapid pulse, rise in venous pressure, and loss of consciousness. If air embolism occurs, the source of air entry must be immediately rectified. The patient should be turned on his left side with his head down.[8] This causes the air to rise in the right atrium, preventing it from entering the pulmonary artery. Oxygen is then administered and the physician notified.

Catheter Embolism

Catheter embolism may occur during the insertion of a through-the-needle catheter if strict adherence to the proper procedure is not followed. The catheter should never be pulled back through the needle. If it becomes necessary to remove the catheter, the entire unit should be removed and a new catheter inserted. Catheter embolism may also occur during the insertion of an over-the-needle catheter if the needle is either partially or totally withdrawn and then reinserted. If the catheter is sheared off and embolized, the intervention of cardiac catheterization with shearing the catheter under the fluoroscope may be necessary.

Pulmonary Edema

Overloading the circulation is a real hazard to the elderly patient and to patients with impaired renal and cardiac function. Fluids too rapidly infused increase the venous pressure, with the possibility of cardiac dilation and subsequent pulmonary edema.

Preventive Measures
These measures should be taken to prevent pulmonary edema.

1. Infusions should be maintained at the flow rate prescribed.

2. Positive pressure, using the pressure-chamber administration sets, should never be applied by the nurse to infuse solutions. If the patient requires fluids at such rapidity that positive pressure is required, infusion then becomes the physician's responsibility.

3. Controlled-volume infusion sets give added protection by preventing large quantities of fluid from being accidentally infused. These sets control the volume from 10 to 150 mL.

4. Solutions not infused within the 24-hour period ordered should be discarded and not infused with the following day's solutions; fluids administered in excess of the quantity ordered can overtax the homeostatic controls, increasing the danger of pulmonary edema.

The attending nurse must be alert to any signs or symptoms suggestive of circulatory overloading. Venous dilation, with engorged neck veins, increased blood pressure, and a rise in venous pressure, should alert the nurse to the danger of pulmonary edema. Rapid respiration and shortness of breath may occur. The infusion should be slowed to a minimal rate and the physician notified. Raising the patient to a sitting position may facilitate breathing.

Speed Shock

Speed shock is the term used to denote the systemic reaction that occurs when a substance foreign to the body is rapidly introduced into the circulation. Caution must be observed in the administration of IV push injections. Rapid injection permits the concentration of a medication in the plasma to reach toxic proportions, flooding the organs rich in blood—the heart and the brain. As a result, syncope, shock, and cardiac arrest may occur.[1]

Preventive Measures

Certain precautions can minimize the potential danger of speed shock.

1. By reducing the size of the drop, pediatric-type infusion sets provide greater accuracy, thereby reducing the risk of rapid administration. These sets are valuable when solutions containing potent drugs must be maintained at a minimal rate of flow.

2. Electronic flow-control devices control the rate of infusion, an asset imperative to the administration of IV medications.

3. On initiating the infusion, ascertain that the solution is flowing freely before adjusting the rate. Movement of a cannula in which the aperture is partially obstructed by the wall of the vein can cause an increase in the flow, contributing to the danger of speed shock.

REFERENCES

1. Adriani, J. (1962). Venipuncture. *American Journal of Nursing 62*, 66–70.
2. Bennett, J. V., & Brachman, P. S. (1986). *Hospital infections* (2nd ed., pp. 562, 563, 567–569). Boston: Little, Brown.
3. Druskin, M. S., & Siegel, P. D. (1963). Bacterial contamination of indwelling intravenous polyethylene catheters. *Journal of the American Medical Association, 185*, 966–968.

4. *Revised intravenous nursing standards of practice.* (1990). *Journal of Intravenous Nursing,* (suppl.), S42, S43.

5. Fonkalsrud, E. W., Pederson, B. M., Murphy, J., & Beckerman, J. H. (1968). Reduction of infusion thrombophlebitis with buffered glucose solutions. *Surgery, 63,* 280–284.

6. Hickan, J. B., & Sieker, H. O. (1959). Pulmonary embolism and infarction. *Disease-A-Month,* January.

7. McNair, T. J., & Dudley, H. A. F. (1959). The local complications of intravenous therapy. *Lancet, 2,* 365–368.

8. Metheny, N. M. (1992). *Fluid and electrolyte balance* (2nd ed., pp 164–165). Philadelphia: J. B. Lippincott.

9. Tarail, R. (1950). Practice of fluid therapy. *Journal of the American Medical Association, 171,* 45–49.

10. Tropp, J. (Speaker). (1992). Central venous thrombosis. Audiotape of presentation to Annual Meeting of Intravenous Nurses Society, May, 1992. Audio Transcripts Ltd, Alexandria, VA 40-729–92.

BIBLIOGRAPHY

Benezra, D., Kiehn, T. E., Gold, J. W. M., et al. (1988). Prospective study of infections in indwelling central venous catheters using quantitative blood cultures. *American Journal of Medicine, 85*(4), 495–498.

Black, R. (1988). Vein extravasation: A severe complication of I.V. therapy. *Parenterals, 6*(4), 1–2, 5–8.

Faehnrich, J. (1984). Extravasation. *Journal of the National Intravenous Therapy Association, 7*(1), 49–52.

Maki, D. (1982). Infections associated with intravascular lines. In J. S. Remington & M. N. Swartz (Eds.). *Current clinical topics in infectious diseases* (pp. 3, 309–363). New York: McGraw-Hill.

Warren, J. (1984). Edema: A serious I.V. complication. *Journal of the National Intravenous Therapy Association, 7*(4), 277–278.

REVIEW QUESTIONS

1. Thrombophlebitis involves what two injuries to the vein?
   a. inflammation
   b. irritation
   c. thrombosis
   d. infection

2. Factors that may contribute to thrombophlebitis include which of the following?
   a. viscosity of solution
   b. pH of solution
   c. type of cannula
   d. all of the above

3. To prevent septicemia, which of the following precautions are needed?
   a. Examine solutions carefully.
   b. Observe maximum hang time.
   c. Mix solutions at bedside.
   d. Mix solutions in laminar flow.

4. In the event of a suspected air embolism, the appropriate nursing intervention is to:
   a. turn patient on left side, head down.
   b. turn patient on right side, head down.
   c. turn patient on left side, head raised.
   d. turn patient on right side, head raised.

5. To prevent the incidence of pulmonary edema, it is necessary to do which of the following?
   a. Maintain prescribed rate of flow.
   b. Avoid positive pressure.
   c. Administer total volume within 24-hour time frame.
   d. Avoid negative pressure.

6. To minimize the danger of speed shock, it is necessary to:
   a. control volume
   b. avoid free flow
   c. catch up all solutions
   d. use positive pressure

7. Symptoms of air embolism include which of the following?
   a. cyanosis
   b. drop in blood pressure
   c. weak, rapid pulse
   d. drop in venous pressure

8. Extravasation may be evidenced by which of the following?
   a. increasing edema at site
   b. decreasing edema at site
   c. blanching
   d. red streak along wall of vein

9. To confirm an infiltration, apply a tourniquet proximal to the injection site tightly enough to restrict what type of flow?
   a. arterial
   b. venous
   c. atrial
   d. pulmonary

10. Factors predisposing the patient to incidence of septicemia include all of the following EXCEPT?
    a. age less than 1 year or more than 60
    b. presence of granulocytopenia
    c. increased red blood cell count
    d. loss of skin integrity

CHAPTER 10

Sources of Contamination and Principles of Prevention

COMPLICATIONS OF INTRAVENOUS THERAPY

Scientific, technologic, and medical advances have extended the lifesaving capabilities of IV therapy. However, despite these advances, IV-associated morbidity and mortality continue to increase.

The literature is full of warnings citing IV fluids and administration sets as potential vehicles for transmission of infection in hospitals. Cases of septicemia and fungemia have been directly traced to contamination of in-use IV apparatus and solutions.[5,7] In 1969, 33 patients with fungal septicemia had been seen over an 18-month period in one university hospital. This complication was the primary cause of death in 13 patients. A correlation with prolonged IV catheterization was found.[5]

From 1970 to 1971, 150 cases of bacteremia associated with IV therapy occurred in eight United States hospitals. These were associated with the IV fluids of a major manufacturer; gram-negative bacteria were found contaminating sterile equipment. As a result, the Centers for Disease Control and Prevention (CDC) performed a study of all commercial IV systems in use in hospitals. The study showed a minimum of 6% prevalence of contamination within tubing and bottles after infusion equipment had been in use.[4] Conditions were shown to exist that potentially contributed to contamination: the characteristics of the apparatus itself and the manipulation of sets and solutions by hospital personnel.

Much has been published concerning the alarming escalation of IV therapy complications, but many health care personnel remain ignorant of the potential dangers. In hospitals using IV teams, communication is better and personnel are more cognizant of complications and their warning signs. Intravenous care delivered by a team of dedicated professionals has been demonstrated to greatly reduce potential problems.

Principles of aseptic technique relevant to infusion therapies should be an integral component of the training programs of hospitals and health care organizations in which IV therapy is provided. A working knowledge of the epidemiology of nosocomial infections helps to instill a greater awareness of the importance of aseptic technique in the prevention of infection.

Sharon M. Weinstein: PLUMER'S PRINCIPLES & PRACTICE OF INTRAVENOUS THERAPY, FIFTH EDITION, © 1993 J. B. Lippincott Company

SOURCES OF BACTERIA

Three main sources yield the bacteria responsible for IV-associated infection: the air, the skin, and the blood. Microorganisms (flora and fauna) characteristic of a given location are referred to accordingly, thus the terms *skin flora*, *intestinal flora*, and so on. Table 10-1 lists microbial pathogens associated with infusion-related septicemia.

TABLE 10-1
Microbial Pathogens Associated with Infusion-Related Septicemia

Source of Septicemia	*Major Pathogens*
Conventional infusion therapy Cannula	Coagulase-negative *Staphylococcus* (>50%) *Staphylococcus aureus* Enterococcus *Klebsiella-Enterobacter* *Serratia marcescens* *Candida* species *Pseudomonas aeruginosa* *Pseudomonas cepacia* *Corynebacterium* species (diphtheroids), JK-1

Contaminated infusate	Tribe Klebsielleae (90%)
	    Klebsiella
	    Enterobacter*
	    Serratia
	P. cepacia*
	Citrobacter freundii
	Flavobacterium

Hyperalimentation, Hickman-Broviac catheters (most, catheter-related)	Coagulase-negative *Staphylococcus* (>50%) *Candida* species, *Torulopsis glabrata* *S. aureus* *Klebsiella-Enterobacter* Enterococcus
Contaminated blood products (contaminated infusate)	Pseudomonads other than *P. aeruginosa* (>50%)* *S. marcescens* Achromobacter *Salmonella choleraesuis* Citrobacter *Flavobacterium*
Arterial pressure monitoring	*P. cepacia** *Serratia* *P. acidovorans* *P. aeruginosa* Enterobacter *Flavobacterium* *Candida* (very rare)
Regional intra-arterial cancer chemotherapy (catheter-related)	*S. aureus*

* Septicemia caused by *E. cloacae*, *E. agglomerans*, or *P. cepacia*, in particular, should prompt investigations for contaminated infusate.

Source: Adapted from Maki, D. G. (*1976*). Growth properties of microorganisms in infusion fluid and methods of detection. In I. Phillips, P. D. Meers, & P. F. D'Arcy (Eds.). *Microbiological hazards of infusion therapy*, Lancaster, England: MTP Press.

The Air

The number of microbes per cubic foot of air varies, depending on the particular area involved. Where infection is present, bacteria escape in body discharges, contaminating clothing, bedding, and dressings. Activity, such as making a bed, sends bacteria flying into the air on particles of lint, pus, and dried epithelium.[15] Increased activity causes a rise in the number of airborne particles and provides an environment that interferes with aseptic technique and potentially contributes to contamination. Airborne microorganisms may be plentiful in patient areas and utility rooms. These contaminants find easy access to unprotected IV fluids.

The Skin

The skin is the main source of bacteria responsible for IV-associated infection. The bacteria found on the skin are referred to as *resident* or *transient*. Resident bacteria are those normally present, and they are relatively constant in a given individual. They adhere tightly to the skin, and usually include *Staphylococcus albus* as well as diphtheroids and *Bacillus* species.[15] Because not all bacteria are removed by scrubbing, meticulous care must be observed to avoid touching sterile equipment.

The transient bacteria are responsible for infection carried from one person to another. Touch contamination is a potential hazard of infection because hospital personnel move about frequently, touching patients and objects. Frequent handwashing is imperative.

The skin of the patient offers fertile soil for bacteria growth. It has been estimated that a minimum of 10,000 organisms are present per square centimeter of normal skin.[36] A square centimeter is equal to 0.155 square inches. Organisms such as *Staphylococcus epidermidis*, *Staphylococcus aureus*, gram-negative bacilli (especially *Klebsiella*, *Enterobacter*, and *Serratia*), and enterococci are ubiquitous on the skin of hospitalized patients.[21]

The Blood

The blood may harbor potentially dangerous microorganisms. Therefore, care must be taken to prevent bacterial contamination from blood spills when drawing samples and performing venipuncture. However, more likely to be a problem in blood is the hepatitis virus and the acquired immunodeficiency syndrome (AIDS) retrovirus. Hepatitis is transmitted by blood containing the hepatitis B virus and unidentified viruses non-A, non-B. Screening blood donors became a reality in 1970 when a test for the surface antigen (HBsAG) became available, reducing the occurrence of posttransfusion hepatitis.

The hepatitis virus is easily transmitted and can be destroyed only by heat or gas sterilization. Proper care of cannulas, syringes, and IV sets is imperative. Adequate precaution and warning on blood samples that may possibly be contaminated with hepatitis virus are necessary to prevent the spread of any infection among hospital employees.

Acquired immunodeficiency syndrome is caused by the retrovirus HTLV-111, which destroys the body's immune system, leaving the patient vulnerable to infection and other diseases. The AIDS epidemic, first recognized in 1981, seriously affected the nation's blood supply and complicated transfusion therapy.[16] The AIDS test to detect the presence of antibodies to the virus HTLV-111 in potential donors became available in the spring of 1985.

The subject of transfusion-transmitted disease is addressed in detail in Chapter 21. See box, Precautions to Prevent Transmission of HIV for the Occupational Safety and Health Administration (OSHA) guidelines.

FACTORS INFLUENCING THE SURVIVAL OF BACTERIA

Infection depends on the ability of bacteria to survive and proliferate. The factors that influence their survival are: (1) the specific organisms present, (2) the number of such organisms, (3) the resistance of the host, and (4) the environmental conditions.[24]

The Specific Organisms

Bacteria are referred to as *pathogenic* or *nonpathogenic*. Pathogenic bacteria are capable of producing disease. All bacteria should be considered pathogenic. Reports show that bacteria previously considered nonpathogenic may produce infection. In one study, *Serratia* was implicated in 35% of cases of gram-negative septicemia resulting from IV therapy.[1, 23]

Bacteria are classified as *gram-positive* and *gram-negative*. In recent years gram-negative bacteria have replaced gram-positive bacteria as the leading cause of death from septicemia.[26] The single most important reason for the intensity of the problem is probably the increased usage of antibiotics highly effective against gram-positive organisms but only selectively effective against gram-negative organisms. With the competitive inhibition of gram-positive bacteria eliminated, the more resistant gram-negative organisms have proliferated in the hospital environment.[20]

Number of Organisms

The number of contaminants present influences the probability of production of an infection. The power of bacteria to proliferate must not be underestimated. It is simply *not true* that a small amount of bacteria from touch contamination is harmless. Contamination of IV fluids and bottles with even a few organisms is extremely dangerous, because some fungi and many bacteria can proliferate at room temperature in a variety of IV solutions to more than 10^5 organisms/mL within 24 hours.[8]

Host Resistance

The resistance of the host influences the development and course of septicemia. Underlying conditions such as diabetes mellitus, chronic uremia, cirrhosis, cancer, and leukemia may adversely affect the patient's capacity to resist infection. Treatments such as immunosuppressive drugs, corticosteroids, anticancer agents, and extensive radiation therapy may depress immunologic response and permit the invasion of infection. Therapy may mask infection so that septicemia may be unrecognized until autopsy.[1]

Environmental Factors

Environmental factors that affect the survival and propagation of bacteria in IV fluids are (1) the pH, (2) the temperature, and (3) the presence of essential nutrients in the infusion.

Some organisms grow rapidly in a neutral solution and are less likely to grow in an acid medium. Buffering of acidic dextrose solutions has been recommended for preven-

Precautions to Prevent Transmission of HIV*

Universal Precautions

Because medical history and examination cannot reliably identify all patients infected with human immunodeficiency virus (HIV) or other blood-borne pathogens, blood and body-fluid precautions should be consistently used for *all* patients. This approach, previously recommended by the CDC and referred to as *universal blood and body-fluid precautions* or *universal precautions*, should be used in the care of *all* patients, especially those in emergency care settings in which the risk of blood exposure is increased and the infection status of the patient is usually unknown.

BARRIER PRECAUTIONS

Health-care workers should always use appropriate barrier precautions to prevent exposure of skin and mucous membranes when contact with blood or other body fluids of any patient is anticipated.

1. Gloves should be worn when touching blood and body fluids, mucous membranes, or nonintact skin of all patients, for handling items or surfaces soiled with blood or body fluids, and for performing venipuncture and other vascular access procedures.
2. Gloves should be changed after contact with each patient.
3. Masks and protective eyewear or face shields should be worn during procedures that are likely to generate droplets of blood or other body fluids to prevent exposure of mucous membranes of the mouth, nose, and eyes.
4. Gowns or aprons should be worn during procedures likely to cause splashes of blood body fluids.

HAND WASHING

1. Hands and other skin surfaces should be washed immediately and thoroughly if contaminated with blood or other body fluids.
2. Hands should be washed immediately after gloves are removed.

PROTECTION AGAINST INJURY

1. All health care workers should take precautions to prevent injuries caused by needles, scalpels, and other sharp instruments or devices
   (a) During procedures
   (b) When cleaning used instruments
   (c) During disposal of used needles
   (d) When handling sharp instruments after procedures
2. To prevent *needlestick injuries*, needles should not be recapped, purposely bent or broken by hand, removed from disposable syringes, or otherwise manipulated by hand.
3. After they are used, disposable syringes and needles, scalpel blades, and other sharp items should be placed in puncture-resistant containers for disposal. The puncture-resistant containers should be located as close as practical to the use area.
4. Large-bore reusable needles should be placed in a puncture-resistant container for transport to the reprocessing area.

SALIVA

Although saliva has not been implicated in HIV transmission, to minimize the need for emergency mouth-to-mouth resuscitation, mouthpieces, resuscitation bags, or other ventilation devices should be available for use in areas in which the need for resuscitation is predictable.

EXUDATE

Health care workers who have exudative lesions or weeping dermatitis should refrain from all direct patient care and from handling patient-care equipment until the condition resolves.

PREGNANCY

1. Pregnant health care workers are not known to be at greater risk of contracting HIV infection than health care workers who are not pregnant.
2. If a health-care worker develops HIV infection during pregnancy, the infant is at risk of infection resulting from perinatal transmission.
3. Because of this risk, pregnant health care workers should be especially familiar with and strictly adhere to precautions to minimize the risk of HIV transmission.

ISOLATION

1. Implementing universal blood and body-fluid precautions for *all* patients eliminates need for use of the isolation category of "blood and body-fluid precautions" previously recommended by the CDC for patients known or suspected to be infected with blood-borne pathogens.
2. Isolation precautions (*e.g.*, enteric, AFB) should be used as necessary if associated conditions, such as infectious diarrhea or tuberculosis, are diagnosed or suspected.

(continued)

Precautions to Prevent Transmission of HIV* (continued)

Precautions for Invasive Procedures

In this document, an invasive procedure is defined as surgical entry into tissues, cavities, or organs, or repair of major traumatic injuries.

1. In an operating or delivery room, emergency department, or outpatient setting, including both physicians' and dentists' offices
2. Cardiac catheterization and angiographic procedures
3. A vaginal or cesarean delivery or other invasive obstetric procedure during which bleeding may occur
4. The manipulation, cutting, or removal of any oral or perioral tissues, including tooth structure, during which bleeding occurs or the potential for bleeding exists

   The universal blood and body-fluid precautions listed previously, combined with the precautions listed in the following section, should be the minimum precautions for *all* such invasive procedures.

BARRIER PROTECTION

1. All health care workers who participate in invasive procedures must routinely use appropriate barrier precautions to prevent skin and mucous membrane contact with blood and other body fluids of all patients.

2. Gloves and surgical masks must be worn for all invasive procedures.
3. Protective eyewear or faceshields should be worn for procedures that commonly result in the generation of droplets, splashing of blood or other body fluids, or the generation of bone chips.
4. Gowns or aprons made of materials that provide an effective barrier should be worn during invasive procedures that are likely to result in the splashing of blood or other body fluids.
5. All health care workers who perform or assist in vaginal or cesarean deliveries should wear gloves and gowns when handling the placenta or the infant until blood and amniotic fluid have been removed from the infant's skin. They should also wear gloves during post-delivery care of the umbilical cord.
6. If a glove is torn or a needle stick or other injury occurs, the glove should be removed and a new glove used as promptly as patient safety permits. The needle or instrument involved in the incident should also be removed from the sterile field.

---

* (OSHA Instruction CPL-2-2.44A, Office of Health Compliance Assistance)

---

tion of phlebitis,[9] but at the same time, the neutral environment provided by the buffer may enhance the survival and proliferation of bacteria.

The temperature of the fluid may affect the ability of bacteria to multiply. At room temperatures, strains of *Enterobacter cloacae*, *Enterobacter agglomerans*, and other members of the tribe Klebsiellae proliferate rapidly in commercial solutions of 5% dextrose in water.[4,21] Total parenteral nutrition fluids should be used as soon as possible after preparation, and when it becomes necessary to store them temporarily they should be refrigerated at 4°C; at this temperature growth of *Candida albicans* is suppressed.[21]

The presence of certain nutrients is essential to the growth of bacteria. Blood and crystalloid solutions provide nutrients that broaden the spectrum of pathogens capable of proliferation. Maki and associates stated that the administration of blood or reflux of blood into the infusion system may provide sufficient nutrients to broaden this spectrum.[21] The American Association of Blood Banks requires blood to be stored at a constant controlled refrigeration of 1°C to 6°C.

It has been reported that saline solutions are likely to contain enough biologically available carbon, nitrogen, sulfur, and phosphate together with traces of other material to support, under favorable conditions, the survival and multiplication of any gram-negative bacillus introduced to as many as a million organisms per milliliter.[25]

FACTORS CONTRIBUTING TO CONTAMINATION AND INFECTION

Local complications of phlebitis and infection, as well as systemic complications and septicemias, are hazards of prolonged IV therapy that complicate recovery. Extrinsic contamination may occur through the administration sets, the medication sites, and supplementary apparatus such as extension tubes, containers of fluid, and cannulas. Each time a medication is added, a container is changed, or supplementary equipment is added, the likelihood of contamination increases.

Breaks in aseptic technique contribute to contamination. Too much reliance on antibiotics has fostered a decline in aseptic technique. Instead of overcoming contamination, antibiotic therapy has simply changed the spectrum of organisms from gram-positive to gram-negative.[23] Antibiotic therapy may have contributed to the development and increasing incidence of gram-negative septicemia. In some instances, toxemia and shock seemed to be temporarily intensified, presumably by the sudden destruction and lysis of gram-negative bacteria and the liberation of endotoxin.[1]

Faulty Handling

Faulty handling and procedures contribute to contamination. Containers of parenteral fluid are accepted as being sterile and nonpyrogenic on arrival from the manufacturer. The potential risk of contamination occurring in transit or in use is frequently overlooked by hospital personnel. However, through faulty handling or carelessness, glass containers may become cracked or damaged and plastic bags punctured. Bacteria and fungi may penetrate a hairline crack in an IV container, even though the crack is so fine that fluid is not lost from the container. Robertson reported two cases in which fluid contaminated with fungi was inadvertently administered; the containers were cracked.[29] These two patients were treated with amphotericin B (Fungizone), and recovery was complete.

Intravenous solutions of dextrose, as well as providing carbon and an energy source, include the extra nutrients needed to support the growth of 10 million organisms per milliliter. If the fluid is not examined closely, its opalescence may be overlooked, and subsequent infusion of a few hundred milliliters of such contaminated fluid will result in deep shock or possibly death.[25]

Before use, containers of fluid should be examined, preferably against a light and dark background, for cracks, defects, turbidity, and particulate matter; plastic containers should be squeezed to detect any puncture hole. Accidental puncture may occur without being evident and provide a point of entry for microorganisms.[21,34] Any container with a crack or defect must be regarded as suspect and not used. Any glass container lacking a vacuum when opened should not be used.

Airborne Contamination

Studies by Hansen and Hepler showed that IV fluids in an open IV stream (without an air filter) may become contaminated by airborne microbes when the container vacuum is replaced by unsterile air.[14] When a 1L glass container is opened, approximately 100 mL of air rushes in to replace the vacuum. In areas with a high concentration of airborne particles, contamination of unprotected fluids is a potential risk. The sterile environment of a laminar flow hood prevents this problem.

Discarding Outdated Intravenous Solutions

Several studies have demonstrated that IV fluids and sets often become contaminated while in use.[4,5,7] The longer the container is in use, the greater the proliferation of bacteria and the greater the infection should contamination inadvertently occur. The risk of infusing outdated fluids can be avoided by adhering to special limits, supported by a strong monitoring policy. Every container should be labeled with the time it is opened. The CDC guidelines and Intravenous Nurses Society (INS) Standards should be followed.

Admixtures

Allowing untrained hospital personnel to add drugs to IV containers potentially contributes to the risk of contamination. This risk is reduced when admixtures are prepared under laminar flow hoods by trained personnel adhering to strict aseptic technique as provided by a pharmacy additive program. The necessity for nurses and physicians to prepare admixtures in an emergency does arise. All personnel involved in the preparation and administration of IV drugs should receive special training in the preparation of admixtures and the handling of IV fluids and equipment. Adherence to strict aseptic methods is vital. It must be understood that touch contamination is the primary source of infection and that although laminar flow hoods prevent airborne contamination, they do not ensure sterility when a break in aseptic technique occurs.

Manipulation of In-Use Intravenous Equipment

Intravenous fluids can be inadvertently contaminated by faulty techniques in the manipulation of equipment. In open systems, where solutions are not protected by air filters, the simple procedure of hanging the container may be taken for granted and the risk of contamination overlooked. When an administration set is inserted into the container and the container is inverted, the fluid tends to leak out the vent onto the unsterile surface of the container. Regurgitation of the contaminated fluid into the container occurs when the container vents. Instructions in the use of the equipment often go unread and unheeded. Squeezing the drip chamber of the administration set before inserting it into the container and releasing it when the container is inverted will prevent regurgitation of fluid and minimize the risk of contamination.

Injection Ports

Meticulous aseptic technique must be observed in the use of injection ports because they are a potential source of contamination when used to "piggyback" infusions. The injection port location, at the distal end of the tubing, exposes it to patient excreta and drainage, which enhance the growth of microorganisms and contribute to contamination. The injection port must be *scrubbed* at least 1 minute with an accepted antiseptic; 70% isopropyl alcohol is commonly used. Scrubbing the injection cap for 30 seconds with an antimicrobial (povidone–iodine) solution provides very good protection. The needle should be firmly engaged up to the hub in the injection site and securely taped to prevent an in-and-out motion of the needle from introducing bacteria into the infusion. The use of needleless systems minimizes risk. (See Chapter 12.)

Three-Way Stopcocks

Three-way stopcocks are potential mechanisms for transmission of bacteria to the host because their ports, unprotected by sterile covering, are open to moisture and contaminants. Connected to central venous catheters and arterial lines, they are frequently used for drawing blood samples. Aseptic practices are vital in preventing the introduction of bacteria into the line. A sterile catheter plug attached at the time the stopcock is added and changed after each use will reduce the risk of contamination. Whenever fluid leakage is discovered at injection sites, connections, or vents, the IV set should be replaced.

Cannula-Associated Infection

Following insertion of a plastic cannula into a vessel, a loosely formed fibrin sheath forms around the intravascular portion of the device within 24 to 48 hours (Figure 10-1), forming a nidus within which microorganisms can multiply and that shields them to an extent from host defenses and antibiotics. Thrombogenesis of cannula materials may play a role in vulnerability to cannula-related infections. Again, careful adherence to policies and procedures, based on Standards of Practice, with respect to site rotation and indwell time, may reduce the inherent problems of cannula-associated infection.

Most device-related septicemias are actually caused by the patient's own skin flora or by microorganisms transmitted from the hands of the health care professional.

Antibiotic Lock Technique

The antibiotic lock technique has met with favorable response from the health care community as a means to lessen the potential for central venous cannula-related infection in the immunocompromised patient. Vancomycin, amphotericin-B, and fluconazole have

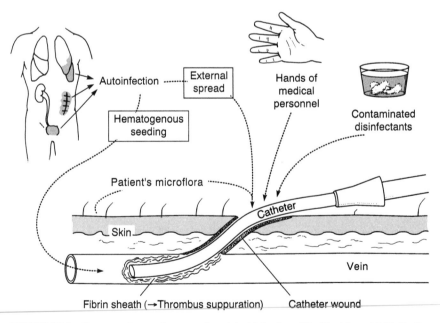

FIGURE 10-1 Sources of vascular cannula-related infection. (Modified from Maki, D. G. [1976]. In I. Phillips, P. D. Meers, & P. F. D'Arcy [Eds.]. *Microbiological hazards of infusion therapy* [p. 106]. Lancaster, England: MTP Press.)

all been successfully used as flush solutions. A small amount of concentrated antibiotic/antifungal agent is instilled within the catheter and capped (Table 10-2).

Skin Preparation

Microbes on the hands of health care personnel contribute to hospital-associated infection. Too often breaks in sterile technique occur from failure to wash the hands before changing containers or sets or preparing admixtures. Besides the usual skin flora, antibiotic-resistant gram-negative organisms frequently contaminate the hands of hospital personnel.[21]

To maintain asepsis, the CDC recommends that the hands be thoroughly washed for insertion of central venous catheters.[3] OSHA guidelines support the use of sterile gloves.

Adequate and reliable preparation of the patient's skin and maintenance of asepsis is imperative when a catheter is used for IV therapy. The skin, the first defense barrier of the body, is broken, providing a vulnerable port for the migration of bacteria. Skin flora has been implicated as a source of contamination of catheters. In a study made of 118 patients receiving IV therapy through an indwelling polyvinyl catheter, 53 catheters were found to be contaminated with bacteria; in 28 of these, the organisms were comparable to those cultured from the skin of the patient before the skin was cleaned with iodine.[2]

Frequently the question arises of whether or not to shave the skin. The need to remove the hair is not substantiated by scientific evidence; antiseptics used to clean the skin also clean the hair. Shaving may produce microabrasions, which enhance the proliferation of bacteria.[21]

Alcohol 70% is frequently used to prepare the skin site for venipuncture. Studies show that ethyl alcohol, 70% by weight, is an effective germicide for the skin when *applied with friction for 1 minute;* INS Standards support its use. It is as effective as 12 minutes of scrubbing and reduces the bacterial count by 75%.[36] Since a minimum of 10,000 organisms/cm^2 are present on normal skin, the count would be reduced to 2500. Too frequently the use of alcohol consists of a quick wipe, which fails to reduce the bacterial count significantly.

Iodine and iodine-containing disinfectants are still the most reliable agents for preparing the skin for venipuncture because they provide bactericidal, fungicidal, and sporicidal activity. Because of occasional patient allergy to iodine, the possibility of sensitivity should be investigated before its use. Tincture of iodine (2% iodine in 70% alcohol) is inexpensive and well tolerated. Solution should be liberally applied, allowed to dry for at least 30 seconds, and washed off with 70% alcohol. Both agents should be applied with friction, working from the center of the field to periphery.[21] Iodophor preparations, when used for patients with sensitive skin, should not be washed off

---

TABLE 10-2
Antibiotic Lock Technique

Indications
    Immunocompromised patients receiving parenteral nutrition
Dosage
    _____ flush, 1 mg/mL
    Instill 3 mL or 5 mL in catheter after flushing with saline solution to
       clear line

because the sustained release of free iodine may be necessary for germicidal action. Iodophor preparations require 30-second contact time.

Quaternary ammonium compounds such as aqueous benzalkonium chloride are inactivated by organic debris and are ineffective against gram-negative organisms and should not be used for skin disinfection.[21]

The tourniquet itself may very well provide a source of cross-infection and contamination because it is used repeatedly from patient to patient and handled just before venipuncture. This possibility should be kept in mind and the tourniquet disinfected periodically; consideration should be given to the use of start-kits.

Once the venipuncture is completed and it is within the lumen of the vein, the cannula must be securely anchored; to-and-fro motion of the catheter in the puncture wound may irritate the intima of the vein and introduce cutaneous bacteria. Thought should be given to the possible contamination of the adhesive tape used to secure the cannula. Rolls of tape last indefinitely and may be a source of contamination; they are transported from room to room, placed on patients' beds and tables, and frequently roll to the floor. Furthermore, before venipuncture, strips of tape often are torn off the roll and placed in convenient locations on the bed, table, and uniform. These facts should be kept in mind. Adhesive tape should not be applied over the puncture wound. The puncture wound must be considered an open wound and asepsis must be maintained.

CARE OF THE VENOUS ACCESS DEVICE

The CDC recommend the use of a topical antibiotic or antiseptic ointment at the IV site after cannula insertion. The wound should be protected by a sterile dressing. Dressing change should be consistent with INS Standards. The same applies to catheter site rotations. Frequent observations should be made for signs of malfunction of the cannula; infiltration; and phlebitis characterized by erythema, induration, or tenderness. Such signs require immediate removal of the cannula. Fuchs has noted that the major factor influencing the frequency of catheter colonization is the presence of other catheter complications such as subcutaneous infiltration and phlebitis.[10] He defined *colonization* as positive culture of the catheter tip without evidence of local or systemic infection.

Irrigation of a plugged catheter may embolize small catheter thrombi, some of which are infected. Contamination of the catheter may result from a break in aseptic technique, from contaminated fluid or set, from bacterial invasion of the puncture wound, or from clinically undetected bacteremia arising from an infection in a remote area of the body, such as a tracheostomy, the urinary tract, or a surgical wound. The clot around or in the catheter serves as an excellent trap for circulatory microorganisms and as a nutrient for bacterial proliferation.

INTRAVENOUS-ASSOCIATED INFECTIONS

Intravenous-associated sepsis is not always accompanied by phlebitis. Symptoms of infection consist of chills and fever, gastric symptoms, headache, hyperventilation, and shock. Should infection develop from an unknown source in a patient receiving IV therapy, the IV system should be suspected and the entire system, including the cannula, removed. The catheter and the infusion fluid should be cultured.

The following procedure should be used for culturing the catheter.[11]

1. Cleanse the skin about the cannula site with alcohol, allowing the alcohol to dry before removing the cannula.

2. Maintaining asepsis, remove the catheter and with sterile scissors snip 1 cm of the catheter tip into blood culture or other appropriate culture medium.

The following procedure should be used for culturing the infusion fluid.[11]

1. Aseptically withdraw 20 mL fluid from the IV line: 1 mL is used to prepare a pour plate; the remaining fluid is used to inoculate two blood culture containers.

2. Add to the remaining IV fluid in the container an equal volume of brain–heart infusion broth enriched with 0.5% beef extract. Inoculate at 37°C; this is a more sensitive culture for detecting low-level contamination.

All containers of fluid previously administered to the patient should be suspected and, if possible, retained and cultured. All information and identification, including the lot number of the suspected solution, should be recorded on the culture requisition and the patient chart. The United States Food and Drug Administration, the CDC, and the local health authorities should be notified if contamination during manufacturing is suspected; fluids bearing implicated lot numbers should be stored for investigation.

PARTICULATE MATTER

The literature concerning particulate matter in infusions and its clinical significance is increasing. Many articles indicate that IV-administered particles can cause pathogenic states.[32] *Particulate matter* is defined as the mobile, undissolved substances unintentionally present in parenteral fluids.[18] Such foreign matter may consist of rubber, glass, cotton fibers, drug particles, molds, metal, or paper fibers.

Vascular Route of Infused Particles

The pulmonary vascular bed acts as a filter for infused particles. Particles introduced into the vein travel to the right atrium of the heart, down through the tricuspid valve, and into the right ventricle. From there they are pumped into the pulmonary artery and on through branches of arteries that decrease in size until the particles are trapped in the massive capillary bed in the lungs, where the capillaries measure 7 to 12 μm in diameter.

Five microns, the size of an erythrocyte suspended in fluid, has been suggested as the largest allowable size for a particle in the pulmonary capillary bed.[12] Particles larger than 5 μm are recognized as potentially dangerous because they are likely to become lodged. Particles as large as 300 μm can pass through an 18-gauge cannula, and much larger particles may pass through an indwelling catheter with a larger lumen. Table 10-3 lists particle size comparisons. If occlusion of a small arteriole inhibits oxygenation or normal metabolic activities, cellular damage or tissue death may result. Where there is ample collateral circulation, the occlusion would have no appreciable biologic effect. However, a particle that is not biologically inert may incite an inflammatory reaction, a neoplastic response, or an antigenic, sensitizing response.[17]

Particles may gain access to the systemic circulation, where occlusion of a small arteriole in the brain, kidney, or eye can be serious, in one of the following ways:

TABLE 10-3
Particle Size Comparisons

Microns		Inches
175	=	.007
150	=	.006
125	=	.005
100	=	.004
75	=	.003
50	=	.002
25	=	.001

Source: Contamination Control Laboratories. *Particle Size Comparisons* (information circular). Livonia, MI, 1970.

Note: One micron equals 40 millionths of an inch (approx.). A human hair is approximately 125 μm in thickness. Bacteria range in size from 0.3 to 0.5 μm. We cannot see a particle or hole smaller than 20 μm. A hole 25 μm in diameter in a HEPA filter is more than 75 times larger than the contaminants and bacteria passing through.

1. The pulmonary vascular bed does not filter out all particles. Prinzmetal and associates demonstrated that glass beads up to 390 μm may pass through the pulmonary capillary bed and reach the systemic circulation.[28]

2. Large arteriovenous shunts have been demonstrated to exist in the human lung.[13, 19] Particles bypass the pulmonary capillary bed and enter the systemic circulation, where a systemic occlusion could be serious.

3. Particles larger than 5 μm may reach the systemic circulation by interarterial injection or infusion.

Sources of Contamination

Studies have shown that particulate contamination is present in all IV fluids and administration sets.[6] The United States Pharmacopeia has established an acceptable limit of particles for single-dose infusion as not more than 50 particles/mL that are equal to or larger than 10.0 μm, and not more than 5 particles/mL that are equal to or larger than 25.0 μm in effective linear dimension (see Chapter 19). Great efforts are being made by manufacturers to produce high-quality IV injections. Their efforts are defeated by numerous manipulations before final infusion.

Medication Additives

Drugs constitute a major source of contamination. Improper technique in the preparation of drugs results in the formation of insoluble particles. An IV additive service is recommended.

Glass Ampules

Glass ampules may be responsible for the injection of thousands of glass particles into the circulation. Turco and Davis, in a study prompted by the frequency of high-dose administration of furosemide, showed that a dose of 400 mg, which at that time required the breaking of 20 ampules, could add 1085 glass particles larger than 5 μm to the injection.[33] A dose of 600 mg, requiring 30 ampules, could result in 2387 particles larger than 5 μm.

Antibiotic Injectables

Studies have been performed in relation to particulate matter in commercial antibiotic injectable products.[22] They showed particulate contamination levels of bulk-filled antibiotics to be two to ten times greater than those of stable antibiotic solutions and lyophilized antibiotics. Filtration is impossible because packaging by the sterile bulk-fill method involves extracting and processing the antibiotic in sterile bulk powder form and then aseptically placing the bulk antibiotic into dry presterilized vials. In the lyophilized and the stable liquid packaging processes, the particulate matter can be terminally removed by filtration directly into presterilized vials. The majority of the antibiotics are packed by the bulk-fill method.

Particulate matter in IV injections may be responsible for much of the phlebitis that so often occurs with the infusion of these drugs. Russell listed the major pathologic conditions caused by particulate matter as (1) direct blockage of vessels, (2) platelet agglutination leading to formation of emboli, (3) local inflammation caused by impaction of particles, and (4) antigenic reactions with subsequent allergic consequence.[30]

Intravenous Fluids

Walter noted that critically ill patients who had received large amounts of IV fluid died of pulmonary insufficiency characterized by increased venous pressure and pulmonary hypertension. He observed that the lungs looked like leather and speculated that the cause of death might be the result of accumulated matter from the many liters of infused fluids.[35]

Reducing the Level of Contamination

Because particulate matter infused through IV fluids may produce pathologic changes that can have an adverse effect on critically ill patients, every effort must be made to reduce the particulate count in IV injections. Nurses and doctors in general have been unaware of the potential dangers that exist and have unknowingly added to the contamination. Official agencies have developed standards for an acceptable limit for particles in IV fluids. Industry has provided the medical profession with filters to limit direct access of bacteria, fungi, and particulate matter to the bloodstream.

Filters

A filter aspiration needle specially designed to remove particulate matter from IV medicaments is available. With this device attached to a syringe, the medication is drawn from the vial or glass ampule filtering out the particles. The filter needle must then be discarded to prevent the particles trapped on the filter from being injected when the medication is added to the IV fluid.

Final Filters

The National Coordinating Committee on Large Volume Parenterals* has recommended the in-line filter that is both particulate and microbe retentive for the following: hyperali-

---

* National Coordinating Committee on Large Volume Parenterals, cosponsored by the United Pharmacopeial Convention and the Food and Drug Administration under FDA contract with U.S.P.C. Ref. No.:79–01, Nov. 30, 1979.

mentation patients and immunodeficient or immunocompromised patients. The particulate-retentive IV filter is generally recommended for patients receiving IV infusions with many additives, when drugs requiring constitution are known to be heavily particulated, or to minimize particulate matter in infusions to which additives have been introduced.

Intravenous Nurses Society policy advocates the routine use of 0.2-μm air-eliminating filters in delivering routine IV therapy because these filters remove particulates, bacteria, and air, and some remove endotoxins as well.[27]

Filters are manufactured in a variety of forms, sizes, and materials. Some block the passage of air under normal pressure when wet. Used in conjunction with electronic infusion devices (EIDS), they play an important role in preventing air from being pumped into the bloodstream should the fluid container become empty.

A knowledge of filter characteristics, use, and proper handling is important for patient safety. Faulty handling can cause plugging of the filter, resulting in the patient not receiving prescribed fluids and the necessity of performing a venipuncture to insert a new line. A ruptured filter may go undetected and introduce filter fragments, bacteria, and possibly air into the IV system. A thorough discussion of IV filtration and its benefits may be found in Chapter 12.

CULTURING

Culture Profile

When line sepsis is suspected, three blood cultures should be drawn, ideally from separate venipuncture sites. Deep candidal sepsis—systemic candidiasis—is often associated with negative blood cultures. It is common practice in a number of clinical settings to develop a culture profile for the patient with suspected sepsis and to routinely culture, in intensive care units, blood of patients receiving multiple infusion therapies. Quantitative blood cultures, using pour plates, provide an excellent method for diagnosis of catheter-related infection.

Semiquantitative Technique for Culturing Cannulas

Before removing a cannula, the skin around the insertion site is cleansed with an alcohol-impregnated pad to reduce contaminating skin flora and to remove any residual antibiotic ointment. After drying, the cannula is withdrawn, taking care to avoid contact with the surrounding skin. If pus can be expressed from the cannula wound, it is Gram's stained and cultured separately. For short indwelling catheters, the entire length of the cannula is cut from the skin-catheter junction (Figure 10-2) using sterile scissors. With longer catheters, a 2-inch segment is cultured: the tip and the intracutaneous segment. Segments are cultured as soon as possible following removal and within 2 hours. In the laboratory, the segment is rolled back and forth across the surface of a 100-mm 5% blood agar plate four times. Plates are then incubated aerobically at 37°C for at least 72 hours. This technique has outstanding sensitivity and specificity in the diagnosis of cannula-related infections. Table 10-4 lists criteria for defining a nosocomial bacteremia as cannula related.

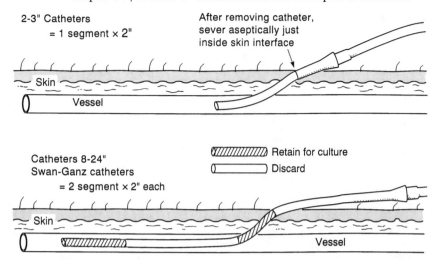

FIGURE 10-2   Segments of vascular cannulas cultured semiquantitatively. (From Maki DG, et al. [1977]. *Journal of Surgical Research, 22,* 513. Reprinted with permission of D. G. Maki and Little, Brown & Co. © 1986)

PRACTICE SETTING

The practice setting in which care is delivered should have no bearing at all on the quality of IV care provided. Many professionals believe that susceptibility to infection is minimized by the provision of care in a patient's place of residence. This theory is based on the fact that the patient is accustomed to the flora in his own environment. In any clinical environment, principles of asepsis must be adhered to in an effort to minimize the risk of IV catheter-related infection and to ensure a high level of IV patient care.

TABLE 10-4
Criteria for Defining a Nosocomial Bacteria
Cannula-Related Infection

- Isolation of the same species in significant numbers on semiquantitative culture of the cannula and from blood cultures obtained by separate venipunctures with negative culture of infusate

- Clinical and microbiologic data disclosing no other apparent source of septicemia

- Clinical features consistent with bloodstream infection

REFERENCES

1. Altemeier, W. A., Todd, J. C., & Inge, W. W. (1967). Gram-negative septicemia: A growing threat. *Annals of Surgery, 166,* 530–542.
2. Banks, D. C., Cawdreys, H. M., Yates, D. B., & Harries, M. G. (1970). *Lancet 1,* 443.
3. Centers for Disease Control. (1982). Guidelines for prevention of intravascular infection. *Journal of the National Intravenous Therapy Association, 5*(1), 39–50.
4. Centers for Disease Control. (1971). Nosocomial bacteremias associated with intravenous fluid therapy. *Morbidity and Mortality Weekly Report, 20*(Special Suppl.), no. 9.
5. Curry, C. R., & Quie, P. G. (1971). Fungal septicemia in patients receiving parenteral hyperalimentation. *New England Journal of Medicine, 285,* 1221.
6. Davis, N. M., Turco, S., & Sivielly, E. (1970). A study of particulate matter in I.V. infusion fluids. *American Journal of Hospital Pharmacy, 27,* 822–826.
7. Deeb, E. N., & Natsios, G. A. (1971). Contamination of intravenous fluids by bacteria and fungi during preparation and administration. *American Journal of Hospital Pharmacy, 28,* 764.
8. Felts, S. K., Shaffner, W., Melly, M. A., & Koenig, M. G. (1972). Sepsis caused by contaminated intravenous fluids: Epidemiological clinical and laboratory investigation of an outbreak in one hospital. *Annals of Internal Medicine, 77,* 881.
9. Fonkalsrud, E. W., Murphy, J., & Smith, F. G., Jr. (1968). Effect of pH in glucose infusions on development of thrombophlebitis. *Journal of Surgical Research, 8,* 539.
10. Fuchs, P. C. (1971). Indwelling intravenous polyethylene catheters: Factors influencing the risk of microbial colonization and sepsis. *Journal of the American Medical Association, 216,* 1447–1450.
11. Goldmann, D. A., Maki, G. D., Rhame, F. S., & Kaiser, A. B. (1973). Guidelines for infection control in intravenous therapy. *Annals of Internal Medicine, 79,* 849.
12. Groves, M. J. (1965). Particles in intravenous fluids (letter). *Lancet 2,* 344.
13. Hales, M. R. (1956). Multiple small arteriovenous fistulae of the lungs. *American Journal of Pathology, 32,* 927.
14. Hansen, J. S., & Hepler, C. D. (1973). Contamination of intravenous solutions by airborne microbes. *American Journal of Hospital Pharmacy, 30,* 326–331.
15. Hirshfield, J. W. (1941). Bacterial contamination of wounds from the air, from the skin of the operator, and from the skin of the patient. *Surgery, Gynecology and Obstetrics, 73,* 72–78.
16. Inderlied, C. B., & Young, L. S. (1985). Clinical microbiology of acquired immune deficiency syndrome (AIDS). *Journal of Medical Technicians, 2*(3), 167, 169.
17. Jonas, A. M. (1967). Potentially hazardous effects of introducing particulate matter into the vascular system of man and animals. In *Safety of large volume parenteral solutions* (Proceedings of National Symposium of the US Food and Drug Administration, Washington, DC, 1966). Washington, DC: Government Printing Office.
18. Kruger, E. O., & Riggs, T. H. (1968). Objectives: Pharmaceutical Manufacturers Association Parenteral Particulate Matter Committee. *Bulletin of the Parenteral Drug Association, 22,* 99–103.
19. Liebow, A. A., Hales, M. R., & Lindskog, G. B. (1949). Enlargement of the bronchial arteries and their anastomoses with the pulmonary arteries in bronchiectasis. *American Journal of Pathology, 25,* 211–231.
20. Lillehei, R. C., Dietzman, R., Moras, S., & Block, J. H. (1967). Treatment of septic shock. *Modern Treatment, 4*(2), 32–346.
21. Maki, D. G., Goldman, D. A., & Rhama, F. S. (1973). Infection control in intravenous therapy. *Annals of Internal Medicine, 79,* 869, 870, 872, 875, 876, 878, 880.
22. Masuda, J. V., & Beckerman, J. H. (1973). Particulate matter in commercial antibiotic injectable products. *American Journal of Hospital Pharmacy, 30,* 72–76.
23. McDonough, J. J. (November, 1971). Preventing contamination in I.V. therapy. *Hospital Physician,* 70.
24. McGaw Laboratories. (1969). *McGaw technical information bulletin #16.* Glendale, CA.
25. Maki, D. G. (1976). Growth properties of microorganisms in infusion fluid and methods of detection. In I. Phillips, P. D. Meers, and P. F. D'Arcy (Eds.), *Microbiological hazards of infusion therapy.* Lancaster, England: MTP Press.
26. Motsay, G. J., Dietzman, R. H., Ersek, R. A., & Lillehei, R. C. (1970). Hemodynamic alterations and results of treatment in patients with Gram-negative septic shock. *Surgery 67,* 577–583.
27. *Revised intravenous nursing standards of practice.* (1990). *Journal of Intravenous Nursing,* (Suppl.), p. S57.
28. Prinzmetal, M., Ornitz, E. M., Jr., Simkin, B., & Bergman, H. C. (1948). Arteriovenous anastomoses in liver, spleen, and lungs. *American Journal of Physiology, 152,* 48–52.
29. Robertson, M. H. (1970). Fungi in fluids—A hazard of intravenous therapy. *Journal of Medical Microbiology, 3,* 99.

30. Russell, J. H. (1970). Pharmaceutical application of filtration, part 2. *American Journal of Hospital Pharmacy, 28,* 125–126.
31. Thomas, C. L. (Ed.). (1973). *Taber's cyclopedic medical dictionary.* Philadelphia: F. A. Davis.
32. Turco, S., & Davis, N. M. (1973). Clinical significance of particulate matter—A review of literature. *Lippincott's Hospital Pharmacy, 8,* 137.
33. Turco, S., & Davis, N. M. (1972). Glass particles in intravenous injections. *New England Journal of Medicine, 287,* 1264–1265.
34. Viaflex containers. (1972). *Medical Letter on Drugs and Therapeutics, 14,* 69–71.
35. Walter, C. W. (1967). *FDA Symposium on Safety of Large Volume Parenteral Solutions.* Washington, DC: US Government Printing Office.
36. Walter, C. W. (1956). *The aseptic treatment of wounds.* New York: Macmillan.

BIBLIOGRAPHY

Bivins, B. A., Rapp, R. P., Deluca, P. P., McKean, H., & Ward, O. G., Jr. (1979). Fluid inline filtration: A means of decreasing the incidence of infusion phlebitis. *Surgery, 85*(4), 388–394.
Buxton, A. E., Highsmith, A. K., Garner, J. S., West, C. M., Stamm, W. E., Dixon, R. E., & McGowan, J. E. (1979). Contamination of intravenous infusion fluid; effects of changing administration sets. *Annals of Internal Medicine, 90,* 764–768.
Contamination Control Laboratories. (1970). *Particle size comparisons* (information circular). Livonia, MI.
Crossley, K., & Matsen, J. M. (1972). The scalp-vein needle: A prospective study of complications. *Journal of the American Medical Association, 220,* 985.
Davis, N. M., & Turco, S. (1971). A study of particulate matter in I.V. infusion fluids—phase 2. *American Journal of Hospital Pharmacy, 28,* 620–623.
Dudrick, S. J. (1974). Article in *Hospital Tribune.* University and Hospital Edition of *Medical Tribune and Medical News, 8*(3), 1.
Jemison-Smith, P. (1984). Understanding the acquired immune deficiency syndrome. *Journal of the National Intravenous Therapy Association, 7*(2), 115.
Moseley, R. V., & Doty, D. B. (1970). Death associated with multiple pulmonary emboli soon after battle. *Annals of Surgery, 171,* 336.
National Coordinating Committee on Large Volume Parenterals. (March, 1976). Recommendations to pharmacists for solving problems with large volume parenterals. *American Journal of Hospital Pharmacy, 33,* 231–236.
Thomas, E. T., Evers, W., & Racz, C. B. (1970). Post infusion phlebitis. *Anesthesia and Analgesia, 49,* 150–159.

REVIEW QUESTIONS

1. Primary sources of bacteria responsible for IV-associated infections include all EXCEPT:
   a. air
   b. skin
   c. blood
   d. mucous membrane

2. A virus that is easily transmitted through blood and may be destroyed by heat or gas is:
   a. hepatitis
   b. HIV
   c. chlamydia
   d. serratia

3. Conditions that adversely affect a patient's capacity to resist infection include all of the following EXCEPT:
   a. chronic uremia
   b. diabetes insipidus
   c. diabetes mellitus
   d. cancer

4. Immune response is depressed by all of the following treatments EXCEPT:
   a. immunosuppressive drugs
   b. corticosteroids
   c. radiation
   d. hypothermia

5. Extrinsic contamination may occur in all of the following areas EXCEPT:
   a. administration sets
   b. additive ports
   c. manufacturing process
   d. cannulas

6. The use of iodophor preparations for skin prep before venipuncture is based on what theory?
   a. disinfectant quality
   b. release of free iodine
   c. presence of skin germs
   d. prevention of cross-infection

7. Improper taping of the cannula may result in which of the following?
   a. mechanical irritation
   b. chemical irritation
   c. incompatibility
   d. bacteremia

8. Particulate matter may be removed from an infusate or infusion in progress by all of the following EXCEPT:
   a. filter needles
   b. inline filters
   c. blood filters
   d. injection ports

9. Sources that contribute to particulate contamination include all of the following EXCEPT:
   a. drugs
   b. rubber closures
   c. flash chambers
   d. glass ampules

10. The governmental agency that has developed guidelines to prevent transmission of the HIV virus is:
    a. OSHA
    b. AABB
    c. AAMI
    d. ECRI

CHAPTER 11

Laboratory Tests

In the past, IV departments included the collection of venous blood samples as one of their functions. Since IV therapy has become highly specialized and requires more of the nurse's time, the collection of venous blood now is often allocated to a team of technicians. There are still many instances in which the IV nurse will be involved: in critical care units; when veins have become exhausted; when the patient is to receive an IV infusion; and when the specimen is to be obtained from a central venous cannula that is to be removed, from a multilumen central venous cannula, from a Hickman-Broviac catheter, or from an implanted vascular access device.

Definite advantages are gained when this nurse is involved in collecting venous blood.[1] The nurse, understanding the importance of the preservation of veins for infusion therapy, is cautious when choosing veins and in applying blood-drawing techniques.[2] Frequently, one venipuncture permits both the withdrawal of blood and the initiation of the infusion, thereby preserving veins, reducing discomfort, and avoiding undue distress of the patient.[3] The patient–blood identification is of paramount importance in preventing the error of infusing incompatible blood. Because the department assumes responsibility for patient–blood identification in administering blood and is aware of existing hazards, its personnel are well qualified and trained in the collection of samples for typing and crossmatching.

The nurse in any clinical setting is often faced with the problem of collecting blood with little or no knowledge of the tests to be performed other than the amount of blood needed and the type of tube required. This chapter is intended primarily to provide the nurse with information concerning the most commonly performed laboratory tests— their purpose and normal values, and the collection and proper handling of the specimens. No attempt is made to explain laboratory procedures.

COLLECTION OF BLOOD

The collection of blood samples for certain tests must meet special requirements. Some tests call for whole blood, whereas others require components such as plasma, serum, or cells. The proper requirements must be met to prevent erroneous or misleading laboratory analysis.

Serum consists of plasma minus fibrinogen and is obtained by drawing blood in a dry tube and allowing it to coagulate. Serum is required by the majority of laboratory tests in common use.

Sharon M. Weinstein: PLUMER'S PRINCIPLES & PRACTICE OF INTRAVENOUS THERAPY, FIFTH EDITION, © 1993 J. B. Lippincott Company

Plasma consists of the stable components of blood minus the cells and is obtained by using an anticoagulant to prevent the blood from clotting. Several anticoagulants are available in color-coded tubes. Choice of the anticoagulant depends on the test to be performed. Most of the anticoagulants, including sodium or potassium oxalate, citrate, and ethylenediaminetetraacetic acid (EDTA), prevent coagulation by binding the serum calcium. Other anticoagulants, such as heparin, are valuable in specific tests but are not commonly used. Heparin prevents coagulation for only limited periods of time.

Whole blood is required for many tests, including blood counts and bleeding time. Potassium oxalate is commonly used to preserve whole blood.

Hemoconcentration through venous stasis should be avoided or inaccurate results will occur in some tests. Hemoconcentration increases proportionally with the length of time the tourniquet is applied. Once the venipuncture has been made, the tourniquet should be removed. This is a simple but important precaution, ignored by many. Carbon dioxide and pH are examples of tests affected by hemoconcentration. If the tourniquet is required to withdraw the blood, it should be noted on the requisition that the blood was drawn with stasis.

Hemolysis causes serious errors in many tests in which lysis of the red blood cells permits the substance being measured to escape into the serum. When erythrocytes rich in potassium rupture, the serum potassium level rises, giving a false measurement. To avoid hemolysis, the following special precautions should be observed:

1. Dry syringes and dry tubes must be used.
2. Excess pressure on the plunger of the syringe should be avoided; such pressure collapses the vein and may cause air bubbles to be sucked from around the hub of the needle into the blood.
3. Clotted blood specimens should not be shaken unnecessarily.
4. Force should be avoided in transferring blood to a container or tube; force of the blood against the tube results in rupture of the cells. In transferring blood to a vacuum tube, no needle larger than 20 gauge should be used.

Intravenous Solutions

Intravenous solutions may contribute to misleading laboratory interpretations. Blood samples should never be drawn proximal to an infusion but preferably from the contralateral extremity. If the solution contains a substance that may affect the analysis, an indication of its presence should be made on the requisition—for example, potassium determination during an infusion of electrolyte solution.

Special Handling

Special handling is required with some samples when a delay is unavoidable. Some determinations, such as the pH, must be done within 10 minutes after the blood is drawn. When a delay is inevitable, the sample is placed in ice, which partially inhibits *glycolysis*, the production of lactic acid by the glycolytic enzymes of the blood cells, resulting in a rapid lowering of pH on standing.

Blood gases also require special handling and must be analyzed as soon as blood is collected. When the carbon dioxide content of serum is to be determined, the blood must completely fill the tube or carbon dioxide will escape. Several procedures are currently in use; in each, the escape of carbon dioxide must be prevented.

Fasting

Because absorption of food may alter the blood, some tests depend on the patient's fasting. Blood glucose and serum lipid levels are increased by ingestion of food. Serum inorganic phosphorous values are depressed after meals.

Promptness of Examination

Immediate dispatch of blood samples to the laboratory is vital to the accurate determination of some blood tests; promptness in examining blood samples is necessary in the analysis of labile constituents of blood. In certain tests, such as potassium, the substance being measured diffuses out of the cells into the serum being examined and gives a false measurement. To prevent this rise in serum concentration, the cells must be separated from the serum promptly.

Infected Samples

Special caution must be observed in the care of all blood specimens because blood from all patients is to be considered infective. Specimens should not be allowed to spill on the outside of the containers. Contaminated material should be placed in bags and treated according to institutional policies for disposal of infectious material. Cannulas should not be recapped or broken but disposed of intact in cannula-proof containers. All personnel handling blood should wear gloves.

Emergency Tests

Blood tests ordered as emergencies must be sent directly to the laboratory. Red cellophane tape or other alert-type stickers, according to facility preference, may be used to indicate a state of emergency. Tests most likely to be designated as emergencies include amylase, blood urea nitrogen (BUN), carbon dioxide, potassium, prothrombin, sodium, sugar, and blood typing.

VENIPUNCTURE: SAMPLING

A venipuncture, when skillfully executed, causes the patient little discomfort. The numerous blood determinations necessary for diagnosis and treatment make good technique imperative.

The one-step entry technique should be avoided because too often it results in through-and-through punctures, contributing to hematoma formation. The needle should be inserted under the skin and then, after relocation of the vein, into the vessel.

The veins most commonly used are those in the antecubital fossa. The median antecubital vein, though not always visible, is usually large and palpable. Because it is well supported by subcutaneous tissue and least likely to roll, it is often the best choice for venipuncture. Second choice is the cephalic vein. The basilic vein, though often the most prominent, is likely to be the least desirable. This vein rolls easily, making the venipuncture difficult, and a hematoma may readily occur if the patient is allowed to flex his or her arm; flexing the arm squeezes the blood from the engorged vein into the tissues.

Sufficient time should be spent in locating the vein before attempting venipuncture. Whenever the veins are difficult to see or palpate, the patient should lie down. If the patient is seated, the arm should be well supported on a pillow.

Complications

Hematomas

Hematomas are the most common complication of routine venipuncture for withdrawing blood, and they contribute more to the limitation of available veins than any other complication. They may result from through-and-through puncture to the vein or from incomplete insertion of the needle into the lumen of the vein, which allows the blood to leak into the tissues through the bevel of the needle. In the latter case, correction may be made by advancing the needle into the vein. At the first sign of uncontrolled bleeding, the tourniquet should be released and the needle withdrawn.

Hematomas also result from the application of the tourniquet after an unsuccessful attempt has been made to draw blood. The tourniquet should never be applied to the extremity immediately after a venipuncture.

Hematomas most frequently result from insufficient time spent in applying pressure and from the bad habit of flexing the arm to stop the bleeding. Once the venipuncture is completed, the patient should be instructed to elevate the arm; elevation causes a negative pressure in the vein, collapsing it and facilitating clotting. With cardiac patients, elevation of the arm should be avoided. Constant pressure is maintained until the bleeding has stopped. Pressure is applied with a dry sterile sponge; a wet sponge encourages bleeding. Band-Aids do not take the place of pressure and, if ordered, are not applied until the bleeding has stopped. Ecchymoses on the arm indicate poor technique or haphazard manner.

Bloodborne Disease

Special caution must be exercised in the care of needles used to draw blood from patients suspected of harboring microorganisms. Contaminated needles should be placed immediately in a separate container for disposal. A vacuum tube with stopper provides adequate protection against accidental puncture from the contaminated needle until proper disposal can be made. Any needle puncture should be reported at once.

Other Complications

Other complications of venipuncture include syncope, continued bleeding, and thrombosis of the vein.

Syncope is rarely encountered when the clinician is confident, skillful, and reassures the patient.

Continued bleeding is a complication that may affect the patient receiving anticoagulants, the patient with a blood dyscrasia, or the oncology patient undergoing chemotherapy. To prevent bleeding and to preserve the vein, pressure to the site may be required for an extended period. The nurse should remain with the patient until the bleeding has stopped.

Thrombosis in routine venipuncture occurs from injury to the endothelial lining of the vein during the venipuncture. Antecubital veins may be used indefinitely if the clinician uses good technique.

THE VACUUM SYSTEM

The vacuum system has increased the efficiency of the process. It consists of a plastic holder into which screws a sterile disposable double-ended needle. A rubber-stoppered vacuum tube slips into the barrel. The barrel has a measured line denoting the distance the tube is inserted into the barrel; at this point the needle becomes embedded in the stopper. The stopper is not punctured until the needle has been introduced into the vein.

After entry into the vein, the rubber-stoppered tube is pushed the remaining distance into the barrel. As the needle is pushed into the vacuum tube, a rubber sheath covering the shaft is forced back, allowing the blood to flow. The tourniquet is released and several specimens may be obtained by simply removing the tube containing the sample and replacing it with another tube. As the tube is removed, the rubber sheath slips back over the needle, preventing blood from dripping into the holder.

If the vein is not located, removing the tube before the needle is withdrawn will preserve the vacuum in the tube.

At times it becomes necessary to draw blood from small veins. If suction from the vacuum tube collapses the vein, difficulty will be encountered in drawing the blood. By pressing the finger against the vein beyond the point of the needle or by placing the bevel of the needle lightly against the wall of the vein, suction is reduced and the vein allowed to fill. In the latter process, particular caution should be exercised to prevent injury to the endothelial lining of the vein. The pressure is intermittently applied and released, filling and emptying the vein. A small-gauge winged infusion needle with vacuum adapter may also be used; the smaller needle reduces the amount of suction and may prevent collapse of the vein. A syringe is often used to draw blood from small veins because the amount of suction can be more easily controlled.

VENOUS SAMPLING: CENTRAL

Occasionally it is desirable to draw blood samples through the central venous catheter. Such occasions include difficulty in obtaining an adequate vein, cases in which the avoidance of stress is imperative, and situations in which blood tests are ordered frequently and repeatedly.

Aseptic technique is vital in preventing the introduction of bacteria into the catheter. A sterile IV catheter cap reduces the risk of bacterial invasion.

Procedure

Follow this procedure in drawing blood by way of the central venous catheter from a patient not on drug therapy:

1. Put on gloves. Clamp off the infusion.
2. Remove catheter plug and, with a sterile syringe, withdraw 4 mL blood; discard it.
3. Using a sterile syringe, withdraw the required amount of blood. If difficulty is encountered in drawing blood samples, raise patient's arm to shoulder level or higher to reduce axillary pressure on catheter.
4. Recap stopcock with a sterile plug.
5. Open clamp and flush catheter with about 5 mL infusion fluid to maintain catheter patency.
6. Adjust flow to prescribed flow rate. After contact with patient, remove gloves and wash hands.

If the patient is receiving drug therapy, follow the same procedure, except *use a hemostat* to stop the infusion temporarily; after the blood is drawn, the control clamp maintains the prescribed rate of flow without readjustment. Note: Only a jawless clamp should be used on a silastic tunneled catheter.

Precaution

Patients receiving vasopressors may not tolerate an interruption of medication. Check with the charge nurse before stopping the infusion; extra caution may be required.

WITHDRAWING BLOOD AND INITIATING AN INFUSION _____

Drawing blood samples and initiating an infusion can be efficiently accomplished by a single venipuncture in the following way:

1. Put on gloves. Fill IV set with solution.
2. Regulate the flow to a minimum rate.
3. Clamp tubing manually by kinking between third and little fingers.
4. Hold adapter between the forefinger and second finger, leaving the hand free for holding the syringe and cannula and collecting blood.
5. Draw blood.
6. Remove syringe; attach the infusion set to the cannula, releasing little finger; solution will flow at the previously adjusted rate.
7. Secure cannula with a piece of tape.
8. Attach syringe to needle, previously imbedded in stopper of vacuum tube, and transfer blood. Vacuum will cause tube to fill—never apply force. Use needle no larger than 20 gauge; lysis of cells can occur.
9. Remove gloves and wash hands.

COMMONLY USED LABORATORY TESTS _____

Laboratory tests are performed (1) routinely because they indicate relatively common disorders, (2) for diagnostic purposes, (3) for following the course of a disease, and (4) for regulating therapy. Standard laboratory values are listed in Table 11-1; examples of conversions of those values to Système International (SI) units are given in Table 11-2.

Blood Cultures

In cases of suspected bacteremia, blood cultures are performed to identify the causative microorganisms. Isolation of the organism is necessary to enable the physician to direct proper antimicrobial therapy. Blood cultures are performed during febrile illnesses or when the patient is having chills with spiking fever. Intermittent bacteremia accompanies such infections as pyelonephritis, brucellosis, cholangitis, and other infections. In such cases, repeated blood cultures are usually ordered to be performed when the fever spikes. In other infections, such as subacute bacterial endocarditis, the bacteremia is more constant during the 4 to 5 febrile days. Usually four or five cultures are obtained over a span of 1 to 2 days, and antimicrobial therapy is initiated with the realization that the majority of cultures will be found to harbor the offending microorganism. If anti-

(text continues on page 123)

TABLE 11-1
Laboratory Values

Laboratory Test	*Normal Values*
Blood Chemistry/Electrolytes	
Blood urea nitrogen* (BUN)	7–18 mg/100 mL
Creatinine, serum*	0.7–1.5 mg/100 mL
Creatinine clearance‡	Male: 110–150 mL/min Female: 105–132 mL/min
BUN : Creatinine ratio*	10 : 1
Hematocrit*	Male: 44%–52% Female: 39%–47%
Hemoglobin†	Male: 13.5–18.0 g/dL Female: 12.0–16.0 g/dL
Red blood cells†	Male: 4600–6200/mm³ Female: 4200–5400/mm³
Complete blood count (CBC)	
Total leukocytes‡	4500–11,000/mm³
Myelocytes‡	0
Band neutrophils‡ (bands)	150–400/mm³ (3%–5%)
Segmented neutrophils‡ (segs)	3000–5800/mm³ (54%–62%)
Lymphocytes‡	1500–3000/mm³ (25%–33%)
Monocytes‡	300–500/mm³ (3%–7%)
Eosinophils‡	50–250/mm³ (1%–3%)
Basophils‡	15–50/mm³ (0%–0.75%)
Platelets‡	150,000–300,000/mm³
Reticulocytes†	0.5%–1.5%
Red cell volume†	Male: 20–36 mL/kg Female: 19–31 mL/kg
Plasma volume†	Male: 25–43 mL/kg Female: 28–45 mL/kg
Clotting time†	8–18 min
Prothrombin time†	11–15 s
Partial thromboplastin time†	Standard: 68–82 s Activated: 32–46 s
Plasma thrombin time†	13–17 s
Fibrinogen†	160–415 mg/dL
Osmolality, serum*	280–295 mOsm/kg
Amylase, serum‡	25–125 mU/mL
Glucose, serum*	70–110 mg/100 mL
Serum electrolytes	
Sodium*	135–145 mEq/L
Potassium*	3.5–5.5 mEq/L

Calcium*	Total
	   8.5–10.5 mg/100 mL or 4.0–5.5 mEq/L
	Ionized
	   About 50% of total value

Magnesium*	1.5–2.5 mEq/L or 1.8–3.0 mg/100 mL
Chloride*	100–106 mEq/L
Carbon dioxide (CO_2) content*	24–30 mmol/L

(continued)

TABLE 11-1 *(Continued)*

Laboratory Test	Normal Values
Phosphorus*	Adults 3.0–4.5 mg/100 mL (1.8–2.6 mEq/L) Children 4.0–7.0 mg/100 mL (2.3–4.1 mEq/L)
Zinc*	77–137 μg/100 mL (by atomic absorption)
Lithium*	0.8 mEq/L (therapeutic level 8–12 hr after administration)

Serum proteins
  Total*
  Albumin*
  Globulin*
	
	6.0–8.0 g/100 mL
	3.5–5.5 g/100 mL
	1.5–3.0 g/100 mL

Lactate* (arterial blood)	1.5 mEq/L (approximately 10 mg/100 mL)
Ketones, serum*	Often >50 mg/100 mL in diabetic ketoacidosis Usually <20 mg/100 mL in salicylate intoxication
Salicylates, serum*	Therapeutic range 20–25 mg/100 mL Toxic range >30 mg/100 mL
Anion gap*	12–15 mEq/L
Aspartate aminotransferase‡ (AST)	7–40 mU/mL (37°C)
Alanine aminotransferase‡ (ALT)	5–35 mU/mL (37°C)
Alkaline phosphatase‡	20–90 mU/mL (30°C)

Bilirubin, serum
  Total‡
  Direct‡
  Indirect‡
	
	0.3–1.1 mg/dL
	0.1–0.4 mg/dL
	0.2–0.7 mg/dL (total minus direct)

Lactate dehydrogenase‡ (LDH)	100–190 mU/mL (37°C)

Urine Chemistry/Electrolytes

Electrolytes*
(May be of limited value due to recent administration of diuretics. Measurement of urinary electrolytes without knowledge of dietary intake is of limited value.)

Sodium*	80–180 mEq/24 hr (varies with Na^+ intake)
Potassium*	40–80 mEq/24 hr (varies with dietary intake)
Chloride*	110–250 mEq/24 hr
Calcium*	100–150 mg/24 hr (if on average diet) Varies with dietary intake
Osmolality*	Typical urine is 500–800 mOsm/L (extreme range is 50–1400 mOsm/L) Usually about 1.5–3 times greater than serum osmolality
Specific gravity*	1.002–1.030 (most random samples have a value of 1.012 to 1.025)
pH*	4.5–8.0

Arterial Blood Gases

pH*	7.34–7.45
$PaCO_2$*	38–42 mm Hg
PaO_2*	80–100 mm Hg
Bicarbonate*	22–26 mEq/L
Base excess*	−2 to +2

*Metheny, N. M. (1987). *Quick reference to fluid balance* (pp. 47–55). Philadelphia: J. B. Lippincott.

†American Association of Blood Banks. (1985). Technical manual (9th ed., pp. 493–494). Arlington, VA.

‡Tenenbaum, L. (1989). *Cancer chemotherapy: A reference guide.* Philadelphia: W. B. Saunders.

TABLE 11-2
Examples of Conversions to Système International (SI) Units

Component	System	Present Reference Intervals	Present Unit	Conversion Factor	SI Reference Intervals	SI Unit Symbol
Alanine aminotransferase (ALT)	Serum	5–40	U/L	1.0	5–40	U/L
Albumin	Serum	3.9–5.0	mg/dL	10	39–50	g/L
Alkaline phosphatase	Serum	35–110	U/L	1.00	35–110	U/L
Aspartate aminotransferase (AST)	Serum	5–40	U/L	1.00	5–40	U/L
Bilirubin	Serum					
Direct		0–0.2	mg/dL	17.10	0–4	μmol/L
Total		0.1–1.2	mg/dL	17.10	2–20	μmol/L
Calcium	Serum	8.6–10.3	mg/dL	0.2495	2.15–2.57	mmol/L
Carbon dioxide, total	Serum	22–30	mEq/L	1.00	22–30	mmol/L
Chloride	Serum	98–108	mEq/L	1.00	98–108	mmol/L
Cholesterol	Serum					
Age <29 yr		<200	mg/dL	0.02586	<5.15	mmol/L
30–39 yr		<225	mg/dL	0.02586	<5.80	mmol/L
40–49 yr		<245	mg/dL	0.02586	<6.35	mmol/L
>50 yr		<265	mg/dL	0.02586	<6.85	mmol/L
Complete blood count	Blood					
Hematocrit						
Men		42–52	%	0.01	0.42–0.52	1
Women		37–47	%	0.01	0.37–0.47	1
Hemoglobin						
Men		14.0–18.0	g/dL	10.0	140–180	g/L
Women		12–16	g/dL	10.0	120–160	g/L
Red cell count						
Men		$4.6–6.2 \times 10^6$	/mm^3	10^6	$4.6–6.2 \times 10^{12}$/L	
Women		$4.2–5.4 \times 10^6$	/mm^3	10^6	$4.2–5.4 \times 10^{12}$/L	
White cell count		$4.5–11.0 \times 10^3$	/mm^3	10^6	$4.5–11.0 \times 10^9$/L	
Platelet count		$150–300 \times 10^3$	/mm^3	10^6	$150–300 \times 10^9$/L	
Cortisol	Serum					
8 AM		5–25	μg/dL	27.59	140–690	nmol/L
8 PM		3–13	μg/dL	27.59	80–360	nmol/L
Cortisol	Urine	20–90	μg/24 hr	2.759	55–250	nmol/24 hr
Creatine kinase	Serum					
High CK group (black men)		50–520	U/L	1.00	50–520	U/L
Intermediate CK group (nonblack men, black women)		35–345	U/L	1.00	35–345	U/L
Low CK group (nonblack women)		25–145	U/L	1.00	25–145	U/L
Creatinine kinase isoenzyme, MB fraction	Serum	>5	%	0.01	>0.05	1
Creatinine	Serum	0.4–1.3	mg/dL	88.40	35–115	μmol/L
Men		0.7–1.3	mg/dL	88.40		
Women		0.4–1.1	mg/dL	88.40		
Digoxin, therapeutic	Serum	0.5–2.0	ng/mL	1.281	0.6–2.6	nmol/L

(continued)

TABLE 11-2 *(Continued)*

Component	System	Present Reference Intervals	Present Unit	Conversion Factor	SI Reference Intervals	SI Unit Symbol
Erythrocyte indices	Blood					
Mean corpuscular volume (MCV)		80–100	microns^3	1.00	80–100	fL
Mean corpuscular hemoglobin (MCH)		27–31	pg	1.00	27–31	pg
Mean corpuscular hemoglobin concentration (MCHC)		32–36	%	0.01	0.32–0.36	1
Ferritin	Serum					
Men		29–438	ng/mL	1.00	29–438	μg/L
Women		9–219	ng/mL	1.00	9–219	μg/L
Folate	Serum	2.5–20.0	ng/mL	2.266	6–46	nmol/L
Follicle-stimulating hormone (FSH)	Serum					
Children		12 or <	mIU/mL	1.00	12 or <	IU/L
Men		2.0–10.0	mIU/mL	1.00	2.0–10.0	IU/L
Women, follicular		3.2–9.0	mIU/mL	1.00	3.2–9.0	IU/L
Women, midcycle		3.2–9.0	mIU/mL	1.00	3.2–9.0	IU/L
Women, luteal		2.0–6.2	mIU/mL	1.00	2.0–6.2	IU/L
Gases arterial	Blood					
pO$_2$		80–95	mm Hg	0.1333	10.7–12.7	kPa
pCO$_2$		37–43	mm Hg	0.1333	4.9–5.7	kPa
Glucose	Serum	62–110	mg/dL	0.05551	3.4–6.1	mmol/L
Iron	Serum	50–160	μg/dL	0.1791	9–29	μmol/L
Iron-binding capacity	Serum					
TIBC		230–410	μg/dL	0.1791	41–73	μmol/L
Saturation		15–55	%	0.01	0.15–0.55	1
Lactic dehydrogenase	Serum	120–300	U/L	1.00	120–300	U/L
Luteinizing hormone	Serum					
Men		4.9–15.0	mIU/mL	1.00	4.9–15.0	IU/L
Women, follicular		5.0–25	mIU/mL	1.00	5.0–25	IU/L
Women, midcycle		43–145	mIU/mL	1.00	43–145	IU/L
Women, luteal		3.1–31	mIU/mL	1.00	3.1–31	IU/L
Magnesium	Serum	1.2–1.9	mEq/L	0.4114	0.50–0.78	mmol/L
Osmolality	Serum	278–300	mOsm/kg	1.00	278–300	mmol/kg
Osmolality	Urine	None defined	mOsm/kg	1.00	None defined	mmd/kg
Phenobarbital, therapeutic	Serum	15–40	μg/mL	4.306	65–175	μmol/L
Phenytoin, therapeutic	Serum	10–20	μg/mL	3.964	40–80	μmol/L
Phosphate (phosphorus, inorganic)	Serum	2.3–4.1	mg/dl	0.3229	0.75–1.35	mmol/L
Potassium	Serum	3.7–5.1	mEq/L g/mL	1.00	3.7–5.1	mmol/L
Protein, total	Serum	6.5–8.3	g/dL	10.0	65–83	g/L
Sodium	Serum	134–142	mEq/L	1.00	134–142	mmol/L
Theophylline, therapeutic	Serum	5–20	μg/mL	5.550	28–110	μmol/L
Thyroid-stimulating hormone (TSH)	Serum	0–5	μIU/mL	1.00	0–5	mIU/L
Thyroxine	Serum	4.5–13.2	μg/dL	12.87	58–170	nmol/L

(continued)

TABLE 11-2 *(Continued)*

Component	System	Present Reference Intervals	Present Unit	Conversion Factor	SI Reference Intervals	SI Unit Symbol
T_3-uptake ratio	Serum	0.88–1.19	l	1.00	0.88–1.19	1
Tri-iodothyronine (T_3)	Serum	70–235	ng/mL	0.01536	1.1–3.6	nmol/L
Triglycerides	Serum	50–200	mg/dL	0.01129	0.55–2.25	mmol/L
Urate (uric acid)	Serum					
Men		2.9–8.5	mg/dL	59.48	170–510	μmol/L
Women		2.2–6.5	mg/dL	59.48	130–390	μmol/L
Urea nitrogen	Serum	6–25	mg/dL	0.3570	2.1–8.9	mmol/L
Vitamin B_{12}	Serum	250–1000	pg/mL	0.7378	180–740	pmol/L

(From Fischbach, F. T. [1992]. *A manual of laboratory and diagnostic tests* [4th ed., pp. 951–955]. Philadelphia: J. B. Lippincott.

microbial therapy is administered before the blood culture or before the patient's admittance to the hospital, the bacteremia may be suppressed, rendering isolation difficult.

Penicillinase may be ordered to be added to the blood culture medium to neutralize the existing penicillinemia and to recover the organism. Usually antimicrobial therapy must be withheld to await report of culture to make a precise diagnosis. The penicillinase is added to the culture medium before or immediately after the blood sample is drawn.

Some bacteriology laboratories routinely culture blood under both aerobic and anaerobic conditions. If this is not done routinely and bacteremia with strict anaerobes is suspected, the laboratory should be notified because a special culture broth is necessary.

Extreme care must be observed in preparing the area for venipuncture because the skin affords a fertile field for bacterial growth. *Staphylococcus albus*, diphtheroids, and yeast (common skin or environment contaminants) usually indicate contamination, whereas *Staphylococcus aureus* presents a greater problem by indicating either a contaminant or the presence of a serious pathogen.

Procedure

Several procedures are currently in use. Newer methods for collecting the blood sample use special vacuum tubes containing prepared culture media. The amount of blood required depends on the laboratory and procedure used. All require thorough preparation of the puncture area with an effective antiseptic. An iodine preparation followed by 70% isopropanol is a highly recommended preparation; question the patient about iodine sensitivity. Gloves should be worn by all personnel performing venipuncture.

MEASUREMENTS OF ELECTROLYTE CONCENTRATION

Electrolyte imbalances are serious complications in the critically ill patient. Such imbalances must be recognized and corrected at once. Frequently electrolyte determinations are ordered on an emergency basis. Accurate measurement is essential and to a large degree depends on the proper collection and handling of blood specimens.

Potassium

Potassium is an electrolyte essential to body function. Approximately 98% of all body potassium is found in the cells; only small amounts are contained in the serum.

The kidneys normally do not conserve potassium. When large quantities of body fluid are lost without potassium replacement, a severe deficiency occurs. Chronic kidney disease and the use of diuretics may cause a potassium deficit. Adrenal steroids play a major role in controlling the concentration of potassium: hyperadrenalism causes increased potassium loss, with deficiency resulting; steroid therapy promotes potassium excretion.

An elevated potassium level results from potassium retention in renal failure or in adrenal cortical deficiency. Hypoventilation and cellular damage also result in an elevated potassium level.

Because intracellular ions are not accessible for measurement, determination must be made on the serum. Because the concentration of potassium in the cells is roughly 15 times greater than that in the serum, the blood for potassium determination must be carefully drawn to prevent hemolysis.

Blood Collection
Blood (2 mL) is drawn in a dry tube and allowed to clot or, preferably, placed under oil; oil minimizes friction and hemolysis of the red blood cells. The blood should be sent to the laboratory immediately because potassium diffuses out of the cells and gives a falsely high reading.
Normal serum range is 3.5 to 5.0 mEq/L.[2,4]

Sodium

The main role of sodium is the control of the distribution of water throughout the body and the maintenance of a normal fluid balance.

The excretion of sodium is regulated to a large degree by the adrenocortical hormone aldosterone. Water excretion is regulated by antidiuretic hormone (ADH), and as long as these two systems are in harmony, the sodium and water remain in isosmotic proportion. Any change in the normal sodium concentration indicates that the loss or gain of water and sodium is in other than isosmotic proportion. Increased sodium levels may be caused by excessive infusions of sodium, insufficient water intake, or excess loss of fluid without a sodium loss, as in tracheobronchitis. Decreased sodium levels may be caused by excessive sweating accompanied by intake of large amounts of water by mouth, adrenal insufficiency, excessive infusions of nonelectrolyte fluids, or gastrointestinal suction accompanied with water by mouth.

Blood Collection
Blood (3 mL) is drawn carefully to prevent hemolysis and placed in a dry tube or a tube with oil.
Normal serum range is 135 to 145 mEq/L.[1]

Chlorides

Chlorides are usually measured along with other blood electrolytes. The measurement of chlorides is helpful in diagnosing disorders of acid–base balance and water balance of the body. Chloride has a reciprocal power of increasing or decreasing in concentration whenever changes in concentration of other anions occur. In metabolic acidosis, a reciprocal rise in chloride concentration occurs when the bicarbonate concentration drops.

Elevation in the blood chloride level occurs in such conditions as Cushing's syndrome, hyperventilation, and some kidney disorders. A decrease in blood chloride levels may occur in diabetic acidosis, heat exhaustion, and following vomiting and diarrhea.

Blood Collection
Venous blood (5 mL) is withdrawn and placed in a dry tube to clot.
Normal serum range is 97 to 110 mEq/L.

Calcium

Calcium, an essential electrolyte of the body, is required for blood clotting, muscular contraction, and nerve transmission. Only ionized calcium is useful but, because it cannot be satisfactorily measured, the total amount of body calcium is determined; 50% of the total is believed to be ionized.[2] In acidosis there is a higher level of ionized calcium; in alkalosis, a lower level.

Hypocalcemia (decrease in normal blood calcium) occurs whenever impairment of the gastrointestinal tract, such as sprue or celiac disease, prevents absorption. Deficiency also occurs in hypoparathyroidism and in some kidney diseases and is characterized by muscular twitching and tetanic convulsions.

Hypercalcemia (excess of calcium in the blood) occurs in hyperparathyroidism and in respiratory disturbance where carbon dioxide blood content is increased, such as in respiratory acidosis.

Blood Collection
Venous blood (5 mL) is placed in a dry tube and allowed to clot. Analysis is performed on the serum.
Normal serum range in adults is 8.9 to 10.3 mg/100 mL.[1] The range is slightly higher in children.

Phosphorus

Phosphorus metabolism is related to calcium metabolism and the serum level varies inversely with calcium.

Increased concentration of phosphorus may occur in such conditions as hypoparathyroidism, kidney disease, or excessive intake of vitamin D. Decreased concentrations may occur in hyperparathyroidism, rickets, and some kidney diseases.

Blood Collection
Because red blood cells are rich in phosphorus, hemolysis of the blood must be avoided. Analysis is performed on the serum; 4 mL blood is placed in a dry tube to clot.
Normal serum range is 2.5 to 4.5 mg/100 mL.[1] In infants in the first year, the range is up to 6.0 mg/100 mL.

VENOUS BLOOD MEASUREMENTS OF ACID–BASE BALANCE

Acid–base balance is maintained by the buffer system, carbonic acid–base bicarbonate at a 1 to 20 ratio. When deviations occur in the normal ratio, a change in pH results and is accompanied by a change in bicarbonate concentration.

Carbon Dioxide Content

Carbon dioxide content is the measurement of the free carbon dioxide and the bicarbonate content of the serum, which provides a general measure of acidity or alkalinity. An increase in carbon dioxide content usually indicates alkalosis; a decrease indicates acidosis. This test, along with clinical findings, is helpful in surmising the severity and nature of the disorder. Measurement of pH is necessary for accuracy—a change in carbon dioxide does not always signify a change in pH because pH depends on the ratio and not the carbon dioxide content. When the carbon dioxide and pH are known, the buffer ratio can be determined.

An elevated carbon dioxide content is present in metabolic alkalosis, hypoventilation, loss of acid secretions such as occurs in persistent vomiting or drainage of the stomach, and excessive administration of corticotropin or cortisone. A low carbon dioxide content usually occurs in loss of alkaline secretions such as in severe diarrhea, certain kidney diseases, diabetic acidosis, and hyperventilation.

Blood Collection
Several procedures are now in use: collection in a heparinized syringe with immediate placement on ice, collection in a heparinized vacuum tube, or collection in a dry tube without an anticoagulant. The procedure used depends on the laboratory's routine. The containers must always be filled with blood to prevent carbon dioxide from escaping. In all methods, it is important that the patient avoid clenching the fist; excess muscular activity of the arm can increase the carbon dioxide level in the blood.

Normal serum range is 22 to 31 mEq/L.[1]

Acidity (pH) Content

The pH, a symbol for acidity, indicates the serum concentration of hydrogen ions. The pH becomes lower in acid conditions such as hypoventilation, diarrhea, and diabetic acidosis. The pH rises in alkaline conditions such as hyperventilation and excessive vomiting.

Blood Collection
The blood is collected *without stasis* in a heparinized 2-mL syringe; the syringe is then capped. The blood may be drawn with a small-vein needle, the needle discarded, and the tubing tied off. The specimen is left in the syringe and packed in ice. Loss of carbon dioxide from contact with the air is thus avoided and excess production of lactic acid by enzymic reaction reduced. Blood (5 mL) may also be collected in a green-stoppered vacuum tube containing heparin.

Normal blood range is 7.35 to 7.45.

Blood tests used to evaluate fluid and electrolyte status may be found in Table 11-3.

ENZYMES

Amylase

Amylase determination is helpful in the diagnosis of acute pancreatitis or the acute recurrence of chronic pancreatitis. Amylase is secreted by the pancreas; a rise in the serum level occurs when outflow of pancreatic juice is restricted. This test is usually

(*text continues on page 131*)

TABLE 11-3
Blood Tests Used to Evaluate Fluid and Electrolyte Status

Test	Usual Reference Range	Comments
Serum Potassium	3.5–5.0 mEq/L (3.5–5.0 mmol/L)	Alterations in acid–base balance significantly affect potassium distribution: • Acidosis results in a shift of potassium out of the cells, causing the serum potassium concentration to increase. • Alkalosis results in a shift of potassium into the cells, causing a decrease in serum potassium concentration. • On the average, every 0.1 unit change in arterial pH causes a reciprocal change of 0.5 mEq/L in plasma potassium concentration. • Insulin promotes entry of extracellular potassium into cells and thus temporarily lowers the serum potassium concentration. There are a number of causes of factitious hyperkalemia. • Tight tourniquet around an exercising extremity (as in opening and closing the hand) can elevate potassium as much as 2.7 mEq/L. • Hemolysis of sample releases potassium from blood cells into the serum, thus elevating the serum potassium level • Leukocytosis in range of 70,000 per cubic millimeter, as in leukemia, or platelet counts greater than one million per cubic millimeter (Leukocytes and platelets, which are rich in potassium, may release their large intracellular potassium stores during the clotting process.)
Serum Sodium	135–145 mEq/L (135–145 mmol/L)	Serum sodium level is closely related to body water status: • For the adult, it can be roughly estimated that each 3 mEq elevation of serum sodium above normal range represents a deficit of approximately 1 L of body water. • An elevated plasma glucose level pulls water out of the cells into the extracellular fluid; by dilution, this lowers the plasma sodium concentration. In theory, every 62 mg/dL increment increase in plasma glucose will draw enough water out of the cells to dilute the plasma sodium concentration 1 mEq/L. For example, if the plasma glucose is 1000 mg/dL (930 mg/dL above normal), the plasma sodium should fall 15 mEq/L. This expected change does not always occur, however, because of the effect of osmotic diuresis associated with hyperglycemia. • The measured plasma sodium concentration may be artifactually reduced when marked hyperlipidemia is present.

(continued)

TABLE 11-3 *(Continued)*

Test	Usual Reference Range	Comments
Serum Calcium	Total Calcium: 8.9–10.3 mg/dL (2.23–2.57 mmol/L) Total calcium in serum is the sum of the ionized (47%) and nonionized 53% calcium components. The nonionized portion consists of calcium bound to albumin (40%) and the portion (13%) chelated to anions (such as citrate and phosphate).	• Total calcium is the test performed in most clinical settings. To evaluate the actual calcium level, the clinician must first know the serum albumin level to apply the following rule: In the noncritically ill, the total serum calcium may be corrected for variations in the serum albumin by estimating that a change in the serum albumin of 1.0 g/dL (10 g/L) will change the total serum calcium by 0.8 mg/dL (0.2 mmol/L). • The above estimation is not valid when situations are present that affect pH (which changes the percentage of ionized calcium) or the quantity of substances available to bind with calcium is altered. Alkalosis increases the binding of calcium to albumin, as does an increased free fatty acid level (common in stressed patients). Other factors that can acutely lower ionized calcium are increased levels of lactate, bicarbonate, citrate, phosphate, and some substances in radiographic contrast media.
	Ionized Calcium: 4.6–5.1 mg/dL (1.15–1.27 mmol/L)	Many laboratories now have the capability to directly measure the ionized calcium level. This is desirable, especially in critically ill patients, since it is the ionized calcium that is physiologically active and thus clinically important. One should be aware that variations in the sample collection technique can affect the results. For example, acid–base changes from prolonged tourniquet application and variations in the amount of heparin in the collecting syringe can both artifactually alter the measured Ca^{++}.
Serum Magnesium	1.3–2.1 mEq/L (0.65–1.05 mmol/L	Hemolysis of the sample will invalidate the results by releasing magnesium from the red blood cells into the serum (recall that magnesium is primarily an intracellular ion).
Serum Chloride	97–110 mEq/L (97–110 mmol/L)	• Less than normal concentration indicates hypochloremia (commonly associated with hypokalemia and metabolic alkalosis). • Greater than normal concentration indicates hyperchloremia, which may be associated with excessive administration of isotonic saline.
Carbon Dioxide Content	22–31 mEq/L (22–31 mmol/L)	• This test measures total bicarbonate and carbonic acid in venous blood and is a general measure of the degree of alkalinity or acidity. (It should not be confused with the partial pressure of carbon dioxide, pCO_2, obtained from arterial blood gas analysis.) • A level below normal indicates metabolic acidosis. • In the absence of chronic obstructive pulmonary disease, an elevated level indicates metabolic alkalosis.

(continued)

TABLE 11-3 *(Continued)*

Test	Usual Reference Range	Comments
Serum Phosphate	2.5–4.5 mg/dL (0.81–1.45 mmol/L)	• Hemolysis of the sample will invalidate the results by releasing phosphate from the red blood cells into the serum (recall that phosphate is primarily an intracellular ion). • Phosphate levels are evaluated in relation to calcium levels since there is an inverse relationship between the two (*eg*, an increased phosphorus level causes the calcium level to decrease). • Phosphate levels normally higher in children than adults. • Drugs containing high phosphate levels may temporarily increase the serum phosphate level for several hours after the dose. • Insulin promotes entry of extracellular phosphorus into cells. • Intravenous glucose running before or at the time of the test causes a lowered serum phosphorus level (due to carbohydrate metabolism).
Plasma Ammonia	11–35 µmol/L (Reported values vary according to laboratory.)	• The body is less able to handle high ammonia levels when the serum potassium is low or when alkalosis is present. • Ammonia level varies with protein intake and is affected by some antibiotics.
Serum Osmolality	280–295 mOsm/kg Can be measured by lab or can be calculated by the following formula: $pOsm = 2(Na) + \dfrac{G}{18} + \dfrac{BUN}{2.4}$	• Serum osmolality is determined mainly by serum sodium concentration (recall that serum sodium makes up 90% of the osmotic pressure generated by plasma). • Finding is increased in dehydration (hypernatremia). • Finding is decreased in overhydration (hyponatremia). • Finding is increased in hyperglycemia and in presence of elevated BUN.
Anion Gap	12–15 mEq/L $AG = Na - (Cl = HCO_3)$	• Anion gap is useful in ascertaining cause of metabolic acidosis. • A level greater than 15 mEq/L indicates presence of excessive organic acids (as in diabetic ketoacidosis, lactic acidosis, uremic renal failure, and salicylate intoxication). • Normal anion gap acidosis may be due to diarrhea, ureterostomies, excessive chloride administration, and distal tubular acidosis.
BUN	8–25 mg/dL (2.9–8.9 mmol/L)	• Elevated BUN can be due to reduced renal blood flow secondary to fluid volume deficit (causing reduced urea clearance). • Excessive protein intake can elevate BUN by increasing urea production.

(continued)

TABLE 11-3 *(Continued)*

Test	Usual Reference Range	Comments
		• Increased catabolism due to trauma, starvation, bleeding into the intestines, or catabolic drugs can also increase the BUN by increasing urea production. • A low BUN is often associated with overhydration and may also be associated with low protein intake.
Creatinine	0.6–1.5 mg/dL (53–133 μmol/L)	• As an indicator of renal disease is more specific and sensitive than BUN since nonrenal causes of elevation are few. • Test is useful in evaluating renal dysfunction when a large number of nephrons have been destroyed (not increased above normal until at least half of nephrons are nonfunctioning). • In patients with large muscle mass or acromegaly, it may be slightly above normal. • A slightly elevated creatinine level may occur in severe fluid volume depletion, which results in a reduction in glomerular filtration rate.
BUN : Creatinine Ratio	10:1 (approximate)	• This ration is useful in evaluating hydration status. • When the ratio increases in favor of the BUN (ratio >10:1), conditions such as hypovolemia, low perfusion pressures to the kidney, or increased protein metabolism may be present. • When the ratio is <10:1, conditions such as low protein intake, hepatic insufficiency or repeated dialysis may be present. • When both the BUN and creatinine levels rise, maintaining the 10:1 ratio, the problem is likely intrinsic renal disease (although it may also be seen when fluid volume depletion results in reduction in the glomerular filtration rate).
Hematocrit (%)	Male: 44–52 Female: 39–47	• Hematocrit determines the percentage of red blood cells in plasma. • Changes are interpretable in terms of fluid balance only when no changes in the red blood cell mass (such as bleeding or hemolysis) are occurring. • Hematocrit is elevated in fluid volume deficit (because red blood cells are contained in a relatively smaller plasma fluid volume). • Hematocrit is decreased in fluid volume excess (because the red blood cells are contained in a relatively larger plasma fluid volume).
Fasting Plasma Glucose	65–110 mg/dL (3.58–6.05 mmol/L)	A markedly elevated glucose level in blood stream causes osmotic diuresis and resultant fluid volume deficit. • Results will be elevated above baseline if patient is receiving parenteral glucose (regardless of site from which the specimen is drawn.)

(continued)

TABLE 11-3 *(Continued)*

Test	Usual Reference Range	Comments
Plasma Lactate	0.3–1.3 mEq/L (0.3–1.3 mmol/L)	• Lactic acidosis is considered to be present if the plasma lactate level is greater than 4 to 5 mEq/L. • Most cases of lactic acidosis are due to marked tissue hypoperfusion. • False low values occur with high lactic dehydrogenase levels; elevations may occur with exercise, alcohol, glucose, and sodium bicarbonate infusions.
Albumin	3.5–4.8 g/dL (35–48 g/L)	• Decreased serum albumin level causes reduced colloidal osmotic pull in intravascular space, allowing fluid to shift to the interstitial space and produce edema. • It is important to know the albumin level when evaluating total calcium values.

(From Metheny, N. M. [1992]. *Fluid and electrolyte balance* [2nd ed., pp. 30–33]. Philadelphia: J. B. Lippincott.)

performed on patients with acute abdominal pain or on surgical patients in whom questionable injury may have occurred to the pancreas. Amylase levels usually remain elevated for only a short time—3 to 6 days.

Blood Collection

Venous blood (6 mL) is allowed to clot in a dry tube.

Normal serum range is 4 to 25 U/mL. The range may depend on the normal values established by clinical laboratories because the method may be modified.

Lipase

Lipase determination is used for detecting damage to the pancreas and is valuable when too much time has elapsed for the amylase level to remain elevated. When secretions of the pancreas are blocked, the serum lipase level rises.

Blood Collection

The test is performed on serum from 6 mL clotted blood. *Normal serum range* is 2 U/mL or less.

Phosphatase, Acid

Acid phosphatase is useful in determining metastasizing tumors of the prostate. The prostate gland and carcinoma of the gland are rich in phosphatase but do not normally release the enzyme into the serum. Once the carcinoma has spread, it starts to release acid phosphatase, increasing the serum concentration.[2] In addition to carcinoma of the prostate, other conditions that produce increased serum acid phosphatase levels are Paget's disease, hyperparathyroidism, metastatic mammary carcinoma, renal insufficiency, multiple myeloma, some liver disease, arterial embolism, myocardial infarction, and sickle cell crisis.[2]

Blood Collection
Blood (5 mL) is allowed to clot in a dry tube. Hemolysis should be avoided. Analysis should be done immediately, or the serum should be frozen.
   Normal serum range. (1) Male: Total, 0.13 to 0.63 Sigma U/mL. (2) Female: Total, 0.01 to 0.56 Sigma U/mL. (3) Prostatic: 0 to 0.5 Fishman-Lerner U/100 mL.[1]

Phosphatase, Alkaline

Alkaline phosphatase is a useful test in diagnosing bone diseases and obstructive jaundice. In bone diseases, the small amount of alkaline usually present in the serum rises in proportion to the new bone cells. When excretion of alkaline phosphatase is impaired, as in some disorders of the liver and biliary tract, the serum level rises and may give some evidence of the degree of blockage in the biliary tract.[2]

Blood Collection
Blood (5 mL) is drawn and the test is performed on the serum. Sodium sulfobromophthalein dye should be avoided.
   Normal serum range is 13 to 39 U/mL.[1]

TRANSAMINASE

The transaminases are enzymes found in large quantities in the heart, liver, muscle, kidney, and pancreas cells. Any disease that causes damage to these cells will result in an elevated serum transaminase level; clinical signs and other tests are used in diagnosis.

Aspartate Aminotransferase (AST)

(Also known as SGOT [serum glutamic-oxaloacetic transaminase].)
   The AST level is used to distinguish between myocardial infarction and acute coronary insufficiency without infarction. It is also useful as a liver function test in following the progression of liver damage or in ascertaining when the liver has recovered.

Blood Collection
The test is performed on serum from 5 mL clotted blood.
   Normal serum range is 10 to 40 U/mL. In myocardial infarction, the level is increased four to ten times, whereas in liver involvement a high of ten to 100 times normal may occur. The serum level remains elevated for about 5 days.

Alanine Aminotransferase (ALT)

(Also known as SGPT [serum glutamic-pyruvic transaminase].)
   Alanine aminotransferase is another transaminase that is more specific for hepatic malfunction than AST.

Blood Collection
The test is performed on serum from 5 mL blood. *Normal serum range* is 6 to 36 Karmen U/mL.[2]

Serum Lactate Dehydrogenase (LDH)

The transaminase LDH is present in all tissues and in large quantities in the kidney, heart, and skeletal muscles. Elevated serum levels usually parallel the AST levels. Elevation occurs in myocardial infarction and may continue through the sixth day. Elevations have been found in lymphoma, disseminated carcinoma, and some cases of leukemia.

Blood Collection
Blood (3 mL) is collected and allowed to coagulate. Care must be taken to avoid hemolysis because only a slight degree may give an incorrect reading.
    Normal serum range is 60 to 120 U/mL.[1]

LIVER FUNCTION TESTS

Albumin, Globulin, Total Protein, and A/G Ratio

These tests may be useful in diagnosing kidney and liver disease or in judging the effectiveness of treatment. The chief role of serum albumin is to maintain osmotic pressure of the blood; globulin assists. The globulin molecule, being larger than the albumin, is less efficient in maintaining osmotic pressure and does not leak out of the blood. With the loss of albumin through the capillary wall, the body compensates by producing more globulin. The osmotic pressure is reduced and may result in some edema. Certain conditions, such as chronic nephritis, lipoid nephrosis, liver disease, and malnutrition result in a lowered albumin concentration.[2]

Blood Collection
The test is performed on serum from 6 mL clotted blood.
    Normal serum range. (1) Total protein, 6.0 to 8.0 g/100 mL. (2) Albumin, 3.2 to 5.6 g/100 mL. (3) Globulin, 1.3 to 3.5 g/100 mL.

Bilirubin (Direct and Indirect)

The bilirubin test, which is becoming less common, differentiates between impairment of the liver by obstruction and hemolysis. Bilirubin arises from the hemoglobin liberated from broken-down red blood cells. It is the chief pigment of the bile, excreted by the liver. If the excretory power of the liver is impaired by obstruction, there is an excess of circulatory bilirubin and it is free of any attached protein. Measurement of free bilirubin (direct) usually indicates obstruction.

When increased red blood cell destruction (hemolysis) occurs, the increased bilirubin is believed to be bound to protein (indirect).

A *total bilirubin* determination detects increased concentration of bilirubin before jaundice is seen.

Blood Collection
The test is performed on serum from 5 mL clotted blood.
    Normal serum range is 0.1 to 1.0 mg/100 mL.[2]

Cephalin Flocculation

This test is being replaced in many hospitals by more specific tests. In diagnosing liver damage, it frequently detects damage before jaundice becomes evident. It is also useful in following the course of liver disease such as cirrhosis. The serum of patients with damaged liver cells flocculates a colloidal suspension of cephalin and cholesterol, whereas the serum of normal patients does not clump the suspension. Abscesses and neoplasms do not damage liver cells and therefore give negative results.[2]

Blood Collection
The test is performed on serum from 5 mL clotted blood.
Normal serum range is either negative or 1 +. Reports are delayed 24 to 48 hours.

Cholesterol

Cholesterol, a normal constituent of the blood, is present in all body cells. In various disease states the cholesterol concentration in the serum may be raised or lowered. Cholesterol is transported in the blood by the LDLs (low-density lipoproteins) (60%–75%) and HDLs (high-density lipoproteins) (15%–35%).

Blood Collection
The test is performed on serum from 5 mL clotted blood.
Normal serum range is 120 to 260 mg/100 mL.

Prothrombin Time

The prothrombin time, considered one of the most important screening tests in coagulation studies, indirectly measures the ability of the blood to clot. During the clotting process, prothrombin is converted to thrombin. It is thought that when the prothrombin level is reduced to below normal, the tendency for the blood to clot in the blood vessel is reduced. It is an important guide in controlling drug therapy and is commonly used when anticoagulants are prescribed. The prothrombin content is reduced in liver diseases.

Blood Collection
Venous blood (4 mL) is collected, added to the coagulant, and quickly mixed. It is important to avoid clot formation and hemolysis. The blood should be examined as soon as possible.
The *normal value* is between 11 and 18 seconds, depending on the type of thromboplastin used.

High-density Lipoprotein (HDL)
A high level of HDL is indicative of a healthy metabolic system in a patient free of liver disease.

Very-low-density Lipoproteins (VLDL) and Low-density Lipoproteins (LDL)
VLDL is a major carrier of triglyceride. Degradation of VLDL leads to a major source of LDL.

Thymol Turbidity

Thymol turbidity detects damaged liver cells and differentiates between liver disease and biliary obstruction. Turbidity is usually increased when the serum of patients with liver damage is mixed with a saturated solution of thymol. Turbidity is usually normal in biliary obstruction without liver damage.

Blood Collection
The test is performed on serum from 5 mL clotted blood. *Normal serum range* is 0 to 4 U.[1]

KIDNEY FUNCTION TESTS

Creatinine

The creatinine test measures kidney function. Creatinine, the result of a breakdown of muscle creatine phosphate, is produced daily in a constant amount in each individual. A disorder of kidney function prevents excretion and an elevated creatinine value gives a reliable indication of impaired kidney function. A normal serum creatinine value does not indicate unimpaired renal function, however.

Blood Collection
The test is performed on serum from 6 mL clotted blood.
    Normal serum range is 0.6 to 1.3 mg/100 mL.

Blood Urea Nitrogen (BUN)

The BUN is a measure of kidney function. Urea, the end product of protein metabolism, is excreted by the kidneys. Impairment in kidney function results in an elevated concentration of urea nitrogen in the blood. Rapid protein metabolism may also increase the urea nitrogen above normal limits. The *non-protein nitrogen* is a similar test for measuring kidney function.

Blood Collection
The test is performed on blood or serum. Blood (5 mL) is added to an oxalate tube and shaken or placed in a dry tube to clot.
    Normal range is 8 to 25 mg/100 mL.

BLOOD SUGAR TESTS

The test for blood sugar is used to detect a disorder of glucose metabolism, which may be the result of any one of several factors, including (1) inability of pancreas islet cells to produce insulin, (2) inability of intestines to absorb glucose, and (3) inability of liver to accumulate and break down glycogen.

An elevated blood sugar level may indicate diabetes, chronic liver disease, or overactivity of the endocrine glands. A decrease in blood sugar may result from an overdose of insulin, tumors of the pancreas, or insufficiency of various endocrine glands.

Fasting Blood Sugar

A fasting blood sugar test requires that the patient fast for 8 hours.

Blood Collection
Venous blood (3–5 mL) is collected in an oxalate tube and shaken to prevent microscopic clots.

Normal serum range is 70 to 100 mg/100 mL (true blood sugar method). The normal value depends on the method of determination. Values greater than 120 mg/100 mL on several occasions may indicate diabetes mellitus.

Postprandial Blood Sugar Determinations

The postprandial sugar test is helpful in diagnosing diabetes mellitus. Blood is drawn 2 hours after the patient has begun to eat. If the blood sugar value is above the upper limits of normal for fasting, a glucose tolerance test is performed.

Glucose Tolerance

The glucose tolerance test is indicated

1. When the patient shows glycosuria
2. When fasting or 2-hour blood sugar concentration is only slightly elevated
3. When Cushing's syndrome or acromegaly is a questionable diagnosis
4. To establish cause of hypoglycemia

Blood Collection
A fasting blood sugar sample is drawn. The patient drinks 100 g glucose in lemon-flavored water (some laboratories use 1.75 g glucose/kg ideal body weight). Blood and urine samples are collected at 30, 60, 90, 120, and 180 minutes after ingestion of glucose.

Normal (true blood sugar) values are: (1) Fasting blood sugar below 100 mg/100 mL. (2) Peak below 160 mg/100 mL in 30 or 60 minutes. (3) Two-hour value returning to fasting level. The values depend on the standards used.

BLOOD TYPING

Blood typing is one of the most common tests performed on blood, being required by all donors and by all patients who may need blood. The ABO system denotes four main groups: O, A, B, and AB. The designations refer to the particular antigen present on the red cells: group A contains red cells with the A antigen, B with B antigen, AB with A and B antigens, and O red cells contain neither A nor B antigens.

When red cells containing antigens are placed with serum containing corresponding antibodies under favorable conditions, agglutination (clumping) occurs. Therefore, an antigen is known as an agglutinogen and an antibody as an agglutinin.

An individual's serum contains antibodies that will react to corresponding antigens not usually found on the individual's own cells. For instance, serum of group O contains antibodies A and B, which will react with the corresponding antigens A and B found on the red cells of group AB.

Although agglutination occurs in antigen–antibody reaction in the laboratory, hemolysis occurs in vivo; antibody attacks red cells, causing rupture with liberation of hemoglobin. Hemolysis results from infusing incompatible blood and may lead to fatal consequences.

Rh Factor

The antigens belonging to the Rh system are D, C, E, c, and e; they are found in conjunction with the ABO group. The strongest of these factors is the $Rh_o(D)$ factor, found in about 85% of the white population. Therefore the $Rh_o(D)$ factor is often the only factor identified in Rh typing. When not present, further typing may be done to identify any of the less common Rh factors.

Blood Collection

Venous blood is collected and allowed to clot. Usually one tube (10 mL) will set up 4 to 5 U blood. Positive patient identification must be made before the blood is drawn; the name and number on the identification bracelet must correspond to that on the requisition and label. Identity should never be made by addressing the patient by name and awaiting the response. The label is placed on the blood tube at the patient's bedside.

Blood Grouping

Various methods are used in typing blood, but all involve the same general principle: The patient's cells are mixed in standard saline serum samples of anti-A and of anti-B. The type of serum, A or B, which agglutinates the patient's cells indicates the blood group. As a double check, the patient's serum is mixed with saline suspensions of A and of B red cells. The ABO group is determined on the basis of agglutination or absence of agglutination of A and of B cells.

Coombs' Test

Not all antibodies cause agglutination in saline; some merely coat the red blood cells by combining with the antigen, which is not a visible reaction. The Coombs' test is performed to detect antibodies that cannot cause agglutination in saline; these are known as *incomplete antibodies*. Antihuman globulin serum is used. This serum is obtained by the immunization of various animals, usually rabbits, against human gamma globulin by the injection of human serum, plasma, or isolated globulin. This antiserum, when added to sensitized red blood cells (erythrocytes coated with incomplete antibody), causes visible agglutination.

The Coombs' test is performed in two ways. The *direct Coombs' test* is performed when the patient's red blood cells have become coated in vivo. This test is a valuable procedure in

1. Diagnosis of erythroblastosis fetalis. The erythrocytes of the baby are tested for sensitization.
2. Acquired hemolytic anemia. The patient may have produced an antibody that coats his or her own cells.
3. Investigation of reactions. The patient may have received incompatible blood that has sensitized his red blood cells.

The *indirect Coombs' test* detects incomplete antibodies in the serum of patients sensitized to blood antigens. It involves use of the patient's serum, in contrast to the use of the patient's red blood cells in the direct Coombs' test. When pooled, normal erythrocytes containing the most important antigens are exposed in a test tube to the patient's serum and to Coombs' serum, agglutination of the red blood cells occurs and indicates the incomplete antibody present. This test is valuable in

1. Detecting incompatibilities not found by other methods
2. Detecting weak or variant antigens
3. Typing with certain antiserums, such as anti-Duffy or anti-Kidd, which require Coombs' serum to produce agglutination
4. Detecting antiagglutinins produced by exposure during pregnancy

REFERENCES

1. Castleman, B., & McNeeley, B. (January 2, 1986). Case records of the Massachusetts General Hospital: Normal laboratory values. *New England Journal of Medicine, 314*, 39–49.
2. Garb, S. (1976). *Laboratory tests in common use* (6th ed., pp. 23–123). New York: Springer.
3. Grove-Rasmussen, M., Lesses, M. F., & Anstall, H. B. (1961). Transfusion therapy. *New England Journal of Medicine, 264*, 1089.
4. Fischbach, F. (1992). *A manual of laboratory and diagnostic tests* (4th ed., pp. 370, 371). Philadelphia: J. B. Lippincott.

REVIEW QUESTIONS

1. Serum consists of:
   a. plasma minus fibrinogen
   b. plasma plus fibrinogen
   c. plasma minus fibrin
   d. plasma plus fibrin

2. Glycolysis refers to production of glycolytic enzymes causing which of the following?
   a. rise in pH on standing
   b. drop in pH on standing
   c. rise in blood pressure
   d. orthostatic hypotension

3. Hemolysis refers to:
   a. lysis of cells
   b. lysis of enzymes
   c. clysis of cells
   d. clysis of enzymes

4. Pressure should be applied to a puncture site:
   a. for 1 minute
   b. for 3 minutes
   c. until bleeding stops
   d. until bleeding slows

5. The most important factor in drawing blood for blood grouping and typing is:
   a. preservation of specimen
   b. method used
   c. positive identification
   d. use of OSHA standards

6. BUN is a measure of what function?
   a. liver
   b. kidney
   c. cardiac
   d. lung

7. Which of the following is closely related to body water status?
   a. potassium
   b. calcium
   c. magnesium
   d. sodium

8. Amylase determination is useful in diagnosis of which of the following diseases?
   a. acute gastritis
   b. acute pancreatitis
   c. metastasizing tumors of prostate
   d. primary alkalosis

9. Acid–base balance is maintained by what system?
    a. buffer
    b. neutral
    c. pulmonary
    d. cardiac

10. Red blood cells are rich in:
    a. calcium
    b. magnesium
    c. phosphorus
    d. sodium

PART III

Principles of Equipment Selection and Application

CHAPTER 12

Intravenous Equipment

Rapidly changing technology has kept pace with the advances in medical science and has provided many improved, sophisticated devices for the administration of IV therapy. Specialized equipment is available to meet the patient's every need: positive-pressure pumps for IV and intra-arterial therapy; controllers and monitors for regulating and monitoring the rate of infusion; ambulatory infusion devices; and air-venting microbe-retentive filters, catheters, and administration sets. A nurse's knowledge of the selection and use of these devices is vital for the patient's comfort and safety.

FLUID CONTAINERS

Sterile evacuated glass containers with premixed fluids first became available in 1929. Later, plastic containers became available for the storage and delivery of blood products. Baxter was the first to develop the plastic bag for parenteral fluids.

The plastic container is easily transported with minimal risk of damage and is easily disposed of. Because it contains no rubber bushings, coring is eliminated and particulate matter is reduced. Air venting is not required; thus, the risk of air embolism and airborne contamination is reduced.

Plastic bags are susceptible to accidental puncture, which creates a port of entry for microorganisms. Because punctures may not be evident, the container should be squeezed before use and visually checked for leakage. Today, plastic containers are used for most infusions unless contraindicated because of the type of drug additive.

DELIVERY SYSTEMS

Three types of infusion systems have been used: (1) the plastic bag and plastic bottle, (2) the closed system, and (3) the open system. The plastic bag and plastic bottle contain no vacuum, and because the containers are flexible and collapsible, they need no air to replace fluid flowing from the containers. All other systems use glass bottles with a partial vacuum requiring air vents. The closed system admits only filtered air to the container; the air vent, containing the filter, is an integral part of the administration set. The open system allows air to enter through a plastic tube in the container and collect in the air space in the bottle.

Methods for adding medications to the fluid containers vary with each system. The plastic bag contains a resealable latex medication port through which the medication is

Sharon M. Weinstein: PLUMER'S PRINCIPLES & PRACTICE OF INTRAVENOUS THERAPY, FIFTH EDITION, © 1993 J. B. Lippincott Company

injected. Because the plastic bag lacks a vacuum, medications must be added with a syringe and needle or additive needle. A unit for creating a vacuum in the container is available to the pharmacist and provides speed and ease to the admixture program. When medications are added to the plastic containers during the infusion, special precautions must be taken to make certain that the clamp on the administration set is completely closed and the flow interrupted before the medication is added. This prevents an un-diluted, toxic dose of medication from entering the administration set and being infused. Medications and solutions should always be mixed thoroughly before administration, regardless of the system used.

In the closed system, medication may be added to the solution bottle during the infusion by using the air vent located in the administration set as a medication port. The 5-μm filter is removed and the syringe is attached. Meticulous care must be observed to maintain sterility of the filter when removing the filter, adding the medication, and replacing the filter. The fluid bottle contains a solid rubber stopper through which medications may be added before infusion.

In the open system, bottles have a removable metal disk under which a sterile latex disk provides a closed method for aseptically adding a medication and for a visible check for vacuum. The vacuum is noted by the depression in the seal and must be present to ensure sterility. Before the latex disk is removed, the medication is added through the outlet port with a syringe and needle; the vacuum draws the medication into the bottle. During infusion, the medication may be added through the designated area on the rubber bushing after the clamp on the administration set has been closed. The medication and solution must be mixed thoroughly by agitating the fluid before administration.

PRESSURE AND INFUSION THERAPY

Pressure is the principle of physics underlying fluid therapy. Pressure enables us to overcome the natural resistance to flow created by the administration set, in-line filters, narrow-gauge needles, and venous or arterial backpressure. The human body adapts to changes in pressure, which enables clinicians to deliver IV therapy safely.

Pressure in the arterial system ranges from 80 mm Hg in the aorta to a low of 5 to 10 mm Hg in the venous return system. Intravenous pressure is created by the weight of a column of fluid in the tubing—the weight is due to gravity—and we know it as *hydrostatic pressure*. Fluid always flows from an area of higher pressure to one of lower pressure. To infuse by gravity, it is necessary to create a pressure only slightly more than normal or 40 mm Hg in a peripheral line.

A number of resistance factors may interfere with or inhibit fluid flow. These factors include the patient's own vascular pressure, internal diameter of the tubing, in-line filters, viscosity of fluid, narrow-gauge needles, and the length of the tubing. Resistance to flow is determined by the smallest component in the IV system; this is usually the cannula.

Electronic infusion devices (EIDs) have incorporated the concept of pressure to deliver precise amounts of drug and solution. Most recently, differential pressure has been a component of such devices. With a range of two or three levels, such equipment may sense a change in pressure, usually 5 psi over baseline, and some devices monitor and read out line pressure. *Operating* or *line pressure* is the pressure generated by a pump to cause fluid to flow at a predetermined rate. *Maximum occlusion pressure* is the limit to operating pressure at which an occlusion alarm is triggered. *Needle pressure* is the same as venous pressure, and, during an infusion, pressure at the tip of the cannula is only slightly more than the pressure within that vein or artery regardless of the output pressure of the pump. The pressure at the needle tip needs to be slightly higher than vascular pressure for fluid to flow. An understanding of pressure and psi is essential to safely use EIDs, filters, and other components of the IV system.

ADMINISTRATION SETS

An important factor in the administration set is the rate of flow that the given set is gauged to produce. Commercial sets vary—they may deliver from 10 to 15 drops/mL, depending on the nature of the fluid. Increased viscosity causes the size of the drop to increase, so that a set that delivers 15 drops/mL may deliver 10 drops/mL when blood is administered. This information is of vital concern to the accurate control of the rate of infusion.

Most conventional sets use the roller clamp or slide clamp for controlling the flow rate (Figure 12-1). Changes in the drop rate invariably occur after the rate is regulated and require time-consuming readjustments of the clamp to establish and maintain flow rates. Alternatives to the roller clamp that save nursing time and that are valuable in maintaining the rate of parenteral solutions are also available.

Another method uses a flow-metering system that eliminates drifting flow rates. The metering device consists of "an adjustable dam" controlled by a knob. Because it is connected on the entry and exit ports, the IV tubing is isolated from the metering device and does not affect changes in the flow rate. The rate can be set and it will stay until the infusion is complete, eliminating "free flow" runaway IVs and helping prevent IV flow–rate variations. Refinements in infusion technology continue to provide alternative means by which rate of flow is regulated.

SPECIAL-USE SETS

Nonpolyvinylchloride IV administration sets are available for gravity infusion and for volumetric pumps. Nitroglycerin, fat emulsions, and other drugs can be administered without altering the dosage of the drug through absorption into the walls of the poly-vinylchloride (PVC) tubing.

It is frequently necessary to maintain the flow at a minimal rate. One method is to reduce the size of the drop by using special sets, originally designed for pediatric infusions. These sets are valuable in parenteral therapy for adults as well because, by reducing the size of the drop, a constant IV flow may be maintained with a minimal amount of fluid. These sets deliver 60 drops/mL; at the rate of 60 drops/min, it would take 1 hour to infuse 60 mL. A variety of commercial sets are available for alternate or simultaneous infusion of two solutions. Some sets contain a filter (Figure 12-2A).

A significant hazard of air embolism may occur when the Y-type administration set is used ignorantly or carelessly with vented containers. Constant vigilance is necessary if both solutions are administered simultaneously. If one container is allowed to empty, large quantities of air can be sucked into the tubing; the empty bottle becomes the vent because of the greater atmospheric pressure in the empty bottle and tube over the pressure below the partially constricted clamp in the tubing of the flowing solution.[7]

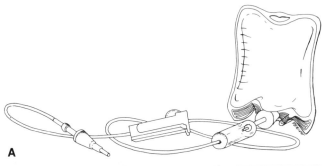

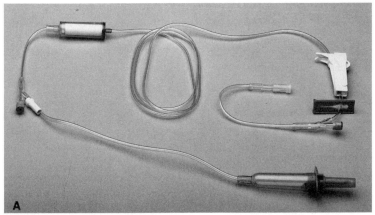

FIGURE 12-1 (A) Standard administration set with in-line filter. (B) Primary venoset, macrodrop. (Courtesy: Abbott Laboratories, North Chicago, IL)

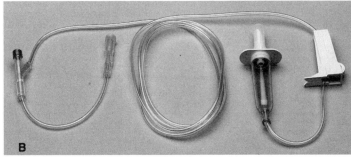

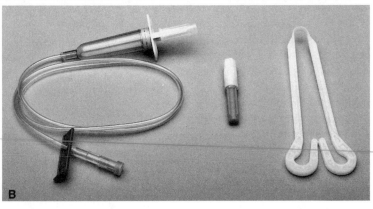

FIGURE 12-2 (A) Primary venoset with IVEX-2 integral filter. (B) Secondary venoset with hook and needle for piggybacking. (Courtesy: Abbott Laboratories, North Chicago, IL)

Positive-pressure sets are designed to increase the rapidity of infusions and are an asset when rapid replacement of fluid becomes necessary. They permit fluid to be administered by gravity, with a built-in pressure chamber available for rapid administration of blood should an emergency arise. When used with the collapsible plastic blood unit, this system avoids the danger of air embolism; because the bag collapses, the need for air is eliminated. In contrast to the collapsible bag, the glass container must be vented to allow the fluid to flow; air pressure must be used when blood or fluid is forced into the bloodstream. As the last portion of blood from the container is forced into the bloodstream, the air under pressure may rapidly enter the vein before the clamp can be applied, resulting in a fatal embolus. According to Adriani, "Air pressure should not be used to force blood and other fluids into the blood stream."[1]

The pump chamber must be filled at all times. The nurse should never apply positive pressure to infuse fluids.

CHECK-VALVE SETS

Sets are available with an in-line check valve, which provides a more convenient and safer method for administering medications and fluids. A secondary infusion or a single dose of medication can be administered "piggyback" into the injection site located below the check valve. The valve automatically shuts off the main-line infusion while the admixture is running and automatically allows the main infusion to start when the medication has run in. This valve prevents mixing of the two fluids, eliminates the risk of air entering the line when the secondary bottle empties, and prevents the cannula from becoming occluded by an interruption in the infusion. Because the rate of flow must be regulated by one clamp, the rate of administration remains the same for both fluids (Figure 12-2A,B).

VOLUME-CONTROLLED SETS

With the increasing use and number of solutions containing drugs and electrolytes, greater accuracy in controlling the volume of IV fluids is necessary. Several available devices permit accurate administration of measured volumes of fluids (Figure 12-3).

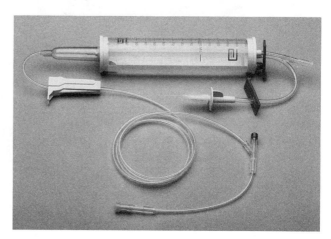

FIGURE 12-3 Volume-controlled infusion set. (Courtesy: Abbott Laboratories, North Chicago, IL)

Sets contain vented, calibrated burette chambers that control the volume from 100 to 150 mL. The burette chamber of some sets contains a rubber float that prevents air from entering the tubing once the infusion is completed.

Some calibrated burette chambers contain a microporous filter to block the passage of air when the chamber empties. Refilling these chambers requires a specific procedure. The word OSCAR will help recall the procedure: O—Open clamp; S—Squeeze drip chamber and hold; C—Close clamp close to drip chamber; A—And; R—Release drip chamber.

PUMP-SPECIFIC SETS

Some sets are made specifically for use with EIDs. These sets also come in a number of configurations. Such sets and their respective electronic delivery systems ensure safe delivery of infusion therapy to patients of all ages in a variety of clinical settings (Figure 12-4).

FINAL INTRAVENOUS FILTERS

Filters prevent passage of undesirable substances into the vascular system (Figure 12-5). Particulate filters of 1 or 5 μm are recommended when IV medications are being prepared. A bacteria-retentive filter, 0.2 μm in range, is recommended for the routine delivery of IV therapies. The time of change should coincide with the changing of the administration set.

Filters today come in diverse configurations, including add-on and integral units. Add-on filters should be securely connected to the administration set and treated as a part

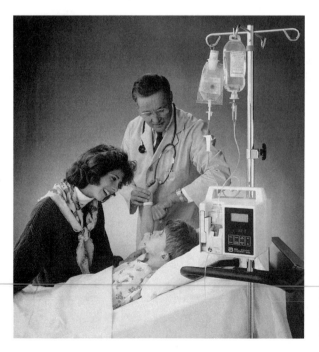

FIGURE 12-4 Infusion therapy delivered via electronic infusion devices (EIDs) enhances the quality of IV care. (Courtesy: Abbott Laboratories, North Chicago, IL)

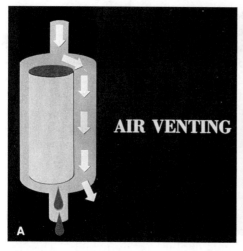

AIR VENTING

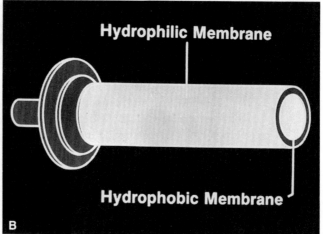

Hydrophilic Membrane

Hydrophobic Membrane

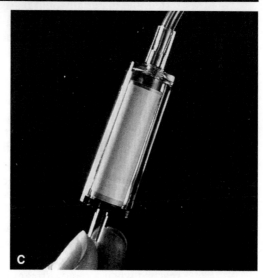

FIGURE 12-5 **(A)** Air-eliminating properties of an IV filter. **(B)** Hydrophilic/hydrophobic membrane properties of an IV filter. **(C)** Optimal IV filter for add-on or in-line use. (Courtesy: Abbott Laboratories, North Chicago, IL)

of that set. Integral filters are attached by the manufacturer to the administration set. To achieve final filtration, the filter should be located as close to the cannula site as possible. A 0.2-μm filter is considered an absolute, bacteria-retentive, air-eliminating filter and decreases the complications of infection and the potential for air embolism.

The industry standard is a membrane filter. Membrane filters are screen-type filters with uniformly sized pores that provide an absolute rating. A 0.2-μm screen-type filter will retain on the flat surface membrane all particles greater than 0.2 μm in size.

The Unites States Pharmacopeia (USP) has established an acceptable limit of particles for single-dose infusion as not more than 50 particles/mL that are equal to or larger than 10.0 μm and not more than 5 particles/mL that are equal to or larger than 25.0 μm in effective linear dimension.

Pressure and Air

All filters have a certain pressure value at which they will allow the passage of air from one side of a wetted hydrophilic membrane to the other. This pressure valve is called the *bubble point* of that particular membrane. Because different filter materials (*eg*, hydrophobic, hydrophilic, depth, screen) have different wetting or nonwetting characteristics, both the pressure value of the material and the test liquid must be specified when bubble points are discussed. Water or saline solution, for example, would be the test fluid of choice when testing hydrophilic membranes for IV filters because solutions given IV are primarily water. Water is inexpensive, can be filtered easily for control of particulates and microorganisms, and is readily available. There are other advantages to using water as a bubble point test fluid. Water will test the wetting characteristics of hydrophilic membrane filters. To further define this point, an explanation of bubble point tests in relation to membranes is required.

Bubble Point Tests
Bubble point tests are conducted in a specific way. The material being tested is first wetted in the solution designated for performing the test. For example, if a flat membrane is being tested, the material would be soaked in the liquid until it has "wetted out." Then the material would be sealed into a holder that has a reservoir constructed over the membrane. More liquid would be poured on top of the membrane. Air pressures would then be applied to the other side of the membrane from below. As the air pressure increased, eventually a *steady* stream of bubbles would be seen rising through the liquid on top of the membrane. The pressure at which this happens is the bubble point of the material. This is called an *open bubble point* because the bubbles can be seen in real time or the time at which the bubble point actually happened.

Testing involves encapsulation of the membrane within an integral housing. Two different types of bubble point tests may be performed: open bubble and closed bubble point. An open bubble point can only be performed if the direction of normal flow is such that the bubbles produced can be seen as they are formed. This means that the housing of the filter must be transparent and the "downstream side" of the membrane can be observed. This test is performed by first flowing the test liquid through the device at low pressures until it is wetted out. Usually, this pressure is the same as that used in administering solution by gravity feed pressures (36 to 39 inches of water). Then, after the membrane is wetted out, air pressure is applied as before. The bubble point has been reached when a steady stream of bubbles is seen on the downstream side of the membrane.

A *closed bubble point* must be performed when the downstream side of the membrane may not be visualized. The general manipulations of the test are the same, but because the bubbles are not visible as they occur, the distal (outlet) port of the device must be observed. When a steady stream of bubbles exits the distal port, this is the closed bubble point. Closed bubble points will result in slightly higher values than open bubble points because the air pressure during the test is steadily increasing, and it will take more time for the air bubbles to escape through the distal port. If the pressure is increased slowly, the test will be more accurate.

Testing of membranes and filter devices used in IV therapy with water is significant. Most hydrophilic membranes incorporate either external (applied after they are made) or internal (in the base formula) wetting agents to render them more wettable with water. It is particularly important in IV therapy because it is critical that the membrane should wet properly so that air will not pass the membrane at low pressures.

The 0.2-μm air-venting filters automatically vent air through a nonwettable (hydrophobic) membrane and permit uniform high gravity flow rates via large wettable (hydrophilic) membranes. They prevent an air block, which could ultimately result in a plugged cannula.

Filters are also rated according to the psi of pressure they will withstand, an important consideration in selecting the proper filter. The filter should withstand the psi exerted by the infusion pump or rupture may occur. If the psi rating of the housing is less than that of the membrane, excess force will break the housing, leaving the filter intact.

Optimal filters should (1) automatically vent air; (2) retain bacteria, fungi, and endotoxins; (3) be nonbinding of drugs; (4) allow high gravity flow rates; and (5) have a pressure tolerance to withstand the psi of the infusion pump. Pressure rating of the housing, when less than that of the filter membrane, may provide added protection.

BLOOD/FLUID WARMERS

Prewarmed blood may be indicated when conditions (such as massive hemorrhage) warrant large and rapid transfusions; cold blood administered under such conditions may produce effects of cardiac and general hypothermia. Boyan cited results of observations made in the operating rooms of Memorial (Sloan-Kettering Cancer Center) Hospital, New York, which showed that the incidence of cardiac arrest during massive blood replacement (3000 mL or more per hour) dropped from 58.3% to 6.8% when cold bank blood was warmed to body temperature during infusion. He stated, "To avoid the effects of cardiac and general hypothermia during massive hemorrhage, cold bank blood should be warmed to body temperature when administered rapidly and in large amounts."[2] Warm blood is usually required in exchange transfusions of newborns and in transfusions of patients with potent cold agglutinins.

Several manufacturing companies have devised units consisting of blood-warming coils that are placed in warm water baths. In one unit, the blood is warmed at an approximate rate of 150 mL/min in the adult coil and at approximately 50 mL/min in the pediatric coil. Some units contain a water bath automatically controlled to maintain a desired temperature of between 39°C and 40°C, warming the blood to about 35°C.

An alternative to the water bath is the dry heat blood warmer. This device contains two warming plates, which hold and warm the disposable plastic warming bag containing integral tubing and a connector on the inlet side for connection to a recipient set. The blood is warmed as it flows from the transfusion administration set through the tubing in the warming bag and through integral tubing to the recipient. It contains a digital temperature display and an audible temperature alarm and shut-off.

Another blood/fluid warmer is a portable solid-state unit. It is particularly useful in emergency rooms, operating rooms, and ambulances because it can be attached to a standard IV pole and does not interfere with nursing care. The warmer uses standard blood tubing, and because there are no connectors and sterilization is not required, potential contamination of the blood is eliminated. The safety features include an independent audio alarm, an automatic power cutoff to the heater, and monitoring lights.

Warming devices must undergo careful and continuing quality control procedures. In many hospitals, this is carried out by the biomedical engineering department.

BLOOD FILTERS

Administration sets with the standard clot filter of 170 μm are available for infusion of blood and blood components. The supplementary filter can be added to an in-use administration set, permitting infusion of blood; easy replacement of the filter, should clogging occur, allows multiple infusions of blood. Several manufacturers design blood filters with a pore size of 40 μm or less to trap microaggregates and protect the lung from this particulate matter. Evidence indicates that cellular degradation develops with storage of banked blood. This debris has been implicated as a cause of respiratory insufficiency when large quantities of stored bank blood are infused. The small-pored filter is recommended when several units of stored bank blood are to be infused.

GRAVITY FLOW

Gravity flow depends on head pressure; roller clamps and screw clamps used to adjust and to maintain rates of flow on gravity infusions vary considerably in their efficiency and accuracy.

Rate minders or flow-control mechanisms may also be used to regulate and adjust flow. The rate minder is added to the IV administration set. The desired flow rate may be preset. Levels of accuracy vary with the type of device used. Factors such as venous spasm, venous pressure changes, patient movement, manipulations of the clamp, and bent or kinked tubing may cause variations in the flow rate.

Either preprinted or self-made time tapes may be used on the IV container to determine consistency with prescribed rate of flow. Attach the time tape to the container and mark hourly increments on the tape or strip, beginning with the time the infusion was hung. Various time tape and preprinted labels are available to assist with this process (Figure 12-6).

ELECTRONIC INFUSION DEVICES

The EIDs are invaluable in neonatal, pediatric, and adult intensive care units, where critical infusions of small volumes of fluid or doses of high-potency drugs are required. These devices have increased the level of safety in parenteral therapy. Today, the risk of air embolism is reduced by alarm systems and by the automatic interruption of the infusion when a container empties. A controlled rate of flow reduces the risk of circulatory overload.

The devices have saved valuable nursing time; uniform control of fluid eliminates the need to count drops and continually adjust flow rates. Plugging of the cannula, which occurs when blood backs into the cannula because of an increase in venous pressure from coughing, crying, or strains, is eliminated. The pressure generated by the EID pump may exceed the maximum venous pressure.

The EIDs are finding increasing uses in keep-open arterial lines and infusion of drugs, blood, and viscous fluids such as hyperalimentation solutions.

Advances in technology have provided us with more sophisticated devices. Many types and models are available. In general, pumps are devices that generate flow under positive pressure. Such devices may be peristaltic, syringe, and pulsatile. Controllers are devices that generate flow by gravity and are capable of either drop counting or vol-

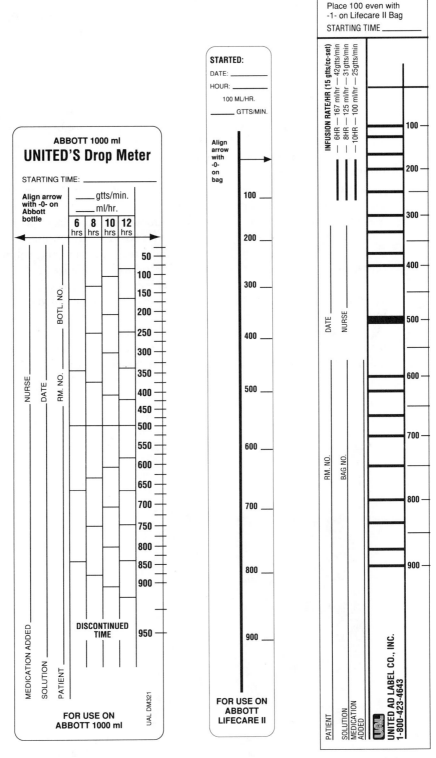

FIGURE 12-6 Time tapes. (Courtesy: United Ad Label Co., Inc., Brea, CA)

umetric delivery.[4] Abbott's LifeCare® 75 BREEZE is a controller that uses a standard administration set, is easily set up, and incorporates graphics on a screen (Figure 12-7).

Pressure exerted by the unit is expressed in psi or mm Hg. One psi and 50 mm Hg exert the same amount of pressure.[4] As already addressed, the psi of an EID is important because it may affect the type of filter being used or the ability of the unit to infuse fluids through arterial lines. The psi should not exceed the pressure the filter can withstand or a rupture may occur; when the pump is used for arterial infusion, the psi must be high enough to overcome arterial pressure. Used in monoplace hyperbaric medicine centers, Abbott's LifeCare® Model 3HB, HYPERBARIC PUMP (Figure 12-8) is the only device of its kind that is capable of pumping up to 2 to 3 atm. Before the development of such a product, infusion therapy during hyperbaric treatments was uncomfortable and caused great pressure along venous walls. The field of external electronic infusion devices includes those that are IV pole dependent yet meet a wealth of needs in the clinical setting. Volumetric pumps such as Sigma International's Sigma 6000 + programmable infusion pump meets a variety of clinical needs and is cost-effective, utilizing standard IV tubing (Figure 12-9). The Gemini PC-1, manufactured with flow and volume ramping capability, and the Gemini PC-2 are in Imed's product line (Figure 12-10). PC-1 and PC-2 do not allow free flow on infusion set removal but still allow users the option of gravity flow. Gemini PC-2 is a multichannel device, capable of simultaneously infusing from and individually monitoring two or more IV lines.

McGaw's 522 Intelligent Pump® (Figure 12-11A) provides volume precision of primary and secondary lines. McGaw's Profile™ 521 *Plus* Intelligent Pump® (Figure 12-11B) is widely used for delivery of nutritional support and IV medications by vol-

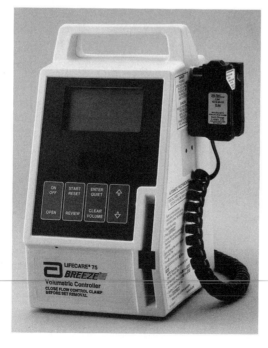

FIGURE 12-7 LifeCare® 75 BREEZE Volumetric Controller. (Courtesy: Abbott Laboratories, North Chicago, IL)

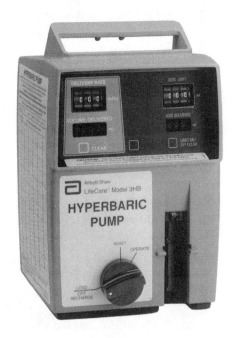

FIGURE 12-8 HYPERBARIC PUMP, Model 3HB. (Courtesy: Abbott Laboratories, North Chicago, IL)

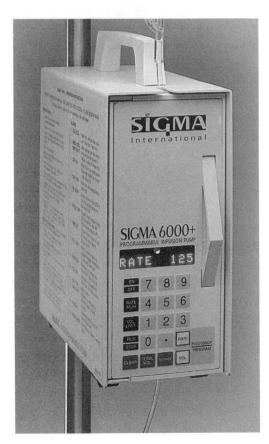

FIGURE 12-9 Sigma International 6000+ (Courtesy: Sigma International, Medina, NY)

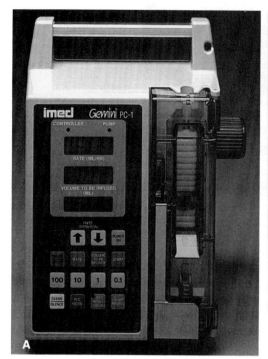

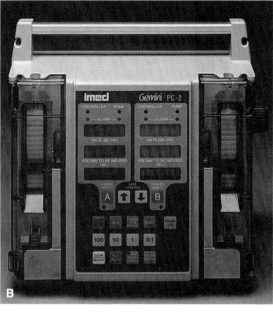

FIGURE 12-10 (**A**) Gemini PC-1. (**B**) Gemini PC-2. (Courtesy: Imed Corp., San Diego, CA)

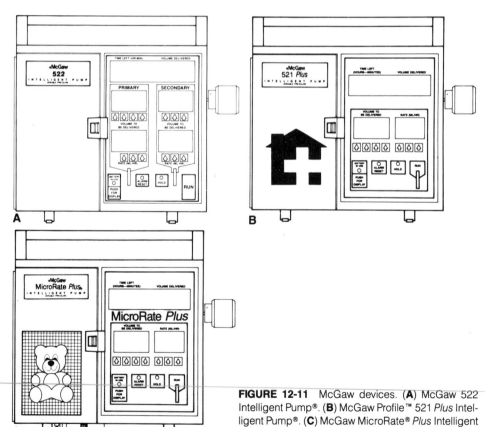

FIGURE 12-11 McGaw devices. (**A**) McGaw 522 Intelligent Pump®. (**B**) McGaw Profile™ 521 *Plus* Intelligent Pump®. (**C**) McGaw MicroRate® *Plus* Intelligent Pump®. (Courtesy: McGaw, Inc., Irvine, CA)

umetric displacement of fluid. McGaw's MicroRate® *Plus* Intelligent Pump® (Figure 12-11C) is designed to meet the needs of the neonatal or pediatric patient.

Abbott Laboratories' LifeCare 4P does not allow free flow when the infusion set is removed and provides optional gravity infusion. It offers progammable secondary and primary flow settings and dosages. The model 4H is capable of delivering nutritional support and IV medications in a flow range of 1 to 350 mL/hr.

A wide assortment of features accompanies EIDs in today's complex health care setting. Nurses must be familiar with the literature and with the device to be used and must take all precautions to ensure safe, efficient operation.

The impact of changing technology has moved us far beyond the basics of instrumentation to a field known as computer-generated technology.

Computer-Generated Technology

Now and into the future, the nursing professional is not as limited by time and space. Research, input, and data will all be computer generated. The computer will be the focal point of the IV drug delivery system. Electronic flow is now the norm rather than the exception. EIDs today are available in a diversity of sizes and technologies and may be found in a broad range of clinical settings. The Omni-Flow Therapist IV Medication Management System by Abbott (Figure 12-12) has a range of 1 to 700 mL/hr, programmable in nine units of measure, with bar codes generated by the pharmacy. It is capable of infusing four medications simultaneously or intermittently (or both) from bags, bottles, or syringes.

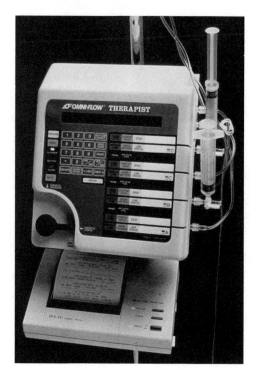

FIGURE 12-12 Omni-Flow Therapist. (Courtesy: Abbott Laboratories, North Chicago, IL)

Product Selection and Evaluation

Selection of equipment is a complex task. Hospitalized patients now receive a multitude of therapies through their intravascular systems. The type of device used to initiate flow depends on the complexity of care, the range of flow needed, pressure, the insertion site, and the delivery rate.

Product selection should be a serious consideration and should be based on needs assessment in the clinical setting. The ability to deliver a specified dose in either $\mu g/kg/min$, $\mu g/kg/hr$, $mg/kg/min$, or $mg/kg/hr$ by entering the appropriate concentration, patient weight, bolus amount, and mass units is a feature often required in the critical care setting. Demands for features such as bolus capabilities, syringe size sensing, and delivery in body weight, mass, continuous, or volume-over-time modes have challenged today's manufacturers to produce the most advanced products ever available.

The product evaluation committee is often involved in the selection of EIDs in the clinical setting. This focus should carry into the alternative care setting as well, so that the EIDs chosen clearly meet the patients' clinical and therapeutic needs while fulfilling a real function as accessories to quality IV nursing care.

ECRI and General Purpose Infusion Pumps

ECRI, formerly the Emergency Care Research Institute, is an independent nonprofit agency dedicated to improving the safety, efficacy, and cost effectiveness of health care technology, facilities, and procedures. Between January 1988 and January 1989, ECRI researchers assessed 14 general purpose infusion pumps from nine manufacturers.[3] Pumps were assessed for the following features:

- Flow range and resolution
- Flow accuracy under optimal conditions
- Flow continuity
- Flow error following 24, 48, and 72 hours
- Occlusion detection
- Accuracy with backpressure
- Effect of fluid–container height
- Operation during transport
- Volume to be infused (VTBI)
- Fluid–container depletion
- Air-in-line detection
- Pump-set malposition
- Keep-vein-open (KVO) rate
- Infusion controller mode
- Resistance to tampering and accidents
- Memory functions
- Alarms
- Battery operation
- Electrical safety

- Electromagnetic interference (EMI)
- Electrostatic discharge (ESD)
- Line voltage variation
- Effects of fluids
- Interference with other equipment
- Quiet operation
- Human factors design
- Ease of servicing

ECRI is involved in developing strict evaluation criteria aimed at helping those of us in the clinical setting to deliver care with a high degree of safety and accuracy. ECRI suggests that the major issues confronting users and purchasers of general purpose infusion pumps are as follows:

- Overall performance
- Free-flow risk versus cost and conditions of acceptability
- Detecting upstream occlusion
- Detecting empty fluid containers
- Special features (including piggybacking, user-selectable occlusion alarm pressure, and pressure monitoring)

AMBULATORY INFUSION DEVICES

Self-care is an important component of our health care delivery system. The development of compact, battery-driven electronic infusion devices has simplified care in diverse ambulatory clinical settings.

External Infusion Pumps

The size, weight, and portability of the unit are important considerations in choosing a system. An active patient must be comfortable wearing the lightest pump possible; a sedentary patient may prefer the advantages of a larger device. Accessories and loading procedures vary with the manufacturer and the product selected. Infusion capacity may dictate the choice of the system. Pump-specific sets may be required, as seen in the patient receiving nutritional support or pain medication.

Integral safety features include the following:

- Occlusion alarm
- Low-volume safety alarm
- Low battery alarm

Competition in this exciting area of growth has stimulated many new companies to enter the electronic infusion market, resulting in greater availability of more sophisticated products for the professional IV nurse.

Advancing technologies enable the user to deliver several modes of therapy, as in the VERIFUSE™ system by BLOCK Medical, Inc. (Figure 12-13), which delivers continuous, continuous with bolus, intermittent, and taper dosages. The VERIFUSE™ is pro-

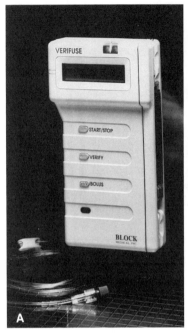

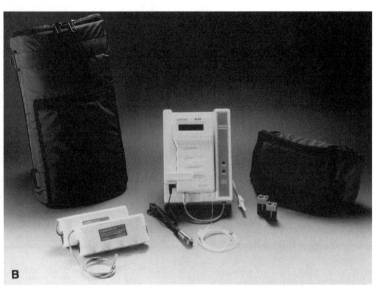

FIGURE 12-13   (A) VERIFUSE multiple therapy infusion pump programs itself by reading a bar code. (B) VERIFUSE components. (Courtesy: BLOCK Medical, Inc., Carlsbad, CA)

grammed by a scanner that reads a bar code. An IBM-compatible software package enables the clinician to produce a bar code that programs the pump for a specific prescription. The software also allows the clinician to communicate with the pump over a telephone line when the pump is used with the Homecase accessory.[5] With four modes of therapy, bar code programming, and remote capabilities, this is just one of a number of devices designed to meet changing needs in infusion delivery.

MedMate™ by Patient Solutions Inc. (Figure 12-14) is an ambulatory system that also provides multiple functions, including intermittent medication delivery with first dose delay and a variable KVO rate, nutritional support with taper flexibility and "end early" option, patient-controlled analgesia with mg or mL programming and bolus

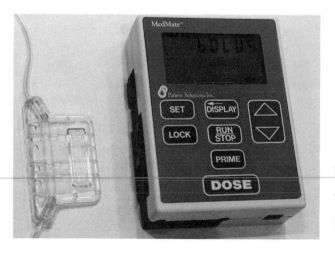

FIGURE 12-14 MedMate™ pump. 78-inch spike set may be used with any standard solution bag; note pumping cartridge. (Courtesy: Patient Solutions, Inc., San Diego, CA)

activity tracking, and continuous fluid therapy with a wide rate range and high resolution flow management.[6]

Pharmacia Deltec's line of ambulatory infusion devices is well-known in the infusion therapy field. The CADD-1® and CADD-PLUS® have been used extensively by many patients. CADD-1 (Figure 12-15) was designed specifically for continuous IV chemotherapy. CADD-PLUS (Figure 12-16) was designed for intermittent or continuous IV antibiotic therapy and can use a removable reservoir adapter and other accessories as needed. The CADD-TPN™ (Figure 12-17) features a programmable taper to eliminate manual rate changes during the infusion cycle. The pump automatically calculates continuous infusion rates for simplicity, and the power pack may be recharged during operation with the AC adapter. Rates up to 400 mL/hr are possible along with the KVO rate at the end of the infusion period. Three programmable lock levels control patient–pump interaction. As with all of their products, Pharmacia Deltec provides a complete line of resources to facilitate introduction of their product line within a setting and for patient–staff education.

Abbott Laboratories' Lifecare® PROVIDER series provides a system for delivery of patient-controlled analgesia, antineoplastic therapy, IV drug administration, and nutritional support. Model 5500 (Figure 12-18) has a flow range of 0.1 to 999 mL/hr and weighs only 14 oz. Driven by two 9V alkaline batteries, it is capable of continuous, continuous with bolus, bolus only, or intermittent delivery.

Becton Dickinson's line of syringe pumps, including rate infuser +, 360 infuser, and rate infuser II (Figure 12-19) has set the industry standard for syringe pumps. Syringe pumps are calibrated in mL/hr, are used with standard disposable syringes, and provide smooth and precise delivery of low volumes of solution to specific patient populations.

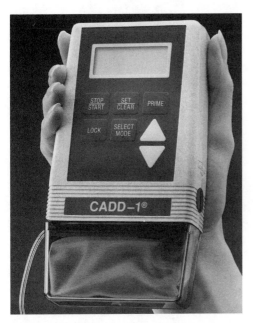

FIGURE 12-15 CADD-1® Ambulatory Infusion Pump. (Property of Pharmacia Deltec Inc., St. Paul, MN)

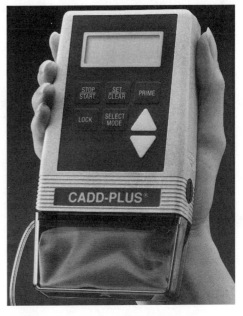

FIGURE 12-16 CADD-PLUS® Ambulatory Infusion Pump. (Property of Pharmacia Deltec Inc., St. Paul, MN)

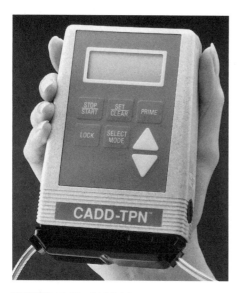

FIGURE 12-17 CADD-TPN™ Ambulatory Infusion System. (Property of Pharmacia Deltec Inc., St. Paul, MN)

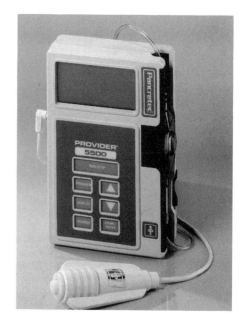

FIGURE 12-18 PROVIDER 5500 Pump. (Courtesy: Abbott Laboratories, North Chicago, IL)

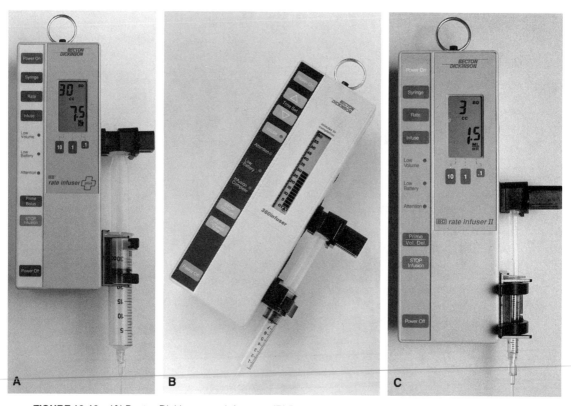

FIGURE 12-19 (**A**) Becton Dickinson rate infuser + . (**B**) Becton Dickinson 360 infuser. (**C**) Becton Dickinson rate infuser II. (Courtesy: Becton Dickinson and Company, Rutherford, NJ)

Elastomeric Devices

Baxter's Intermate® (Figure 12-20) provides fixed rates to ensure accurate dosages and pharmacokinetic consistency. No IV pole or electric cord is needed. The design, in various configurations, is small and lightweight. As a single-use disposable item, it simplifies single-dose infusion therapies.

BLOCK Medical's Homepump™ (Figure 12-21) uses elastomeric strain, which is produced by the pressure of the membrane collapsing to deliver medication. Constant pressure, combined with the capillary orifice, produces a predetermined flow rate/time for delivery of the prescribed medication. Designed to be filled by a pharmacist under a laminar flow hood, flow continuity is in the range of ±15%.

Internal Infusion Pumps

Internal, or implantable infusion pumps, discussed in Chapter 24, are placed beneath the patient's skin, and the inner drug chamber is refilled by percutaneous injection through a self-sealing septum. Such pumps have been implanted in a subcutaneous pocket of the lower abdominal wall for delivery of antineoplastic agents to the liver through the hepatic artery.

Patient Selection and Education

Patients should be carefully evaluated for their ability to comprehend and carry out self-care procedures, especially when EIDs are to be used. The patient should be taught how the pump can be worn, the operating principles, care of the pump and line, technical problems, and troubleshooting techniques. Home teaching checklists addressing pump operation may be found in Chapter 26.

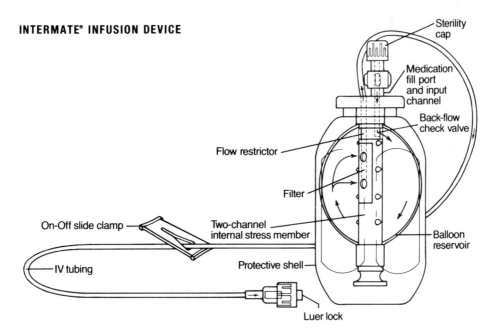

FIGURE 12-20 Baxter Intermate®. (Courtesy: Baxter Healthcare, Deerfield, IL)

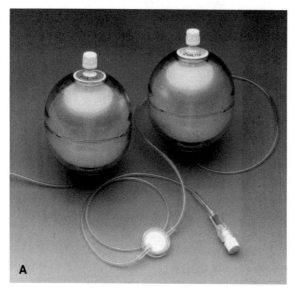

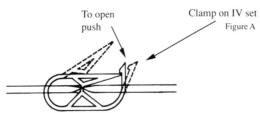

To open push

Clamp on IV set
Figure A

Instructions for Use

- Use aseptic techniques.
- Do not use while showering, bathing, or swimming.
- The Homepump infusion system should be administered at room temperature.

1. Check to be sure the clamp on the IV set is closed. (**Fig. A**)
2. Remove cap at the distal end of the Homepump. (**Fig. B**) Open the clamp to release any air from the line. (**Fig. A**)
3. When fluid has reached the distal end of the Homepump and all air has been eliminated from the tubing, close the clamp. *Note:* It is not required to invert the filter for priming.
4. Attach the end of the IV set to the access site. (*See instructions regarding accessing site provided by your home health care nurse.*)
5. Open the clamp on the IV set to begin the infusion.
6. When the Homepump has dispensed its contents (**Fig. B**), disconnect and dispose of the entire unit in an appropriate manner.
7. Flush access site. (*See instructions for flushing procedure provided by your home health care nurse.*)

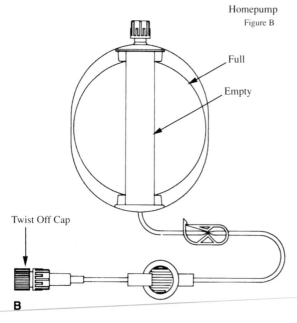

Homepump
Figure B

Full

Empty

Twist Off Cap

FIGURE 12-21 (**A**) 110-mL HOMEPUMP™. 2 mL/hr and 5 mL/hr delivery in a preset continuous flow rate. HOMEPUMP is also available in 200-mL volume with preset flow rate of 175 mL/hr and in 50-mL volume with preset flow rate of 5 mL/hr. (**B**) HOMEPUMP™ instructions for use. (Courtesy: BLOCK Medical, Inc., Carlsbad, CA)

STANDARDS OF PRACTICE FOR FLOW-CONTROL DEVICES

Consistent with Intravenous Nurses Society (INS) Standards of Practice, the rate of IV infusions should be routinely regulated by manual flow-control devices to ensure accurate delivery of the prescribed therapy. Electronic infusion devices should be used when warranted by the patient's age and condition, setting, and prescribed therapy. The nursing professional is responsible and accountable for the use of EIDs. Use of EIDs, deployment of them, selection criteria, and classifications should be outlined in institutional policy and procedure manuals. The nurse's knowledge base concerning EIDs should include at the minimum:

- Indications for use
- Mechanical operation
- Troubleshooting
- psi rating
- Safe usage

PERIPHERAL VASCULAR ACCESS DEVICES

Innovations in catheter technology have produced catheters to meet the patient's every need, from peripheral infusion to the most sophisticated therapy.

Catheters vary in gauge, length, composition, and design. The composition may be PVC, polyurethane, or silicone. Thin-walled catheters provide increased flow rates, which allow smaller sized catheters to be used. Most catheters are radiopaque or contain a stripe of radiopaque material for radiographic visualization.

Catheters may be over-the-needle (ONC), where the catheter, mounted on the needle, is slipped off the needle into the vein and the needle is removed; or inside-the-needle (INC), where the catheter is pushed through the needle until the desired length is in the vein, and the cutting edge is protected by a shield.

Some catheters are provided with wings and all the advantages of a small-vein needle on insertion and on taping. The adapter of the IV set connection is located a few inches from the catheter and provides ease and better technique when changing sets, reducing the potential for mechanical phlebitis and contamination. Such catheters are available with injection sites as an integral part of the catheter; the mixing of drugs or blood components with primary parenteral fluid is reduced to a minimum (0.4 mL), minimizing the potential of incompatibilities.

Over-the-Needle Catheter

The ONC (Figure 12-22) is the most commonly used device for peripheral infusion therapy. The introducer needle, or stylet, is removed once successful cannulation is accomplished. The flexibility of this device, diversity of size and length ranges, and its safety offer patients freedom of movement. Consistent with INS Standards of Practice, the cannula should be placed for a definitive therapeutic or diagnostic indication. Practice dictates using the smallest gauge, shortest length cannula capable of accomplishing the prescribed therapy. All such catheters should be radiopaque and only one device should be used for each attempt at venipuncture. All products should be inspected for integrity before use. Peripheral venous cannulas should be removed every 48 hours and immediately on suspected contamination or complication. Manufacturer's guidelines for the use of their specific products should be adhered to at all times.

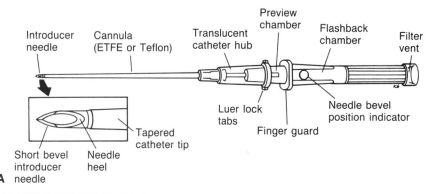

Introducer needle

Cannula (ETFE or Teflon)

Translucent catheter hub

Preview chamber

Flashback chamber

Filter vent

Luer lock tabs

Finger guard

Needle bevel position indicator

Tapered catheter tip

Short bevel introducer needle

Needle heel

A

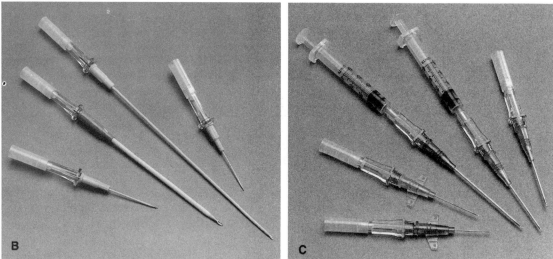

B

C

FIGURE 12-22   (**A**) Over-the-needle IV catheter. (Courtesy: Terumo, Inc., Somerset, NJ) (**B**) ANGIOCATH® IV catheter. (Courtesy: Becton Dickinson Vascular Access, Sandy, UT) (**C**) INSYTE® IV catheter. (Courtesy: Becton Dickinson Vascular Access, Sandy, UT)

Inside-the-Needle Catheters

The INC combines an 8- to 12-inch catheter with an introducer needle, which should be protected by a shield following insertion. Historically, these catheters have been used when venous access has been poor and when administration of caustic drugs or hypertonic solutions is required. They have been replaced in many clinical settings by the peripherally inserted central catheter (PICC).

Winged Infusion Needle

The winged infusion needle (Figure 12-23) is available as an ONC or steel needle. Flexible wings are a part of both devices and are easily grasped during the insertion technique. Once the device is placed within the lumen of the vessel, the wings are flattened against the skin and provide an anchor for stabilization.

Again, manufacturers have kept pace with demands for advanced product concepts, and a variation of the ONC winged infusion needle incorporates a Y-shaped design with a latex cap to permit intermittent infusion of subsequent medications or solutions (Figure

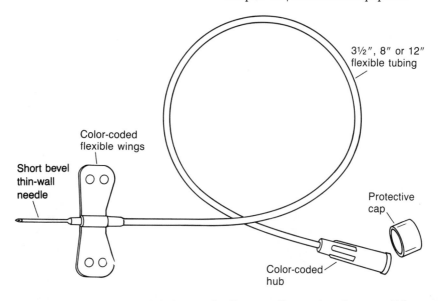

FIGURE 12-23   Winged infusion needle. (Courtesy: Terumo, Inc., Somerset, NJ)

12-24). The thin-walled design of the winged infusion needle facilitates placement; however, the risk of infiltration with the steel needle type deters many professionals from using this product for any use other than short-term.

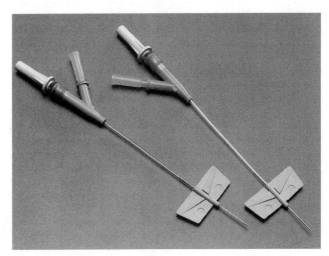

FIGURE 12-24 Angio-Set® IV catheter with built-in extension tubing and adapter in a closed system. (Courtesy: Becton Dickinson Vascular Access, Sandy, UT)

Midline Catheters

Menlo Care, Inc. has developed a midline ONC known as Landmark® (Figure 12-25). Made of Aquavene®, which undergoes a dramatic change in physical properties when in contact with body fluids, the catheter softens by a 50:1 ratio. During the softening process (hydration), Aquavene begins to expand. Expansion occurs like a photo enlargement, that is, the internal diameter, outside diameter, and wall all expand in equal proportion. The complete softening and expansion process takes approximately 90

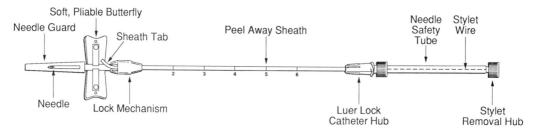

Soft, Pliable Butterfly
Needle Guard
Sheath Tab
Peel Away Sheath
Needle Safety Tube
Stylet Wire
Needle
Lock Mechanism
Luer Lock Catheter Hub
Stylet Removal Hub

FIGURE 12-25   Landmark® Catheter. (Courtesy: Menlo Care, Inc., Menlo Park, CA, Landmark and Aquavene are registered trademarks of Menlo Care, Inc.)

minutes. Aquavene cannulas expand precisely two gauge sizes—they do not continue to expand beyond this fixed unit. Catheter cannulas consist of an Aquavene outer layer and thin polyurethane inner lining. The polyurethane lining is impermeable and prevents hydration from the inner lumen. The outer Aquavene layer hydrates by absorbing water and electrolytes from the blood and plasma. This type of product permits long-term placement when venous access is limited or when therapy is ordered for a specific period of time. Considered a peripheral venous catheter according to the INS standards, professionals are encouraged to develop policies and procedures relevant to indwell time consistent with those Standards of Practice and institutional guidelines.

LATEX INJECTION PORTS

The latex injection port or catheter cap (Figure 12-26) may be used to adapt any indwelling device to an intermittent infusion device. Available either as an individual unit, or incorporated within the design of an ONC or winged infusion set, the use of the latex injection port has simplified the administration of intermittent therapies. Intermittent

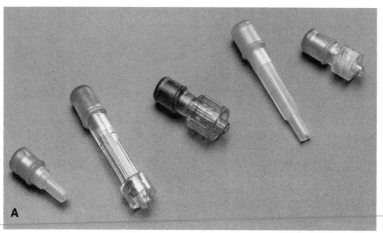

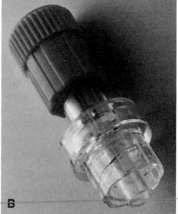

A

B

FIGURE 12-26   (**A**) PRN Adapters, used to convert indwelling IV catheters or infusion sets to intermittent administration devices. (Courtesy: Becton Dickinson Vascular Access, Sandy, UT) (**B**) Burron Safsite® injection cap. (Courtesy: Burron Medical Inc., Bethlehem, PA)

devices may also be called "heparin locks," "INTS," or "PRN Adapters" because heparin or saline is routinely instilled into the cap and its housing to maintain patency. Most products now include a Luer lock device to prevent accidental dislodgement of the cap.

Burron Medical features the Safsite® injection cap. Becton Dickinson's Vascular Access Division provides a number of injection caps to meet all clinical needs.

The Click-Lock™ is a product of ICU Medical and was the first positive locking IV catheter–connecting device (Figure 12-27). It uses a removable stainless steel needle in a clear plastic housing that snap locks onto the injection port. The Piggy Lock™ is a universal IV connection device used when piggybacking medications on primary IV lines. Piggy Lock™ is used to lock on "Y" sites above and below an EID.

NEEDLELESS SYSTEMS

The newest technology is that of the needleless system, which has revolutionized infusion therapy. Consisting of a blunt-tipped plastic insertion device and an injection port that opens and immediately reseals, this system was developed to reduce the incidence of accidental needlestick injuries and to promote safety in infusion practice. Again, diverse systems are available to meet clinical needs in many settings.

Baxter Healthcare's InterLink™ IV Access System (Figure 12-28) eliminates needlestick risks in a wide range of applications, requiring minimal change in technique. The system includes a vial access cannula for single-dose vial access and a lever lock cannula securely locking all injection site connections.

Auto-LOCK™ is a protected needle offered by BLOCK Medical, Inc. (Figure 12-29). It minimizes exposure to needlesticks and prevents accidental disconnects on critical lines. Compatible with most standard intermittent infusion devices, it offers undedicated components and promotes flexibility. Replacement needles are available and allow users to reuse Auto-LOCK housings while changing the needle.

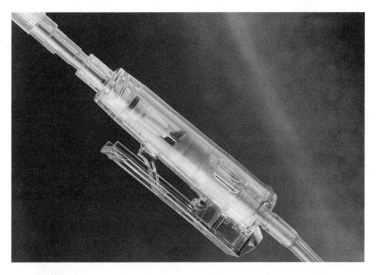

FIGURE 12-27   Click-Lock™ locking (junction securement) device. (Courtesy: ICU Medical, Irvine, CA)

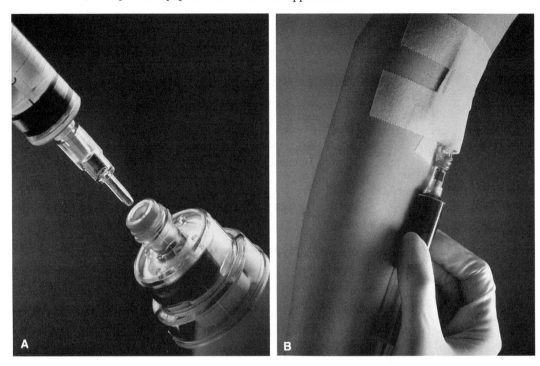

FIGURE 12-28 (**A**) InterLink™ IV Access System components. (**B**) Venous sampling using the InterLink™ IV Access System. (Courtesy: Baxter Healthcare, Deerfield, IL)

Abbott Laboratories provides a LifeShield needleless system with prepierced reseals and a blunt cannula (Figure 12-30).

The Centurion® Kleen-Needle® system provides several sets with and without preattached latex caps. A multiple port manifold with one-way valves simplifies dosing of intermittent medications (Figure 12-31).

Quest Medical features a product known as the "No Needles" set (Figure 12-32) in which all ports are Luer lock, back-check valves prevent retrograding of drug or solution, syringes may be left attached throughout a procedure, and one-handed injection is possible. The set is adaptable to a wide number of clinical settings, including anesthesia.

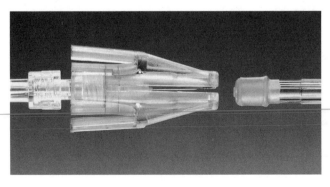

FIGURE 12-29 Auto-LOCK™ is a positive locking needle system designed to prevent accidental disconnects. (Courtesy: BLOCK Medical, Inc., Carlsbad, CA)

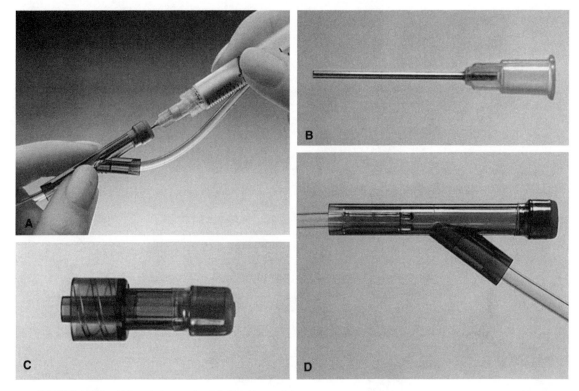

FIGURE 12-30 Abbott Laboratories LifeShield needleless system with prepierced reseals and blunt cannula. (Courtesy: Abbott Laboratories, North Chicago, IL)

INTRAVENOUS ACCESSORIES

In addition to the plethora of injection caps, latex ports, and needleless systems available, today's manufacturers also provide the safety of self-contained IV start kits like SafeStart™ by Becton Dickinson's Vascular Access (Figure 12-33) and IV loops, extension sets, Y adapters, obturators, and T connectors (Figure 12-34). IV systems such as Abbott's ADD-Vantage® unit dose system (Figure 12-35) have simplified the administration of IV piggyback medications. While standard systems still exist, the ADD-Vantage unit incorporates a single-dose method of touch-free drug delivery.

LAMINAR FLOW HOOD

The laminar flow hood minimizes the potential for airborne contamination during admixture of IV solutions. The laminar flow hood incorporates a clean environment. Vertical and horizontal hoods are available—the horizontal hood is used for routine drugs and solutions; the vertical hood or biologic class II safety cabinet is used for admixture of antineoplastic agents (See Chapter 24). The laminar flow clean bench is usually described as a work bench or similar enclosure characterized by its filtered air supply. The clean bench was developed as an adjunct to clean room technology—the need to protect the product from contamination.

(*text continues on page 174*)

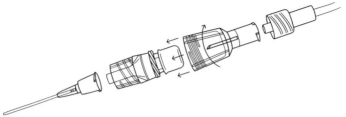

The CENTURION® Kleen-Needle®
System is safe, simple and
adaptable to the I.V. lines and
administration sets that are
currently in use.

FIGURE 12-31 Centurion® Kleen-Needle® needleless system. (Courtesy: Tri-State Hospital Supply, Howell, MI)

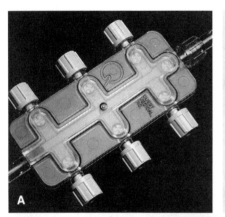

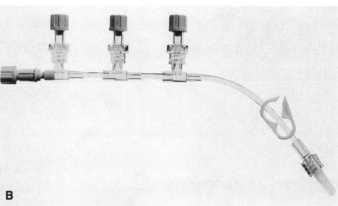

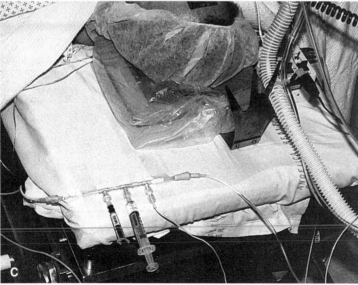

FIGURE 12-32 "No Needles" set. Check-valve extension sets (**A** and **B**) simplify drug administration with syringes and/or pumps (**C**). (Courtesy: Quest Medical, Inc., Dallas, TX)

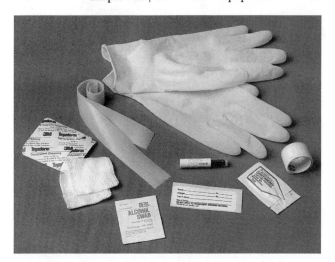

FIGURE 12-33 SafeStart™ IV Start Pak™ components, with gloves. (Courtesy: Becton Dickinson Vascular Access, Sandy, UT)

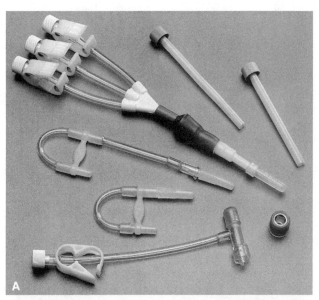

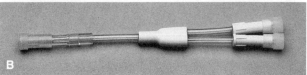

FIGURE 12-34 (**A**) IV accessories. (Courtesy: Becton Dickinson Vascular Access, Sandy, UT) (**B**) Y connector. (Courtesy: Abbott Laboratories, North Chicago, IL)

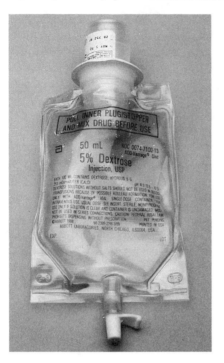

FIGURE 12-35 ADD-Vantage® system for single-dose drug delivery. (Courtesy: Abbott Laboratories, North Chicago, IL)

This is accomplished by ensuring that the product is exposed only to HEPA-filtered air (high efficiency particulate air capable of trapping 9997 to 9999 of every 10,000 particles of a diameter greater than and less than 0.3 μm).

In the horizontal hood, room air is drawn into the base of the hood by the motor/blower and through a washable, reusable prefilter. The air is then pushed up the rear of the hood and passed through a HEPA filter. HEPA-filtered air is directed horizontally across the work surface toward the operator. In the vertical hood, the cabinet is described as protective equipment featuring a front access opening with carefully maintained inward airflow. This class II, type B cabinet was designed to meet the requirement of the National Cancer Institute (NCI). All of the exhaust air is taken directly from the work area (direct exhaust) and pulled through a dedicated exhaust duct into the facility's separate exhaust system to a fan on the roof. The 30% recirculated air is HEPA filtered immediately below the work surface, before it is recirculated. All unfiltered air in the cabinet flows under negative pressure in dedicated ducts. All positive-pressure areas are free of particulate contamination because of the location of the supply HEPA filter.

REFERENCES

1. Adriani, J. (1962). Venipuncture. *American Journal of Nursing, 62,* 70.
2. Boyan, C. P. (1964). Cold or warmed blood for massive transfusion. *Annals of Surgery, 160,* 282.
3. ECRI. (1989). Emergency Care Research Institute Health Devices. Plymouth Meeting, PA. *Infusion Pumps, 18*(3-4), 92–133.
4. *Revised intravenous nursing standards of practice. (1990). Journal of Intravenous Nursing,* (Suppl.), S37, S58.
5. Product Literature, BLOCK Medical, Inc.
6. Product Literature, Patient Solutions, Inc.
7. Tarail, R. (1950). Practice of fluid therapy. *Journal of the American Medical Association, 171,* 45–49.

BIBLIOGRAPHY

Falchuk, K. H., Peterson, L., & McNeil, B. J. (1985). Microparticulate-induced phlebitis: Its prevention by inline filtration. *New England Journal of Medicine, 312*(2), 78–82.

Frey, A. M. (1986). Taking the confusion out of multiple infusion. *Journal of the National Intravenous Therapy Association, 9*(6), 460–463.

Hadaway, L. C. (1989). Evaluation and use of advanced I.V. technology. Part I: Central venous access devices. *Journal of Intravenous Nursing, 12*(2), 73–82.

Quercia, R. A., Hills, S. W., Klimer, J. J., et al. (1986). Bacteriologic contamination of intravenous infusion delivery systems in an intensive care unit. *American Journal of Medicine, 80*(3), 364–368.

Ritter, H. T. M. (1990). Evaluating and selecting general-purpose infusion pumps. *Journal of Intravenous Nursing, 13*(3), 156–161.

REVIEW QUESTIONS

1. The IV container most widely used today unless contraindicated because of the type of drug additive is made of:
   a. silastic
   b. prolastic
   c. plastic
   d. glass

2. The filter attached to a vented medication-additive, IV set is what μm in size?
   a. 0.2
   b. 0.5
   c. 1.0
   d. 1.2

3. The limit to operating pressure at which an alarm is triggered on an electronic infusion device is known as what type of pressure?
   a. system
   b. needle
   c. occlusion
   d. resistance

4. The United States Pharmacopeia (USP) has established an acceptable limit of particles for single-dose infusion not to exceed how many particles per mL equal to or greater than 10.0 μm?
   a. 20
   b. 40
   c. 50
   d. 60

5. Which of the following is NOT an example of filter material?
   a. hydrophobic
   b. hydrophilic
   c. depth
   d. bubble point

6. An alternative to the water bath is:
   a. dry heat blood warmer
   b. warming bag
   c. hypothermia
   d. cell grader

7. 50 mm Hg is equivalent to how many psi?
   a. 12
   b. 30
   c. 50
   d. 62

8. The rate of IV infusions should be routinely regulated by:
   a. electronic flow control
   b. manual flow control
   c. rate minders
   d. elastomerics

9. Which of the following systems was developed to reduce the incidence of needlestick injuries?
   a. needleless
   b. elastomerics
   c. Luer locks
   d. universal connection

10. The laminar flow unit designed to meet the requirements of the National Cancer Institute is the:
    a. class I
    b. class I, type B
    c. class II
    d. class II, type B

CHAPTER 13

Rate of Administration

A primary consideration in the administration of fluids by the parenteral route is the rate of flow. An established rate of flow is a component of a complete physician's order. The nurse who initiates the infusion or who maintains it is responsible for regulating and maintaining the appropriate rate of administration consistent with the physician's order and the patient's clinical condition.

DETERMINING FACTORS

To determine the flow rate intelligently, the nurse must have a knowledge of parenteral solutions, their effect, and rate of administration. The nurse must also understand other factors that influence the speed of the infusion. These factors include (1) body surface area, (2) condition of the patient, (3) age of the patient, (4) composition of the fluid, and (5) the patient's tolerance to the infusion.

Body Surface Area

The body surface area is proportionate to many essential physiologic processes (organ size, blood volume, respiration, and heat loss) and therefore to the total metabolic activity. It provides a helpful guide for determining the amount of fluids and electrolytes and for computing the rates of infusion. The larger an individual, the more fluid and nutrients are required and the faster they can be used. The usual infusion rate is 3 mL/m² body surface per minute (see nomograms for determining surface area, Figure 18-1). This rate applies to maintenance and replacement fluids. However, the speed must be carefully adjusted to each individual.

Condition of Patient

Because the heart and the kidneys play a vital role in the utilization of infused solutions, the cardiac and renal status of the patient affects the desired rate of administration. An expanded blood volume may occur when fluids, rapidly infused, overtax an impaired heart and renal damage causes retention of fluid. Patients suffering from hypovolemia must receive plasma and blood rapidly, but the desired speed of the infusion may be affected by impairment of the homeostatic controls. Therefore, the rate should be specified by the physician. Vital signs must be carefully observed and the speed of the infusion decreased as the blood pressure rises.

Sharon M. Weinstein: PLUMER'S PRINCIPLES & PRACTICE OF INTRAVENOUS THERAPY, FIFTH EDITION, © 1993 J. B. Lippincott Company

Age of Patient

Because the elderly usually have some degree of cardiac and renal damage, fluids are administered slowly to prevent an increase in venous pressure that could result in pulmonary edema and cardiovascular disturbances.[1] Infants and small children are particularly susceptible to pulmonary edema when excessive quantities of fluid or rapidly infused fluids expand the vascular system. The rate of administration must be determined by the physician and all precautions observed to ensure steady maintenance at the required rate of flow. If difficulty is encountered in controlling a constant rate, it should be reported and corrected at once.

The special pediatric infusion sets that deliver a smaller size drop (60 drops/mL) provide precision control of the rate of flow. Various mechanical controlling devices are available to assist the nurse in maintaining a constant accurate flow rate (see Chapter 12). Intravenous Nurses Society Standards advocate the use of EIDs when warranted by the patient's age and condition, setting, and prescribed therapy.[2]

Composition of Fluid

The composition of the fluid affects the rate of flow. When the solution is used as a vehicle for administering drugs, the speed of the infusion depends on the drug and the effect the physician wishes to produce. Because of its deleterious effect on the heart when infused at a rapid rate, potassium should be administered with caution. About 20 to 40 mEq potassium in a liter of solution infused over an 8-hour period is an average rate for administering potassium parenterally.[1]

Concentration of solutions must be considered because the flow rate may alter the desired effect. When dextrose is administered for caloric benefits, it is infused at a rate that will ensure complete utilization. Dextrose has been administered at a maximum speed of 0.5 g/kg body weight per hour without producing glycosuria in a normal individual. At this rate, it would take approximately 1.5 hours to administer a liter of 5% dextrose to an individual weighing 70 kg or twice as long for a liter of 10% dextrose. This maximum rate is faster than usual and is not customarily used except in an emergency.

When a diuretic effect is desired, a more rapid infusion is necessary. If the solution is too rapidly infused for complete metabolism, the glucose accumulates in the bloodstream, increases the osmolality, and acts as a diuretic.

When oliguria or anuria occurs, the status of the kidneys must be determined before solutions containing potassium can be administered. Urinary suppression may be due to a blood volume deficit or to kidney damage. An initial hydrating solution, to test kidney function, is usually administered at a rate of 8 mL/m² body surface per minute for 45 minutes.[1] If urinary flow is not accomplished, the rate is slowed to about 2 mL/m² body surface per minute for another hour. If urinary output has not occurred after this period, it is presumed that kidney damage is present.[1]

Tolerance

Tolerance to solutions varies with individuals and influences the rate of infusion. A 5% solution of alcohol has been administered at the rate of 200 to 300 mL/hr to sedate without intoxication in an average adult. However, when such a solution is to be administered, the rate must be titrated to the individual and prescribed by the physician.

COMPUTATION OF FLOW RATE

Frequently, the physician orders a total volume of fluid to be infused over a 24-hour period. If the nurse knows the volume and the flow rate of the administration set in use, he or she can easily compute the required rate of flow. A quick, easy formula for computing flow rate in drops (gtt) per minute is:

$$\frac{\text{gtt/mL of given set}}{60 \ (\text{min in hr})} \times \text{total hourly volume} = \text{gtt/min}$$

If a set delivers 15 gtt/mL and 240 mL is to be infused in 1 hour:

$$\frac{15}{60} \times 240 = \frac{1}{4} \times 240 = 60 \ \text{gtt/min}$$

Whenever a set is used that delivers 15 gtt/mL, merely divide the hourly volume to be infused by 4 and the number of drops per minute will be obtained.

If the set delivers 10 gtt/mL, divide the number of milliliters to be infused by 6 for drops per minute:

$$\frac{10}{60} \times \text{hourly volume} = \frac{1}{6} \times \text{hourly volume} = \text{gtt/min}$$

Manufacturers of parenteral solutions have devised convenient calculators to assist the nurse in accurate rate determinations.

A Baxter Minislide* has provided the nurse with a handy, quick device for computing fluid rates. It consists of a slide rule containing four scales:

Top, scale A: total milliliters to be infused

Bottom, scale D: flow rate in drops per minute

The insert slides between scales A and D and contains:

Scale B: number of drops per milliliter (10–60) a given set delivers

Scale C: time in hours for infusion

The flow rate or the infusion time at the prescribed rate may be determined by sliding the insert until the number of drops that the set delivers is aligned with total milliliters to be infused. Opposite the time (hours) for infusion, see drops required per minute; opposite the prescribed flow rate, see the infusion time (hours).

The opposite side of the Minislide contains the Cohn Fluid Calculator.[†] Because the body surface area is an important criterion for determining the rate of infusion, this calculator is helpful for determining the surface area and the total amount of fluid required. Total milliliters to be infused in 24 hours is determined by sliding the insert until the weight of the patient in kilograms is reached; consideration is given to the body size of the patient—thin, average, or obese. Once the weight in kilograms is set, the surface area in square meters and the total amount of fluid to be infused in 24 hours is indicated. Other solution manufacturers have produced similar guides.

No guide to safe flow rates is as important as is the patient's reaction to the infusion, which should, therefore, be checked frequently.

---

* Baxter Healthcare Corp., formerly Travenol Laboratories, Inc., Deerfield, IL. Designed by Bertram D. Cohn, MD, FAAP, FACS.

† Copyright 1978, American Slide-Chart Corp., Wheaton, IL. Designed by Harry F. Weisberg, MD.

FACTORS AFFECTING FLOW RATE

The infusion should be checked frequently to maintain the required rate of flow. Because of certain factors, the rate is subject to change.

Height of the Solution Bottle

Intravenous fluids run by gravity. Any change in gravity by raising or lowering the infusion container will change the rate of flow. When patients receiving infusions are ambulated or transported to ancillary departments, the containers should be retained at the same height, or the speed of the infusion should be readjusted to maintain the prescribed rate of flow.

Clot in the Cannula

Any temporary stoppage of the infusion, such as a delay in hanging subsequent solutions, may cause a clot to form in the lumen of the cannula, partially or completely obstructing it. Clot formation may also occur when an increase in venous pressure in the infusion arm forces blood back into the cannula. This results from restriction of the venous circulation and is most commonly caused by (1) the blood pressure cuff on the infusion arm, (2) restraints placed on or above the infusion cannula, and (3) the patient's lying on the arm receiving the infusion.

Change in Position of the Cannula

A change in the cannula's position may push the bevel of the cannula against or away from the wall of the vein. Special precautions should be taken to prevent speed shock or overloading of the vascular system by making sure that the solution is flowing freely before adjusting the rate.

Other Changes

Stimulation of the vasoconstrictors from any infusion of cold blood or irritating solution may cause venous spasm, impeding the rate of flow. A warm pack placed on the vein proximal to the infusion cannula will offset this reaction.

Trauma to the Vein

Any injury, such as phlebitis or thrombosis, that reduces the lumen of the vein will decrease the flow of the solution.

Clogged Vent

A clogged air vent in the administration set used with air-dependent containers will cause the infusion to stop.

If there is any question as to the rate of administration, the nurse should check with the physician. This applies to IV administration of drugs in solution. The rates should also be established on patients receiving two or more infusions simultaneously. Any change in the rate from that normally used should be ordered by the attending physician.

The nurse should never exert positive pressure (manual pressure) to infuse solutions or blood.

REFERENCE

1. Metheny, N. M. (1992). *Fluid and electrolyte balance* (2nd ed., pp 22–23). Philadelphia: J. B. Lippincott.

2. *Revised intravenous nursing standards of practice.* (1990). *Journal of Intravenous Nursing.* (Suppl.), S58.

BIBLIOGRAPHY

Barsan, W. G., Hedges, J. R., Nishiyama, H., et al. (1986). Differences in drug delivery with peripheral and central venous injections: Normal perfusion. *American Journal of Emergency Medicine,* 4(1), 1–3.

Trissel, L. A. (1988). *Handbook on injectable drugs* (5th ed.). Bethesda, MD: American Society of Hospital Pharmacists.

Weinstein, S. M. (1990). Math calculations for intravenous nurses. *Journal of Intravenous Nursing,* 13(4), 231–236.

Weinstein, S. M. (1991). *Nurses' handbook of intravenous medications.* Philadelphia: J. B. Lippincott.

REVIEW QUESTIONS

1. The usual infusion rate for maintenance and replacement of fluids is how many mL/m^2 body surfate per minute?
   a. 2
   b. 3
   c. 4
   d. 5

2. The most commonly occurring danger of too rapid infusion of fluid is which of the following?
   a. congestive heart failure
   b. pulmonary edema
   c. water intoxication
   d. circulatory overload

3. Which of the following factors affect flow rate?
   a. height of container
   b. change in position of needle
   c. trauma to vein
   d. temperature of solution

4. Glucose has what type of effect when infused too rapidly?
   a. diuretic
   b. hypotonic
   c. dehydrating
   d. osmotic

5. Which of the following provides a guide for determining the amount of fluids and electrolytes needed?
   a. body weight
   b. height
   c. body surface area
   d. degree of hydration

6. Kidney status must be determined before administration of which of the following?
   a. sodium
   b. calcium
   c. phosphate
   d. potassium

7. Administration of which of the following solutions provides sedation?
   a. invert sugar
   b. 5% alcohol
   c. 5% ammonium chloride
   d. 0.45% sodium chloride

8. An administration set that delivers 60 gtt/mL delivers how many mL/min?
   a. 10
   b. 12
   c. 15
   d. 60

9. Decreased rate of flow may be caused by:
   a. phlebitis
   b. thrombosis
   c. infection
   d. clogged air vent

10. Factors that influence the rate of flow include:
   a. surface area of body
   b. clinical condition
   c. composition of fluid
   d. age of the patient

Central Venous Catheterization

Advantages of central venous catheterization include (1) placement, usually by percutaneous puncture; (2) a lower risk of infection; and (3) catheter tip placement in the superior vena cava.

The tip placement allows for rapid dilution of the infusate, thus reducing the risk of phlebitis and vein sclerosis. The tip placement also allows for monitoring central venous pressure.

VASCULAR ANATOMY _____

A review of the vascular system is essential in providing care to the patient with central venous access. Vessels involved include the cephalic, basilic, axillary, jugular, subclavian, and innominate veins as well as the superior vena cava (Figures 14-1 and 14-2).

The Cephalic Vein

The cephalic vein ascends along the outer border of the biceps muscle to the upper third of the arm. It passes in the space between the pectoralis major and deltoid muscles. It terminates in the axillary vein, with a descending curve, just below the clavicle.

The cephalic vein is occasionally connected with the external jugular or subclavian vein by a branch that passes from it upward in front of the clavicle.[3]

The Basilic Vein

The basilic vein is larger than the cephalic. It passes upward in a smooth path along the inner side of the biceps muscle and terminates in the axillary vein.[3]

The Axillary Vein

The axillary vein starts upward as a continuation of the basilic vein, increasing in size as it ascends. It receives the cephalic vein and terminates immediately beneath the clavicle, at the outer border of the first rib. At this point it becomes the subclavian vein.[3]

The External Jugular Vein

The external jugular vein is easily recognized on the side of the neck. It follows a descending inward path to join the subclavian vein above the middle of the clavicle.[3]

Sharon M. Weinstein: PLUMER'S PRINCIPLES & PRACTICE OF INTRAVENOUS THERAPY, FIFTH EDITION, © 1993 J. B. Lippincott Company

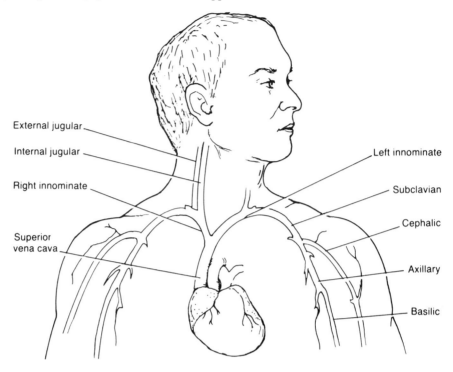

FIGURE 14-1 Central venous catheters are inserted through the subclavian and internal or external jugular veins.

The Internal Jugular Vein

The internal jugular vein descends first behind and then to the outer side of the internal and common carotid arteries. The carotid plexus is situated on the outer side of the internal carotid artery. The internal jugular vein joins the subclavian vein at the root of the neck. At the angle of junction, the left subclavian receives the thoracic duct while the right subclavian receives the right lymphatic duct.[3]

The Subclavian Vein

The subclavian vein, a continuation of the axillary, extends from the outer edge of the first rib to the inner end of the clavicle, where it unites with the internal jugular to form the innominate vein.

Valves are present in the venous system until approximately an inch before the formation of the innominate vein.[3]

The Right Innominate Vein

The right innominate vein is about an inch long. It passes almost vertically downward and joins the left innominate just below the cartilage of the first rib.[3]

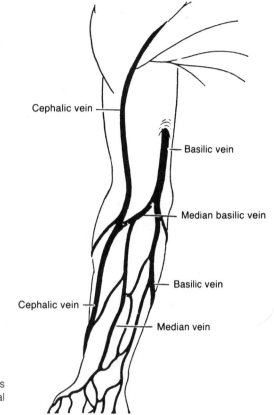

Cephalic vein

Basilic vein

Median basilic vein

Basilic vein

Cephalic vein

Median vein

FIGURE 14-2 The cephalic and basilic veins are used for peripheral insertion of central venous catheters.

The Left Innominate Vein

The left innominate vein is about 2.5 inches in length and larger than the right. It passes from left to right across the upper front chest, in a downward slant. It joins the right innominate to form the superior vena cava.[3]

The Superior Vena Cava

The superior vena cava receives all blood from the upper half of the body. It is comprised of a short trunk 2.5 to 3 inches in length. It begins below the first rib close to the sternum on the right side, descends vertically slightly to the right, and empties into the right atrium of the heart.[3]

CENTRAL VENOUS PRESSURE

Peripheral insertions of central venous catheters were first used for monitoring *central venous pressure*, which denotes the pressure in the right atrium or vena cava of the venous blood as it returns from all parts of the body. The pressure varies among individuals, usually ranging between 4 and 11 cm H_2O in the vena cava; the pressure in the right atrium is usually 0 to 4 cm H_2O.[6] The normal range has little significance because the true value lies in the change or lack of change after attempts to alter the blood volume or to improve cardiac action. Because central venous pressure relates to a fully sufficient circulation, it facilitates assessment of both the blood volume and the ability of the heart to tolerate an increased volume, thereby providing a valuable guide for fluid administration. It requires no laboratory personnel and no expensive equipment; it is simple in technique; and, once set up, it may be monitored quickly and as often as required.

Because central venous pressure relates to an adequate circulatory blood volume, it depends on:[6]

1. Blood volume
2. Status of the myocardium
3. Vascular tone

Circulatory failure may result from deficiency in any one or a combination of these essential factors.

Blood Volume

Changes in blood volume alter the tone of the blood vessels and the ability of the heart to circulate the blood. A reduced blood volume results in less pressure at the right atrium, indicated by a drop in central venous pressure; an increased blood volume produces more pressure at the atrium, with a rise in central venous pressure.[6]

In managing an inadequate circulation, one must first establish a normal blood volume. If the inadequate circulation is due to deficiency in the blood volume, manipulation is made by administering expanders, or in the case of increased volume, phlebotomy.

If the circulation still remains insufficient, it becomes necessary to look at the remaining two essential components—status of the myocardium and vascular tone.

Status of the Myocardium

The myocardial status may be affected by disease, drugs, fluids, or anesthesia. Because the central venous pressure is a measure of the capacity of the myocardium as well as the blood volume, it is invaluable in monitoring the effects of anesthesia and surgery on elderly patients with arteriosclerosis or patients with myocardial insufficiency. The central venous pressure rises if the heart muscle is impaired—the pressure of the volume of blood at the heart increases because the heart muscle is no longer able to pump an adequate flow of blood out of the right atrium.[6] A high central venous pressure may suggest cardiac failure.[6] This is one of the most common causes of an elevated central venous pressure in shock.

Drugs or chemicals are administered to improve myocardial response, thus increasing cardiac output and lowering the central venous pressure.

Vascular Tone

The third essential component, the vascular tone, depends on the arterial pressure and on external and internal pressures on the veins. The arterial pressure arises from the contractile force of the left ventricle and is transmitted through the capillaries to the veins.

The external pressures on the vein result from the muscular and fascial pumping action in the extremities, the intra-abdominal pressure from straining and distention, and the intrathoracic pressure from contraction of the diaphragm and chest wall. Central venous pressure of patients on positive-pressure respirators is usually increased by 4 cm; patients on negative pressure show a decreased central venous pressure.[7]

The internal pressure on the veins is caused by the blood volume, myocardial response, and sympathomimetic amines (epinephrine, norepinephrine). By stimulating contraction of the venous wall, vasopressors decrease the capacity of the venous system and improve vascular tone.

Clinical Applications

Hypotension
The parameters used in evaluating a patient in shock consist of:

1. Blood pressure
2. Rate and quality of pulse
3. Skin temperature and color
4. Urinary output
5. Peripheral venous filling
6. Blood pH

Blood Volume
Prolonged hypovolemia may cause poor tissue perfusion with the inherent risk of renal and myocardial complication; uncorrected hypovolemia can eventually lead to shock and death. Blood volume is not necessarily reflected by the blood pressure. In cardiogenic shock, the blood volume is increased and the blood pressure is low. In septic shock, hypotension accompanies a normal blood volume.

Various methods are used to detect change in a patient's blood volume: hematocrit, change in patient's weight, and blood volume computations. Central venous pressure is a parameter used to assess blood volume. It is an important guide during the following:

1. *Surgery,* when there is a risk of overloading an anesthetized, traumatized patient who is continuously losing blood
2. *Shock,* when origin is unknown
3. *Massive fluid replacement* in open heart surgery and in critical cases, such as severely burned patients, where circulatory overload is a hazard
4. *Anuria* or *oliguria,* when questionable cause is dehydration

Total Parenteral Nutrition
Subclavian insertions were first used for administration of total parenteral nutrition. This subject is thoroughly discussed in Chapter 20.

Cancer Therapy
With the advent of tunneling techniques, antithrombogenic catheter materials, new device designs, and lowered infection rates, central venous catheters became popular for many other uses. The administration of long-term antineoplastic agents, blood or blood components, and antibiotics, as well as venous sampling, is frequently done with a central catheter device in cancer patients.

Limited Venous Access
In any hospital patient requiring a venous access whose peripheral veins cannot be cannulated, a long-term catheter may be used.

Home Intravenous Therapy
Many home patients have been taught to self-administer their continuous or intermittent medications through a central device.

CENTRAL VENOUS PRESSURE MONITORING

Central venous pressure monitoring is achieved by attaching an IV set to a three-way stopcock and to an extension tube with a radiopaque catheter of approximately 24 inches. A vertical length of infusion tubing that serves as the manometer is connected to the stopcock and attached to the IV stand against a marked centimeter tape. Central venous pressure sets are available with disposable water manometers, graduated in units. The zero mark on the tape is adjusted to the level of the patient's right atrium (Figure 14-3). The pressure is measured at either the superior vena cava by introducing the catheter through the antecubital, jugular, or subclavian vein, or at the inferior vena cava through the femoral vein.

The superior vena cava is most commonly used. Complications have been associated with inferior vena caval catheters. Use of the femoral vein and the long duration of time the catheter is in the vein enhance the risk of thrombotic complications. A second disadvantage is the fact that abdominal distention interferes with monitoring an accurate right atrial pressure.

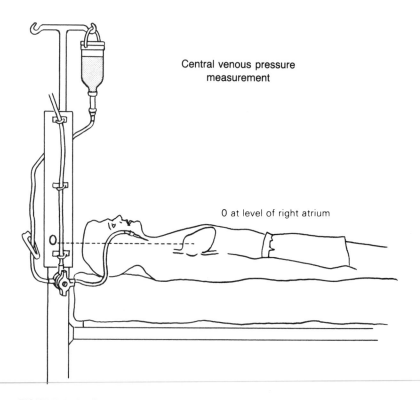

Central venous pressure
measurement

0 at level of right atrium

FIGURE 14-3 Central venous pressure measurement with zero point of manometer at level of right atrium. (From Metheny, N. M. [1992]. *Fluid and electrolyte balance* [p. 26]. Philadelphia: J. B. Lippincott.)

Equipment

With a central venous catheter in place, the following equipment is needed for monitoring central venous pressure:

IV pole

Solution as ordered

IV or transfusion tubing

Central venous manometer set

Venous pressure level (optional)

Armboard with cover

Adhesive tape

Procedure

Connecting pressure manometer to central venous catheter.

1. Wash hands thoroughly and dry.
2. Close three-way stopcock.
3. Hold and squeeze drip chamber while inserting tubing spike into upright bottle or hanging plastic bag. The use of a tubing with a Luer lock connector will aid in the prevention of a connection separation, which could result in an air embolism.
4. Release squeeze, allowing drip chamber to fill one-quarter to one-third full. Prefilling drip chamber prevents air bubbles from entering the system.
5. If the manometer is to be permanently attached to the IV pole, tape centimeter strip onto IV pole with zero point adjusted to the midatrial level. Patient should be in a supine position with the bed flat. Use venous pressure level for accuracy. Midatrial level is at a point approximately equidistant from the sternum and the back. Tape stopcock to pole at a level below patient's right atrium. Do not tape directly on the stopcock. Tape upper end of manometer taut to IV pole.

    If the manometer contains clips and will be removed for each reading, secure manometer to IV pole. When this type of manometer is used, placing a waterproof "X" on the side of the patient's chest at midatrial level will ensure that all readings are taken with zero point at the same level.
6. Adjust stopcock to allow solution to flow into manometer, filling it halfway.
7. Adjust stopcock to flush remainder of tubing.
8. Connect manometer system to central venous catheter.
    a. Use strict aseptic techniques while disconnecting present IV system and connecting manometer system.
    b. Be sure to use air embolism precautions when the catheter is open to air (see air embolism, under the Complications section of this chapter).
    c. Secure catheter hub–tubing connection with tape to aid in prevention of connection separation.
    d. Secure arm to covered armboard. Motion of catheter on flexion of the arm increases the potential risk of phlebitis. A kinked catheter results in unreliable readings and leads to clogging of the lumen.

Central Venous Pressure Measurement

The pressure is usually read at half-hour or hourly intervals. The patient must be quiet, not coughing or straining, and in a supine position with the zero point on the manometer at the midatrial level. The procedure is as follows:

1. Turn stopcock so solution flows from the container to the manometer.
2. When manometer level reaches 30 cm, turn stopcock to stop flow from the container and direct manometer flow to the patient.
3. The fluid level will drop rapidly, reaching the reading level in about 15 seconds. The central venous pressure is measured at the high point of the fluctuation.
4. Readjust the stopcock so the infusion resumes.
5. Document readings.

The catheter is presumed to be in the thoracic cavity when manometer fluid fluctuates 3 to 5 cm during breathing, and coughing and straining cause the column of water to rise. If the catheter is inserted too far and reaches the heart, higher pressure waves synchronous with the pulse will be seen.[6,8]

PATIENT PREPARATION

To allay fears and to obtain patient cooperation, explain the reasons for the insertion and the procedure.

Position During Insertion

If a subclavian entry is to be used, explain to the patient that he or she will be positioned flat in bed with the head lowered and knees bent, to increase the blood supply to the vein, and that a rolled towel will be placed under the back between the shoulder blades to make it easier for the physician to enter the vein. Prior explanation will obtain patient cooperation when the uncomfortable position must be maintained.

Gowns and Masks

Explaining that the nurse and the physician will both wear gowns and masks to keep normal bacteria away from the area will allay apprehension. If the patient will be required to wear a mask, having him or her wear one before the procedure will give reassurance that a mask does not really interfere with breathing.

The Valsalva Maneuver

Practicing the Valsalva maneuver before the insertion will obtain patient cooperation when he or she is asked to hold the breath and "bear down" at the time the catheter is open to the air.

Becoming Acquainted with the Device

If a tunneled catheter or implanted venous access or pump device is being inserted, seeing and touching the device that will remain in their bodies is reassuring to most patients. Any limitations of activity the device will create should be thoroughly discussed. If the patient will be required to give any self-care, this should be completely explained and agreed to by the patient before insertion.

Consent Form

A patient consent form must be signed before any central venous catheter or device insertion.

Blood Studies

Preinsertion blood studies include platelet count, prothrombin time (PT), and partial thromboplastin time (PTT). Any abnormal result may require correction with vitamin K, fresh frozen plasma, or platelet concentrates before insertion is attempted.

Premedication

Depending on the type of device, insertion site, and individual patient needs, some form of sedation may be required before the procedure. This should be explained to the patient.

CENTRAL VENOUS CANNULATION

Any central venous catheter has its inherent risks. *If peripheral veins are obtainable and adequate for the desired treatment, a central venous catheter should not be inserted.*

Contraindications

Contraindications for any type of central venous catheter insertion may include:

1. Abnormal coagulation studies
2. Septicemia
3. Anomalies of the central venous vascular structures
4. Thrombosis of the innominate or subclavian veins, or of the superior vena cava
5. Superior vena cava syndrome

Catheter Tip Placement

The preferred tip placement is usually at the junction of the superior vena cava and the right atrium. If the tip lies in the right atrium, atrial arrhythmias may occur as a result of catheter irritation. For various reasons it is not always possible to advance the catheter far enough to achieve the desired tip location. Depending on the specific purpose of the catheter, innominate or subclavian catheter tip placement may be adequate.

Infection Control

Aseptic technique will minimize the risk of infection in the patient in whom a central line is to be placed. If the patient cannot be masked during the procedure, the head should be turned away from the insertion area. The skin should be cleansed consistent with institutional policy and Centers for Disease Control and Prevention (CDC) and Intravenous Nurses Society (INS) guidelines. Determine the type of catheter material before the use of acetone for defatting the skin; materials such as Silastic are often eroded by contact with acetone solutions.[5] Dress the site in the usual manner and provide catheter maintenance consistent with institutional policy.

Air Embolism Precautions

The risk of air embolism is ever present during catheter insertion because central venous pressure can be negative. Placing the patient in Trendelenburg position will increase the pressure. If possible, the patient should perform the Valsalva maneuver whenever the catheter is opened to the air.[2] If the catheter stylet has been removed, the hub should be occluded with either a syringe or the gloved finger to prevent air entry.

Patient Positioning

During a central venous catheter insertion, the patient is placed in Trendelenburg position. This not only increases central venous pressure, but it also distends the vein and facilitates entry. When the subclavian approach is used, a rolled towel is placed along the spinal cord to hyperextend the neck and elevate the clavicle. For the jugular approach, the head is turned to the opposite direction and extended. This stretches and stabilizes the vein and accentuates the muscular landmarks. During a cephalic or brachial insertion, abduction of the arm may be required to pass the catheter past the shoulder area.

INSERTION SITES

There are basically three approaches for central venous catheter insertions. The veins used for entry are the subclavian and the internal or external jugular veins for central insertion, and the cephalic or basilic vein for peripheral insertion.

CENTRAL INSERTION

The subclavian vein is frequently the entry of choice. It requires the shortest length catheter because it uses the most central veins, thus creating a high blood flow around a large portion of the catheter. This results in minimal catheter irritation or obstruction. All these factors lower the risk of complications, resulting in a longer catheter life.

Subclavian Vein

A subclavian entry is a medical act; major complications can occur during or from this insertion. (See Complications section of this chapter.)

The subclavian entry may be performed by the infraclavicular or the supraclavicular approach. In both approaches, the cannula is inserted under the clavicle, aiming for the jugular notch. For the infraclavicular approach, the cannula is inserted at approximately the midpoint of the clavicle. For the supraclavicular approach, the cannula is frequently inserted at the base of the triangle formed by the sternal and clavicular heads of the sternocleidomastoid muscle.

Contraindications
Contraindications for the subclavian approach may include:
1. Radiation burns at intended insertion site
2. Fractured clavicle
3. Hyperinflated lungs
4. Malignancy at the base of the neck or apex of the lungs

Internal Jugular Vein

The insertion of central venous catheters into the internal jugular vein is usually a medical act. Many physicians select the internal jugular vein as a first choice of site for the insertion of a central venous catheter.

The constant anatomic location of the internal jugular vein makes its cannulation easier than that of the subclavian vein. The right internal jugular vein is usually chosen because it forms a straighter, shorter line to the superior vena cava. It also avoids the higher left pleura and thoracic duct. This insertion is frequently performed by first locating the vein with a small-gauge needle. After making a small skin incision to facilitate entry, a larger-gauge cannula is inserted, following the same direction as the locator needle, aiming for the ipsilateral nipple.

External Jugular Vein

The external jugular vein is observable and easily entered. Insertion complications are rare, so cannulation can be performed by specialty nurses.

The external jugular vein varies in size and its junction with the subclavian vein is acutely angulated. It contains two pairs of valves. The uppermost pair are 4 cm above the clavicle, the lower pair are located at the vein's entrance to the subclavian vein. Because of these factors, central cannulation can be difficult. Because a short cannula may be easily inserted, central cannulation may be achieved by the use of an introducer with a guidewire. Entry into the superficial vein is performed by directing the cannula toward the ipsilateral nipple.

Objections to Jugular Insertions

The main objections to any jugular cannulation are:

1. *Catheter occlusion* is a persistent problem as a result of head movement.
2. *Vein irritation* is created by the same movements. These factors result in a *shorter catheter life*.
3. It is *difficult to maintain an intact dressing* on the area.
4. The idea of having a catheter in the neck is *esthetically and psychologically disturbing* to many patients and families.

PERIPHERALLY INSERTED CENTRAL CATHETERS

Technology has kept pace with our demands for more sophisticated, long-term peripheral venous access devices. The peripherally inserted central catheter (PICC) line was the first product developed specifically for this clinical application. Examples of PICC lines are shown in Figures 14-4 and 14-5.

Vein Selection

The *basilic vein* is usually the first choice for the peripheral insertion of a central venous catheter. It ascends obliquely in the groove between the biceps brachii and pronator teres and perforates the deep fascia slightly distal to the middle of the upper arm. With the arm held at a 90° angle, it forms the straightest, most direct route into the central venous system.

The *median cubital vein* is the second choice. Ascending on the ulnar side of the forearm, it may be divided into two vessels, one joining the basilic vein and the other the cephalic vein. This vein varies substantially, and the proper branch must be ascertained before venipuncture for PICC placement. The median antecubital basilic is preferred.

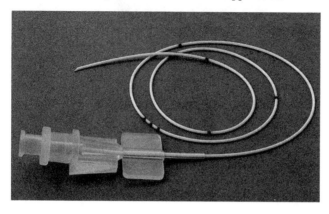

FIGURE 14-4 Lifevac PIC Catheter (Courtesy: Vygon Corporation, East Rutherford, NJ)

The *cephalic vein* runs proximally along the lateral side of the antecubital fossa in the groove between the brachioradialis and the bicep brachii. It becomes a deep vein at the clavipectoral fascia, ending in the axillary vein immediately caudal to the clavicle. It is much more tortuous than the basilic vein and presents a greater potential for catheter tip malposition. It is not preferred because it may also be difficult to thread.

Indications

Placement of a PICC has met with widespread acceptance in the nursing and medical communities. Indications for placement include:

1. Lack of peripheral venous access
2. Infusion of vesicant or irritant drugs
3. Infusion of hyperosmolar drugs
4. Long-term venous access
5. Infusion of antineoplastics agents, blood, or blood components
6. Patient preference
7. Clinician preference

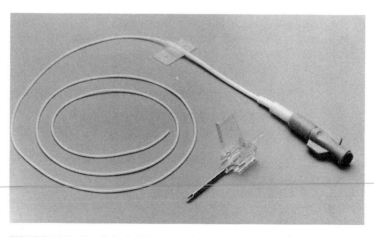

FIGURE 14-5 Per-Q-Cath (Courtesy: Gesco International, San Antonio, TX)

Advantages

The PICC catheter has many advantages over the short-term peripheral catheter and the centrally placed line, including:

1. Elimination or risks associated with central venous catheter placement
2. Potential reduction of catheter sepsis
3. Ease of use
4. Preservation of the peripheral vascular system
5. Decrease in discomfort
6. Reliability

Tip Placement

Placement of a PICC may be in either the superior vena cava, providing a true central line access, and in the axillary or subclavian vein. The physical landmark used for the axillary or subclavian vein is approximately an inch distal from the head of the clavicle.

Superior Vena Cava Tip Placement

This type of placement is preferred for all antineoplastic agents, administration of vesicants, total parenteral nutrition with a final dextrose concentration in excess of 20%, and any sclerosing agents. Measurement for tip placement is from the point of insertion, along the proposed vein track to the third intercostal space.

Subclavian Tip Placement

Subclavian placement is often used for the diversity of IV therapies administered through a conventional short cannula. Measurement of tip placement is from the point of insertion, along the proposed vein track to 1 inch distal to the sternal notch. At this point, the catheter tip should be seated in the median segment of the subclavian vein 2 to 3 cm distal to the junction of the external jugular vein.

Procedure

A physician's order is needed before placement of a PICC line. The patient should be assessed for available venous access, clinical condition, and ability to learn procedures applicable to maintenance.

1. Assemble all supplies/tray (Figure 14-6).
2. Wash hands.
3. Place patient in a supine position with the arm to be accessed extended at 90° to the patient's trunk.
4. Place a tourniquet firmly around the mid upper arm to access insertion site. After selecting the vein, release the tourniquet.
5. Measure the distance from the insertion site to the catheter tip termination point.
6. Open the insertion tray and establish working area.
   a. Drop sterile product onto tray.
   b. Apply first pair of gloves.
   c. Remove items from tray and place them on the sterile field.

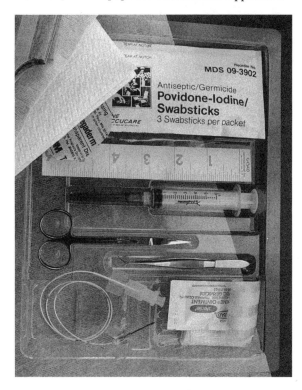

FIGURE 14-6 Per-Q-Cath tray (Courtesy: Gesco International, San Antonio, TX)

7. Prep the site in a 3-inch concentric circle consistent with institutional guidelines and INS Standards of Practice.
8. Drape the patient's arm with the fenestrated drape provided.
9. Prepare the catheter and related items.
   a. Fill a 5-mL syringe with normal saline for injection from the previously prepped vial.
   b. Attach the injection cap to the extension set and prime.
   c. Stretch out the sterile tape measure and place the catheter beside it.
   d. If a guidewire is provided, pull it back beyond the point where trimming will be needed.
   e. Using sterile scissors, trim the catheter at a 45° angle.
   f. Advance the guidewire until it extends 1/4 to 1/2 inch from the tip of the catheter.
   g. At the hub of the catheter, bend the guidewire at a 90° angle to prevent it from advancing beyond the end of the catheter.
   h. Pass the catheter through the introducer needle to the tip of the needle.
   i. Remove the catheter from the needle and loosely attach a syringe; pull back 2 to 3 mL to secure a flush chamber.
10. Administer lidocaine hydrochloride 1% without epinephrine intradermally (optional).
11. Reapply tourniquet.
12. Remove contaminated gloves and reglove.
13. Place a sterile 4 × 4 gauze over the tails of the tourniquet to allow release following successful cannulation.

14. Move the catheter, introducer needle and syringe, and sterile forceps to a point near the intended insertion site.
15. Stabilize the vein below the insertion site and perform venipuncture using shallow angle (Figure 14-7). Following blood return, lower the needle until it is parallel to the vein and advance the introducer needle approximately 1/4 inch to ensure that the entire lumen is well within the wall of the vein.
16. Release the tourniquet, stabilize the introducer needle, and remove the syringe.
17. Remove the introducer needle.
    a. Hold catheter with forceps 1 1/2 inch behind the introducer.
    b. Pull needle along the catheter and out of the insertion site.
    c. Stabilize the catheter at insertion site and pull needle back to the hub of the catheter.
    d. Press wings together and grasp each wing, pulling apart (Figure 14-8).
18. Advance the catheter (guidewire may remain in place for deep peripheral tip placement). If guidewire is removed, attach a syringe of normal saline to the catheter and flush gently.
19. Advance to premeasured length, remove guidewire if needed, and attach extension tubing and injection cap.
20. Check for blood return and establish ease of flushing.
21. Place a steri-strip across the wings to provide stability.
22. Cleanse site, apply skin protectant and place a folded 2 × 2 gauze above the insertion site.
23. Apply transparent dressing (Figure 14-9).
24. Heparinize catheter consistent with manufacturer's recommendations.

Alternatives to Guidewire Technique

Breakaway needle involves venipuncture made with an introducer needle. The catheter, with or without a guidewire, is threaded through the introducer. The introducer is removed from the venipuncture site, broken in half, and peeled away.

Cannula technique involves use of an introducer needle to place a plastic cannula (peel-away sheath) into the vein. The catheter is then threaded through this sheath. The sheath is removed from the insertion site and peeled away from the catheter.

Assess line for evidence of redness, edema, pain, drainage, and a palpable venous cord. Postinsertion complications include:

- Bleeding (unusual after 24 hours)
- Phlebitis
- Cellulitis (tends to spread in a diffuse circular pattern into surrounding tissue)
- Catheter sepsis

Postinsertion Care

A chest x-ray is always done immediately after catheter insertion to rule out pneumothorax and to document tip placement. An isotonic solution is infused until tip placement is confirmed (Table 14-1). The site should be observed for any signs of excess bleeding or swelling. The patient's breathing should be monitored for any signs of respiratory distress. Any unexpected observation should be reported to the physician immediately.

Complications associated with central line placement also apply.

(text continues on page 198)

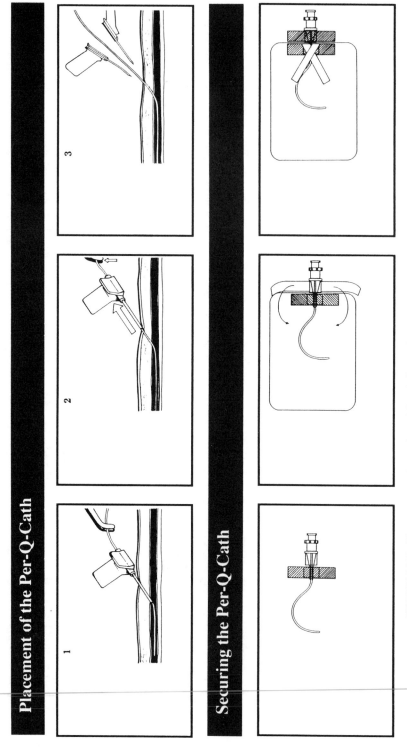

FIGURE 14-7 Placement and securing of Per-Q-Cath. (Courtesy: Gesco International, San Antonio, TX)

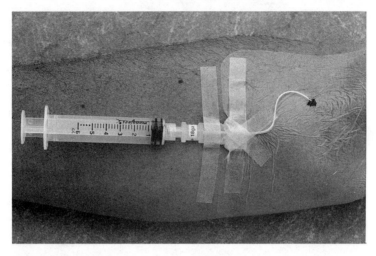

FIGURE 14-8   Transparent dressing applied to PICC insertion site. (Courtesy: Gesco International, San Antonio, TX)

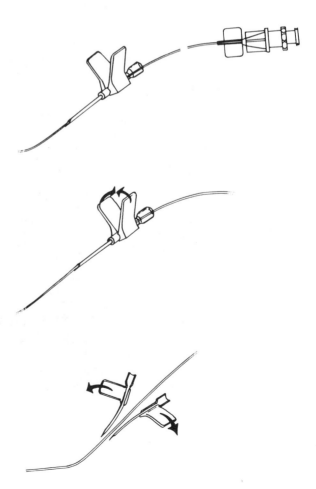

FIGURE 14-9   Breakaway needle design. (Courtesy: Gesco International, San Antonio, TX)

TABLE 14-1
Radiographic Technique for Visualizing the PER-Q-CATH®

The following technique has been found extremely effective in visualizing PER-Q-CATH catheters when verifying placement. (It may be important, since these catheters are not well known in the radiology department, to be sure that they are aware of where the catheter was inserted, the approximate size of the catheter, the proposed route taken, and where you expect the tip to be placed.)

Adult

A 14 × 14 cassette is used with a MR-400 screen and a Bucky tray grid. The KV is increased by 5–10 over the normal shoulder technique. A portable may be done except that definition on film will be compromised. A normal anterior–posterior shoulder position is used but with centering done more toward the sternal area. This position allows visualization of the catheter along the length of the arm, across the axillary and subclavian veins and into the superior vena cava.

Visualization is further enhanced by the use of a 10°–15° oblique angle. In this situation, it does not matter if the oblique is to the right or the left. The result of this procedure is that the catheter tip will be shifted from the mediastinal area into the darkened lung field thereby making tip visualization much easier.

Basic settings for the equipment are as follows:
AVERAGE MALE:
65–75 KV   100 MAS 0.5–1.0 Seconds
AVERAGE FEMALE:
54–65 KV   100 MAS 0.2–0.5 Seconds

Slight adjustments may have to be made depending on the equipment you have, but this will give a beginning reference point.

Pediatric and Neonate

A rib visualization technique is used with a medium to fast screen (a fast screen will give less patient exposure but also less detail). A Kodak O.G., PMG high contrast, or TMG film is used. A KV of 50–60 and setting of 1.0 to 1.5 MAS with a distance of 36–40 inches (the distance may need to be reduced to 30 inches due to the use of overhead warmers).

Contrast Media

If the use of contrast media is felt to be necessary, some feel it could expose the patient to the risk of an adverse reaction. The use of water-soluble radiographic contrast medium containing iohexol may be indicated. This type of contrast solution has shown a lower incidence of adverse reaction. However, due to the PER-Q-CATH's small priming volume, the use of iodized contrast medium (ie, Conray 60, Renografin 60, etc.) may also provide minimal risk of adverse reaction, at a significant reduction in cost. Also, be aware that this exceptionally small amount of media can also be aspirated out of the catheter after the X-ray is taken.

The "Silastic" catheter should never be used for high pressure injection, that is, diagnostic procedure. Be sure that the Radiology Department is aware of the volume of the catheter used so the amount of contrast media infused is not excessive.

(Courtesy: GESCO International, San Antonio, TX.)

PERIPHERAL PORT

The Port-A-Cath® P.A.S. PORT® FLUORO-FREE® Implantable Access System is designed to permit repeated access to the venous system (Figure 14-10). Consisting of a portal with a self-sealing septum, accessible by percutaneous needle puncture, and a catheter for the parenteral delivery of medications and fluids, its use is indicated when patient therapy requires repeated venous access.

Assessment

Before placement, the patient's anatomy should be accessed for evidence of prior trauma to the veins or anatomic irregularities.

Following placement, take these precautions:

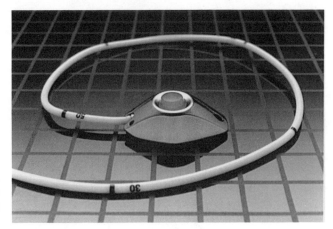

FIGURE 14-10 P.A.S. PORT® Peripheral Venous Access System (Property of Pharmacia Deltec Inc., St. Paul, MN)

1. Do not withdraw blood from or infuse medication into the arm in which the implanted system is placed without using the portal.
2. Do not attempt to measure blood pressure on this arm.

Potential Complications

Potential complications of the peripherally placed port include:

- Air embolism
- Artery or vein puncture
- Brachial plexus injury
- Cardiac arrhythmia
- Cardiac tamponade
- Cardiac puncture
- Catheter disconnection, fragmentation, embolization
- Catheter occlusion, rupture
- Drug extravasation
- Fibrin sheath formation at catheter tip
- Hematoma
- Hemothorax
- Implant rejection
- Infection
- Migration of portal/catheter
- Peripheral nerve damage
- Thoracic duct injury
- Thromboembolism
- Thrombophlebitis
- Thrombosis

System Components

Components include the portal with catheter connector, a 22-gauge PORT-A-CATH needle, one CATH-FINDER® catheter/sensor assembly (consisting of a sensor wire and radiopaque polyurethane catheter). The manufacturer cautions that the assembly must be used only with the Pharmacia Deltec CATH-FINDER Catheter Tracking System Correct placement is seen in Figure 14-11.

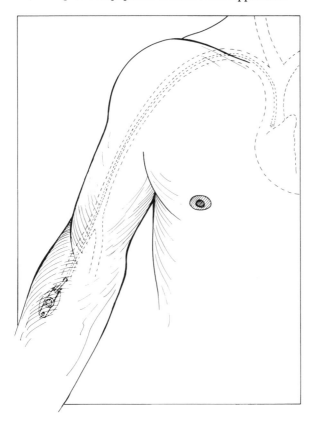

FIGURE 14-11 Placement of the P.A.S. PORT® Peripheral Venous Access System. (Property of Pharmacia Deltec Inc., St. Paul, MN)

Care and Maintenance

Care must be taken when administering fluid through the system because excessive pressure can be generated with all syringes. Pressure in excess of 40 psi may cause catheter rupture with possible embolization. As with any line, appropriate flushing procedures must be implemented to avoid incompatibility with heparin.

A syringe or IV administration set is attached to a 20- or 22-gauge PORT-A-CATH needle, and the needle is primed. The skin is prepped and punctured directly over the septum. Advance the needle slowly through the septum until it makes contact with the bottom of the portal chamber. Do not tilt or rock the needle. Flush with an appropriate solution and administer the injection or infusate. Flush again and administer 5 mL heparinized saline to establish patency. Maintain positive pressure when withdrawing the needle to avoid reflux of blood into the catheter.

COMPLICATIONS OF CENTRAL VENOUS CATHETERIZATION _____

Arterial Puncture

Arterial puncture, one of the most frequently reported complications of subclavian insertions, is usually not a major problem if it is recognized early. The puncture of an artery requires the immediate application of digital pressure for at least 5 minutes. If the patient has a coagulation abnormality, digital pressure must be maintained until all bleeding stops. If the artery puncture is not recognized and treated early, a massive hematoma resulting in tracheal compression or respiratory distress can occur.

Pneumothorax

Pneumothorax, another common complication of subclavian insertion, occurs as a result of pleural puncture; the patient may experience difficult breathing or chest pain. It can be asymptomatic and discovered by radiography. A chest tube may be required to treat the symptoms.

Hemothorax

Hemothorax may result if the subclavian or adjacent veins have been traumatized or transected during the insertion. Symptoms and treatment are the same as for pneumothorax.

Hydrothorax

Hydrothorax results when the IV fluid infiltrates into the chest. The symptoms and treatment are identical to a pneumothorax.

Catheter Embolism

Catheter embolism is always a risk whenever an inside-the-needle (INC) device is inserted or left in situ. During insertion, care must be taken NEVER to withdraw the catheter back through the needle. While the INC is in place, care must be taken to ensure that the needle tip is always protected with a secured tip cover. A severed catheter may require cardiac catheterization to retrieve the embolism. Breakaway needles minimize this hazard.

Air Embolism

Air embolism is always a potential danger whenever any central venous catheter is open to air. This can occur because it is always possible to have negative central venous pressure. During insertion, placing the patient in Trendelenburg position will increase central venous pressure. Placing the sterile gloved finger over the catheter hub, between catheter stylet removal and IV system connection, can prevent air from entering the catheter.

If the patient can cooperate, performing the Valsalva maneuver will increase central venous pressure. However, be sure that the patient takes the deep breath and bears down *before* the disconnection. Performing the disconnection while the patient is inhaling can *increase* the risk of air embolism. During tubing changes, the same precautions are necessary to prevent air embolism. Using junction securement devices can reduce the risk of tubing separations resulting in air embolism.[2, 4]

Air embolism precautions should be taken during catheter removal. The Valsalva maneuver should also be performed at this time. Positioning the patient flat in bed and, immediately on catheter removal, placing a sterile sponge with antimicrobial ointment directly over the puncture site will prevent air from entering the system. This dressing should be left intact for 24 to 48 hours to allow time for tissue healing.

Signs and symptoms of air embolism can include chest pain, dyspnea, hypoxia, apnea, tachycardia, hypotension, or a precordial murmur. Immediate treatment includes placing the patient in a supine position on the left side with the feet elevated. This position is used in an attempt to trap the air in the right atrium, where it can be aspirated with an intracardiac needle.

Catheter-Related Infection

Catheter-related infection is a serious complication of central venous catheters, occurring at the exit site, tunnel, or port pocket. The majority of steps taken in maintenance of the IV system and site are performed to prevent IV-related sepsis.

Whenever a patient with a central venous catheter has an unexpected fever spike, IV-related sepsis must be suspected. The insertion site should be carefully inspected for any signs of infection. A blood culture drawn through the catheter may be ordered. To rule out all sources of contamination, all tubings and containers should be changed immediately and sent promptly to bacteriology for culturing. A complete "fever work-up" must be done to rule out any other obvious source of infection. If the fever remains and no other possible source can be established, catheter removal may be necessary.

Some practitioners perform a catheter exchange with a guidewire. If the blood culture is positive or the semiquantitative culture of the catheter tip yields 15 or more colonies, the new catheter is removed and the patient is considered to have catheter sepsis. If both cultures are negative, then the catheter can be used despite the fever. If septic shock, shaking chills, recent positive blood cultures for *Staphylococcus* or *Candida*, or local infection of the catheter entry site is present, the catheter must be removed immediately.[9] In situ treatment of catheter-related sepsis with a combination of systemic antibiotics and local thrombolytic agents has been reported. Antibiotic lock technique has also been used[10] (See Chapter 10).

Of primary importance in the prevention of IV-related infection is maintaining strict aseptic techniques during insertion, admixture, any line manipulations, and aseptically performing recommended site dressing and tubing changes.

Deep-Vein Thrombosis

Deep-vein thrombosis is not as common with the new catheter materials. The addition of 1000 U heparin per liter of infusate has been recommended as a preventive measure.[9] Thrombosis may be present without any symptoms. Arm and neck pain may suggest the diagnosis. A venogram may be necessary to establish the diagnosis. Signs and symptoms of pulmonary embolism in a patient with a central venous catheter strongly suggests deep-vein thrombosis. Treatment consists of thrombolytic therapy with streptokinase or urokinase.[9]

Thrombus Catheter Occlusion

Thrombus catheter occlusion used to be a frequent cause for catheter removal. A fibrin sheath forms, originating at the intimal injury, either where the catheter enters the vessel or where the catheter tip touches the intima. By 1 to 7 days, an unorganized, unendothelialized fibrin sleeve is apparent on venography.[11] This may result in only a withdrawal occlusion. In this case, it is impossible to withdraw a blood sample, but there is no difficulty with infusion. If there is little or no infusion flow, the patency of the catheter can be restored with the use of a thrombolytic agent. Small-dose vials are available for the declotting procedure.

Preparing the Solution

Urokinase 5000 IU is packaged in a two-chamber vial. The following steps are used to prepare the solution:

1. Remove protective cap and turn plunger–stopper a quarter turn, press to force diluent into lower chamber.
2. Roll and tilt to dissolve; avoid shaking solution.
3. Sterilize stopper top with alcohol.
4. Insert needle through the center of stopper until tip is barely visible. Invert vial and withdraw dose.

Declotting the Catheter

An aliquot of solution equal in volume to the luminal volume of the catheter is used for each injection. Catheter declotting, with urokinase, may be achieved by the following steps, wearing gloves:[1]

1. Using air embolism precautions, aseptically disconnect the IV tubing at the catheter hub and attach an empty 10-mL syringe.
2. Gently attempt to aspirate blood. If aspiration is not possible, remove the syringe.
3. Attach a 1-mL tuberculin syringe filled with prepared urokinase.
4. Slowly and gently inject amount equal to volume of catheter.
5. Remove syringe and connect empty 5-mL syringe.
6. Wait at least 5 minutes before attempting to aspirate drug and residual clot.
7. Repeat aspiration attempts every 5 minutes.
8. If the catheter cannot be opened within 30 minutes, cap the catheter and allow drug to remain for 30 to 60 minutes.
9. A second urokinase injection may be required and may be repeated as long as systemic thrombolysis is not induced.
10. When patency is restored, aspirate 4 to 5 mL blood to ensure removal of all drug and clot residual.
11. Remove blood-filled syringe and connect 10-mL syringe with 0.9% sodium chloride and gently flush to ensure patency.
12. Remove syringe and aseptically reconnect sterile IV tubing to catheter hub.

Care and Maintenance

Risks and complications associated with central venous catheterization may be reduced when a team of qualified nursing specialists assumes responsibility for assisting with insertions, maintaining lines, and providing ongoing IV care. Astute nursing assessment and a comprehensive understanding of the vascular access device (VAD) in place may avert complications such as dislodgement, migration, pinch-off syndrome, and skin erosion.

Electronic Infusion Devices

Electronic instrumentation should be used to maintain flow accuracy and catheter patency. The diversity of electronic infusion devices today ensures availability for patients with central venous access devices.

When a positive-pressure instrument is used, the pressure must not exceed that which is recommended for the type of catheter or electronic infusion device in use.

Catheter Clamps

Smooth-jaw clamps are used when tunneled silicone catheters are placed to prevent damage to the catheter material. Ideally, the clamp is applied to the distal two-thirds portion of the external catheter. If clamp damage should occur, catheter repair is easily facilitated in this area. Clamp sites should be alternated to prevent a weakened area on the catheter itself. Second generation Silastic catheters use integral, soft-jaw clamps.

Catheter Repair

A sterile repair kit, specific to the individual type of catheter, should be readily available. Repairing the external portion of a tunneled catheter is a sterile procedure requiring surgical gloves, mask, and cap. It may be performed by the following steps.

Equipment

Sterile repair kit containing (1) replacement silicone rubber segment with Luer lock connector, (2) silicone rubber splice sleeve, (3) splice segment, (4) Luer lock cap, (5) tube of medical adhesive, and (6) blunt 18-gauge needle.

Sterile drapes, gloves	Guarded hemostat
3-mL syringe	Tongue blade
4 × 4 inch sterile sponges	Povidone–iodine solution
Small beaker for alcohol	Alcohol
Scalpel blades	Heparin flush
Iris scissors	Tape

Procedure

1. Surgically prep catheter and create sterile field. Put on gloves.
2. Clean powder from gloves with 4 × 4 inch sponge and alcohol.
3. Load adhesive into syringe barrel, then insert plunger and attach blunted needle.
4. If catheter is not clamped, clamp with guarded hemostat near chest wall.
5. Cut off the existing damaged catheter 15 to 20 cm from chest wall.
6. Insert splice segment into lumen of catheter (lubricate with alcohol if necessary but be sure all alcohol is removed or evaporated before proceeding).
7. Trim repair segment to desired length and slip onto the splice segment protruding from the implanted catheter. Do not remove the larger splice sleeve loose mounted on the repair segment.

8. Inject adhesive on the outside of the tubing in the area of the splice segment and slide the larger splice sleeve over the area of the splice segment. Inject adhesive underneath each end of splice sleeve. Roll between fingers to extrude excess adhesive and wipe excess adhesive away.

9. A sterile field is no longer required. Splint the repaired joint by taping the area to a tongue blade.

10. Remove clamp and *gently* flush with heparin. Excessive pressure may rupture joint.

The catheter may be used for infusion after a few hours. The splint may be removed after 48 hours, when the joint will have achieved full mechanical strength.

Some manufacturers provide catheter repair kits that may be used to repair most catheters (Figure 14-12).

0.2-μm Air-Eliminating Filter

Taping a Luer lock air-eliminating filter directly to the catheter hub will reduce the risk of connection separation and air infusion that could result in a fatal embolism. If a separation occurs distal to the filter, this device will prevent air infusion and an inadvertent bleed. The 0.2-μm filter can also prevent any particulate matter, fungi, bacteria, and endotoxins from entering the system through the filter.

Intravenous Containers and Admixtures

All recommendations for peripheral containers or admixtures should be strictly adhered to for central catheter usage. To prevent risks of contamination, all manipulation for admixture and container changes must be performed with strict adherence to aseptic technique.

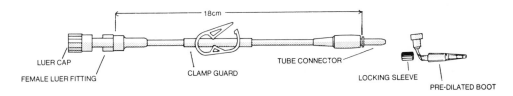

AS EASY AS 1...2...3

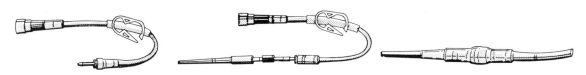

1. JUST SLIDE BOOT OVER CATHETER   2. SLIP SLEEVE INTO POSITION   3. SLIDE BOOT OVER SLEEVE AND CATHETER IS REPAIRED

FIGURE 14-12 Universal catheter repair kit. (Courtesy: GISH Biomedical, Inc., Santa Ana, CA). The Hemed™ catheter repair kit consists of a catheter repair assembly, boot dilator, and locking sleeve.

Tubing Changes

All tubings should be aseptically changed according to INS Standards of Practice.[4] It is extremely important to remember that there is always the possibility of negative pressure with a central catheter. Therefore, the risk of an air embolism is always present when the catheter is open to the air. If the patient cannot perform the Valsalva maneuver, consider using an extension tubing with a clamp that can be closed during the tubing change. Many practitioners use this system especially for critically ill patients. Care must be taken to maintain the sterility of the extension tubing during each IV tubing change. The extension tubing is changed at least weekly.

Between changes of components the system should be maintained as a closed system. All entries into the system should be made through injection ports that have been disinfected immediately before use.

Looping the tubing and taping it to the chest wall will prevent any related stress to the connection or insertion site when the tubing is pulled or inadvertently stretched. All connections should use junction securement devices or Luer locking connections, consistent with INS Standards of Practice.[4]

REFERENCES

1. Bjeletich, J. (1987). Declotting central venous catheters with urokinase in the home by nurse clinicians. *Journal of the National Intravenous Therapy Association, 10*(6), 428–430.
2. Coppa, G. F., Gouge, T. H., et al.(1981). Air embolism: A lethal but preventable complication of subclavian vein catheterization. *Journal of Parenteral and Enteral Nutrition, 5*, 166–168.
3. Gray, H. (1977). *Anatomy, descriptive and surgical* (Rev. American ed. from the 15th English ed.). New York: Crown.
4. *Revised intravenous nursing standards of practice.* (1990). *Journal of Intravenous Nursing,* (Suppl.). S45–48, S40.
5. Maki, D. G., & Band, J. D. (1981). A comparative study of polyantibiotic and iodophor ointments in prevention of vascular-catheter-related infection. *American Journal of Medicine, 70*, 739–744.
6. Metheny, N. M. (1992). *Fluid and electrolyte balance* (2nd ed., pp 25, 26). Philadelphia: J. B. Lippincott.
7. Hudak C., Gallo B., Benz J. (1990). *Critical care nursing.* (5th ed., p 123). Philadelphia: J. B. Lippincott.
8. Ryan, G. M., & Howland, W. S. (1966). An evaluation of central venous pressure monitoring. *Anesthesia and Analgesia, 45*, 754–759.
9. Ryan, J. A., Jr., & Gough, J. A. (1984). Complications of central venous catheterization for total parenteral nutrition. *Journal of the National Intravenous Therapy Association, 7*(1), 29–35.
10. Schuman, E. S., Winters V., Gross, G. F., and Hayes, J. F. (1985). Management of Hickman catheter sepsis. *American Journal of Surgery, 149*, 627.
11. Fischer, J. E. (1991). Total parenteral nutrition. (2nd ed., pp 36–37). Boston: Little Brown and Co.

BIBLIOGRAPHY

Bradham, G. B., & Walsh, N. (1965). Silastic for intravenous intubation. *Journal of S.L. Medical Association, 61*, 165.
Brendel, V. (1983). Current concepts in the care of central line catheters. *Journal of the National Intravenous Therapy Association, 6*, 272–274.
Camp-Sorrell, D. (1990). Advanced central venous access. *Journal of Intravenous Nursing, 6*, 361–365.
Gilligan, J. E., Phillips, P. J., et al.(1979). Streptokinase and blocked central venous catheter. *Lancet, 2*, 1189.
Hoshal, V. L. Jr., Ause, R. G., et al. (1971). Fibrin sleeve formation on indwelling subclavian central venous catheters. *Archives of Surgery, 102*, 353–358.
Hurtubise, M. R., Bottino, J. C., and Lawson, M. (1980). Restoring patency of occluded central venous catheters. *Archives of Surgery, 115*, 212–213.
Lindblad, B. (1982). Thromboembolic complications and central venous catheters (letter). *Lancet, 2*, 936.

Maki, D. G., Weise, C. E., and Sarafin, H. W. (1977). A semiquantitative culture method for identifying intravenous-catheter-related infection. *New England Journal of Medicine, 296*, 1305–1309.

Mansell, C. W. (1983). Peripherally inserted central venous catheterization by I.V. nurses: Establishing a precedent. *Journal of the National Intravenous Therapy Association, 6*, 355–356.

Nursing Photobook. (1980). *Managing I.V. Therapy.* Horsham, PA: Intermed Communications, Inc.

Ostrow, L. S. (1981). Air embolism and central venous lines. *American Journal of Nursing, 81*, 2036.

Peters, W. R., Bush, W. H., et al. (1973). The development of fibrin sheath on indwelling venous catheters. *Surgery, Gynecology and Obstetrics, 137*, 43–47.

Rubin, R. N. (1983). Local installation of small doses of streptokinase for treatment of thrombotic occlusions of long-term access catheters. *Journal of Clinical Oncology, 1*, 572.

Sriram, K., Kaminski, M. V., et al. (1982). A safe technique of central venous catheterization. *Journal of Parenteral and Enteral Nutrition, 6*, 245–248.

Stephens, W., & Lawler, W. (1982). Thrombus formation and central venous catheters. *Lancet, 2*, 664.

REVIEW QUESTIONS

1. The ideal tip location for a central venous catheter is which of the following?
   a. junction of superior vena cava and right atrium
   b. junction of inferior vena cava and right atrium
   c. in the right atrium
   d. in the internal jugular

2. When measuring central venous pressure, zero point on the manometer is adjusted to the level of:
   a. patient's heart
   b. right atrium
   c. left lung
   d. sternum

3. The vein of choice for insertion of a PICC is:
   a. basilic
   b. axillary
   c. median carpal
   d. innominate

4. The Valsalva maneuver is used to minimize the risk of:
   a. serratia
   b. air embolism
   c. septic shock
   d. speed shock

5. Clinical parameters used to evaluate a patient in shock include all of the following EXCEPT:
   a. blood pressure
   b. rate/quality of pulse
   c. temperature
   d. urinary output

6. Measurement of central venous pressure is an important guide during all of the following EXCEPT:
   a. surgery
   b. shock
   c. anuria
   d. polyuria

7. Alternatives to guidewire insertion technique for the PICC catheter include which of the following?
   a. laser
   b. breakaway needle
   c. cannula technique
   d. fluoro

8. All connections should use all of the following systems EXCEPT:
   a. taping
   b. junction securement
   c. Luer locking
   d. slide clamps

9. Repair of an external tunneled catheter is what type of procedure?
   a. clean
   b. sanitary
   c. sterile
   d. nonsterile

10 Main objections to jugular cannulation include all of the following EXCEPT:
   a. catheter occlusion
   b. vein irritation
   c. difficulty in assessing sterility
   d. difficulty in maintaining dressing

CHAPTER 15

Advanced Vascular Access

Vascular access has become a highly complex area of nursing specialization. With newer and more advanced therapies available to patients with diverse clinical needs, the infusion therapy nursing specialist must remain cognizant of changes in this exciting field. Manufacturers have kept pace with demands for more sophisticated products specific to various therapeutic modalities. In all clinical settings, a working knowledge of advanced vascular access is an essential part of IV nursing care.

CENTRAL VENOUS ACCESS DEVICES

Central venous catheterization is an integral component of the care of critically ill patients, allowing hemodynamic monitoring as well as administration of fluids, blood products, medications, and nutritional solutions. Central venous catheterization is now also an integral component of the care of patients in alternative settings, freeing the patient for months or a lifetime of nutritional support and related therapies.

Central venous access devices include tunneled lines, implanted ports, pumps, and reservoirs, and a diversity of central venous catheter products including single-, double-, and triple-lumen catheters with and without J wires, with and without introducer needles, and with and without peel-away sheaths. Each product is aimed at simplifying infusion therapy in a safe, efficient manner.

Quality central venous care mandates the development of policies and procedures based on Intravenous Nurses Society (INS) Standards of Practice and the Oncology Nursing Society (ONS) Recommendations for Nursing Practice for venous catheters. A clinical practicum and evaluation tool should be developed to ensure safe practice by those professionals responsible for accessing and maintaining long-term venous access.

RECOMMENDATIONS FOR NURSING PRACTICE

(Source: Oncology Nursing Society, reprinted with permission)

I. Venous catheters

The nursing care of patients with venous catheters is complex, and numerous controversial issues surround the care of these catheters. While much research is in progress, current study results have not conclusively resolved these practice issues.

Sharon M. Weinstein: PLUMER'S PRINCIPLES & PRACTICE OF INTRAVENOUS THERAPY, FIFTH EDITION, © 1993 J. B. Lippincott Company

The recommendations in this document are consistent with the literature cited to date and are deemed reasonable in the absence of definitive studies. Healthcare professionals who work with venous catheters should study new information as it becomes available.

A. Policies

1. The registered professional nurse is designated as qualified to care for patients with short-term or long-term venous catheters after adequate educational preparation according to the individual care setting's policies and procedures.

2. After adequate educational preparation, the registered professional nurse should demonstrate knowledge and skills in the following areas:
   a) Patient preparation for catheter placement
   b) Immediate post-procedural care of the patient,
   c) Methods of accessing short-term and long-term venous catheters
   d) Methods of maintaining patency of short-term and long-term venous catheters
   e) Care of the exit site
   f) Recognition of complications associated with short- and long-term venous catheters
   g) Management of a severed or damaged catheter
   h) Management of an occluded catheter
   i) Management of a migrated catheter
   j) Management of a thrombosed catheter
   k) Management of catheter where there is no blood return
   l) Management of chemotherapy extravasation (see *ONS Cancer Chemotherapy Guidelines*, Module V—*Recommendations for the Management of Extravasation and Anaphylaxis*, 1988.)
   m) Documentation procedures
   n) Policies and procedures on patient education

3. A mechanism for annually evaluating the registered professional nurse's knowledge and skill in caring for patients with short-term or long-term venous catheters should be established by the administrative authorities of the institution.

4. Ongoing participation in continuing education on venous catheter care is recommended to maintain a current knowledge base.

5. Only registered professional nurses or physicians with specialized training should care for patients with short-term or long-term venous catheters.

6. Personnel who insert short- or long-term venous catheters should be familiar with the specific equipment used as well as the proper selection of insertion site and catheter type, size, and length.

7. Proper aseptic technique must be used in caring for short-term and long-term venous catheters.

8. Patients with short-term and long-term venous catheters should be cared for within the framework of the nursing process and taught self-care management of the device.

9. Patients should be informed of the therapeutic benefits and risks of a short-term or long-term venous catheter in the degree of detail they desire.

10. The individual care setting should have written policies and procedures on:
   a) Short-term and long-term venous catheter placement
   b) Infection control practices for short-term and long-term venous catheters
   c) Short-term and long-term venous catheter care
   d) Declotting the long-term venous catheter
   e) Management of a damaged long-term venous catheter
   f) Management of a migrated catheter
   g) Extravasation of chemotherapy

B. Outcomes
   1. Only adequately prepared registered professional nurses who are skilled in caring for patients with short-term or long-term venous catheters will assume responsibility for the care of the device to insure quality patient care and maintain the highest standards of patient and personnel safety.
   2. The patient will verbalize the consequences of the treatment decision to have a short-term or long-term venous catheter.
   3. The sterility of the short-term or long-term venous catheter system will be maintained.
   4. The patient and/or significant other will be able to manage the short-term or long-term venous catheter.

C. Procedures
   (Review product information supplied by the manufacturer to become familiar with the specifics of the catheter before using.)
   1. Short-term venous catheters
      a) Patient preparation and short-term venous catheter placement
         (1) Perform a pre-placement assessment of the patient to determine if a short-term venous catheter is appropriate, including any or all of the following characteristics:
            (a) Short-term treatment with chemotherapy (45–60 days)
            (b) Short-term infusions of vesicant chemotherapy
            (c) Single bolus injections of chemotherapy
            (d) Brief life expectancy
            (e) Frequent venous access requirements
            (f) Limited venous access availability
            (g) Patient's desire for venous catheter
            (h) Total parenteral nutrition
            (i) Pain management
            (j) Hydration
            (k) Antibiotic therapy
            (l) Other supportive therapies

(text continues on page 214)

Long-Term Catheter Practicum

Long-Term Venous Catheters

PART I—CLINICAL PRACTICUM EVALUATION

As part of the nurse's evaluation, the preceptor will verify the nurse's performance of basic skills with a long-term venous catheter by indicating whether the nurse completes the following steps.

Skill	Met	Not Met
A. Patient Preparation		
1. Performs preplacement assessment of patient		
2. Explains procedure to patient and/or significant others		
3. Performs preplacement preparation		
4. Performs postoperative assessment of patient and catheter		
5. Confirms position of catheter prior to initiating treatment		
B. Accessing the Long-Term Venous Catheter		
1. Organizes catheter care to minimize entry into system		
2. Maintains strict aseptic technique		
3. Never leaves catheter open to air		
4. Uses only smoothed edged clamps or latex- or plastic-covered clamps		
5. Protects catheter prior to clamping		
6. Tapes catheter securely to patient's body		
7. Washes hands		
8. Prepares appropriate equipment		
9. Applies gloves		
10. Accesses catheter		
C. Blood Drawing		
1. Follows procedures for accessing system		
2. Removes at least 5 mL blood/solution and discards		
3. Clamps catheter at appropriate times		
4. Withdraws desired amount of blood		
5. Flushes catheter with 10 mL normal saline		
6. Using alcohol swab, removes any blood from catheter hub		
7. Heparinizes catheter or connects an appropriate solution		

(continued)

Long-Term Venous Catheters (continued)

Skill	Met	Not Met

D. Maintaining Patency

1. Heparinizes catheter with correct dose of heparin at appropriate frequency

E. Injection Cap Change

1. Washes hands
2. Prepares appropriate equipment
3. Applies gloves
4. Cleanses catheter
5. Changes injection cap with appropriate frequency

F. Exit Site Care

1. Washes hands
2. Prepares appropriate equipment
3. Carefully removes old dressing
4. Inspects exit site
5. Applies sterile gloves
6. Cleanses exit site
7. Applies appropriate dressing

G. Damaged Catheter

1. Clamps catheter proximal to severance
2. Obtains repair kit and follows direction to repair catheter

H. Occlusion

1. Diagnoses occlusion
2. Obtains physician order to instill urokinase
3. Verifies catheter placement prior to beginning procedure
4. Checks patient's platelet count prior to beginning procedure
5. Accesses long-term venous catheter
6. Prepares urokinase
7. Instills urokinase
8. Aspirates catheter

I. Documentation/Patient Education

1. Documents all procedures
2. Teaches patient and/or significant others short-term venous catheter care

(continued)

Long-Term Venous Catheters (continued)

PART II—CLINICAL PRACTICUM EVALUATION

The nurse performs the following activities at a satisfactory level. If there has not been an opportunity to carry out a particular activity, indicate N/A (not applicable) in the space provided. Under "Comment" give examples of how the nurse met each objective or performed each activity.

Behavior	Met	Not Met
1. Participates in interdisciplinary planning related to insertion and care of the patient's long-term venous catheter (*eg*, physician, social service, home care) *Comment:*		
2. Anticipates complications associated with long-term venous catheters and takes action to prevent/minimize complications *Comment:*		
3. Involves patient and/or significant others in care planning and establishes interventions specific to the individual needs of the patient *Comment:*		
4. Instructs patient and/or significant others how to care for the long-term venous catheter including: a. care of the exit site b. flushing the catheter and heparinization c. changing the injection cap d. possible complications *Comment:*		
5. Demonstrates knowledge of the principles of infection control related to long-term venous catheters *Comment:*		
6. Demonstrates knowledge and skill in the assessment, management, and follow-up care of the extravasation of chemotherapy *Comment:*		
7. Demonstrates knowledge of the assessment and management of a damaged long-term venous catheter *Comment:*		

(continued)

Long-Term Venous Catheters (continued)

Behavior	Met	Not Met
8. Demonstrates knowledge of the assessment and management of an occluded long-term venous catheter Comment:		
9. Demonstrates knowledge of the assessment and management of a migrated long-term venous catheter Comment:		
10. Demonstrates knowledge of the assessment and management of a thrombosed, long-term venous catheter Comment:		
11. Demonstrates knowledge of the assessment and management of a long-term, venous catheter that has lost blood return Comment:		

(Reproduced with permission of Oncology Nursing Society.)

CATHETER MATERIALS

The ideal material for a central venous catheter would inhibit thrombus formation, be easily insertable, and be radiopaque.

Deep-Vein Thrombosis

Deep-vein thrombosis from central venous catheters has many contributing factors. Any foreign material in the bloodstream becomes coated with a protein and fibrin deposit. Internal coagulation is activated, causing platelet activation, and platelets adhere to the catheter. Damage to endothelial cells at the puncture site enhances platelet activation. Patients requiring central venous catheters often have activated coagulation systems because of trauma or severe disease, both of which also promote the development of central venous catheter thrombosis. Thrombosis may be limited to a fibrin sheath formation or may be severe enough to cause vein occlusion. It may have no clinical significance or it may result in a fatal pulmonary embolism.[15]

The majority of central venous catheters are made of polyvinyl chloride (PVC), Teflon (™DuPont), polyurethane, or silicone (Table 15-1).

Polyvinyl Chloride

PVC was the first catheter material. High incidences of thrombosis have been associated with this material.[10] Today, most central venous catheters are made of less thrombogenic materials.

TABLE 15-1
Catheter Materials

PVC/Teflon

- Stiff
- Causes damage to the tunica intima
- Increased risk of platelet aggregation and subsequent thrombus formation
- Increased risk of perforation of vessel wall
- Limited to subclavian or jugular insertion due to lack of flexibility

Polyurethane

- Rigid during insertion but softens at body temperature
- Less thrombogenicity
- Can be used at all sites

Silicone Elastomer/Silastic

- Very flexible
- Minimal thrombus formation
- Biocompatible
- Good for long-term use
- Dramatic fibrin sheath formation when particulate matter is present; rinse gloves and catheter before insertion

Elastomeric Hydrogel

- Available in peripheral lines; central lines in production
- Combines stretchable polymer with hydrophilic substance (water absorbing and similar to extended-wear contact lenses)
- Rinse with normal saline; easier to insert

Teflon

Teflon catheters are easily inserted because they are relatively stiff. However, they are reported to have a high incidence of thrombus formation.[10]

Polyurethane

Polyurethane is only moderately firm, so it is not as easily inserted. Thrombus formation is reported to be less than with Teflon. Hydromer-coated polyurethane catheters reportedly have a low incidence of thrombus formation.[2]

Silicone

Silicone catheters are very soft, much like a wet noodle, so they require special mechanisms for insertion. They are reported to have the lowest incidence of thrombus formation.

Radiopaque Catheters

Radiopaque catheters are available in all materials. This property is required to affirm catheter tip placement after insertion.

BONDED CATHETERS

The most frequent life-threatening complication of central venous catheters is septicemia. Most related septicemias derive from invasion of the catheter wound by organisms from the patient's cutaneous microflora. Studies involving a triple-lumen poly-

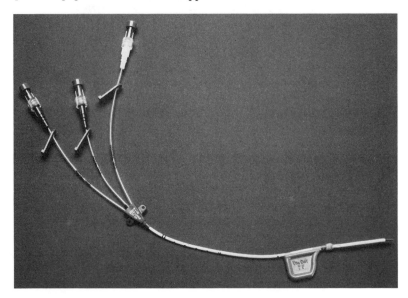

FIGURE 15-1   Vita Cuff® is composed of two concentric layers of material; used with Arrow's triple-lumen catheter. (Courtesy: Arrow International, Inc., Reading, PA)

urethane central venous catheter in which the entire catheter is impregnated with silver sulfadiazine and chlorhexidine proved favorable. It is believed that use of such a bonded catheter may substantially reduce the incidence of catheter-related infection, can extend the time that such lines may safely remain in place, and is cost efficient.[11] Known as Vita Cuff®, the product is available as a stand-alone to be used with Arrow's single-, double-, and triple-lumen catheters, percutaneous sheath introducers, and hemodialysis catheters (Figure 15-1).

The cuff is composed of two concentric layers of materials: an inner silicone sleeve that secures the cuff in place around a catheter, and an outer collagen matrix. The collagen matrix is made from purified type I bovine tendon collagen. Silver ions are chelated to the collagen matrix. Silver possesses a broad antimicrobial spectrum and has been used extensively in topical antimicrobial preparations in burn patients.

The cuff, with introducer attached, is placed around a catheter before catheter insertion. The catheter is inserted percutaneously to the desired level. Then, the cuff is placed subcutaneously with the introducer, which is then separated from the cuff. Following insertion, subcutaneous tissue grows into the collagenous matrix, anchoring the catheter and creating a barrier against invasion by extrinsic organisms. Significant antimicrobial activity associated with the Arrow catheter has been demonstrated using zone of inhibition bioassays against the following organisms:

- *Escherichia coli*
- *Pseudomonas aeruginosa*
- *Staphylococcus epidermidis*
- *Klebsiella pneumoniae*
- *Candida albicans*

CATHETER DESIGNS

The design of the device is frequently related to the properties of the catheter material. The design also dictates insertion methods.

Inside-the-Needle Catheter

The inside-the-needle catheter (INC) is often made of polyurethane or PVC.

Device Components
The unit consists of a stainless steel needle attached to a plastic sheath containing a catheter with or without a stylet and needle tip cover (Figure 15-2).

Insertion Technique
The venipuncture is performed with the stainless steel needle. The catheter is advanced through the needle. The needle is drawn back over the catheter and its tip protected with a cover (Figure 15-3).

Device Features
Because of its stiffness, the catheter is easy to insert a short distance into the vein. When attempting to thread a long catheter, difficulty may be encountered because of the stiffness. If this occurs, the stylet (if present) can be partially withdrawn to soften the catheter. A smooth insertion requires a vein without sharp twists or curves. The INC is always a single-lumen catheter. If not used according to manufacturer's instructions, this device has a high risk of catheter embolism. During insertion the catheter must NEVER be drawn back through the needle. The sharp needle can easily sever the catheter with a resultant embolism. Because the sharp needle must remain over the catheter, there is always the risk of catheter severance if manufacturer's instructions as to needle point protection are not followed. The INC is a *short-term* inpatient central venous catheter. It was not designed for long-term or home care usage.

Catheter with Removable Introducer

Catheters with removable introducers are frequently made of polyurethane.

Device Components
The unit consists of an introducer catheter or syringe and needle and a catheter with stylet.

Insertion Technique
The venipuncture is performed with the needle and syringe. The syringe is removed and the catheter threaded through the needle. The needle is withdrawn from the vein and removed from the catheter by splitting the needle into two parts (Figure 15-4).

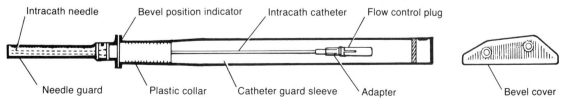

FIGURE 15-2 Components of an inside-the-needle catheter (INC). Intracath™. (Courtesy: Becton Dickinson Vascular Access, Sandy, UT)

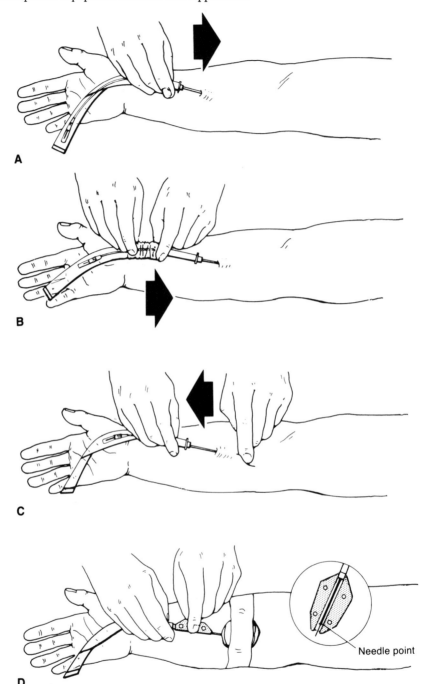

FIGURE 15-3 Insertion technique with INC. (**A**) Venipuncture is performed with the stainless steel needle. (**B**) The catheter is advanced through the needle. (**C**) The needle is withdrawn over the catheter. (**D**) The needle tip is protected with the cover. (Courtesy: Becton Dickinson Vascular Access, Sandy, UT)

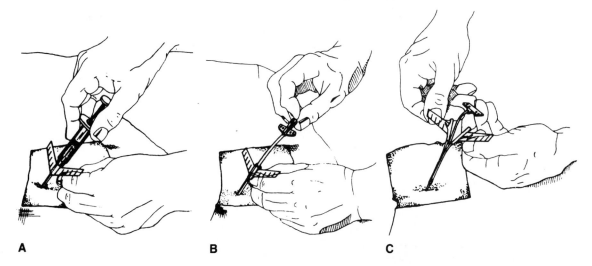

A   **B**   **C**

FIGURE 15-4   Insertion technique for catheter with removable introducer. (**A**) Venipuncture is performed with the introducer needle and syringe. (**B**) The syringe is removed and the catheter threaded through the needle. (**C**) The needle is withdrawn from the vein and removed from the catheter by splitting into two parts. (Courtesy: Luther Medical Products, Inc., Santa Ana, CA)

Device Features

A catheter with a removable introducer is a single-lumen catheter with a fairly easy method of insertion. Because the device is usually made of polyurethane, it is softer than Teflon and easier to thread through twists and curves. Removal of any sharp needle eliminates the risk of catheter embolism. Because thrombus formation can be a problem with polyurethane, this may not be the catheter of choice for long-term therapy. However, minimal thrombus formation has been reported with hydromer-coated polyurethane and long-term usage.

Catheter with Introducer and Guide Wire

A catheter with an introducer and guide wire allows for the insertion of a multiple-lumen silicone catheter.

Device Components

The unit consists of a syringe and needle or an over-the-needle catheter (ONC), long central catheter, and a guide wire (Figure 15-5).

Insertion Technique

The venipuncture is performed with the syringe and needle or ONC. The syringe or stylet is removed. The guide wire is threaded through the short catheter or needle, and the short catheter or needle is withdrawn. The puncture site may be enlarged with a no. 11 scalpel blade. The long catheter is threaded over the guide wire (Figure 15-6), and the guide wire withdrawn, leaving the long catheter in the vein.

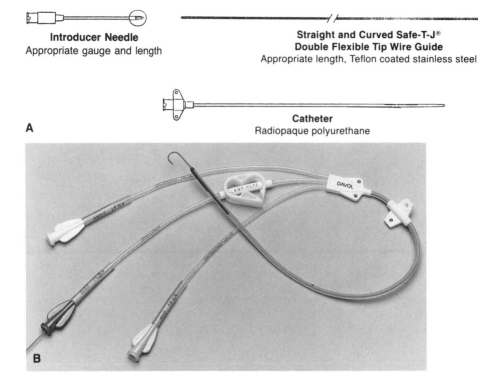

Introducer Needle
Appropriate gauge and length

Straight and Curved Safe-T-J®
Double Flexible Tip Wire Guide
Appropriate length, Teflon coated stainless steel

Catheter
Radiopaque polyurethane

A

B

FIGURE 15-5 (**A**) Components of a catheter with introducer and guide wire. (Courtesy: Cook Critical Care, Bloomington, IN) (**B**) Groshong OTG catheter (Courtesy: Davol, Inc. Subsidiary CR Bard Inc., Salt Lake City, UT)

Device Features
The silicone catheter has the lowest reports of thrombus formation. The design allows for multiple-lumen catheter placement. It requires a fairly complex method of insertion with a large amount of "in-and-out" manipulation in the vein. The silicone catheter is an excellent *long-term* central catheter for both inpatient and home care use.

Indwelling Tunneled Catheter

The indwelling tunneled catheter is made of polymeric silicone.

Device Components
This single- or double-lumen catheter contains a Dacron cuff. The external end has a "ring" with a threaded Luer lock adapter covered with a Luer lock cap. An integral clamp may be present (Figure 15-7). One version of this catheter has a closed tip and a lateral two-way valve. The valve opens outward for infusion and inward for blood sample drawing. This model does not require heparin flush to maintain catheter patency.

Insertion Technique
The insertion may be performed by cutdown or percutaneous puncture. This is performed under fluoroscopy, usually in a minor surgery operating room.

The catheter is placed by locating the subclavian vein, forming a tunnel from the vein to an area between the sternum and the nipple, pulling the catheter through the tunnel,

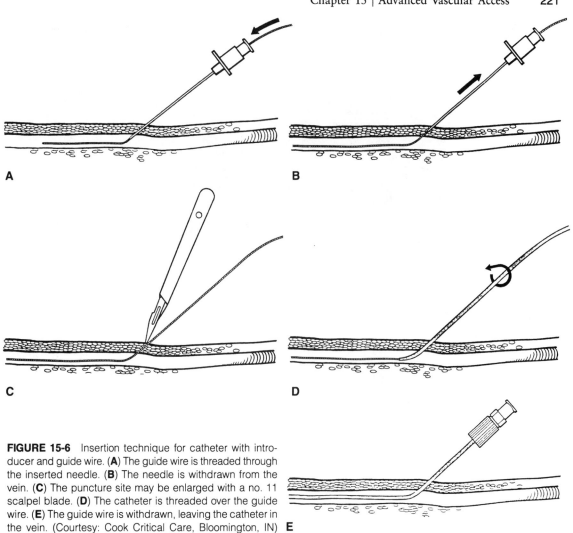

FIGURE 15-6 Insertion technique for catheter with introducer and guide wire. (**A**) The guide wire is threaded through the inserted needle. (**B**) The needle is withdrawn from the vein. (**C**) The puncture site may be enlarged with a no. 11 scalpel blade. (**D**) The catheter is threaded over the guide wire. (**E**) The guide wire is withdrawn, leaving the catheter in the vein. (Courtesy: Cook Critical Care, Bloomington, IN)

inserting it into the vein, and threading it until the tip is in the superior vena cava (Figure 15-8).

Device Features
Fibrous tissue forms around the Dacron cuff. The cuff and tunnel anchor the catheter and help prevent infection. Because the material is polymeric silicone, this catheter has reports of a low incidence of thrombus formation. It is a perfect central venous catheter for home IV therapy. This catheter is also inserted for long-term inpatient use.

Totally Implanted Venous Access Device

Totally implanted devices for repeated venous access eliminate the need for frequent venipunctures.

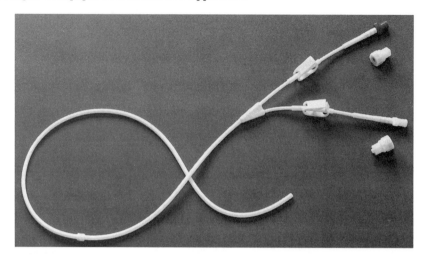

FIGURE 15-7   Dual-lumen Hickman catheter. (Courtesy: Davol, Inc., Subsidiary CR Bard Inc., Salt Lake City, UT)

Device Components

The unit consists of a silicone catheter attached to a reservoir with a self-sealing septum. At the present time there are four manufacturers of this device (Figures 15-9 through 15-12). Units are available with single or double lumens. Special noncoring needles are required to access these devices.

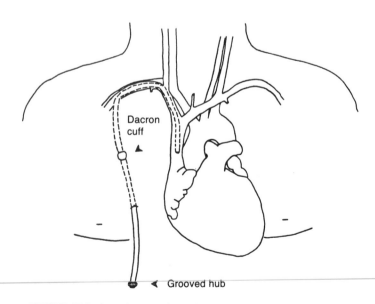

FIGURE 15-8   Insertion technique of indwelling tunneled catheter. A tunnel is formed from the vein to an area between the sternum and the nipple. The catheter tip is placed in the superior vena cava.

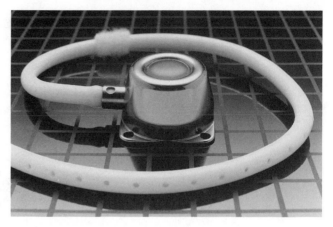

FIGURE 15-9 PORT-A-CATH® Implantable Peritoneal Access System (Property of Pharmacia Deltec, Inc., St. Paul, MN)

Insertion Technique

The unit is surgically placed under local or general anesthesia. The insertion technique is similar to that used for implanted tunneled catheters. The catheter is placed in the subclavian vein and threaded into the vein until the tip lies in the superior vena cava. This position is confirmed by fluoroscopy. A pocket is made for the reservoir. The reservoir is sutured in the pocket. Because the center of the port will be punctured repeatedly, when the pocket is closed the suture line is lateral, medial, superior, or inferior to the port septum (Figure 15-13).

Device Features

This device has reports of a low incidence of thrombus formation from the silicone catheter. When not in use, the only care required is a monthly heparin flush. The fact that this is totally implanted, leaving no catheter exiting from the chest, makes it a favorite device with many patients. It is an "artificial vein" perfect for any patient receiving *long-term periodic* infusion therapy in the home or in the hospital.

Totally Implanted Pump

Totally implanted pumps are designed for continuous, low-volume, long-term ambulatory therapy. They may be used for arterial or venous infusion and tissue perfusion.

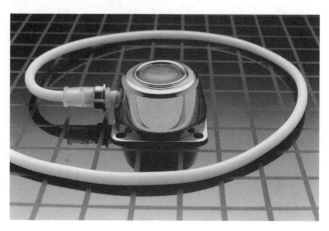

FIGURE 15-10 PORT-A-CATH® Implantable Access System (Property of Pharmacia Deltec, Inc., St. Paul, MN)

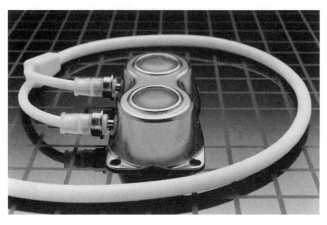

FIGURE 15-11 PORT-A-CATH®
Dual-Lumen Implantable Access
System (Property of Pharmacia
Deltec, Inc., St. Paul, MN)

Device Components

The device consists of two chambers separated by flexible metal bellows. One chamber is the drug reservoir; the other contains the charging fluid in a completely sealed compartment. The vapor pressure of the charging fluid exerts a constant pressure on the bellows, forcing the drug out of the reservoir through an outlet filter and flow restrictor into a silicone catheter (Figure 15-14). When the pump is refilled, the increasing pressure within the drug chamber exerts a pressure on the charging fluid, causing the fluid vapor to condense to its liquid state, thereby storing energy for the next pumping cycle.

Various models are available. The basic device has one catheter. One model also has a direct access port that bypasses the reservoir for administering bolus injections. Another model has double catheters, which can be used to administer a drug to more than one site.

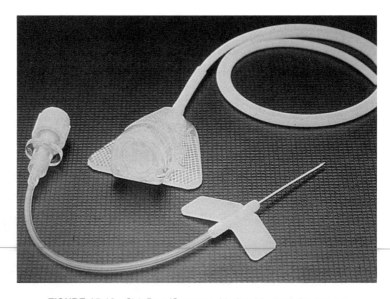

FIGURE 15-12 SidePort (Courtesy: Norfolk Medical, Skokie, IL)

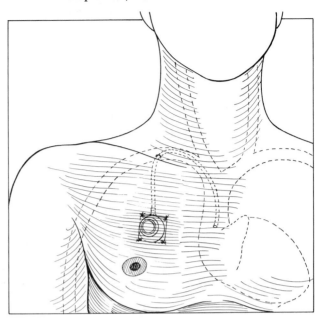

FIGURE 15-13 Placement of the PORT-A-CATH® Implantable Access System (Property of Pharmacia Deltec, Inc., St. Paul, MN)

Insertion Technique

The pump is implanted in the operating room under fluoroscopy. To activate the charging fluid, the pump must be heated for 30 minutes at 30°C to 40°C before implantation. This is done with a heating pad. The insertion technique is the same as that for the implanted venous access. The pocket is frequently located below the umbilicus on the abdomen.

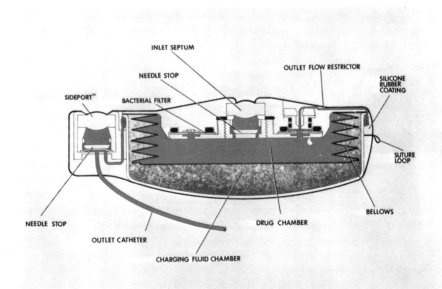

FIGURE 15-14 Components of the implanted pump. Infusaid™. (Courtesy: Intermedics Infusaid, Inc., Norwood, MA)

Device Features
Several factors will influence the pump flow rate. If the catheter site is arterial and *arterial blood pressure increases significantly*, the flow rate can decrease by as much as 15%. *Hypotension* can increase the rate by as much as 6%. When the patient moves from one *altitude* to another, the rate can increase by as much as 38%. *Fever* can increase flow rate by as much as 13%. The *amount of drug in the reservoir* will affect the flow rate. The pump flow rate is established with the reservoir half full. At full volume the rate will be approximately 3% faster and at low volume 3% slower than the mean flow rate.[7]

The silicone catheter results in a low incidence of thrombus formation. This is an excellent method for *continuous long-term administration* of *low-volume* narcotics or chemotherapeutic agents to cancer patients. Because there are no external parts, it requires no care between port refills.

Contraindications
Contraindications for the implanted pump include:

1. All but very small volumes of drugs

2. A body size not large enough for the size and weight of the pump

3. Patients with severe emotional, psychiatric, or neurologic disturbances

4. Patients who travel extensively or frequently and experience altitudinal changes[7]

CATHETER SITE CARE

A regular, standardized site inspection, disinfection, and dressing change should minimize catheter-related sepsis. Catheter site care and dressing change should be performed consistent with institutional policy and dressing material. If the dressing becomes wet, soiled, or loose, it should be changed immediately. Aseptic technique must be maintained during the procedure.

Nontunneled Catheter

Many variations are acceptable for performing site care and changing central venous catheter dressings. However, they are all based on the same principles. On a routine basis, the old dressing must be removed; both site and catheter carefully inspected, cleaned, and disinfected; an antimicrobial ointment applied; and an occlusive dressing secured. The person performing the care thoroughly washes the hands and wears sterile gloves and a mask. If the patient cannot be masked, the face should be turned away from the dressing site.

Equipment
The use of a prepackaged dressing kit will ensure the immediate availability of all required supplies. It will also help to ensure that all persons performing the care are using a standard procedure.

Procedure
1. Prepare a clean table for a work area.

2. Prepare the patient in a comfortable position on the bed.

3. Put on the mask, wash hands thoroughly, and dry. Put on gloves.

4. Carefully, remove old dressing. Removing the tape from the outside edges inward toward the center will prevent stress at the insertion site. The site should be carefully inspected for any signs of discharge or leakage. The catheter should be inspected to ensure (a) that the sutures are intact, (b) that the length of the external portion has not increased, (c) that any needle protective cover is in place and locked, and (d) that the catheter and hub are intact.

   If the hands should become contaminated during the dressing removal, they must be rewashed. If the procedure is performed with two pairs of gloves, the first pair is worn to remove the old dressing.

5. Open kit. The overlay will provide a sterile field.

6. Put on the sterile gloves.

7. The site and the portion of the catheter close to the site should be cleansed of all debris. Polyurethane and silicone catheters should not come in contact with 100% acetone, which could weaken the material and cause leakage. Concentrated acetone may also cause skin irritation, which can increase the risk of infection. Some practitioners use a combination of dilute acetone and alcohol for cleansing purposes. The cleansing is performed in a circular fashion, starting at the center and working outward. The cleansing agent must be allowed to dry before the disinfection is started.

8. Disinfection may be done with (a) 1% or 2% tincture of iodine followed by a complete removal with alcohol or (b) povidone–iodine solution. Povidone–iodine must not be removed with alcohol. The skin prep is applied in the circular method as described for cleansing. The nurse must not forget to disinfect the portion of the catheter that is close to the insertion site. Allow the agent to dry.

9. Apply antimicrobial ointment sparingly directly to the insertion site. Povidone–iodine is recommended for central catheter sites.

10. Placing a sterile 2 × 2 inch sponge directly over the ointment will ensure that the ointment stays at the site. A sterile sponge may be placed under the catheter and hub for patient comfort.

11. If the tape causes skin damage, tincture of benzoin may be used to protect the exposed skin. Be sure that it dries before applying the tape.

12. An adhesive cover is applied to maintain an occlusive dressing. Several types are available. Foam adhesive bandage or transparent tape is frequently used. The sterile tape is placed directly over the site with the catheter exiting from the bottom of the tape. This position is important to prevent stress at the catheter hub–tubing connection when the patient moves. Be sure this connection is outside the tape to facilitate tubing changes.

13. The catheter hub–tubing connection is inspected to be sure that it is locked and taped. The tubing is looped and taped to the chest wall to prevent stress at the connection or insertion site when the tubing is pulled or stretched.

14. The dressing change label is signed, dated, and applied to the dressing (Figure 15-15A).

15. Transparent dressings may be used (Figure 15-15B).

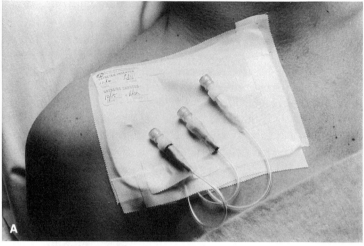

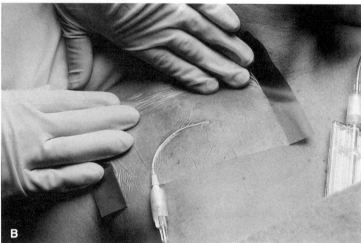

FIGURE 15-15 (**A**) Connections are taped and the site is labeled. (**B**) Transparent dressings may also be used. (Courtesy: Acme United Corp., Fairfield, CT)

Tunneled Catheters

The dressing change procedure may be modified for the tunneled catheter. If the patient is immunosuppressed or if site healing is not complete, the same care given to the nontunneled catheter may be used for this catheter. If the patient is not immunosuppressed and site healing is complete, site care may be limited to daily inspection and cleansing with soap and water while bathing.

Totally Implanted Devices

Totally implanted devices do not require any site care because the entire device is under the skin.

CATHETER MAINTENANCE

Heparin Flush

After using the catheter and at routine intervals, flushing with heparin solution will maintain catheter patency. For tunneled or nontunneled catheters, the frequency and heparin strength vary considerably among institutions. The volume of heparin needs to be only slightly more than the volume of the catheter—2.5 to 5 mL should be sufficient. Many practitioners have found that every-other-day flushes maintain catheter patency. The strength of heparin may depend on the condition of the patient, usually 10–100 U/mL.

Prefilled Heparin Flush Syringe
Using a prefilled heparin syringe reduces the risk of touch contamination during preparation and ensures administration of the correct dosage of heparin. Saline flush may also be used.

Gauge and Length of Needles
Whenever injections are made into injection ports or intermittent injection caps, using a short needle prevents the risk of accidental puncture of the tubing or catheter. Small-gauge needles prevent large holes in the cap or injection port, which can result in fluid leakage or an entry point for air or bacteria.

Aids for Preventing Catheter Clotting
While the nurse injects the heparin flush, the clamp is applied before the syringe is completely empty. The syringe and needle are removed while pressure is applied on the plunger. This prevents reflux of blood into the lumen, which could result in catheter clotting.

When the catheter is not in use, taping the hub to the chest wall above heart level will minimize blood pressure at the catheter tip.

Automated Flushing

Auto-SASH™ by BLOCK Medical, Inc. is a one-piece closed system for IV site flushing that presents a safe, convenient alternative to the more traditional needle/syringe technique (Figure 15-16). Using only one connection to the patient's IV site, Auto-SASH reduces the potential for touch contamination and possible infection. Patients with limited vision or limitations of manual dexterity can easily be taught to self-flush their lines using this device. Auto-SASH contains three fluid reservoirs inside a protective outer casing. The reservoirs are filled with two doses of saline and one dose of heparin flush. Once connected to the IV line, pressing the appropriate button will deliver up to a 3-mL volume of saline or heparin to the IV line. The system is compatible with any gravity IV set, disposable infusion device, or electronic pump. Stability, once filled, is estimated at up to 28 days for 10 U/mL and 100 U/mL dilutions.

Discontinuing Infusion

When an infusion is completed, an injection cap and heparin flush are used to maintain catheter patency. A normal saline flush is given before the heparin to rinse the IV fluid from the catheter. If the catheter is of a material that cannot be clamped without possible

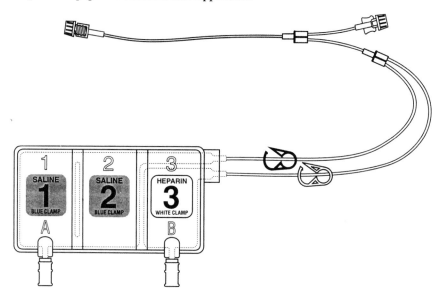

FIGURE 15-16 Auto-SASH, closed system for IV site flushing. Individual reservoirs hold two doses of saline and one dose of heparin sodium. (Courtesy: BLOCK Medical, Inc., Carlsbad, CA)

damage and there is no extension tubing that can be clamped, the patient must perform the Valsalva maneuver at any time the catheter is open to the air.

The following steps may be used to discontinue the infusion, connect an injection cap, and flush with normal saline and heparin.

Equipment

    Smooth blade catheter clamp (1)

    Luer lock injection cap (1)

    10 mL syringe (1)

    22 gauge × 1 inch needle (1)

    Sodium chloride 0.9% 10 mL (1)

    Prefilled syringe with heparin flush (1)

    Povidone–iodine swab (3)

    Alcohol sponge (1)

    Sterile 2 × 2 inch sponge (1)

    Tape

    Sterile gloves one pair (optional)

Procedure

    1. Wash hands thoroughly and dry.

    2. Aseptically open all sterile supplies.

    3. Prepare air-purged 10 mL 0.9% sodium chloride syringe with a 22-gauge × 1 inch needle.

4. Prepare air-purged heparin flush.
5. Shut infusion off and clamp catheter.
6. Remove old tape from catheter filter–IV tubing connection.
7. Cleanse connection with povidone–iodine swab for 30 seconds.
8. Place connection on sterile 2 × 2 inch sponge and allow to dry.
9. Put on gloves, they may be used at this time. Pick up connection by holding catheter hub with the sterile sponge.
10. Aseptically disconnect and discard infusion tubing.
11. Aseptically connect and lock injection cap.
12. Remove clamp.
13. Cleanse rubber end of injection cap with povidone–iodine for 30 seconds. Allow to dry.
14. *Carefully* insert needle of syringe with normal saline flush into center of injection cap. Do not exert force. If an obstruction is felt, realign needle angle.
15. Inject normal saline flush.
16. While still holding catheter hub, remove empty syringe. Recleanse injection cap end with povidone–iodine for 30 seconds; allow to dry.
17. *Carefully* insert needle of heparin flush. Do not force insertion. If an obstruction is felt, realign needle angle.
18. Inject heparin flush. Before the syringe is completely empty, close catheter clamp.
19. Remove syringe and needle, applying pressure on plunger during withdrawal.
20. Remove clamp.
21. Secure injection cap to catheter with a strip of tape.
22. Tape catheter hub on the chest wall above heart level.

Routine Flushing

Routine flushing is required to maintain patency of unused catheters. If the catheter has more than one lumen, remember to flush each unused lumen. Either heparin or saline may be used.

The following steps may be used to perform heparin flush without changing the intermittent injection cap.

Equipment
  Smooth-blade catheter clamp (1)
  Prefilled syringe with heparin dosage (1) (Figure 15-17)
  Povidone–iodine swab (1)
  Tape

Procedure
  1. Wash hands thoroughly and dry.
  2. Prepare air-purged heparin flush.

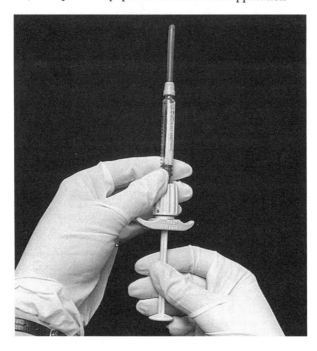

FIGURE 15-17 Wyeth's Tubex Injector, loaded for instillation of saline or heparin in lock. (Courtesy: Wyeth-Ayerst Laboratories, Philadelphia, PA)

3. Remove tape holding end of catheter to chest wall.

4. Cleanse rubber end of injection cap with povidone–iodine for 30 seconds. Allow to dry.

5. While stabilizing the catheter hub, carefully insert needle of heparin flush syringe into center of cap. If an obstruction is felt, do not apply force but realign needle angle.

6. Gently inject heparin flush. Clamp the catheter before the syringe is completely empty.

7. Apply pressure on plunger while removing syringe and needle.

8. Remove clamp.

9. Tape catheter hub on chest wall above heart level.

Changing Intermittent Injection Cap

The injection cap must be changed at routine intervals. If the catheter is flushed every other day, cap changing may be coordinated with each third flushing (every 6 days). Using an intermittent injection cap that has a very small amount of dead space eliminates the need to preflush the cap. This minimizes the risk of touch contamination.

If the catheter contains more than one lumen, remember to change the caps on all unused lumens. If the catheter is made of a material that cannot be clamped without catheter damage, be sure that the patient is flat in bed and performs the Valsalva maneuver at any time the catheter is open to the air.

The following steps may be used to change the intermittent injection cap at the time of heparin flushing.

Equipment

    Smooth-blade catheter clamp (1)

    Prefilled syringe with heparin dosage (1)

    Luer lock intermittent injection cap (1)

    Sterile 2 × 2 inch sponge (1)

    Povidone–iodine swabs (2)

    Tape

Procedure

1. Wash hands thoroughly and dry.
2. Aseptically prepare sterile supplies. Put on gloves.
3. Prepare air-purged heparin flush.
4. Remove tape holding catheter to chest wall. Remove tape securing cap to catheter.
5. Cleanse cap–catheter connection point with povidone–iodine for 30 seconds. Place on sterile sponge and allow to dry.
6. Close clamp.
7. Pick up catheter hub protected by sterile sponge. Be careful not to touch the cleansed connection.
8. *Carefully* unlock, remove, and discard old cap.
9. Holding the new cap by the rubber injection end, connect and lock to catheter.
10. Secure connection with a strip of tape.
11. Remove clamp.
12. Cleanse rubber end of injection cap with povidone–iodine for 30 seconds. Allow to dry.
13. *Carefully* insert needle of heparin flush into center of rubber end. Do not force insertion. If an obstruction is felt, realign needle angle.
14. Gently inject heparin. Before the syringe is completely empty, close clamp.
15. Apply pressure on plunger while withdrawing syringe and needle.
16. Remove clamp.
17. Tape catheter hub on the chest wall above heart level.

Venous Sampling

Many central venous catheters are placed on patients without available peripheral veins or to minimize peripheral venipunctures. Therefore, drawing blood specimens through central catheters is common practice. Three basic methods are used with tunneled and nontunneled catheters: (1) drawing specimens from a continuous infusion line maintaining the closed system, (2) drawing specimens from a continuous infusion line by opening the system, and (3) drawing specimens from a catheter with an in-place intermittent injection cap.

If the system does not have the possibility of catheter clamping, the patient must be placed flat in bed and perform the Valsalva maneuver whenever the catheter is open to the air. If this is not done, air embolism is always possible.

Prothrombin Time and Partial Thromboplastin Time Tests and Heparin

Any blood specimen drawn through a central catheter that has been flushed with heparin or that has heparin as a solution additive should not be used for prothrombin time or partial thromboplastin time testing. Heparin adheres to the catheter and can result in falsely elevated values for these tests.

Catheter Withdrawal Occlusion

The inability to withdraw blood through a central venous catheter even though infusion creates no difficulties is frequently encountered. It has been postulated that the formation of a fibrin sheath over the catheter tip allows infusion but inhibits blood withdrawal.[9] Having the patient cough or move into various positions may be helpful. Sometimes the problem will be intermittent; after an hour's wait, blood specimens can be obtained without difficulty. At other times and in some patients, it may continue to be impossible to withdraw blood through the central venous catheter. Flushing the catheter with normal saline before blood withdrawal appears to be helpful.

Patient Identification

Before drawing any blood specimens the patient must be accurately identified. This should be done by the patient's hospital identification band. Asking the patient to state his or her name may supplement but should never be substituted for some form of written identification on the patient.

Labeling Specimen Tubes

Before drawing the blood specimen, all tubes should be labeled with the patient's full name, room number, hospital identification number, and the initials of the person drawing the blood. This is done to prevent mislabeling, which can result in inadequate or inappropriate treatment.

Drawing Blood Specimens from Continuous Infusion Line Maintaining a Closed System. This procedure requires an injection port between the filter and the catheter. It may be performed by using the following equipment and procedure.

Equipment

Vacuum tube holder (1)

Multiple draw needle: 22 gauge × 1 inch (1)

Appropriate number and type vacuum tube(s) for tests

0.9% sodium chloride 10 mL (2)

10-mL syringe (2)

Needles: 22 gauge × 1 inch (2)

Povidone–iodine swab (3)

Alcohol sponge (1)

Procedure

1. Put on gloves. Strict aseptic technique must be used throughout the entire procedure.

2. Prepare two air-purged 10 mL 0.9% sodium chloride syringes with 22 gauge × 1 inch needles.

3. Prepare vacuum tube holder, needle, and tube. Do not fully insert tube into needle because vacuum will be lost.

4. Shut off infusion for 1 minute before drawing blood specimens to prevent blood contamination with infusion fluid. This is especially important when total parenteral nutrition is infusing.

5. Close clamp distal to injection port (Figure 15-18A).

6. Cleanse injection port with povidone–iodine for 30 seconds. Allow to dry.

7. Hold injection port while performing all entries and withdrawals. Aseptically insert needle of first normal saline flush directly into center of port. Gently inject solution to flush extension tubing (if used) and catheter of infusate (Figure 15-18B).

8. Withdraw syringe full (10 mL) of blood and fluid mixture. Remove and discard syringe and needle.

9. Recleanse injection port with povidone–iodine for 30 seconds. Allow to dry.

10. Aseptically insert needle of vacuum tube unit into center of injection port.

11. Fully insert tube into needle. Allow tube to fill with blood.

12. Remove tube. Continue to insert, allow to fill, and remove required tube(s) for blood specimen(s). Be sure to mix, by gentle rotation, all specimens drawn in tubes with an anticoagulant.

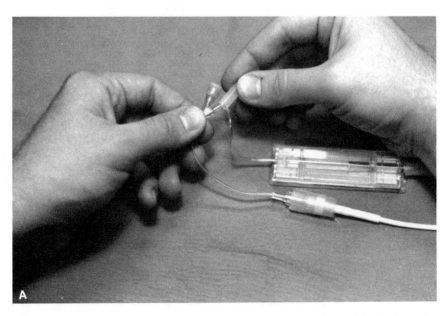

FIGURE 15-18 Procedure for drawing blood specimens from continuous infusion line maintaining a closed system. (**A**) The clamp distal to the injection port is closed. (**B**) Normal saline is injected to clear system of infusate. (**C**) Allow vacuum tube to fill with blood.

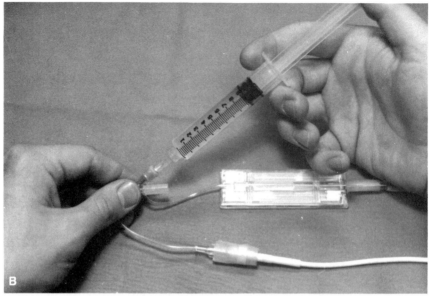

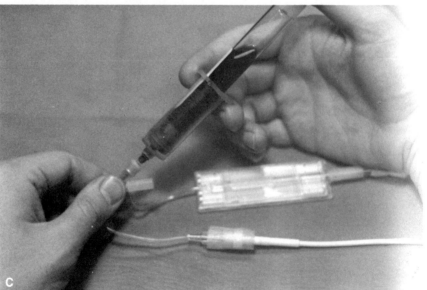

FIGURE 15-18   (*Continued*)

13. Remove holder, tube, and needle.

14. Recleanse injection port with povidone–iodine for 30 seconds. Allow to dry.

15. Aseptically, insert needle of second syringe with 0.9% sodium chloride into center of injection port. Gently flush to rinse blood cells from the catheter.

16. Open clamp and regulate infusion drip rate.

Drawing Blood Specimens from Continuous Infusion Line by Opening the System.
This procedure requires a catheter that can be clamped because the catheter will be

opened to the air several times. An extension tubing that contains a clamp may be aseptically Luer locked and taped to the catheter hub as a substitute. Extreme care must be taken to maintain sterility when the extension tubing is used for this purpose. This procedure should be performed in correlation with the tubing change to avoid reconnecting a used tubing after the blood specimens are drawn.

The following equipment and steps may be used to perform the venous sampling.

Equipment

    Catheter clamp or in-site extension tubing with clamp (1)

    Appropriate number and type vacuum tubes for tests

    Syringe large enough to hold required amount of blood (1)

    10-mL syringes (2)

    Needles: 20 gauge × 1 inch (3)

    0.9% sodium chloride 10 mL (2)

    Povidone–iodine swab (1)

    Alcohol sponge (1)

    Sterile 2 × 2 inch sponge (1)

    Appropriate infusion tubing (1)

    Luer lock 0.2-μm air-eliminating filter (1)

Procedure

1. Put on gloves. Strict aseptic technique must be maintained throughout the entire procedure.
2. Prepare fresh IV system, flush tubing and filter.
3. Prepare two air-purged syringes of 10 mL 0.9% sodium chloride.
4. Shut infusion off for 1 minute. Close clamp.
5. Remove old tape at catheter–tubing or filter connection.
6. Cleanse connection for 30 seconds with povidone–iodine swab. Place on sterile sponge to dry.
7. Pick up connection by protecting catheter hub with sterile sponge.
8. Disconnect and discard infusion system.
9. Continue to hold hub with sterile sponge during all connection and disconnection manipulations. Connect first air-purged syringe of 0.9% sodium chloride.
10. Open clamp. Gently inject flush to rinse catheter, and extension tubing, if used.
11. Withdraw 10 mL blood and fluid mixture. Close clamp.
12. Disconnect and discard syringe.
13. Connect large syringe, open clamp, and.withdraw required amount of blood for all ordered tests.
14. Close clamp. Disconnect syringe filled with blood. A second person may be required to add needle and fill specimen tube(s). Be sure to mix by gentle rotation all tubes with an anticoagulant.

15. Connect second air-purged syringe with 0.9% sodium chloride. Open clamp and inject flush to rinse blood from catheter.

16. Close clamp, remove syringe. Connect, lock, and tape Luer lock connection of IV tubing or filter to catheter. Open clamp. Reestablish infusion flow rate.

17. Tape tubing to chest wall to prevent relayed stress to the connection if the tubing is pulled or stretched.

Drawing Blood Specimens from Catheters with Injection Cap in Place.   This procedure is frequently performed, especially with multiple-lumen catheters. The most proximal lumen is usually reserved for this purpose. By using the distal lumen(s) for infusions, the fluid is downstream from the site where the blood will be drawn. This decreases the risk of blood contamination with the infusate if the solution cannot be turned off or can be turned off only for a very short period of time.

When inserting needles into an intermittent injection cap, force should never be applied. If an obstruction is felt, realigning the angle of the needle will facilitate entry.

Blood may be drawn from a central catheter with an injection cap in place by using the following equipment and steps.

Equipment
Vacuum tube holder (1)

Multiple-sample needle: 22 gauge × 1 inch (1)

Appropriate number and type vacuum tubes for tests

0.9% sodium chloride 10 mL (2)

10-mL syringes (2)

Needles: 22 gauge × 1 inch (2)

Prefilled syringe with heparin dosage (1)

Povidone–iodine swabs (4)

Alcohol swab (1)

Tape

Procedure
1. Put on gloves. Aseptic technique must be maintained throughout the entire procedure.

2. Prepare two air-purged 10-mL 0.9% sodium chloride flushes. Prepare air-purged heparin flush.

3. Prepare vacuum tube holder and needle with first tube. Do not fully insert tube into needle because vacuum will be lost.

4. Cleanse rubber end of injection cap with povidone–iodine for 30 seconds. Allow to dry.

5. Hold catheter hub without touching end of injection cap during all needle entries and withdrawals. Insert needle of first air-purged syringe with normal saline flush into center of rubber cap.

6. Inject flush to rinse heparin from catheter.

7. Withdraw 10 mL blood and solution mixture. Remove and discard needle and syringe.

8. Recleanse rubber end of injection cap with povidone–iodine for 30 seconds. Allow to dry.

9. Insert needle of vacuum tube unit into center of injection cap. Fully insert tube into needle. Allow tube to fill with blood. Remove tube.

10. Insert, allow to fill, and remove required specimen tubes. Be sure to mix by gentle rotation all tubes with an anticoagulant.

11. Recleanse rubber end of injection cap with povidone–iodine for 30 seconds. Allow to dry.

12. Insert needle of second syringe with normal saline flush into center of injection cap.

13. Inject flush to rinse blood from catheter. Remove syringe and needle.

14. Recleanse rubber end of injection port with povidone–iodine for 30 seconds. Allow to dry.

15. Insert needle of heparin flush into center of injection cap.

16. Gently inject heparin. Before the syringe is completely empty, clamp tubing. Apply pressure on plunger while withdrawing needle and syringe.

17. Remove clamp and tape catheter hub on chest wall above heart level.

18. Remove gloves and wash hands.

TUNNELED CATHETERS

Originally available as a Broviac catheter and later modified with a larger diameter by Hickman and associates, today's tunneled right atrial catheter is made of silicone and is available in a single-, double-, and triple-lumen configuration (Figure 15-19). Many tunneled lines feature an integral catheter clamp and a reinforced segment of catheter to reduce the risk of silicone fatigue following repeated clamping.

Insertion is performed as a surgical procedure, through a cutdown in which the vein

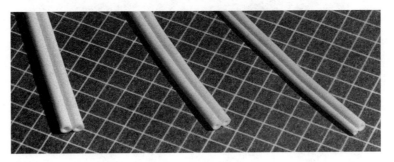

FIGURE 15-19 Dual-lumen Hickman catheters (Courtesy: Davol, Inc., Subsidiary CR Bard Inc., Salt Lake City, UT)

is isolated and the catheter is inserted. After locating the catheter tip in the central vein, the remaining portion is threaded or tunneled into the subcutaneous tissue 3 to 5 cm to an exit site outside the skin. Typical exit sites are below the nipple, in the abdomen, or in the groin. A Dacron cuff is an integral part of the tunneled line and extends from the exit site. Granulation tissue forms around the cuff in 10 to 14 days, preventing migration of microorganisms into the catheter pathway.

When a dual-lumen catheter is used, the lumens should be labeled to indicate the purpose and function of each port.

Manufacturers have continued to provide more advanced product options. In addition to the Hickman and Broviac catheters and their multiple-lumen styles, the Groshong catheter (Davol) offers an alternative. The Groshong catheter is distinguished by the construction of a rounded, blunt catheter tip that incorporates a three-way valve. A three-position pressure-sensitive valve (Figure 15-20) that remains closed at normal vena caval pressure restricts either entrainment of air into the venous system or backflow of blood from the catheter. Application of a vacuum with a syringe allows the valve to open inward for blood aspiration. Positive pressure into the catheter by the infusion forces the valve to open outward. Advantages of this type of catheter include:

- Decreased risk of bleeding or air emboli
- Elimination of catheter clamping
- Elimination of the use of heparin in the catheter
- Reduction of flushing between use

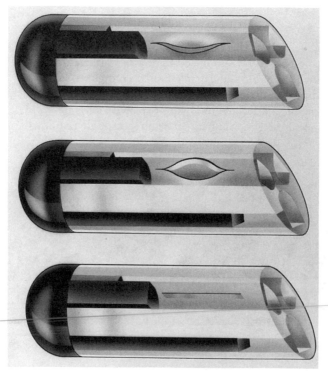

FIGURE 15-20   Groshong valve. (Courtesy: Davol, Inc., Subsidiary CR Bard Inc., Salt Lake City, UT)

For the valve to function properly, catheter tip position is critical. The tip must be situated in the midsuperior part of the vena cava.[12] If the tip is in the right atrium, thrombus formation around the tip could result, followed by malfunction and loss of valve competence. Occasional use of a fibrinolytic agent may restore valve function. Clamping and flushing with heparin similar to the procedure followed with nonvalved catheters may be needed.

The Hemed central venous catheter (GISH Biomedical, Inc.) is a long-term tunneled catheter composed of biocompatible silicone and available in single- and dual-lumen configurations. A locking clip holds the dilator and sheath together as a unit during surgical insertion. GISH Biomedical also manufactures a CathCap Catheter System in which a prefilled povidone–iodine cap immerses and bathes the hub while the cap serves as a barrier against airborne, waterborne, and touch-contamination microorganisms.

Tunneled Catheter Repair

Although conventional methods of catheter repair using adhesives have been available for some time, emergency, temporary repair may be accomplished as follows:

1. Clamp the catheter between the chest wall and the tear.
2. Clean the torn area with povidone–iodine solution.
3. Using sterile scissors, cut off the damaged portion.
4. Insert a blunt-end needle (14 or 16 gauge) into the distal end of the catheter.
5. Insert an injection cap in the hub of the needle and heparinize the catheter.
6. Secure the needle and catheter with silk suture material.
7. Release the clamp.
8. Determine patency by flushing with saline solution.

Permanent repair may be needed and is accomplished by splicing a new section of catheter with an end connector to the remainder of the line. GISH Biomedical also provides a nonadhesive repair kit. Developed specifically to be used with GISH Biomedical's central catheter line, the kit may also be used for other tunneled and central venous catheters. Key components of the kit are featured in Figure 15-21.

Clinicians have indicated that several items, not included in the repair kits, but recommended during the repair of Hemed™ Catheters are as follows:

isopropyl alcohol	swab
povidone–iodine	4″ × 4″ gauze
padded/jawless clamp	heparin flush
surgical gloves	sterile drapes
syringe	aseptic garments (*ie*, mask)

The padded clamp is placed between the damaged area and the body exit site, at least 2½″ from the damaged area, to facilitate repair. Using the GISH method:

1. Cleanse and drape the body exit site area. Using sterile technique, carefully cut off the damaged portion of the catheter, allowing at least 2½″ between the cut end and the clamp to permit catheter repair. Discard the damaged tubing and the old Luer.

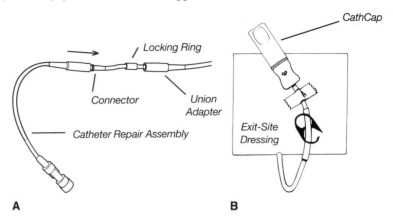

FIGURE 15-21 Hemed™ central venous access catheter nonadhesive repair kit. (Courtesy: GISH Biomedical, Inc., Santa Ana, CA). (**A**) The union adapter and locking ring are unique to the GISH repair kit. (**B**) Repaired catheter with exit-site dressing in place.

2. The union adapter slides onto the remaining tubing, tapered end first; 1/2″ of tubing should extend beyond the tabbed union adapter.

3. Grasp the adapter tab with one hand and the union adapter and silicone tubing with the other hand. The adapter tab is removed with a slight twist while pulling.

4. The locking ring easily slides over the extended catheter tubing.

5. Remove the end cap and carefully insert the straight end of the guidewire through the Luer fitting on the catheter repair assembly, consistent with GISH recommendations for the use of its products, specifically as they apply to the use of the guidewire assembly.

6. Slip the catheter tubing onto the connector of the catheter repair assembly. The tubing should be positioned approximately two-thirds up the connector.

7. The GISH locking ring is advanced onto the connector until it is against the flange. The locking ring will pull the catheter tubing up over the flange.

8. The union adapter is then advanced over the locking ring and the flange and adjusted for a tight fit.

9. Grasp the tubing on both sides of the repair site and pull gently to remove any kinks in the tubing under the union adapter.

10. The manufacturer warns the clinician to aspirate the repaired catheter before use to remove any air.

Regardless of the type of repair product utilized, it is imperative that the clinician familiarize herself with the manufacturer's recommendations for use. A working knowledge of the intricacies of the catheter itself and repair methodologies will ensure safe practice and return a damaged catheter to patency.

IMPLANTED PORTS

Implanted ports are designed to permit repeated access to the vascular system. In general, the portal consists of one or two self-sealing silicone septa, accessible by percutaneous needle puncture, and a single- or dual-lumen catheter. For the patient in need of long-term vascular access, the implanted port system is ideal. As with any central venous access system, potential complications exist, including:

- Air embolism
- Artery or vein puncture
- Arteriovenous fistula
- Brachial plexus injury
- Cardiac arrhythmia
- Cardiac puncture
- Cardiac tamponade
- Catheter disconnection/ fragmentation/embolization
- Catheter occlusion
- Catheter rupture
- Drug extravasation

- Erosion of portal/catheter through skin and/or blood vessel
- Fibrin sheath formation
- Hematoma
- Hemothorax
- Implant rejection
- Infection/sepsis
- Migration of portal/catheter
- Pneumothorax
- Thoracic duct injury
- Thromboembolism
- Thrombosis

The implanted port may be used for arterial access or implanted into the epidural space, peritoneum, pericardia, or pleural cavity (Figure 15-22). Vascular access ports may be side entry or top entry. In a side-entry port, the needle is inserted almost parallel to the reservoir. In a top-entry port, the needle is inserted perpendicular to the reservoir. Only noncoring needles should be used to access the port. A noncoring needle has an angled or deflected point that slices the septum on entry. When removed, the septum reseals itself. Noncoring needles are available in straight and 90° angle configurations, with or without extension sets. Some clinicians recommend the use of an

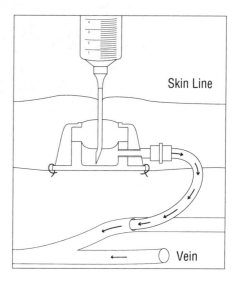

FIGURE 15-22 Accessing the PORT-A-CATH® Implantable Access System (Property of Pharmacia Deltec, Inc., St. Paul, MN)

ONC for continuous access to an implanted port. A winged noncoring needle, such as the Gripper™ by Pharmacia Deltec, is also helpful and relatively easy to stabilize (Figure 15-23).

Sterile Technique

Because this device is placed for long-term usage, extreme care must be taken to maintain sterile technique while performing any manipulations.

Needles

To prevent septum damage, only noncoring needles may be used for cannulation of the device. Straight needles are used for heparin flush, bolus injection, or blood drawing. Needles bent to a 90° angle are used for continuous or frequent intermittent infusions. The bent needle may also be used for heparin flush, bolus injection, or blood drawing. Noncoring needles are also available with a permanently attached extension tubing and clamp.

Needles are available, with metal or plastic hubs, in gauges 24 to 19, and in lengths from 0.5 inch to 2.5 inches. The needle length required will depend on how superficial or deep the septum is implanted. The gauge will depend on the type and rate of infusate to be given. Packed red cells may require a 19-gauge needle, whereas a 24-gauge needle may be adequate for flushing.

The needle must be held securely against the needle stop during all procedures to avoid injecting the drug into the subcutaneous tissue. Do not use an angular motion or twist the needle once in the septum. This action will cut the septum and create a drug leakage path. If the heparin flush is given without an extension tubing, 3 mL heparin (100 U/mL) is used. If an extension tubing is used, 5 mL heparin may be required.

Access of the side port is similar (Figure 15-24).

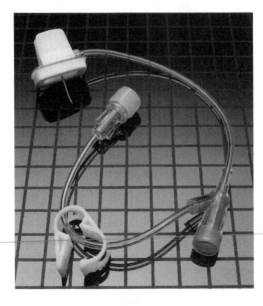

FIGURE 15-23 PORT-A-CATH® Gripper™ Needle. Access of implanted ports is facilitated by the use of a needle with gripping device. (Property of Pharmacia Deltec, Inc., St. Paul, MN)

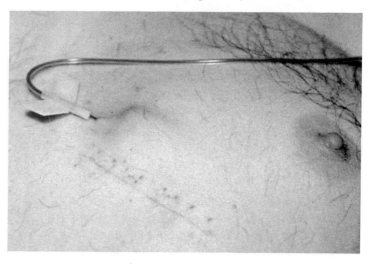

FIGURE 15-24 Access side port. (Courtesy: Norfolk Medical, Skokie, IL)

Heparin Flush

Implanted catheters require heparin flushing after each use and monthly when not in use. This is almost universally done with 3 to 5 mL of 100 U/mL heparin.

The heparin flush may be performed by the following steps:

Equipment

   Sterile noncoring needle (1)

   Sterile syringe with 3 mL heparin flush (100 U/mL)

   Sterile gloves (1 pair)

   Sterile towel (1)

   Sterile fenestrated drape (optional)

   Povidone–iodine swabs (3)

Procedure

1. Identify septum by palpating the outer perimeter of the port. Confirm septum location.
2. Wash hands thoroughly and dry.
3. Aseptically prepare sterile supplies on opened sterile towel.
4. Put on sterile gloves. Observing sterile technique, perform *three* separate skin preps with povidone–iodine. Start at center of septum and work outward toward the periphery of the port.
5. Place fenestrated drape over prepped area (optional). The availability of a sterile field at the insertion site will decrease risk of touch contamination during the procedure.
6. Attach syringe with heparin flush to noncoring needle and eliminate air from

syringe and needle. A straight or 90° angled needle may be used for heparin flush.

7. *While stabilizing the port*, using a *perpendicular angle*, insert needle into septum until the needle stop is felt.

8. Inject flush no faster than 5 mL/min.

9. Withdraw needle while *maintaining stability of the port*.

10. Examine the site closely for any signs of infiltration or leakage. Apply sterile dressing if necessary.

Connecting Implanted Catheter to Continuous Infusion System

When a continuous infusion is to be started, the device is cannulated with an extension tubing connected between the needle and the infusion tubing. If frequent intermittent infusions are given, the needle and extension tubing are left in place and the extension tubing covered with an intermittent injection cap. This prevents the need for frequent septum punctures.

Equipment

Electronic infusion device (optional)

Appropriate infusion tubing

Luer lock air-eliminating 0.22-μm filter (1)

Luer lock extension tubing with clamp or stopcock (1)

Admixture or infusion solution

Noncoring 90° angled needle

Sterile towel (1)

Sterile fenestrated drape (optional)

Sterile 10-mL syringe with 0.9% sodium chloride

Sterile strip of tape (1)

Povidone–iodine swabs (3)

Povidone–iodine ointment (optional)

Sterile gloves (1 pair)

Sterile 2 × 2 inch sponges (2)

Sterile transparent tape dressing (1)

Procedure

1. Identify septum by palpating the outer perimeter of the port. Confirm septum location.

2. Wash hands thoroughly and dry.

3. Prepare solution container, tubing, and filter. Flush system. If infusion pump is used, be sure psi is less than 15 to prevent possibility of catheter rupture.

4. Aseptically prepare all sterile supplies on opened sterile towel.

5. Put on sterile gloves. Using sterile technique perform *three* separate site preps

with povidone–iodine. Start at the center of the septum and work outward beyond the periphery of the port.

6. Place fenestrated drape over prepped area (optional).

7. Attach 10-mL syringe with 0.9% sodium chloride to extension tubing.

8. Firmly lock noncoring 90° angle needle to extension tubing.

9. Flush extension tubing and needle with the 0.9% sodium chloride. Close stopcock or clamp.

10. *While stabilizing the port*, using a perpendicular angle, insert needle into septum until the needle stop is felt. Digital pressure on top of the needle at the bend point will facilitate septum entry.

11. Open stopcock or clamp, stabilize port, and inject normal saline to affirm needle placement. Carefully observe site for any signs of infiltration. If desired, a small amount of blood may be withdrawn to affirm septum entry.

12. Close stopcock or clamp and remove syringe.

13. Securely connect and lock prepared infusion system to the extension tubing. The use of Luer locks and taping connections will reduce the risk of separation.

14. Open stopcock or clamp and start the infusion.

15. If the needle does not lie flush with the skin, place a sterile sponge under needle or needle hub.

16. If povidone–iodine ointment is to be used, apply to insertion site. The use of an ointment at this access point may create increased risk of needle movement with resultant dislodgement and can prevent direct observation of the insertion site.

17. Placing a strip of sterile tape over the needle at the insertion site can help prevent needle dislodgement.

18. Using aseptic technique, apply sterile transparent tape dressing over the site and a portion of the extension tubing. Using clear sterile tape allows for site inspection without removing the dressing.

19. Loop the tubing and tape on the skin to prevent stress at the needle site if the tubing is stretched or pulled.

Discontinuing Infusion

A continuous infusion may be discontinued by the following steps:

1. Shut infusion off. Close clamp on extension tubing or turn stopcock off.

2. Aseptically disconnect IV tubing from stopcock or extension tubing.

3. Aseptically connect air-purged syringe with 10 mL 0.9% sodium chloride. Open clamp or stopcock. Inject sodium chloride to flush system. Close clamp or stopcock.

4. Remove empty syringe. Connect air-purged syringe with 5 mL (100 U/mL) heparin. Open clamp or stopcock. Inject heparin flush.

5. Stabilize the needle while removing the clear tape and any sponges.

6. Remove the needle while *maintaining* stability.

7. Examine injection site for any signs of swelling or fluid seepage.

8. Apply a sterile dressing if necessary.

Administering a Bolus Injection

A bolus injection may be given by the following steps:

Equipment

Sterile noncoring needle (1)

Sterile extension tubing with clamp or two-way stopcock (1)

Sterile syringes 10 mL (2)

Sterile syringe 5 mL (1)

Sterile syringe appropriate size for drug (1)

Sterile needles: 22 gauge × 1 inch (4)

Sodium chloride 0.9% 20 mL

Heparin flush 5 mL (100 U/mL)

Drug to be injected

Sterile gloves (1 pair)

Sterile towel (1)

Sterile fenestrated drape (optional)

Povidone–iodine swabs (3)

Alcohol sponge (1)

Procedure

1. Identify septum by palpating the outer perimeter of the port. Confirm septum location.

2. Wash hands thoroughly and dry.

3. Open sterile towel and aseptically prepare all sterile supplies.

4. Put on sterile gloves. Observing sterile technique perform *three* separate skin preps with povidone–iodine. Start at center of septum and work outward toward the periphery of the port.

5. Place fenestrated drape over prepped area (optional). The availability of a sterile field at the needle insertion site will decrease risk of touch contamination during the procedure.

6. Using sterile technique, prepare two air-purged syringes with 10 mL normal saline, one air-purged syringe with 5 mL heparin flush, and an air-purged syringe with drug to be injected.

7. Connect extension tubing or stopcock to first syringe with 0.9% sodium chloride and noncoring needle. Flush the system. Close clamp or turn stopcock off.

8. While stabilizing port, using a perpendicular angle insert needle into septum until needle stop is felt. Open clamp or turn stopcock on. Inject sodium chloride. To prevent needle dislodgement during any injection, the needle should be

stabilized either digitally or with a 90° angle needle by the use of a sterile strip of tape.

9. Turn stopcock off or clamp extension tubing, disconnect empty syringe, and connect air-purged syringe with drug. Turn stopcock on or open tubing clamp, inject drug at recommended rate but no faster than 5 mL/min.

10. Turn stopcock off or clamp extension tubing, disconnect empty syringe, and connect second air-purged 10-mL syringe of 0.9% sodium chloride. Turn stopcock on or open tubing clamp, inject flush.

11. Turn stopcock off or clamp extension tubing, disconnect empty syringe, and connect air-purged syringe with heparin flush. Turn stopcock on or open tubing clamp, and inject heparin flush.

12. Remove needle while *maintaining stability of the port.*

13. Examine site closely for any signs of infiltration or leakage. Apply sterile dressing if necessary.

Venous Sampling

Blood samples may be drawn as a separate procedure, at the time of a bolus injection, or during continuous infusion. To draw a blood sample as a separate procedure or at the time of a bolus injection:

1. Follow all steps including the first flush with 0.9% sodium chloride given for a bolus injection (steps 1 through 7).

2. Using the empty syringe, draw back 10 mL blood and saline mixture. Close stopcock or clamp and remove and discard syringe with blood.

3. Attach fresh sterile syringe, open stopcock or clamp, and withdraw required amount of blood for ordered specimen. Close stopcock or clamp and remove syringe.

4. Immediately attach second syringe with 10 mL 0.9% sodium chloride. Open stopcock or clamp and flush device. Close stopcock or clamp.

5. If bolus injection is to be given, proceed with bolus procedure after first 0.9% sodium chloride flush (steps 8 through 11).

6. If the catheter will not be used, perform heparin flush by the following steps.
   a. Remove empty syringe and connect air-purged heparin syringe.
   b. Inject flush at 5 mL/min.
   c. Remove needle while *maintaining positive pressure* (Figure 15-25). Inspect site closely for any signs of infiltration or leakage. Sterile dressing may be applied to site if necessary.

Drawing Blood Samples during Continuous Infusion

1. Shut off infusion.

2. Close clamp on extension tubing.

3. Aseptically disconnect system at extension tubing–IV system connection. Blood samples should be drawn in coordination with tubing and filter changes. This prevents unnecessary manipulation of the system and prevents the risk of contamination that is present if the same tubing is reconnected.

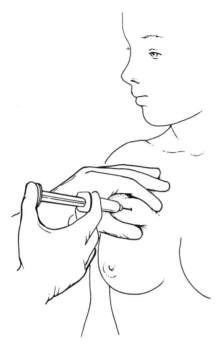

FIGURE 15-25   Withdraw needle while maintaining positive pressure.

4. Aseptically connect air-purged syringe with 10 mL 0.9% sodium chloride. Open clamp. Inject normal saline to flush infusate from septum and catheter.

5. Using empty syringe, withdraw 10 mL blood and saline mixture. Close clamp.

6. Aseptically remove and discard syringe with blood and connect empty syringe. Make sure the syringe is large enough to collect all blood required for specimens.

7. Open clamp and withdraw required amount of blood. Close clamp.

8. Aseptically remove syringe with blood, attach air-purged syringe with 10 mL sodium chloride.

9. Open clamp and inject to flush blood from the catheter and septum.

10. Close clamp. Remove syringe. Reconnect sterile IV system and lock and tape connections.

11. Reestablish flow rate.

Tubing and Dressing Changes

Tubing and filter down to the extension tubing should be changed consistent with institutional guidelines and INS standards.

MRI® Port

The MRI® Port, designed by Davol, Cranston, Rhode Island, is designed to eliminate interference caused by metal ports during magnetic resonance imaging or computerized tomography.

IMPLANTED PUMPS

The implanted pump provides long-term venous or arterial access, a safe means of treatment for those with chronic diseases, direct infusion that can be targeted at a tumor or organ, a decreased infection rate, and enhanced patient mobility.

Criteria for use of implanted pumps include the following:

- Histologically proven primary or metastatic hepatic cancer
- Absence of extrahepatic disease or malignant ascites
- Measurable hepatic disease
- Satisfactory condition for major surgery
- Absence of acute infection/prolonged fever

Insertion is performed during laparotomy in which the infusion catheter is threaded through a gastric artery to a common hepatic artery. The catheter is then sutured in place and the feeding arteries are ligated. A pump pocket is prepared, and the pump is sutured to the underlying fascia. An infusate is injected into the pump reservoir and remains in place for 4 to 6 postoperative days. Then, the pump is emptied and filled with an initial dose of chemotherapy.

Patient Identification Card

When the pump is implanted, the surgeon should fill out the Patient Registration and Implantation Record. The manufacturer will issue the patient a wallet-sized identification card containing information pertinent to the implanted pump. The physician should fill in the space provided for any medical emergency instructions. This card should be carried by the patient at all times.

Postimplantation Care

Patients should be monitored carefully after implantation to confirm proper pump performance, wound healing, and favorable response to therapy. The pump should not be used for the administration of drugs for several days after implantation to allow for adequate wound healing:[7]

Patient Instructions

The patient should be instructed to:[7]

1. Avoid traumatic physical activity to prevent tissue damage around the implant site.
2. Avoid long hot baths, saunas, and other activities that increase body temperature and result in increased drug flow.
3. Consult the physician during febrile illness to assess the effects of increased drug flow.
4. Consult the physician before air travel or change of residence to another geographic location. Adjustments in drug dosage may be required to compensate for an anticipated change in drug flow.
5. Avoid deep sea or scuba diving.

6. Report any unusual symptoms or complications relating to the specific drug therapy or the device.

7. Return at the prescribed time for pump refill.

Pump Refill Procedure

The pump will require refills at specific intervals of time. The intervals will depend on the volume of the reservoir and the rate of administration.

The pump may be refilled by the following steps:[7]

Equipment

Sterile fenestrated drape (1)	Sterile extension tubing with clamp (1)
Sterile towel (1)	Sterile gloves (1 pair)
50-mL syringe with drug solution (1)	Sterile 2 × 2 inch sponge (1)
Sterile empty 50-mL syringe (1)	Povidone–iodine swabs (3)
Sterile noncoring needle (1)	Heating pad (1)

Procedure

1. Warm 50-mL syringe with drug solution to 15°C to 35°C with the heating pad.

2. Identify the outer perimeter of the pump by palpating the pump pocket. Locate pump septum.

3. Wash hands thoroughly and dry.

4. Using sterile technique, place all sterile items on opened sterile towel.

5. Put on sterile gloves.

6. Disinfect pump site with povidone–iodine. Use *three* separate preps. Start at the center of the pump and work outward beyond the periphery of the pump.

7. Place fenestrated drape over prepped pump site. Sterile template may be aligned over septum.

8. *Securely* connect *barrel* of empty 5-mL syringe and extension tubing to the noncoring needle. Close clamp.

9. Using a perpendicular angle, insert needle into center of septum.

10. Open clamp. Lower syringe barrel to below patient level and allow pump to empty (Figure 15-26A).

11. Close clamp. Record returned volume, adding 1 mL for amount of drug remaining in extension tubing. Disconnect and discard syringe barrel.

12. *Securely* attach air-purged syringe with drug solution to extension tubing. Open clamp.

13. Using both hands, inject 5 mL of solution into pump. Release pressure and allow drug to return to syringe. This test confirms proper needle placement. Continue to inject and check needle placement at 5-mL increments until syringe is emptied (Figure 15-26B).

14. Pull needle out quickly and apply digital pressure with sterile sponge. If necessary, apply a sterile adhesive bandage.

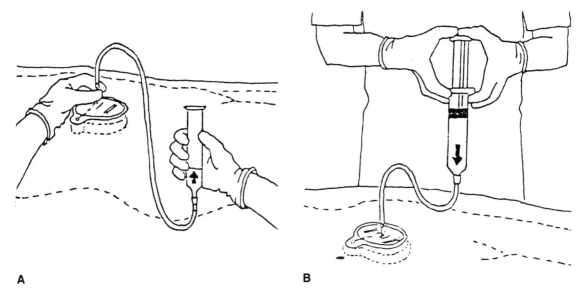

FIGURE 15-26 Pump refill procedure. (**A**) The syringe barrel is lowered to allow the pump to empty. (**B**) Using both hands, 5 mL is injected into the pump. (Courtesy: Intermedics Infusaid, Inc., Norwood, MA)

Important Considerations

Never attempt to aspirate fluid from the pump. This will cause blood to be drawn back into the catheter, resulting in occlusion. If no fluid is returned into the syringe barrel, either the septum has not been penetrated or the pump is completely empty of infusate. To test for septum penetration, remove the syringe barrel and connect 5- mL syringe with normal saline. Inject the solution and release the plunger to allow the fluid to return to the syringe. If the fluid does not return, again attempt to locate and penetrate the septum, using 5 mL normal saline to test penetration. If you are not successful, the physician should be notified because pump failure may have occurred. Accurate fill and refill records are essential to ensure that the pump is refilled at the required intervals; these records also document appropriate pump functioning.

Bolus Injection Through the Side Port

A bolus injection may be given through the side port of the implanted pump by the following steps:[7]

Equipment

Sterile 5-mL syringes (2)

Sterile syringe appropriate size for drug to be injected (1)

Sterile needles 22 gauge × 1 inch (3)

Noncoring needle (1)

Stopcock or extension tubing with clamp (1)

0.9% sodium chloride 10 mL (1)

Drug to be injected (1)

Sterile towel (1)

Sterile fenestrated drape (1)

Sterile gloves (1 pair)

Alcohol sponge (1)

Povidone–iodine swabs (3)

Procedure

1. Identify the outer perimeter of the pump by palpating the pump pocket. Locate the *side port* septum.
2. Wash hands thoroughly and dry.
3. Using sterile technique, place all sterile items on opened sterile towel.
4. Put on sterile gloves.
5. Disinfect side port septum with povidone–iodine. Use *three* separate preps. Start at the center of the side port and work outward beyond the periphery of the port.
6. Place fenestrated drape over prepped area.
7. Using sterile technique, prepare two syringes with 5 mL 0.9% sodium chloride. Prepare drug to be injected in separate syringe.
8. Connect first normal saline syringe to stopcock or extension tubing and noncoring needle. Secure all connections. Flush system with solution. Close clamp or stopcock.
9. While stabilizing port, insert noncoring needle into *side port* septum at a perpendicular angle.
10. Open stopcock or clamp. Inject saline to flush catheter and confirm needle placement. Close stopcock or clamp.
11. Disconnect and discard syringe. Connect syringe with drug. Open stopcock or clamp. Inject drug at manufacturer's recommended rate, but do not exceed 10 mL/min. Close stopcock or clamp. Disconnect and discard syringe.
12. Connect second syringe with normal saline flush. Open stopcock or clamp. Flush catheter. Close clamp.
13. Stabilize port while gently withdrawing needle.
14. Carefully check area for any signs of infiltration or leakage. A sterile dressing may be applied if necessary.

CATHETER DECLOTTING

Clots develop when thrombin, an enzyme made from prothrombin, converts fibrinogen to fibrin, a collagen. The fibrin forms the clot. Activated plasminogen forms plasmin, an enzyme that dissolves the clot and keeps fibrinogen from reforming fibrin; this process is known as *fibrinolysis.*

Within the lumen of a right atrial catheter, clot or fibrin sheath occludes the line, and fibrinolytic agents are often used to restore patency. Urokinase dissolves clots by stimulating the conversion of plasminogen to plasmin, triggering fibrinolysis. When urokinase is used as directed for IV catheter clearance, therapeutic serum levels are not observed, because only minute amounts of the drug enter the bloodstream.

To declot catheters using a fibrinolytic agent, perform the following procedure:

1. Connect a 10-mL syringe to the catheter. Put on gloves.

2. Gently attempt to aspirate blood from the catheter.

3. If occlusion is present and cannot be aspirated, attach a 5-mL syringe filled with urokinase in a concentration equal to the volume of the catheter:

   - 11 Fr. Hickman = 0.8–0.9 mL

   - 6 Fr. = 0.5–0.7 mL

   - Port-A-Cath = 1.3 mL

4. Slowly and gently inject the drug into the lumen of the catheter.

5. Cap the catheter and wait 10 minutes.

6. Attempt to aspirate drug and residual clot with a 10-mL syringe. If unsuccessful, reattempt every 10 minutes.

7. After 30 minutes, wait 30 additional minutes before trying again.

8. If unsuccessful, draw the urokinase from the catheter, clamp it, and remove the syringe.

9. Place a sterile, Luer lock cap on the catheter and unclamp it.

10. Wait 1 hour and repeat procedure.

INTRAOSSEOUS ACCESS

When factors such as venous collapse in shock, anatomic scarcity of veins, and thrombosis of venous sites preclude the ability to establish peripheral venous access, intraosseous (IO) infusion should be considered. First used in patients in 1934, this technique has endured for nearly 60 years and has recently gained acceptance and interest as a viable alternative to peripheral or central venous access.

Historical Background

Use of the bone marrow for infusion of IV fluids was first proposed by Drinker of Harvard in 1922.[4] During the 1940s, Tocantins and O'Neill became the best known advocates of IO infusions.[19] Principal indications for IO infusion were:

- Pediatric emergencies
- Adults with mutilated skin
- Transportation of uncooperative patients
- Shock

Commonly administered fluids were colloids, crystalline solutions, plasma, blood products, antibiotics, epinephrine, morphine, and glucose. Interest in IO infusions dwindled between 1950 and 1970 because of the development of disposable IV needles and catheters. Since 1976, interest in this route of administration has grown dramatically.

Indications

Indications for the use of IO infusions include anaphylaxis, burns, cardiac arrest, coma, dehydration, drowning, respiratory arrest, septic shock, hypovolemia, diabetic acidosis, status epilepticus, status asthmaticus, sudden infant death syndrome (SIDS), and trauma. Standard protocol calls for the establishment of an IO line in children if percutaneous peripheral venous access cannot be established within 60 to 120 seconds.[1,3] It may be the route of choice in event of cardiac arrest or hypotension.[14]

Anatomy

Bones are vascular structures with dynamic circulation capable of accepting large volumes of fluid and rapidly transporting fluids or drugs to the central circulation.[16] Long bones consist of a shaft called the diaphysis with a very dense cortex, the epiphysis (or the rounded ends of the bone), and the metaphysis (the transitional zone). The epiphysis and the metaphysis have a much thinner cortex and contain cancellous, or spongy, bone. The iliac crest is comprised of a thin cortex and is filled with cancellous bone. The hollow core of the shaft of long bones and the spaces within the cancellous bone are referred to as the medullary space and contain the marrow.

The marrow cavity has been appropriately called the noncollapsible vein.[13,18] The intramedullary space is an integral part of the vascular system and is made up of a vastly interconnected network of venous sinusoids, analogous to a sponge.[17] The marrow is supplied by nutrient arteries that penetrate the cortex of the bone.

Technique

Many sites have been used for IO infusions, including the sternum, the tibia (Figure 15-27), the femur, and the iliac crest. In children under the age of 5, the site of choice is the flat anterior medial surface of the proximal tibia just below the tibial tubercle or the distal tibia, followed by the distal femur.[5] In adults, the iliac crest is the bone of choice.

Strict asepsis is essential and the skin preparation should be consistent with INS Standards of Practice. Local anesthesia may be used for conscious patients.

A sturdy needle with a stylet, such as a standard bone marrow needle, is used. The IO needle is quickly advanced through the skin to the bony cortex. With firm pressure and a rotary motion, the needle is further advanced into the marrow cavity. Insertion resistance decreases as the needle penetrates the cortex, also known as the "trap door effect." The stylet is removed and the correct position is verified by observing the needle standing without support and the ability to aspirate blood and marrow contents. Once these criteria are fulfilled, a continuous infusion can begin.[6] If, however, an attempt is unsuccessful, further attempts must be undertaken in other bones because if IO infusion were established in the same bone, the infused fluid would leak from the original abandoned hole in the cortex.[5,16,17]

Intraosseous Access Needles

The standards throughout the industry for IO access have been the Kormed/Jamshidi bone marrow biopsy needle, the Osgood needle, and the Cook IO infusion needle; these products come in several sizes and with various tips.

The Osteoport, an improved IO access needle, was developed by Von Hoff and his

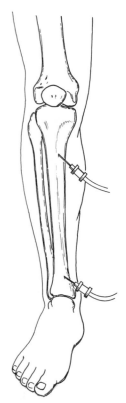

FIGURE 15-27 Possible insertion sites of percutaneous intraosseous infusion device in the lower extremities. (Reproduced with permission of *Journal of Emergency Nursing*)

colleagues and was patented as the intramedullary catheter (Figure 15-28). To decrease the complications of insertion, threads were added to the needle so that the IO needle could be precisely placed within the marrow. To decrease the rate of leakage, a cone was added to provide a tight seal between the bone and the Osteoport. To decrease the rate of osteomyelitis and cellulitis, the Osteoport was made implantable so that there would not be a direct conduit from outside the body into the bone marrow. To increase comfort to the patient, the Osteoport has a low profile and does not require a stiff needle protruding through the skin. For repeated use, the patient will not require repeated bone punctures.[5,20]

The Osteoport is made of medical implant-grade titanium. Thread size and shape are identical to commonly accepted orthopedic devices. The Silastic membrane is made of medically implantable-grade Silastic, commonly used in intravenous catheters and implanted ports.

Primary indications for the Osteoport are patients who require access to the vascular system but have exhausted all other reasonable IV sites. The recommended duration of implant is less than 30 days.[20]

The Osteoport consists of a 1-inch titanium or stainless steel needle with a self-sealing cap. The hollow device, which resembles a partially threaded bolt (see Figure 15-28A) is implanted in a large bone of the hip or leg. Once the incision is closed, the device is ready for use. The implant may be performed under local or general anesthesia.

To initiate the flow of fluids, a needle attached to the IV tubing is inserted through

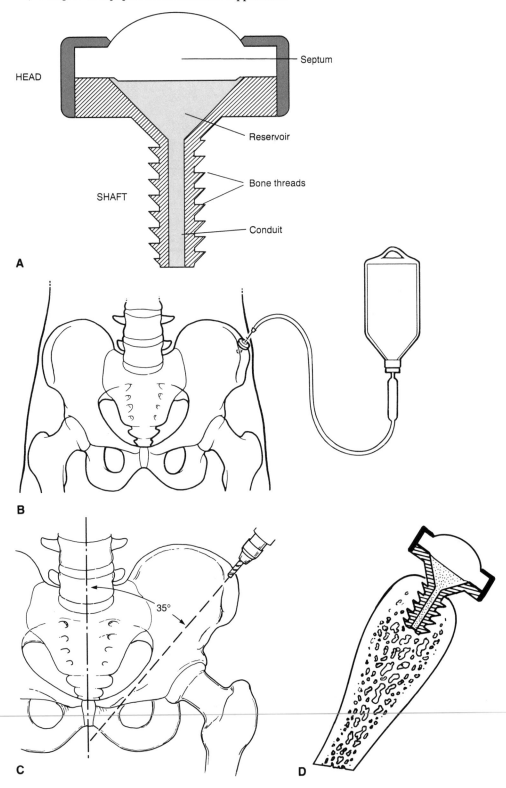

HEAD

SHAFT

Septum

Reservoir

Bone threads

Conduit

A

B

C

35°

D

the skin into the Osteoport's cap. The physician will be able to locate the device by feeling it under the skin. (See Figure 15-28B–D.)

Because it is implanted in bone, the device offers numerous advantages:

- Fluids are rapidly absorbed by the blood from the marrow cavity.
- Clotting and lung puncture problems are eliminated.
- The risk of infection is reduced.

VENTRICULAR RESERVOIRS

The ventricular implanted reservoir is used to provide access directly into the cerebrospinal fluid (CSF) without performing a spinal tap, to measure CSF pressure, to obtain CSF specimens, and to instill medication.[8] Implanted surgically, it is positioned in the right frontal region, into the lateral ventricle, sutured to the pericranium, and covered with a skin flap. (See Chapter 24.)

Major complications include:

- Infection, characterized by tenderness, redness, drainage, fever, neck stiffness, and headache with or without vomiting
- Reservoir malfunction in which the catheter is obstructed from the distal subarachnoid blockage of CSF, causing inability to aspirate or inject the port and slow refilling of the reservoir after manual expression of fluid
- Displacement or migration of the catheter, assessed by slow or absent refilling of the reservoir after manual expression of fluid and confirmed by computed tomography and change in neurologic status

The following procedure applies to accessing and administering medications through the ventricular reservoir:

1. Explain procedure to patient/family.
2. Gather supplies.
3. Obtain vital signs.
4. Place patient in comfortable position; Trendelenburg's is recommended to facilitate gravitational force for specimen collection.
5. Wash hands.
6. Put on gloves and mask.
7. Open packages using aseptic technique; use a sterile field.
8. Scalp hair over the port may be clipped to facilitate access.
9. Swab area vigorously with povidone–iodine in a concentric circle, covering an area 2 inches in diameter.
10. Repeat skin preparation; allow to air dry.
11. Remove and discard gloves.

◄ **FIGURE 15-28** (**A**) Osteoport intraosseous infusion port. (**B**) Intraosseous infusion via Osteoport. (**C**) Needle insertions should be aligned with the central axis of the Osteoport, which is approximately 35° from the longitudinal axis of the body. (**D**) Cross section of the Osteoport sitting in the greater tubercle of the anterior superior iliac spine. (Courtesy: LifeQuest Medical, San Antonio, TX)

12. Apply new sterile gloves.

13. Attach syringe to a 23- or 25-gauge winged infusion set.

14. Using nondominant hand, palpate and stabilize reservoir port (this hand is no longer sterile).

15. Puncture the reservoir obliquely with a 23- or 25-gauge needle.

16. Withdraw 3 mL CSF and detach syringe; place on sterile field.

17. Attach syringe with medication to access needle.

18. Administer medication as ordered over 5 minutes. Monitor patient during administration and immediately thereafter for presence of nausea/vomiting, headache/dizziness.

19. Detach medication syringe and attach syringe with 3 mL reserved CSF.

20. Flush reservoir with CSF.

21. Maintain positive pressure on syringe and withdraw access needle.

22. Apply gentle pressure over the site with sterile gauze.

23. Instruct patient to remain in supine position without a pillow under his head for 30 minutes following this procedure.

24. Discard biohazardous waste consistent with institutional policy.

25. Document in appropriate area of clinical record.

REFERENCES

1. American Academy of Pediatrics and American College of Emergency Physicians. (1989). *Advanced pediatric life support*, pp. 3, 10–11, 39, 76–77, 123.

2. Brendel, V. (1984). Catheters utilized in delivering total parenteral nutrition. *Journal of the National Intravenous Therapy Association, 7*(6), 488–490.

3. Brunette, D. D., & Fischer, R. (1988). Intravascular access in pediatric cardiac arrest. *American Journal of Emergency Medicine, 6*(6), 577–579.

4. Drinker, C. K., Drinker, K. R., & Lund, C. C. (1922). The circulation in the mammalian bone marrow. *American Journal of Physiology, 62*(1).

5. Fuentes-Afflick, E. (1990). Use and management of intraosseous infusions. Presentation to the Bay Area Vascular Access Nurses (BAVAN) Fourth Annual Conference. March 12, 1990, San Francisco, CA.

6. Ho, M. T., & Saunders, C. E. (1990). *Current emergency diagnosis and treatment* (3rd ed.). Norwalk, CT: Appleton & Lange.

7. Intermedics Infusaid Corp. (1983). *Implantable drug delivery system—physician's manual*. Norwood, MA.

8. *Revised intravenous nursing standards of practice*. (1990). *Journal of Intravenous Nursing*, (Suppl.), S73.

9. Lokick, J. J., Bothe, A., Jr., et al.(1985). Complications and management of implanted venous access catheters. *Journal of Clinical Oncology, 3*, 710–717.

10. McIntyre, P. B., Laidlow, J. M., et al. (1982). Thromboembolic complications and central venous catheters (Letter). *Lancet, 2*, 936.

11. Product literature (1990). Arrow Corp. VitaCuff® Technical Report. Arrow-Howes Multi-lumen catheter with antiseptic surface and VitaCuff.

12. Product literature (1991). Davol Inc., subsidiary of C. R. Bard, Inc., PO Box 8500, Cranston, RI. Groshong three-way valve.

13. Rosen, P., Baker, F. J., II, Barkin, R. M., Braen, G. R., Dailey, R. H., & Lewvy, R. C. (1988). *Emergency medicine concepts and clinical practice* (Vol. 1). St. Louis: C. V. Mosby.

14. Rosetti, V. A., Thompson, B. M., Miller, J., Mateer, J. R., & Aprahamian, C. (1985). Intraosseous infusion: An alternative route of pediatric intravascular access. *Annals of Emergency Medicine, 14*, 885–888.

15. Ryan, J. A., Jr., & Gough, J. A. (1984). Complications of central venous catheterization for total parenteral nutrition: The role of the nurse. *Journal of the National Intravenous Therapy Association, 7*(1) 29–35.

16. Spivey, W. H. (1991). Clinical procedure in emergency medicine. In J. Roberts, J. Hedges *Intraosseous infusion* (Chap. 24). Philadelphia: W. B. Saunders.
17. Spivey, W. H. (1987). Intraosseous infusions. *Journal of Pediatrics, 3*(5), 639–643.
18. Standards for CPR and ECC. Part V: Pediatric advanced life support. (1986). *Journal of the American Medical Association, 255*(21), 2961–2969.
19. Tocantins, L. M., O'Neill, J. F., & Price, A. H. (1941). Infusions of blood and other fluids via the bone marrow: Application in pediatrics. *Journal of the American Medical Association, 117,* 1229–1234.
20. Von Hoff, D. D. (in press). Intraosseous infusions: An important but forgotten method of vascular access. *Cancer Investigations Journal.*

BIBLIOGRAPHY

Esparza, D. M., & Weyland, J. B. (1982). Nursing care for the patient with an Ommaya reservoir. *Oncology Nursing Forum, 9*(4), 17–20.

Handy, C. M. (1989). Vascular access devices. *Journal of Intravenous Nursing, 12*(1S), S12–S14.

Manley, L. (1989). Intraosseous infusion: A lifesaving technique that should be used more widely. *Journal of Intravenous Nursing, 12*(6), 367–368.

Newton, R., DeYoung, J. L., & Levin, H. J. (1985). Volumes of implantable vascular access devices and heparin flush requirements. *Journal of the National Intravenous Therapy Association, 8*(2), 137–140.

Winter, V. (1984). Implantable vascular access devices. *Oncology Nursing Forum, 11,* 25–30.

REVIEW QUESTIONS

1. Central venous access devices include all of the following EXCEPT:
   a. tunneled line
   b. implanted port
   c. tunneled port
   d. reservoir

2. The majority of central venous catheters are made of which of the following materials?
   a. polyvinyl chloride
   b. silicone
   c. Teflon
   d. polystyrene

3. The collagen matrix in a bonded catheter is made of what type of material?
   a. purified type I bovine tendon collagen
   b. human collagen
   c. purified type II bovine artery
   d. animal artery

4. The blunt catheter tip with three-way valve is a feature of what type of catheter?
   a. Groshong
   b. Hickman
   c. Broviac
   d. peripherally inserted central catheter

5. Complications associated with the implanted port include all of the following EXCEPT:
   a. speed shock
   b. cardiac tamponade
   c. catheter occlusion
   d. fibrin sheath formation

6. The implanted port may be implanted into all of the following sites EXCEPT:
   a. peritoneum
   b. epidural space
   c. pleural cavity
   d. right atrium

7. Catheter declotting may be performed with the instillation of:
   a. urokinase
   b. saline
   c. 10-U heparin flush
   d. lidocaine

8. IO access has routinely been performed with all of the following EXCEPT:
   a. bone marrow biopsy needle
   b. laser device
   c. Osgood needle
   d. IO port

9. Principal indications for IO infusion include all of the following EXCEPT:
   a. pediatric emergencies
   b. adults with mutilated skin
   c. cancer
   d. shock

10. Major complications with the implanted reservoir include all of the following EXCEPT:
    a. infection
    b. malfunction
    c. displacement
    d. air embolism

CHAPTER 16

Intra-arterial Therapy

Through technical advancement of blood analyzers, it is now possible to obtain measurements of blood levels and pressures of carbon dioxide and oxygen as well as bicarbonate blood levels. Because arterial blood supplies all body tissues, medical practitioners recognized the advantages gained for diagnosis and assessment of treatment if this blood analysis were performed on arterial rather than venous blood. Placement of indwelling arterial catheters to allow for multiple drawings of arterial blood specimens and continuous arterial pressure monitoring is a common IV nursing practice.

OVERVIEW OF ARTERIAL ACCESS

Methods and Purposes

An arterial puncture may be performed with a syringe and needle for a one-time sample of arterial blood for arterial blood gas (ABG) measurement or by insertion of an indwelling catheter to obtain serial or daily ABG samples and constant arterial pressure monitoring.

Sites

The *radial artery* is usually the site of first choice because (1) it is very superficial and easiest to enter; (2) its location at the wrist makes it easy to stabilize for a quick entry; (3) if thrombosis should occur, the ulnar artery will, by collateral circulation, supply blood to the entire hand (shown by the Allen's test); and (4) it is easy to apply a postpuncture pressure dressing at this site.

Second and third site choices vary according to institution and personal preferences.

The *ulnar artery* is usually much deeper and more difficult to stabilize than the radial artery, so, although it may be larger, it is usually not the first choice as an entry site. Further, most authors will agree that if the radial artery has been entered, the ulnar artery of the same arm should not be used.

The *brachial artery* at the antecubital fossa frequently lies deep, close to nerves and tendons, and is difficult to stabilize. If thrombosis should occur in the brachial artery, blood supply to the forearm and hand may be compromised (Figure 16-1).

The *femoral artery* located midway between the anterior superior spine of the ilium and the symphysis pubis (Figure 16-2) is the largest accessible artery and is easily palpated, stabilized, and entered. However, digital pressure is required for postpuncture

Sharon M. Weinstein: PLUMER'S PRINCIPLES & PRACTICE OF INTRAVENOUS THERAPY, FIFTH EDITION, © 1993 J. B. Lippincott Company

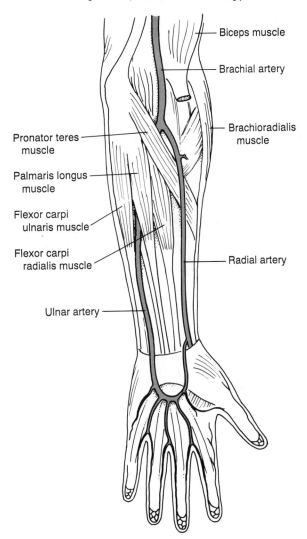

Biceps muscle

Brachial artery

Brachioradialis
muscle

Pronator teres
muscle

Palmaris longus
muscle

Flexor carpi
ulnaris muscle

Flexor carpi
radialis muscle

Radial artery

Ulnar artery

FIGURE 16-1 Anatomic location of
radial, ulnar, and brachial arteries.

pressure. If postpuncture thrombosis should occur in the femoral artery, a limb- or life-threatening condition may result.

ONE-TIME ARTERIAL BLOOD GAS SAMPLING

Patient Preparation

Steps for patient preparation for ABG sampling include the following:

1. The physician's order should include the fraction of inspired oxygen (FIO_2) or room air fraction of oxygen (21% O_2), and the patient should be at this steady state continuously for 15 to 20 minutes before the blood sample is drawn.

2. Unless a postexercise sample is ordered, the patient should be at rest for this period of time.

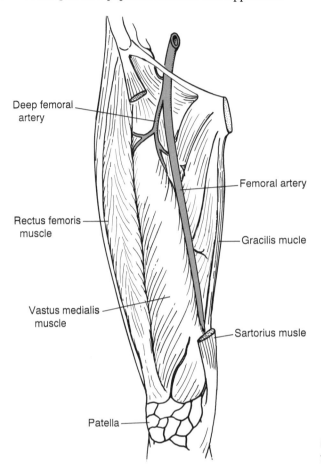

Deep femoral artery

Femoral artery

Rectus femoris muscle

Gracilis mucle

Vastus medialis muscle

Sartorius musle

Patella

FIGURE 16-2 Anatomic location of the femoral artery.

3. The patient's position can result in varied ABG measurements. A supine position may result in more difficult breathing than would sitting upright. The most comfortable position for the patient should be used for all blood sampling procedures.

4. The procedure must be fully explained to the patient because anxiety and fear can cause hyperventilation and alteration of the blood values.

5. The person performing the arterial puncture should be competent because undue trauma will cause pain, often leading to hyperventilation by the patient and resulting in alteration of the blood values.

Equipment

The laboratory requisition form should have all the usual information plus the oxygen status of the patient, time of day (for serial drawings), and, if the patient is on a respirator, all pertinent settings. In some institutions, the patient's temperature and hemoglobin count are also required.

Blood samples can be drawn with existing equipment.

Needed supplies are as follows:

- Gloves
- Airtight syringe (2–10 mL)
- Appropriate size needles (2)
  - For radial or brachial artery: 25 gauge × ⁵/₈ inch or 22 gauge × 1 inch
  - For femoral artery: 22 gauge × 1¹/₂ inch or 20 gauge × 1¹/₂ inch
- Heparin 1 mL (1000 USP U/mL)
- Alcohol swab
- Iodophor prep
- Sterile 2 × 2 inch sponge
- Rubber stopper or syringe cap
- Labeled container with ice (paper cup or emesis basin)
- 1-inch adhesive tape

Note: Prepackaged kits are also available from some manufacturers. They are simple to use, more cost effective, and may be contained in ice.

To heparinize the syringe, attach a needle other than the one to be used for puncture to the syringe, cleanse top of heparin vial or neck of ampule with alcohol swab, and open ampule. Withdraw 1 mL heparin into the syringe, draw plunger back and forth several times to coat plunger with heparin, and rotate plunger to eliminate dry spots. To eliminate any air bubbles, hold the syringe with the needle upright and gently tap sides of syringe, or turn syringe with needle pointed downward and *slowly* invert syringe upright. Discard needle used for heparinization, and place and *secure tightly* needle selected for arterial puncture. With syringe in inverted position, push plunger up and expel all excess heparin. *The only heparin remaining should be in the dead space of the needle and on the walls of the syringe.* Excess heparin or air bubbles will alter the resultant ABG values.

An ABG kit is commonly used for this procedure. Such kits are inexpensive and contain, except for ice and tape, all equipment needed to perform a one-time arterial puncture. If the kit contains a heparinized prefilled syringe, remove syringe cap, place and secure appropriate size needle, wet inner walls of syringe with heparin, and expel excess heparin with the same method used for a syringe that is not prefilled. Most ABG kits contain a plastic bag for the iced blood sample. *An ABG blood sample that has not been immediately placed in ice can have faulty results because red blood cells will continue to metabolize oxygen and give off carbon dioxide.*

Procedure

Radial Puncture
As with any invasive procedure, begin by putting on gloves. Check the site for a palpable pulse and take precautions to monitor the condition of skin, surrounding tissues, and any previous arterial puncture marks. Perform Allen's test to ensure the adequacy of collateral circulation (Figure 16-3).

A rolled towel may be placed under the wrist, causing hyperextension of the hand to stretch and stabilize the artery. The skin is prepped with iodophor, wiping with the circular method and allowing at least a 30-second contact time with the intended puncture site. Gloves should be worn.

A local anesthetic is not always necessary for an arterial puncture with a needle.

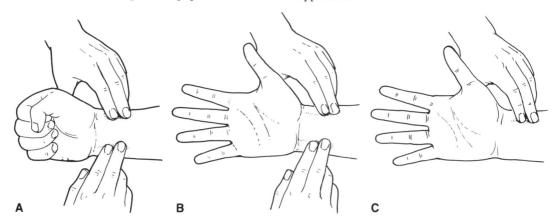

FIGURE 16-3 Perform Allen's test to determine the adequacy of ulnar blood flow before inserting a radial artery catheter: (**A**) Elevate patient's hand. Instruct patient to alternately clench and unclench the elevated hand several times, then occlude both the radial and ulnar arteries and instruct the patient to clench the hand again. (**B**) Lower the patient's hand and ask the patient to relax the hand. Note that the palm is drained of blood and pale. (**C**) While maintaining pressure on the radial artery, release pressure on the ulnar artery and note length of time required for return of color to hand. Use the following gauge to evaluate blood return: 5–7 seconds = ulnar artery is patent providing adequate blood supply to hand; 7–15 seconds = ulnar arterial blood flow is impaired; more than 15 seconds = ulnar arterial blood flow is inadequate, indicating that the radial artery should not be used.

With it, the chances for a quick, successful entry are less, and the anesthetic does not help the discomfort of arterial entry. However, if a difficult entry is anticipated or multiple attempts are necessary, a local anesthetic injected at the intended entry site may eliminate skin discomfort.

To perform the radial puncture, palpate the artery and align two or three fingertips along the direction the artery follows. Hold syringe no higher than a 30° angle with the needle pointed directly toward the artery. With one smooth step, quickly enter skin and artery. Artery pressure will usually cause the blood to spontaneously pulsate back into the syringe. If blood pressure is low or the syringe not free flowing, it may be necessary to withdraw *gently* on the plunger.

The plunger should be withdrawn 1 to 2 mL before the stick. This accomplishes two purposes: (1) if the sample is indeed arterial and not venous, the patient's pressure will cause a brisk and often pulsatile reflux of blood into the syringe (unless the patient is severely hypotensive); and (2) this prevents complications such as arterial spasm and blood hemolysis.

The blood return will stop when the level of the automatic shutoff is reached. If a shutoff feature is not available, 1 to 2 mL blood is sufficient for the blood gas analyzer.

The 2 × 2 inch sterile sponge is folded to form a pressure point and, immediately following the quick withdrawal of the needle and syringe, is applied with digital pressure to the puncture site. Taking precautions not to encircle the entire wrist, the pressure dressing is firmly secured with tape.

If a syringe cap is to be used, remove the needle from the syringe and attach the cap quickly and securely. If a rubber stopper is to be used, stick the needle tip into the center of the stopper. Roll the syringe back and forth between the hands for 5 to 10 seconds to ensure mixing of the blood and heparin. The unit is then placed in the iced container and taken immediately for analysis. A small amount of cold water added to the ice provides for even, cold distribution and facilitates placement of the sample so that all the blood in the barrel is in contact with iced water.

Femoral Puncture

The femoral artery is usually easily palpated with the patient in the supine position. If the patient is very obese, assistance may be needed to hold the abdomen away or the patient's buttocks may be placed on an inverted bedpan. If the abdomen is pendulous, you may tape it up and away to provide easier access and maintain sterility.

Wearing gloves, prepping of patient's skin, and finger prepping are done in the same manner as for a radial artery puncture.

The following two different techniques may be used for a femoral arterial puncture:

1. The artery is located and "fixed" between two fingers, allowing pulsation to be felt on both fingers but at the same time allowing enough room between them for the needle entry. The syringe and needle are held almost straight down. When the puncture is made in this manner, care must be taken not to pierce through the other wall of the artery.

2. The entry may be performed with the same techniques used for a radial artery puncture. Two or three fingertips are placed along the direction of the femoral artery, and the syringe and needle are held no higher than a 30° angle. This method must be used for femoral artery catheter placement and, if used for a one-time needle and syringe sample, there is less chance of artery perforation.

Regardless of the method used, when pulsation is strong, it will be relayed up through the needle and syringe as the needle touches and penetrates the artery. The walls of the femoral artery are usually very thick and resistant to puncture, so feeling pulsations can be a good guide to needle tip placement. When the artery is entered, the blood will usually pulsate back into and fill the syringe without any traction being applied on the plunger.

When the needle and syringe are removed, digital pressure is needed because a pressure dressing with tape is difficult to maintain in the femoral artery area.

Maintain pressure for at least 10 minutes, and 20 minutes or longer in an anticoagulated patient. It is helpful to remember to release pressure slowly. A sudden release often causes undue pressure against the arterial wall and the patient will begin bleeding.

The care of the blood sample is the same as that outlined for a radial artery puncture.

Postprocedure Patient Care

If the oxygen status of the patient has been altered *only* for the blood sampling, presampling status should be resumed as soon as the blood specimen is drawn.

The pressure dressing should be maintained long enough—usually 5 minutes is sufficient—to prevent excessive seepage of blood into the tissues. The pressure dressing must not be so restrictive as to cause blanching or severe restriction of venous blood in the hand. It should be removed when bleeding has stopped and not left on indefinitely. *If the patient is receiving anticoagulation therapy, digital pressure must be used for all arterial punctures. Personal observation and digital pressure must be maintained until all signs of bleeding have stopped or massive hematomas may result.*

Digital pressure is also preferable to the use of a "C-clamp" at the femoral site, because significant occult bleeding into the retroperitoneal space can occur rapidly and might result in unnecessary blood loss and discomfort for the patient.

PLACEMENT OF AN INDWELLING ARTERIAL CATHETER _____

Serial or Daily Arterial Blood Gas Sample Drawing

Frequently, serial or daily ABG sample drawing is necessary. To avoid multiple punctures it may be advisable to place an indwelling catheter to obtain the blood samples.

The *radial artery* is usually the site of first choice because it is the easiest to enter, easiest to maintain with intact sterile dressings, and allows the patient the greatest freedom of movement. It is imperative that Allen's test be performed before placing any indwelling catheter in the radial artery because the long-term placement with decreased blood flow will increase the risk of thrombosis.

The *brachial artery* is rarely used now because the catheters easily become fractured or bent, thus increasing the chance of embolization. The brachial artery also provides inaccurate readings.

The *femoral artery* may be a favorable site because it can accommodate a catheter of substantial diameter to achieve consistent monitoring and sampling of blood. Care must be taken at all times not to leave the patient in bed at a 30° angle or less. Frequent pedal pulse checks for strength of pulsatile flow and color of limb should be maintained and documented. The patient should have a shave prep before the procedure, and a sterile occlusive dressing may then be maintained intact.

Note: If the catheter is to be maintained for a substantial period of time, it is probably more prudent to suture it in place. This is also true with arterial lines to be maintained in the radial artery.

When inserting any indwelling arterial catheter, extra precautions must be taken to wash hands thoroughly. Skin prepping in this instance may include an acetone defatting as well as a complete iodophor prep. In some institutions, sterile gloves are mandatory for this procedure and should always be used by practitioners without expertise where probing is anticipated.

A local anesthetic may be injected at the insertion site, especially if an 18-gauge or larger catheter is being used. It is preferable that only experienced personnel perform this procedure; a successful entry with the first attempt is highly desirable because the availability of suitable arteries is limited.

Catheter Insertion and Sample Drawing

Catheter with Obturator

When using a catheter with obturator, follow the procedure outlined below.

1. Wearing gloves, insert catheter at a 30° angle, using the same techniques as those used to perform venipuncture of a superficial vein without a tourniquet.

2. As the catheter tip touches and enters the artery, pulsation can be felt up through the catheter. The artery walls are thicker and more resistant to entry than vein walls, making this procedure painful if not done quickly and expertly.

3. When the artery is fully entered, blood will pulsate back into the stylet; the catheter is then fully advanced.

4. To maintain a sterile field while removing the stylet and placing the obturator, an iodophor swab or sterile 2 × 2 inch sponge may be placed under the catheter hub.

5. To facilitate the stylet–obturator change, the arterial blood flow may be tempo-

rarily shut off, either by digital pressure at the catheter tip or by adequate placement of a tourniquet proximal to the insertion site.

6. After the obturator is removed from its protective shield, the stylet is removed from the catheter, the obturator is inserted and locked by twisting in place, and arterial pressure is released.

7. Label the arterial entry, and include the date and time of insertion and the initials of the person performing the procedure on the dressing.

8. Document the procedure stating the date, time, type, and gauge catheter used, insertion site, any patient reactions, name of person performing procedure, and pertinent data regarding distal extremity, including color, pulse, warmth.

Arterial Blood Gas Sample.   When an ABG sample is needed:

1. Wearing gloves, prepare heparinized syringe without needle.

2. Apply digital or tourniquet arterial pressure.

3. Place iodophor swab or sterile 2 × 2 inch sponge under catheter hub.

4. Remove obturator.

5. Connect heparinized syringe to catheter hub.

6. Release arterial pressure.

7. Allow syringe to fill with required amount of blood.

8. Reapply arterial pressure.

9. Remove syringe from catheter.

10. Insert and lock new sterile obturator.

11. Release arterial pressure.

12. Cap syringe and treat sample as for a one-time puncture for ABG specimen.

Intermittent Catheter (Heparin Lock)

When using a heparin lock, observe the following method:

1. Wearing gloves, insert catheter using same techniques used for catheter with obturator.

2. Pressure to stop arterial blood flow is not needed because there is no stylet–obturator change.

3. Flush catheter with dilute heparin solution.

4. Dressing, documentation at site, and charting are the same as for catheter with obturator.

Arterial Blood Gas Sample.   When an ABG sample is needed:

1. Wearing gloves, prepare:

   a. Heparinized syringe with 1 inch × 22-gauge needle for the blood sample

   b. Plain syringe with 1 inch × 22 gauge-needle for withdrawal of dilute heparin in heparin lock

   c. Syringe and needle with dilute heparin solution for flushing the catheter after drawing the ABG sample

2. Cleanse injection site of catheter with antiseptic.

3. Securely anchor catheter hub with free hand to prevent excessive pressure at insertion site and insert needle with plain syringe. Withdraw and discard approximately 0.5 mL blood with dilute heparin from catheter.

4. Recleanse injection port and insert needle in syringe heparinized for ABG sample. Allow syringe to fill with enough blood for sample. Remove syringe with needle.

5. Recleanse injection port and still maintaining secure anchorage of catheter hub, insert needle of syringe with dilute heparin and flush catheter. Remove syringe and needle.

6. Treat blood sample in the same manner as for one-time puncture for ABG specimen.

When entering any intermittent catheter with a needle, *extreme care must be taken to use a needle short enough that the needle tip cannot pass beyond the catheter hub* into the catheter itself. If the needle tip does enter the catheter, the catheter can be pierced and broken off by the needle tip with a resultant catheter embolus. The needle gauge must be small enough to allow postpuncture closure of the entry site, otherwise leakage of blood and risk of contamination are increased.

Postarterial Care

Close site monitoring, including the following steps, is required after placement of any type of indwelling arterial catheter:

1. Observe the site for thrombosis of the artery, hematoma formation, perforation of artery, and catheter kinking or dislodgement.

2. Check the hand for adequate blood supply by noting color and temperature.

3. Maintain secure, clean, and intact dressings.

4. Avoid undue stress at insertion site by using the unaffected arm for blood pressure monitoring and venipunctures.

CONSTANT ARTERIAL PRESSURE MONITORING

Placement of Catheter

Constant arterial pressure monitoring requires placement of an indwelling arterial catheter. This procedure allows for:

1. Continuous systolic, diastolic, and mean arterial pressure readings

2. An assessment of the cardiovascular effects of vasopressor/vasodilator drugs during the treatment of shock

3. Simultaneous drawing of arterial blood for ABG measurements

A cardiac monitor with a module for measuring arterial pressure is required. The monitor is connected by cable and a transducer to a special IV setup (Figure 16-4). The IV system consists of a 500-mL bag of normal saline solution that has been heparinized (usually 500–2000 U/500 mL) to inhibit catheter clotting and thrombus formation at the catheter tip. *Klebsiella, Enterobacter,* and *Serratia* species and *Pseudomonas cepacia*

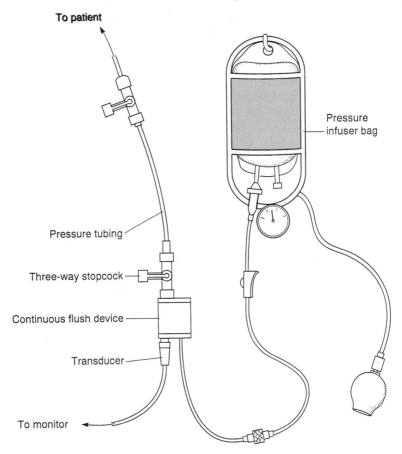

FIGURE 16-4 IV set-up for constant arterial pressure monitoring.

show rapid growth within 24 hours with 5% dextrose in water. The bag is connected to an IV tubing and placed inside a pressure infusor bag with a gauge and inflation bulb, the same one used to pump blood transfusions. Some institutions prefer microdrip tubings, but air bubbles are more persistent with this size drip. Other hospitals prefer macrodrip tubings; this size drip allows a larger volume of fluid to be infused.

The IV tubing is connected by a high-pressure extension tubing, a continuous flush attachment, and three-way stopcocks to a transducer dome. Most of these systems deliver 3 to 5 mL solution. The entire system is flushed. *All connections must be secured and all air bubbles eliminated.* The transducer is covered with the dome and secured on a plate attached to an IV pole at the level of the patient's right atrium. Each manufacturer provides detailed instructions for this setup, which should be read and carefully followed.

Any indwelling catheter may be used for this procedure and the insertion is the same as that shown for serial or daily ABG sample drawing. The catheter is connected to the primed IV tubing by placing an iodophor swab or sterile 2 × 2 inch sponge under the catheter hub, applying digital or tourniquet arterial pressure distal to the site, removing the stylet, connecting and securing the tubing adapter, and releasing arterial pressure. The pressure infusor bag is inflated to 300 mm Hg to automatically deliver a designated volume, depending on the drip size, of fluid per hour.

A sterile dressing is applied to the insertion site and taped securely. The site is labeled to clearly denote arterial access, date, time, type and gauge of catheter, and initials of person performing the insertion. A short handboard may be required to limit wrist motion. If restraints are necessary, they should be applied around the handboard, not the patient's wrist, because this could cause arterial pressure interference and increase the risk of catheter kinking or dislodgement.

Aftercare

Aftercare of the insertion site is the same as that for an indwelling catheter placed for serial or daily ABG drawing.

Arterial Blood Gas Sample

When an ABG sample is needed, a sampling port provides an easy arterial access.

Another method is to attach a three-way stopcock connection as close as possible to the site. Cap the sampling site with a heparin lock (intermittent infusion cap). Remove the cap when sampling and attach appropriate syringe. Turn the stopcock off to pressure or to the sampling site. Gently withdraw the sample and handle consistent with institutional policy. Flush the port and turn the stopcock back to pressure.

Devices such as VAMP™ from Baxter Healthcare allow for better, uncontaminated sampling of blood.

Sampling may be performed with the use of syringes and needles or, to minimize the number of port punctures into a latex port, a pediatric vacuum tube holder (22 gauge × 1 inch needle) and pediatric specimen tubes may be used.

Syringe and Needle Method

The syringe and needle method is performed as follows:

1. Wearing gloves, prepare an empty 3-mL syringe with 22 gauge × 1 inch needle and a heparinized syringe and needle for the ABG sample.
2. Swab injection latex port with antiseptic.
3. Insert needle of empty syringe into port.
4. Turn stopcock ON between catheter and injection port, OFF between catheter and transducer.
5. Allow syringe to fill to rid line of IV fluid and blood mixture.
6. Remove and discard filled syringe.
7. Cleanse injection port.
8. Insert needle of heparinized syringe into injection port and allow syringe to fill to the appropriate level.
9. Remove syringe and needle.
10. Turn stopcock back to operating position and flush tubing until it is clear of blood.

If the injection port has a cap without a latex entry site, the syringes are used without needles, and a new sterile cap must be replaced on the port after each sample drawing.

Pediatric Vacuum Tube Method

For the pediatric vacuum tube method, use the following steps:

1. Wearing gloves, swab injection port with antiseptic.
2. Insert needle connected with pediatric vacuum tube holder and a plain vacuum tube into injection port.
3. Turn stopcock ON between catheter and injection port.
4. Fully insert tube into holder and allow to fill with IV fluid and blood mixture.
5. Remove and discard filled tube.
6. Insert heparinized tube and allow to fully fill.
7. Remove filled heparinized tube (ABG sample) and place in ice.
8. Insert plain vacuum tube, turn stopcock back to operating position, and allow it to fill, rinsing port free of blood. Remove and discard filled tube and holder.
9. Flush remainder of tubing until clear of blood.

The blood specimen is gently rotated to ensure mixing of blood with heparin, placed in a labeled iced container, and sent immediately for analysis.

Malfunctions and Complications

Malfunctions
Common malfunctions occurring in arterial pressure lines include the following:

1. Air bubbles in the system can cause distorted wave patterns. During the original setup, care must be taken that all air bubbles are eliminated and all connections tightly secured. During each manipulation of the system, caution must be taken that air is not allowed to enter the line.
2. Near-exsanguination has been reported from disconnection of the line with the catheter remaining in the artery. Here again, care must be taken that *all* connections are secure during the original setup and at frequent intervals thereafter to avoid this serious malfunction.
3. A "damped" pressure tracing, almost flat, will result if the catheter tip lies against the artery wall or the catheter becomes kinked. Secure catheter hub taping, intact dressings, and proper application of restraints can all help prevent this malfunction.
4. Catheter clotting occurs if the pressure infusor bag is allowed to fall below 300 mm Hg. The pressure must be periodically checked to ensure that it is properly maintained.
5. If the height of the transducer is zero reference point, an abnormally high or low reading will result if the transducer is not maintained at the same level. If the transducer used is the type placed with a plate on an IV pole not attached on the bed, the transducer will not remain at the level of the right atrium when the bed is raised or lowered and abnormal readings will result. One method used to avoid this malfunction is to tape a note on the control switch of the patient's bed.

Complications
Certain complications related to arterial pressure lines are:

1. The incidence of thromboses, hematomas, pseudoaneurysms, and prolonged arterial spasms may be reduced by the clinician's exercising expertise during catheter insertion and by careful monitoring of insertion sites.

2. Infection is a serious threat. Arterial pressure monitoring has been related to as high as 13% of reported outbreaks of nosocomial bacteremia. Incidences of contaminated transducers, transducer domes, and flush solutions have all been well documented. Sterilizing the transducer after each use, using disposable domes, and changing the entire monitoring system except for the catheter every 2 days have all been shown to reduce infection rates. As with any invasive procedure, thorough handwashing before insertion and maintaining of aseptic techniques during setup of the entire system, during insertion, and during all manipulations of the line are mandatory.

SWAN-GANZ CATHETERS

Although the insertion sites for Swan-Ganz catheters are veins, they are included in arterial access because they enter the pulmonary artery and measure arterial pressures. Central venous pressure lines give assessment only of right heart pressure. Swan-Ganz catheters, however, give assessment of both right and left heart pressures so they are frequently used for diagnosis and management of treatment in heart failure resulting from myocardial infarction and cardiogenic shock. In the treatment of cardiogenic shock, the Swan-Ganz catheter not only serves as a guide for IV therapy administration, a site for this administration, and evaluation of any therapeutic drugs given but also provides information regarding the cause of shock.

Basic Swan-Ganz catheters have double or triple lumens. Catheters are approximately 110 cm in length and come in sizes 5 Fr., 6 Fr., 7 Fr. and 7.5 Fr. Each has a balloon tip that is inflated with 0.8 to 1.5 mL air, depending on the size and manufacturer. A double-lumen catheter contains a larger port, which is connected to an IV system and monitor to measure pulmonary artery wedge pressure (PAWP), and a smaller port, with a two-way stopcock for inflation and deflation of the balloon. Triple-lumen catheters contain a third proximal port, which is connected to another IV system and may be used to monitor right atrial pressure.

The *IV system* contains a heparinized bag, pressure infusor bag, pressure tubings with stopcocks, and transducer with cable connected to a monitor. This equipment is the same as that used for arterial monitoring except that for Swan-Ganz catheters the lines may be coded in blue to differentiate them from arterial lines, which may be coded in red.

Insertion

The Swan-Ganz catheter may be inserted either percutaneously or by cutdown in any accessible vein large enough to allow passage of the catheter. As the catheter is threaded and the tip passes the superior vena cava, inflation of the balloon will allow normal blood flow to assist catheter advancement. The tip enters the right atrium and passes through the tricuspid valve, entering the right ventricle. It then passes through the pulmonic valve into the pulmonary artery. Use of a cardiac monitor is essential during this insertion because the pattern shows definite changes with each advancement, thus providing a guide for tip location, and simultaneously allowing for patient monitoring throughout the procedure. The catheter tip placement must be confirmed by radiography.

Pulmonary capillary wedge pressure (PCWP), which reflects left heart pressure, is measured intermittently by inflating the balloon to its recommended level (Figure 16-5).

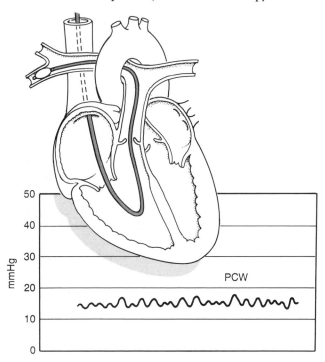

FIGURE 16-5 Pulmonary capillary wedge pressure. The catheter, with balloon inflated, is advanced until it wedges in a small branch of the pulmonary artery. Normal capillary wedge pressure is 5–12 mm Hg.

Care should be taken not to overinflate or to inflate too frequently. Typically, one would inflate every 4 hours, with the pressure maintained no longer than 1 to 2 minutes.

Complications

Possible complications include:

1. Cardiac arrhythmias may occur during insertion. Lidocaine–hydrochloride and defibrillation equipment must be readily available. Serious arrhythmias during insertion are rare.

2. Catheter knotting may occur with the 5 Fr. when it it advanced too far for the chamber whose pressure is being registered.

3. Balloon rupture is possible in a patient without intracardiac shunting of blood.

4. Pulmonary damage may result from pulmonary artery blood flow obstruction caused by peripheral migration of the catheter to a wedged position. This is avoidable with constant monitoring and by following recommendations regarding balloon inflation.

5. Infection is always a threat. The use of disposable equipment has minimized the occurrence of infection. Strict adherence to aseptic technique is mandatory.

ARTERIAL BLOOD GAS PARAMETERS

The purposes of arterial blood gas interpretation are to cope with respiratory imbalances, specifically, to diagnose, regulate oxygen therapy, and assess all other therapy—and metabolic imbalances—in particular, to diagnose and assess the effectiveness of the therapy.

To interpret ABG values, it is necessary to understand the physiologic, chemical, and physical processes that influence each parameter.

pH

pH is the parameter that refers to the degree of acidity or alkalinity of the blood. It is not an absolute measurement but shows an approximation of hydrogen ion concentration. The pH scale is as follows (numbers are inversely related to the degree of acidity): (1) the range compatible with life is roughly 6.8 to 7.8, and (2) the normal range lies between 7.35 and 7.45. A pH increase represents a decrease in acidity and a pH decrease represents an increase in acidity; a pH decrease of 0.3 shows a doubling of hydrogen concentration. Blood pH 7.10 has twice the hydrogen concentration of blood pH 7.40.

Blood pH is directly proportional to the ratio of carbonic acid to bicarbonate (HCO_3^-). When there is 1 part carbonic acid to 20 parts bicarbonate, the resultant pH is 7.35 to 7.45. If only carbonic acid increases or only bicarbonate decreases, the ratio becomes closer (1:5–16) and acidosis results. Conversely, when only carbonic acid decreases or only bicarbonate increases, the ratio widens (1:25–50) and alkalosis results.

Carbonic acid or bicarbonate changes themselves produce no toxic effects; it is the ratio alteration and resultant pH change that interfere severely with enzyme activity.

Hydrogen

Cell metabolism produces hydrogen, which combines with bicarbonate to form carbonic acid. This breaks down into water, which is excreted by the kidneys, and carbon dioxide, which is excreted by the lungs.

Because waste products of metabolism are mainly acidic, people are by nature acid-producing animals. The body generates and processes 15,000 to 20,000 mEq hydrogen daily. The majority (99.8%) is nonfixed or volatile acid, which means it can change into gaseous form. The remainder (0.2%) is fixed or nonvolatile.

Body processing of hydrogen is accomplished without any appreciable change in blood concentration by elimination of volatile acid as carbon dioxide by the lungs, by excretion and reabsorption of fixed acid and bicarbonate by the kidneys, and by chemical buffering.

Buffers

A *buffer* is a solute that resists pH change when acids or bases are added. The buffer base consists of bicarbonate and all nonbicarbonate buffers. The bicarbonate buffer system cannot buffer volatile acids but does buffer approximately 75% of all the fixed acid generated by the body. The nonbicarbonate buffer system consists primarily of proteins, hemoglobin, and phosphate. It buffers volatile, nonfixed, acids.

Bicarbonate

The primary metabolic parameter bicarbonate may be reported as carbon dioxide content, carbon dioxide combining power, carbon dioxide, or standard bicarbonate, any of which refers to the same factor. Bicarbonate is measured by concentration and reported as mEq/L. It is universally related to the quantity of fixed acid *excess* and therefore is more a controlled than a controlling factor.

Sources of fixed acids are: (1) organic and inorganic dietary acids; (2) lactic acid as a by-product of cell metabolism without oxygen; and (3) keto acids as by-products of cell metabolism without glucose or insulin.

The normal excretion rate of fixed acid by the kidneys is 50 mEq each day. However, the excretion and reabsorption of both hydrogen and bicarbonate can be greatly increased or decreased by body demands.

The normal bicarbonate range is 24 ± 3 mEq/L. The minimal stated as being compatible with life is 1 mEq/L, the maximal is 48 mEq/L.

Base Excess

The parameter base excess (BE) is the sum total in concentration of all the buffer anions (bicarbonate and nonbicarbonate) in a sample of whole blood, equilibrated with a normal PCO_2 (40 mm Hg). As base excess is equilibrated with a normal PCO_2, it is not affected by primary respiratory imbalances.

Normal base excess is 48 ± 3 mm/L but is reported as plus or minus zero, with zero representing 48 mm/L. In metabolic acidosis, base excess is minus; in metabolic alkalosis, base excess is plus.

Physics of Gas

So far we have discussed parameters that are measured by concentration. The two respiratory parameters measured by pressure (intensity) warrant a brief review of the physics of gas.

Gas has *volume*, which refers to the space the gas occupies and is measured in centimeters (cc). Gas has *pressure*, which is measured mathematically as force per unit area by noting height to which force can support a column of mercury, and is expressed in millimeters of mercury (mm Hg). Gas has *temperature*, which is generated by gas molecules in constant motion and is measured in degrees centigrade (°C) or Fahrenheit (°F).

Dalton's law regarding the behavior of gas in a mixture, as applied to oxygen in the atmosphere (room air), tells us the following:

1. The total pressure of the gas mixture equals the sum of the partial pressures of each gas, or total pressure of atmosphere (P_{atm}) = partial pressure oxygen (PO_2) + partial pressure nitrogen (PN_2) + partial pressure carbon dioxide (PCO_2).

2. Each gas acts independently, as if it alone occupied the total space.

3. Each gas contribution to the total pressure depends solely on the percentage of the total gas it occupies. The contribution of oxygen to the total atmospheric pressure is 21%. (Other variables not discussed here can exist.)

4. The partial pressure of each gas depends on the number of molecules existing in the fixed space. At high elevations, because the number of oxygen molecules is decreased, PO_2 will be decreased.

5. Each gas is unaffected by any changes in other gas molecules. The PO_2 will not increase or decrease because PCO_2 is increased or decreased.

Partial Pressure Carbon Dioxide

The PCO_2 value reflects the adequacy of alveolar ventilation. It is the primary respiratory parameter.

Carbon dioxide is eliminated by the lungs at the same rate formed by the tissues and at the same time maintains constant blood levels.

Arterial PCO_2 is inversely related to the level of ventilation. With hypoventilation, carbon dioxide is retained and the PCO_2 elevates; with hyperventilation, carbon dioxide is blown off and the PCO_2 decreases.

The PCO_2 normal range is 40 ± 4 mm Hg. The minimal value stated as compatible with life is 9 mm Hg, with the maximal value 158 mm Hg.

Partial Pressure Oxygen

The PO_2 value is also an intensity factor, measured in mm Hg. It tells how fast and for how long oxygen will pass from blood into tissue. The PO_2 is usually not a direct influence in acid–base balance.

Normal PO_2 values are oxygen and age dependent. When the FIO_2 is 21% (room air) and the patient is 60 years of age or less, the PO_2 should be at least 80 mm Hg. With each 10-year advance in age, the normal PO_2 will decrease by 10 mm Hg. If the PO_2 is 50 mm Hg or below in a patient less than 60 years of age, respiratory failure is present. A PO_2 between 50 and 75 mm Hg reflects moderate hypoxemia.

Hypoxemia

Hypoxemia is insufficient oxygenation of the blood and can be measured directly by the PO_2. Hypoxia is insufficient oxygenation of the tissues; it cannot be directly measured but is presumed if the partial pressure oxygen, venous blood (P_vO_2) is 30 mm Hg or below. To avoid hypoxia when hypoxemia is present, either the cardiovascular system must increase the rate of tissue perfusion or the hemoglobin content must be elevated.

Shunting is frequently a cause of hypoxemia. *Shunting* is any impediment in the blood transport system that results in blood not coming in contact with oxygen. This can be seen in vascular lung tumors, a right-to-left intracardiac shunt, or capillary shunting where pulmonary capillary blood comes in contact with totally unventilated alveoli (dead space).

Oxygen Saturation

Oxygen saturation (O_2 Sat) is the parameter that tells the amount of oxygen taken up by hemoglobin when fully saturated. It is a quantity factor and is measured in percentage. It may also be called PO_2%.

The normal adult values are 96% to 97% under age 65 years and 95% to 96% in older patients. Oxygen saturation:

1. Depends on PO_2. When the pressure exceeds a certain value, the amount of oxygen taken in no longer increases.
2. Is altered by pH. If PO_2 remains constant, oxygen saturation will decrease when the pH decreases, and will increase when the pH increases.
3. Is altered by temperature. If the PO_2 is constant, oxygen saturation will decrease when the temperature increases and will increase when the temperature decreases.

This tells us that hyperthermia causes metabolic acidosis and hypothermia causes metabolic alkalosis. In hypothermia, the oxygen need is decreased, but the oxygen is bound so tightly to the hemoglobin that the ability to deliver it is greatly decreased. Inhalation of carbon dioxide may be used to cause acidosis and release the bound oxygen.

Chemoreceptors

Chemoreceptors located peripherally in aortic and carotid bodies and centrally in the brain play a role in body responsive changes to abnormal PCO_2 and PO_2 values. Chemoreceptors signal the brain to stimulate or depress ventilation, according to body needs. The response to an elevated PCO_2 is greater than a decreased PO_2 because PCO_2 elevation is a danger signal of respiratory failure. At high altitudes where oxygen supply is lowered, oxygen need is greater than PCO_2 constancy; the chemoreceptors stimulate hyperventilation to obtain more oxygen, but this hyperventilation results in a decreased PCO_2.

Arterial Blood Gas Normal Values (at sea level)[1]
  pH: 7.35–7.45
   PCO_2: 36–44 mm Hg
   PO_2: 80–95 mm Hg
   O_2 Sat: 95%–96%
  $HCO_3{}^-$: 22–26 mEq/L
   BE: ± 3

FOUR PRIMARY ACID–BASE IMBALANCES

Metabolic Acidosis

Metabolic acidosis is a process resulting from an excess of fixed acids or a primary bicarbonate deficit.
 The primary causes are:

1. Increased production of fixed acids
   a. Keto acids, as seen in diabetic acidosis or starvation, where glucose and insulin are unavailable for cell metabolism
   b. Lactic acid, as seen in cardiopulmonary failure when oxygen is unavailable for cell metabolism
2. Failure of kidneys to excrete fixed acid
3. Primary bicarbonate deficit
   a. Severe diarrhea
   b. Bowel or biliary fistula

This is a metabolic imbalance because bicarbonate is the parameter primarily affected. Acidosis is present because the carbon dioxide level has not changed, but the decrease in bicarbonate has caused the ratio to go closer than 1 part acid to 20 parts base. It can be anywhere between 1:16 and 1:5, depending on the degree of bicarbonate deficit. Because pH is dependent on the acid–base ratio, and this ratio has now narrowed, acidosis is present. Base excess is minus because there is not enough bicarbonate to buffer the fixed acid.

Arterial Blood Gas Values in Metabolic Acidosis
> pH: <7.35
>
> HCO_3^-: <22 mEq/L
>
> PCO_2: normal (40 ± 4 mm Hg)
>
> BE: < −3

If the metabolic acidosis is of renal origin, the kidneys cannot respond. If it is of nonrenal origin, the kidneys will increase the excretion of hydrogen and increase the reabsorption of bicarbonate. This response is slow, but, once started, can be maintained for weeks or months.

The chemoreceptors are sensitive to the increase in hydrogen and will stimulate compensatory hyperventilation to blow off carbon dioxide, decreasing the PCO_2 less than 40 mm Hg to obtain an acid–base ratio closer to normal (1 : 20) needed for a normal pH. This compensatory respiratory response is prompt and predictable—it will occur within minutes but becomes less effective with time. The limit of compensatory hyperventilation is when the PCO_2 reaches 12 mm Hg.

After the kidneys and lungs have responded, bicarbonate will increase to a level closer to normal, PCO_2 will decrease, and the acid–base ratio will come closer to 1:20 with a resultant pH closer to normal. Compensation thus occurs.

With bicarbonate administration, the bicarbonate level will revert to normal, and the lungs will stop hyperventilation. Therefore, PCO_2 will revert to normal, resulting in a 1:20 acid–base ratio and allowing a normal pH (7.35–7.45). Correction thereby is achieved.

Metabolic Alkalosis

Metabolic alkalosis results from a decrease in body content of fixed acids or a primary bicarbonate excess. The primary causes are:

1. Excessive loss of fixed acids by
   a. Prolonged vomiting
   b. Gastric suctioning
   c. Potassium deficit
2. Primary bicarbonate excess by
   a. Excessive administration of sodium bicarbonate or sodium citrate
   b. Chloride deficit, where bicarbonate increases to maintain cation–anion balance
   c. Sodium deficit, with bicarbonate excretion dependent upon sodium

This is a metabolic imbalance because the primary parameter affected is bicarbonate. Alkalosis is present because the acid–base ratio has widened to 1 part acid to 25 to 50 parts base. This ratio results in a pH elevation; because there is an excess of bicarbonate, the base excess is plus.

Arterial Blood Gas Values in Metabolic Alkalosis
> pH: >7.45
>
> HCO_3^-: >26 mEq/L
>
> PCO_2: normal (40 ± 4 mm Hg)
>
> BE: > +3

Whether the kidneys respond to metabolic alkalosis depends on several factors. An increase in bicarbonate causes the excretion of bicarbonate to increase, provided there is no deficit of chloride or potassium. If a chloride depletion is present, bicarbonate will be reabsorbed as the accompanying anion for sodium. Because a bicarbonate increase is usually accompanied by an increase in sodium, a decrease in chloride, and a potassium deficit, bicarbonate is not excreted but reabsorbed.

Compensatory respiratory response to metabolic alkalosis is variable. The degree of hypoventilation that occurs depends on the causative factors. Regardless of the cause, hypoventilation as a compensatory response will rarely be sufficient to bring the PCO_2 above 55 mm Hg because an elevated PCO_2 will cause the chemoreceptors to stimulate breathing to prevent respiratory failure.

When the lungs and kidneys do respond, some compensation will occur—bicarbonate will decrease, PCO_2 will increase, and the acid–base ratio will come closer to 1:20; thus the pH will decrease to a level closer to normal.

Correction occurs with the administration of solutions containing chloride and potassium.

In the assessment and treatment of respiratory imbalances, ABG measurements are an absolute clinical necessity because ventilation is reflected in PCO_2 and oxygenation in PO_2. Furthermore, acute respiratory failure may occur with slight changes in pulse, blood pressure, or alertness until cardiopulmonary collapse occurs.

Respiratory Acidosis

Respiratory acidosis is always caused by carbon dioxide retention from hypoventilation. This is rarely seen without hypoxemia (PO_2 less than 60 mm Hg). The causes of hypoventilation include:

1. Anesthesia, narcotics
2. Central nervous system (CNS) disease such as polio, spinal cord lesions
3. Severe hypokalemia
4. Intrathoracic collection of blood, fluid, or air
5. Pulmonary diseases
   a. Restrictive (congestive heart failure, tumors, atelectasis)
   b. Obstructive (bronchitis, emphysema, asthma, or foreign body)

This process is respiratory because the PCO_2 is the primary parameter involved. Nonfixed, volatile, acid (PCO_2) is in excess but the base (bicarbonate) is normal. The acid–base ratio is closer than 1:20; it is between 1:5 and 1:20, resulting in acidosis.

Arterial Blood Gas Values in Respiratory Acidosis

pH: <7.35

PCO_2: >44 mm Hg

HCO_3^-: normal (24 ± 2 mEq/L)

Because the lungs are always the primary cause of respiratory acidosis, they cannot play any role in compensation. Renal compensation is always slow in onset but very effective once started: generation and reabsorption of bicarbonate will increase, excretion of hydrogen will increase, and the excretion of chloride will increase, resulting in a chloride deficit.

With renal response, bicarbonate will elevate above normal, and PCO_2 will remain unchanged. The acid ratio will be closer to 1:20, allowing for some compensation, with a pH closer to normal.

Correction of respiratory acidosis is possible only by correction of the pulmonary cause. Chloride solutions are usually given to treat the chloride deficit.

Respiratory Alkalosis

Respiratory alkalosis is always caused by a carbon dioxide deficit due to hyperventilation. Factors causing hyperventilation include:

1. Chemoreceptor response to hypoxemia. The chemoreceptors sense the decrease in oxygen and send a message to the brain to stimulate ventilation. This hyperventilation results in carbon dioxide being blown off, thus decreasing PCO_2. This is normal at high altitudes.

2. Respiratory response to metabolic acidosis. This response can persist for several hours or days after the metabolic acidosis is corrected because of higher levels of hydrogen excess in cerebrospinal fluid and the fact that chemoreceptors are more responsive to cerebrospinal fluid than to blood.

3. CNS malfunctions (trauma, infection, brain lesions)

4. Anxiety, pain, fever, shock

5. Anemia, carbon monoxide poisoning

6. Epinephrine, salicylates, and progesterone

7. Improper mechanical ventilation. Any patient with chronic obstructive pulmonary disease who is overcorrected by mechanical ventilation so that the PCO_2 decreases faster than 10 mm Hg/hr will have respiratory alkalosis.

This hyperventilation process is respiratory because PCO_2 is the primary parameter affected. Alkalosis is present because carbon dioxide is decreased and the bicarbonate value is normal, resulting in an acid–base ratio between 1:25 and 1:50. This ratio results in a pH above 7.45.

Arterial Blood Gas Values in Respiratory Alkalosis
    pH: >7.45

    PCO_2: <36 mm Hg

    HCO_3^-: normal (24 ± 2 mEq/L)

Because the lungs are the primary cause of respiratory alkalosis, they cannot respond for compensation. Renal response occurs after several hours or days. The kidneys will decrease excretion of hydrogen and increase excretion of bicarbonate. The urine cannot become more alkaline than pH 7.0. This renal response will create some *compensation*. The bicarbonate value will decrease below 24 mEq/L. The acid–base ratio will come closer to 1:20, allowing the pH to come closer to normal.

Respiratory alkalosis can be corrected by administering chloride solutions to replace the bicarbonate ion load. However, the buffering capacity of the plasma has been compromised as a result of the alkalosis and any additional insult to the balance will be poorly tolerated.

MIXED ACID–BASE IMBALANCES

In the hospital setting, two or more primary imbalances may coexist in the same patient. The following combinations sometimes occur:

1. Metabolic acidosis and metabolic alkalosis appear in a patient with diabetic acidosis who is vomiting.
2. Metabolic acidosis and respiratory acidosis occur in a patient with severe pulmonary edema, followed by cardiogenic shock.
3. Metabolic acidosis and respiratory alkalosis are seen in a patient with both kidney and liver failure.
4. Respiratory acidosis and metabolic alkalosis appear in a patient with chronic respiratory insufficiency who is on a salt-poor diet and taking diuretics.
5. Respiratory alkalosis and metabolic alkalosis are usually seen as a result of mechanical overventilation.

Respiratory acidosis and respiratory alkalosis cannot coexist because a person cannot hypoventilate and hyperventilate at the same time.

REFERENCES

1. Metheny, N. M. (1992). *Fluid and electrolyte balance. Nursing considerations* (2nd ed., pp. 133–135). Philadelphia: J. B. Lippincott.

BIBLIOGRAPHY

Bennett, J. V., & Brachman, P. S. (1986). *Hospital infections* (2nd ed., pp. 572–575). Boston: Little, Brown.
Covey, M., McLane, C., Smith, N., et al. (1988). Infection related to intravascular pressure monitoring: Effects of flush and tubing changes. *American Journal of Infection Control, 16*(5), 206–213.

REVIEW QUESTIONS

1. Before insertion of an indwelling catheter in the radial arterial, the following test should be done:
   a. Abbott's
   b. Allen's
   c. Demer's
   d. Swan's
2. The ABG parameter that reflects ventilation is:
   a. bicarbonate
   b. PO_2
   c. pH
   d. PCO_2
3. The primary metabolic parameter in ABGs is:
   a. bicarbonate
   b. PCO_2
   c. base excess
   d. PO_2
4. The physician's order for ABG sampling should include:
   a. postexercise or at rest
   b. FIO_2
   c. outside air
   d. room air

5. In a patient receiving anticoagulants, the drawing of an ABG sample should include:
   a. personal observation
   b. chest pressure
   c. digital pressure
   d. avoid use of heparin

6. Two methods used ONLY for drawing ABG samples include:
   a. syringe and needle
   b. catheter with heparin lock
   c. needle with heparin lock
   d. peripherally inserted central catheter

7. At the onset of metabolic acidosis, what parameters will be decreased:
   a. pH
   b. bicarbonate
   c. base excess
   d. PO_2

8. At the onset of respiratory acidosis, which of the following will be increased?
   a. PCO_2
   b. PO_2
   c. positive end-expiratory pressure
   d. pulmonary artery wedge pressure

9. Strong traction on the plunger of the syringe to withdraw ABG samples faster may increase the chance of:
   a. air contamination
   b. blood hemolysis
   c. arterial spasm
   d. venous spasm

10. Blood pH is directly proportional to the ratio of:
   a. carbonic acid to bicarbonate
   b. carbonic acid to PCO_2
   c. bicarbonate to carbonic acid
   d. PCO_2 to carbonic acid

PART IV

Application of Intravenous Therapy for Homeostasis

CHAPTER 17

Principles of Fluid and Electrolyte Balance

Over the past 25 years our knowledge of fluid and electrolyte balance has increased to the extent that we now recognize an imbalance as a threat to life. With this increased knowledge has come an increase in the nurse's responsibility in parenteral therapy. Not only is accurate recording of the patient's intake and output important, but so too is the ability to recognize symptoms of imbalance; prompt recognition of an imbalance may indicate adjustment in therapy that may be crucial to the safety of the patient.

Today electrolyte therapy is used extensively. At least 80% of all fluids administered contain some electrolytes. Electrolyte therapy is often a lifesaving procedure; its safe and successful administration is essential. Knowledge of the fundamentals of fluid and electrolyte metabolism contributes to safe electrolyte therapy. This knowledge alerts the nurse to the necessity for accurate fluid and electrolyte administration, the potential dangers of electrolyte therapy, and a change in the patient's condition that could alter the therapy prescribed.

Abnormalities of body fluid and electrolyte metabolism present certain therapeutic problems. When the mechanisms normally regulating fluid volume, electrolyte composition, and osmolality are impaired, therapy becomes complicated. An understanding of these metabolic abnormalities enables the nurse to understand the problems involved. Such problems exist in patients with renal insufficiency, adrenal insufficiency, adrenal hyperactivity, and other kinds of impaired organ function. For example, correction of a severe potassium deficit resulting from vomiting and diarrhea presents a problem in the dehydrated patient. Potassium replacement is imperative. However, potassium administered to patients with renal insufficiency results in potassium toxicity; the kidneys are unable to excrete electrolytes. The adverse effects of excess potassium on the heart muscle are arrhythmia and heart block. The nurse must recognize the importance of both hydrating the patient before potassium can be administered safely and watching for diminished diuresis that could necessitate a change in therapy. Once antidiuresis occurs, the potassium infusion must be interrupted and the physician notified.

Therapeutic problems also exist in patients with impaired liver function. Gastric replacement is necessary when excessive loss of gastric fluid has occurred. Most deficits caused by gastric suction, unless severe, are treated with 0.9% sodium chloride in 5% dextrose in water or 0.33% sodium chloride in 5% dextrose in water. However, severe

Sharon M. Weinstein: PLUMER'S PRINCIPLES & PRACTICE OF INTRAVENOUS THERAPY, FIFTH EDITION, © 1993 J. B. Lippincott Company

loss may call for gastric replacement solutions containing ammonium chloride, which can be potentially dangerous when administered to patients with impaired liver function. Ammonium chloride administered to a patient with severe liver damage may result in ammonia intoxication because of the liver's inability to convert ammonia to hydrogen ion and urea.

These examples illustrate how knowledge of fluid and electrolyte metabolism contributes to safe, successful therapy in the critically ill patient.

FLUID CONTENT OF THE BODY

The total body water content of an individual varies with age, weight, and sex. The amount of water depends on the amount of body fat. Body fat is essentially water free; the greater the fat content, the less is the water content.

In the typical adult patient, approximately 60% of weight consists of fluid (water and electrolytes; Figure 17-1). After age 40, mean values for total body fluid in percentage of body weight decrease for both men and women; the sex differentiation, however, remains. After 60 years of age, the percentage may decrease to 52% in men and 46% in women. With aging, lean body mass decreases in favor of fat. Infants have a high body fluid content, approximately 70% to 80% of their body weight.[4]

Compartments

The total body fluid is functionally divided into two main compartments: the intracellular and the extracellular compartments. The intracellular compartment consists of the fluid inside the cells and comprises about two thirds of the body fluid, or 40% of the body weight. The extracellular compartment consists of the fluid outside the body cells—the plasma representing 5% of the body weight and the interstitial fluid (fluid in tissues) representing 15% of the body weight. Figure 17-2 is a schematic representation of compartments.

In newborn infants the proportion is approximately three-fifths intracellular and two-fifths extracellular. This ratio changes and reaches the adult level by the time the infant is about 30 months old.

There is one additional compartment, the transcellular compartment. The transcellular fluid is the product of cellular metabolism and consists of secretions such as gastrointestinal secretions and urine. Analysis of the secretions may assist the physician in tracing lost electrolytes and prescribing proper fluid and electrolyte replacement.

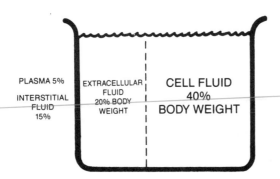

FIGURE 17-1 Total body fluid is 60% of body weight. (From Metheny, N. M. [1992]. *Fluid and electrolyte balance* [2nd ed., p. 4]. Philadelphia: J. B. Lippincott.)

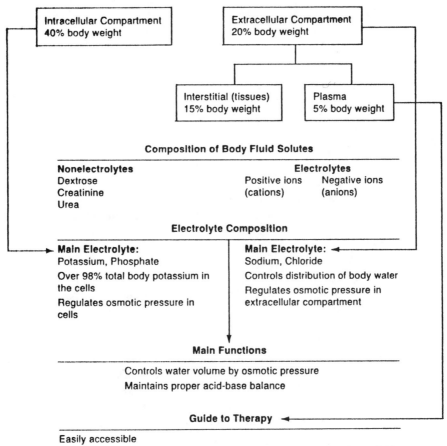

Intracellular Compartment	Extracellular Compartment
40% body weight	20% body weight

Interstitial (tissues)	Plasma
15% body weight	5% body weight

Composition of Body Fluid Solutes

Nonelectrolytes	Electrolytes	
Dextrose	Positive ions	Negative ions
Creatinine	(cations)	(anions)
Urea		

Electrolyte Composition

Main Electrolyte:	Main Electrolyte:
Potassium, Phosphate	Sodium, Chloride
Over 98% total body potassium in the cells	Controls distribution of body water
Regulates osmotic pressure in cells	Regulates osmotic pressure in extracellular compartment

Main Functions

Controls water volume by osmotic pressure
Maintains proper acid-base balance

Guide to Therapy

Easily accessible
Composition of intracellular fluid directly related to that of extracellular fluid
Disturbances in serum related to symptoms

FIGURE 17-2 Total body water composition.

Excessive fluid and electrolyte loss must be replaced to maintain fluid and electrolyte balance in the two main compartments. The amount of body water loss is easily computed by weighing the patient and noting loss of weight: 1 L body water is equivalent to 1 kg, or 2.2 lb, of body weight. Up to 5% weight loss in a child or adult may signify moderate fluid volume deficit—more than 5% may indicate severe fluid volume deficit.[5] Weight changes are also valuable as indicators of body water gains—acute weight gain may indicate water excess.

COMPOSITION OF BODY FLUID

The body fluid contains two types of solutes (dissolved substances): the electrolytes and the nonelectrolytes, as shown in Figure 17-2. The *nonelectrolytes* are molecules that do not break into particles in solution but remain intact. They consist of (1) dextrose, (2) urea, and (3) creatinine.

Electrolytes are molecules that break into electrically charged particles called ions.

The ion carrying a positive charge is called a cation, the ion with a negative charge, an anion. Potassium chloride is an electrolyte that, dissolved in water, yields potassium cations and chloride anions. Chemical balance is always maintained; the total number of positive charges equals the total number of negative charges. The quantity of charges and their concentration is expressed as milliequivalents (mEq) per liter of fluid. Because the number of negative charges must equal the number of positive charges for chemical balance, the milliequivalents of cations must equal the milliequivalents of anions[1] (see Tables 17-1 and 17-2 later in this chapter for an example).

Electrolyte Composition

Each fluid compartment has its own electrolyte composition (see Figure 17-2). The extracellular compartment (plasma and interstitial fluid) contains a high concentration of sodium, chloride, and bicarbonate and a low concentration of potassium. The composition of the intracellular fluid is quite different; the concentrations of potassium, magnesium, and phosphate are high, whereas the sodium and chloride concentrations are relatively low.

Electrolyte composition of the intracellular fluid is in part related to electrolyte composition of the plasma and interstitial fluids. Disturbances in the extracellular fluid are reflected in the patient's symptoms. These facts, combined with the accessibility of plasma, make the analysis of plasma a valuable guide to therapy. Occasionally, however, the electrolyte determination of plasma may be misleading. For example, concentration of potassium in plasma may be high while there is a body deficit. This surplus is due to the shift of potassium from intracellular to extracellular fluid in the process of large potassium losses through the kidneys. Determination of plasma sodium may also present a false picture. In the case of an edematous cardiac patient, the plasma concentration may be low despite excess body sodium because total body sodium is equal to the sum of the products of volume times concentration in the various compartments.

Electrolytes serve two main purposes: (1) to act in controlling body water volume by osmotic pressure and (2) to maintain the proper acid–base balance of the body.

Osmolality

Osmolality is the total solute concentration and reflects the relative water and total solute concentration because it is expressed per liter of serum. The osmotic pressure is determined by the number of solutes in solution. If the extracellular fluid contains a relatively large number of dissolved particles and the intracellular fluid contains a small amount of dissolved particles, the osmotic pressure would cause water to pass from the less concentrated fluid to the more concentrated. Therefore, fluid from the intracellular compartment would pass into the extracellular compartment until the concentration became equal.

The unit of osmotic pressure is the osmole and the values are expressed in milliosmoles (mOsm). Normal blood plasma has an osmolality of about 290 mOsm/kg water. The determination of serum osmolality is sometimes used to detect dehydration or overhydration. Because sodium chloride is the principal solute in the extracellular fluid, the osmolality reading usually parallels the sodium reading or is close to two times the serum sodium plus ten. Therefore, measurement of sodium concentration also indicates the water needs of the body. At times the osmolality reading may falsely indicate dehydration. Because the osmolality is the total solute concentration, nonelectrolytes are included in the reading. An elevated level of blood urea can therefore increase the osmolality without exerting osmotic pressure. A determination of blood urea nitrogen may supply a correction to the osmolality reading in cases of increased serum urea.

Units of Measure

Concentrations of solutes may be expressed in several ways in addition to mEq/L; for example, milligrams per deciliter (mg/dL) or millimoles per liter (mmol/L). Each of these units of measure may be used in a clinical setting. A *milliequivalent* of an ion is its atomic weight expressed in milligrams divided by the valence. This is the measure most often used for expressing small concentrations of electrolytes in body fluids because it emphasizes the principles that ions combine milliequivalent for milliequivalent. *Milligrams per 100 mL (deciliter)* expresses the weight of the solute per unit volume. In those countries in which the *Système Internationale (SI)* is used, electrolyte content in body fluids is expressed in *millimoles*. One *mole* (mol) of a substance is defined as the molecular (or atomic) weight of that substance in grams. For example, a mole of sodium is equivalent to 23 g (the atomic weight of sodium is 23). A *millimole* is one thousandth of a mole, or the molecular or atomic weight expressed in milligrams. Therefore, a *millimole* of sodium equals 23 mg.

Sometimes it is necessary to convert from millimoles per liter to milliequivalents per liter. The following formula applies: mEq/L = mmol/L × valence (Figure 17-3).[4]

Acid–Alkaline (Base) Balance

The alkalinity or acidity of a solution depends on the degree of hydrogen ion concentration. An increase in the hydrogen ions results in a more acid solution; a decrease results in a more alkaline solution. Acidity is expressed by the symbol pH, which refers to the amount of hydrogen ion concentration. A solution having a pH of 7 is regarded as neutral.

The extracellular fluid has a pH ranging from 7.35 to 7.45 and is slightly alkaline. When the pH of the blood is higher than 7.45, an alkaline condition exists; when lower than 7.35, an acid condition exists.

The biologic fluids, both extracellular and intracellular, contain a buffer system that maintains the proper acid–base balance. This buffer system consists of fluid with salts of a weak acid or weak base. A base or hydroxide neutralizes the effect of an acid. These weak acids and bases maintain pH values by soaking up surplus ions or releasing them; acids yield hydrogen ions, bases accept hydrogen ions.

The carbonic acid–sodium bicarbonate system is the most important buffer system in the extracellular compartment. The normal ratio is 1 part of carbonic acid to 20 parts of base bicarbonate, which represents 1.2 mEq carbonic acid to 24 mEq base bicarbonate.[5]

FIGURE 17-3 Millimoles versus milliequivalents for univalent and divalent ions. (From Metheny, N. M. [1992]. *Fluid and electrolyte balance* [2nd ed., p. 6]. Philadelphia: J. B. Lippincott.)

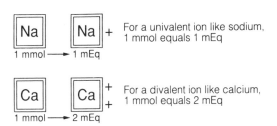

Acid–Base Imbalance

Acid–base imbalances are normally the result of an excess or a deficit in either base bicarbonate or carbonic acid. Deviations of pH from 7.35 to 7.45 are combated by the buffer system and by the respiratory and renal regulatory mechanisms. Two types of disturbance can affect the acid–base balance: respiratory and metabolic. A diagrammatic presentation of the following information is found in Figure 17-4.

Respiratory Disturbances

Respiratory disturbances affect the carbonic side of the balance by increasing or decreasing carbonic acid; when carbon dioxide unites with extracellular fluid, carbonic acid is produced.

Respiratory alkalosis is caused when excess carbon dioxide is exhaled during rapid or deep breathing. Carbonic acid is depleted because of the carbon dioxide loss. Respiratory alkalosis may occur as the result of emotional disturbances, such as anxiety and hysteria, and also from lack of oxygen or from fever.[5]

Symptoms are convulsions, tetany, and unconsciousness. Laboratory determination is a urinary pH above 7 and a plasma bicarbonate concentration less than 24 mEq/L.[5] The body attempts to restore the ratio to normal by depressing the bicarbonate so as to compensate for the deficit in the carbonic acid.

Respiratory acidosis occurs when exhalation of carbon dioxide is depressed; the excess retention of carbon dioxide increases the carbonic acid. It may occur in conditions that interfere with normal breathing, such as emphysema, asthma, and pneumonia.[5]

Symptoms are weakness, disorientation, depressed breathing, and coma. Urinary pH is below 6, and plasma bicarbonate concentration is above 24 mEq/L. The bicarbonate increase is due to the body's attempt to restore the carbonic acid–bicarbonate ratio.[5]

Metabolic Disturbances

Metabolic disturbances affect the bicarbonate side of the balance. Kidney function controls the bicarbonate concentration by regulating the amount of cations (hydrogen, ammonium, and potassium) in exchange for sodium ions to combine with the reabsorbed bicarbonate in the distal tubular lumen. As hydrogen ions are excreted, bicarbonate is generated, maintaining the proper acid–base balance of the blood. Ammonia excretion is increased in response to a high acidity; bicarbonate replaces the ammonia.

Metabolic alkalosis is a condition associated with excess bicarbonate. This condition occurs when chloride is lost. Chloride and bicarbonate are both anions, which must equal the total number of cations. When the chloride anions are lost, the deficit must be made up by an equal number of anions to maintain electrolyte equilibrium; bicarbonate increases in compensation and alkalosis occurs.

Metabolic alkalosis is also associated with decreased levels of intracellular potassium. Potassium escapes from the cell into the extracellular fluid and is lost through the transcellular fluid. When body potassium is lost, the shift of the sodium and hydrogen ions from the extracellular fluid causes alkalosis, while the increase of hydrogen ions in the intracellular fluid causes acidosis of the cells.

Muscular hyperactivity, tetany, and depressed respiration are symptoms of metabolic alkalosis. The muscular hyperactivity and the tetany are symptoms of the deficit in ionized calcium that exists in alkalosis. Laboratory determinations are urinary pH above 7, plasma pH above 7.45, and bicarbonate level above 24 mEq/L.[5]

Treatment consists of the administration of solutions containing chloride to replace bicarbonate ions. Excess of bicarbonate ions is accompanied by potassium deficiency, so potassium must also be replaced.

Metabolic acidosis is a condition associated with a deficit in the bicarbonate concentration. This occurs when (1) excessive amounts of ketone acids accumulate, as in uncontrolled diabetes or starvation; (2) inorganic acids like phosphate and sulfate accumulate, as in renal disease; and (3) excessive losses of bicarbonate occur from gastrointestinal drainage or diarrhea. Acidosis may occur also from IV administration of excessive amounts of sodium chloride or ammonium chloride, causing chloride ions to flood the extracellular fluid.

Stupor, shortness of breath, weakness, and unconsciousness are the symptoms of metabolic acidosis, and laboratory determinations of metabolic acidosis are a urinary pH below 6, plasma pH below 7.35, and plasma bicarbonate concentration below 24 mEq/L.[5]

Treatment and clinical management consist of increasing the bicarbonate level. Solutions of sodium lactate are often used, but because lactate ion must be oxidized to carbon dioxide before it can affect the acid–base balance, it is advisable to use sodium bicarbonate solutions, which are effective even when the patient is suffering from oxygen lack.

HOMEOSTATIC MECHANISMS

The body contains regulating mechanisms that maintain the constancy of body fluid volume, electrolyte composition, and osmolality. These mechanisms consist of the renocardiovascular, endocrine (adrenal, pituitary, and parathyroid), and respiratory systems. The kidneys, skin, and lungs are the main regulating agents.[4,5]

The *kidney* plays a major role in fluid and electrolyte balance. To function adequately, the kidney depends on its own soundness as well as on the coordination of all the regulating organs. The distal renal tubules in the kidney are important in regulating the body fluid. They selectively retain or reject electrolytes and other substances to maintain normal osmolality and blood volume; sodium is retained and potassium is excreted.[1]

The kidneys also play an important part in acid–base regulation. The distal tubule has the ability to form ammonia and exchange hydrogen ion (in form of ammonia) for bicarbonate to maintain the carbonic acid–bicarbonate ratio.

The *lungs* and the *skin* play an important role in fluid balance—the skin in loss of fluid through insensible perspiration and the lungs in loss of fluid by expiration. It has been noted that normal intake of 2500 mL from all sources will deliver a loss of about 1000 mL in breath and perspiration, 1400 mL in urine, and 100 mL in feces.[2]

The *renocardiovascular system* maintains fluid balance by regulating the amount and composition of urine. Plasma must reach the kidneys in sufficient volume to permit regulation of water and electrolyte balance. Renal disease, cardiac failure, shock, postoperative stress, and alarm impair this regulating mechanism.

The *adrenal glands* influence the retention or excretion of sodium, potassium, and water. These glands secrete aldosterone, a hormone that increases the reabsorption of sodium from the renal tubules in exchange for potassium, thus maintaining normal sodium concentration.[5] Any stress, such as surgery, increases the secretion of aldosterone, thus increasing the reabsorption of sodium bicarbonate. Adrenal hyperactivity also increases the secretions of the hormone and causes excess sodium retention. Excess loss of sodium occurs with adrenal insufficiency.

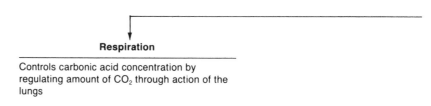

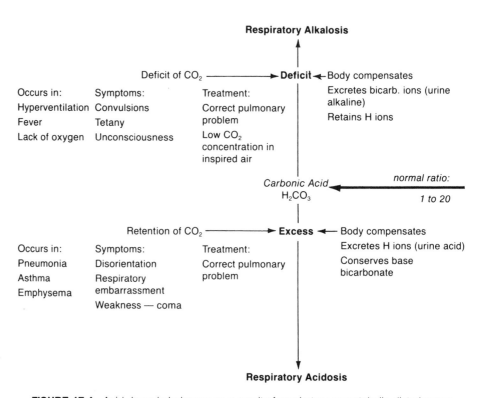

FIGURE 17-4   Acid–base imbalances as a result of respiratory or metabolic disturbances.

The *pituitary gland* is another important organ in the control of fluid and electrolyte balance. The posterior lobe of the pituitary releases antidiuretic hormone (ADH), which inhibits diuresis by increasing water reabsorption in the distal tubule. Increased concentration of sodium in the extracellular fluid stimulates the pituitary to release ADH. This hormone increases the reabsorption of water to dilute the sodium to the normal level of concentration. Increased body fluid osmolality, decreased body fluid volume, stress, and shock are conditions that increase ADH secretion. Increased body fluid volume, decreased osmolality, and alcohol inhibit ADH secretion.[4]

The *parathyroid glands,* pea-sized glands embedded in the corners of the thyroid gland, regulate calcium and phosphate balance by means of parathyroid hormone (PTH). When calcium level is low, PTH secretion is stimulated. When calcium concentration is too high, PTH secretion is depressed so that almost no bone reabsorption occurs.

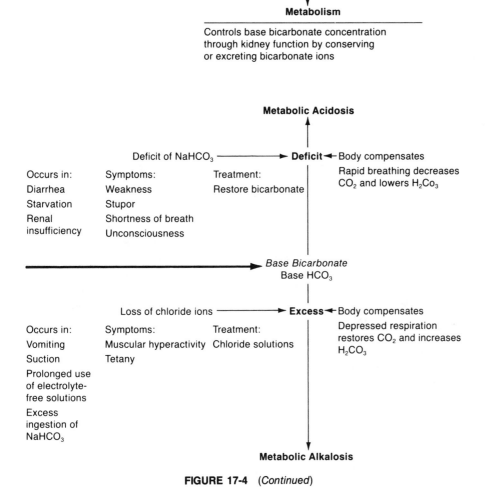

Metabolism

Controls base bicarbonate concentration
through kidney function by conserving
or excreting bicarbonate ions

Metabolic Acidosis

Deficit of NaHCO₃ ⟶ **Deficit** ⟵ Body compensates

			Rapid breathing decreases
Occurs in:	Symptoms:	Treatment:	CO_2 and lowers H_2Co_3
Diarrhea	Weakness	Restore bicarbonate	
Starvation	Stupor		
Renal	Shortness of breath		
insufficiency	Unconsciousness		

Base Bicarbonate
Base HCO₃

Loss of chloride ions ⟶ **Excess** ⟵ Body compensates

			Depressed respiration
Occurs in:	Symptoms:	Treatment:	restores CO_2 and increases
Vomiting	Muscular hyperactivity	Chloride solutions	H_2CO_3
Suction	Tetany		
Prolonged use			
of electrolyte-			
free solutions			
Excess			
ingestion of			
NaHCO₃			

Metabolic Alkalosis

FIGURE 17-4   *(Continued)*

The *pulmonary system* regulates acid–base balance by controlling the concentration of carbonic acid through exhalation or retention of carbon dioxide.

ELECTROLYTES OF BIOLOGIC FLUIDS

Electrolyte content of the intracellular fluid differs from that of extracellular fluid. Because specialized techniques are required to measure electrolyte concentration in the intracellular fluid, it is customary to measure the electrolytes in the extracellular fluid, chiefly plasma. Plasma electrolyte concentrations may be used to assess and manage patients with a diversity of electrolyte imbalances. Although some tests are performed on serum, the terms serum electrolytes and plasma electrolytes are used interchangeably. Table 17-1 lists the electrolytes in intracellular fluid and Table 17-2 lists those in plasma.

TABLE 17-1
Approximation of Major Electrolyte Content in Intracellular Fluid

Electrolytes	mEq/L	Electrolytes	mEq/L
Cations		**Anions**	
Potassium (K$^+$)	150	Phosphates ⎫	
Magnesium (Mg^{2+})	40	Sulfates ⎭	150
		Bicarbonate (HCO$_3^-$)	10
Sodium (Na$^+$)	10	Proteinate	40
Total cations	200	Total anions	200

(From Metheny, N. M. [1992]. *Fluid and electrolyte balance* [2nd ed., p. 5]. Philadelphia: J. B. Lippincott.)

Potassium

Potassium is one of the most important electrolytes in the body. An excess or deficiency of potassium can cause serious impairment of body function and even result in death.

Potassium is the main electrolyte in the intracellular compartment, which houses more than 98% of the body's total potassium. The healthy cell requires a high potassium concentration for cellular activity. When the cell dies, there is an exchange of potassium into the extracellular fluid with a transfer of sodium into the cell. This process also occurs to some degree when cellular metabolism is impaired, as in catabolism (breaking down) of cells from a crushing injury.

Serum concentration of potassium is 3.5 to 5.0 mEq/L.[4] In the cell, the normal concentration is 115 to 150 mEq/L fluid. Variations from either of these levels can produce critical effects. When a repeated potassium level is above 5.6 mEq/L, a potassium excess is indicated; renal impairment will usually be shown by renal function studies. High serum concentrations have an adverse effect on the heart muscle and may cause cardiac arrhythmias; elevation to two to three times the normal level may result in cardiac arrest. The electrocardiogram may detect signs of potassium excess with peaked and elevated T waves; P waves later disappear, and finally, "biphasic deflections [result] from

TABLE 17-2
Plasma Electrolytes

Electrolytes	mEq/L	Electrolytes	mEq/L
Cations		**Anions**	
Sodium (Na$^+$)	142	Chloride (Cl$^-$)	103
Potassium (K$^+$)	5	Bicarbonate (HCO$_3^-$)	26
Calcium (Ca^{2+})	5	Phosphate (HPO$_4^{2-}$)	2
Magnesium (Mg^{2+})	2	Sulfate (SO$_4^{2-}$)	1
		Organic acids	5
Total cations	154	Proteinate	17
		Total anions	154

(From Metheny, N. M. [1992]. *Fluid and electrolyte balance* [2nd ed., p. 5]. Philadelphia: J. B. Lippincott.)

fusion of the QRS complex, RST segment, and the T waves."[5] *Hypokalemia* is the term that expresses serum potassium level below normal; *hyperkalemia* denotes a serum potassium level above normal.

Hypokalemia

Hypokalemia (serum potassium level less than 4 mEq/L) may result when any one of the following conditions occurs: (1) total body potassium is below normal, (2) concentration of potassium in cells is below normal, or (3) concentration of potassium in serum is below normal.[3]

These conditions are often caused by variations in the intake or output of potassium. A decreased intake of potassium from prolonged fluid therapy (lacking potassium replacement) may result in hypokalemia. It may also occur during a "starvation diet" because the kidneys do not normally conserve potassium. An increased loss of potassium usually results from polyuria, vomiting, gastric suction (prolonged), diarrhea, and steroid therapy.[3]

On the other hand, these conditions of potassium deficiency may be unrelated to intake and output. They can be caused by a sudden shift of potassium from extracellular fluid to intracellular fluid, such as that occurring from anabolism (building up of cells), healing processes, or the use of insulin and glucose in the treatment of diabetic acidosis.[3] The shifts resulting from anabolism and healing processes are not usually of severe consequence unless accompanied by intervening factors. In the treatment of diabetic acidosis, the potassium shift may occur suddenly with grave consequences. When cells are anabolized, potassium shifts into the cells. During the use of glucose in the treatment of diabetic acidosis, the glucose in the cells is quickly metabolized into glycogen for storage, causing a sudden shift of potassium from the extracellular fluid to the intracellular fluid.[3] This process results in hypokalemia.

The signs and symptoms of hypokalemia are malaise, skeletal and smooth muscle atony, apathy, muscular cramps, and postural hypotension. Treatment consists of administration of potassium orally or parenterally.

Hyperkalemia

Hyperkalemia may result from renal failure with potassium retention or from excessive or rapid administration of potassium in fluid therapy. It may also occur in conditions unrelated to retention or excessive intake. A sudden shift of potassium from intracellular to extracellular fluid results when catabolism of cells takes place, as in a crushing injury; potassium shifts from cells to plasma.

The signs and symptoms of hyperkalemia are similar to those of hypokalemia. In addition to the signs already listed, the patient may experience tingling or numbness in the extremities, and the heart rate may be slow. A serum potassium level greater than 5.5 mEq/L confirms the diagnosis.

Treatment consists of stopping the potassium intake. Dialysis may be necessary for a long-term renal problem. If the cause is a shift of potassium from cells to plasma, glucose and insulin therapy may be used.

Sodium

Sodium is the main electrolyte in the extracellular fluid; its normal concentration is 135 to 145 mEq/L plasma. The main role of sodium is to control the distribution of water throughout the body and to maintain a normal fluid balance. Alterations in sodium concentration markedly influence the fluid volume: the loss of sodium is accompanied by water loss and dehydration; the gain of sodium, by fluid retention.

The body, by regulating the urinary output, normally maintains a constant fluid volume and isotonicity of the plasma. The urinary output is controlled by ADH, secreted by the pituitary gland. If a hypotonic concentration results from a low sodium concentration, the fluid is drawn from the plasma into the cells. The body attempts to correct this process; the pituitary inhibits ADH and diuresis results, with a loss of extracellular fluid. This loss of fluid increases sodium concentration to a normal level.

If a hypertonic concentration results from increased concentration of extracellular sodium, fluid is drawn from the cells. Again the body reacts, and the pituitary is stimulated to secrete ADH. This causes a retention of fluid that dilutes sodium to normal concentrations.

Therefore, increased sodium concentration stimulates the production of ADH, with retention of water, thus diluting sodium to the normal level; a decrease in sodium concentration inhibits the production of ADH, resulting in a loss of water, which raises the concentration of sodium to the normal level.

In the kidneys, sodium is reabsorbed in exchange for potassium. Therefore, with an increase in sodium there is loss of potassium; with a loss of sodium there is an increase in potassium.

A *sodium deficit* may be present when plasma sodium concentration falls below 135 mEq/L. It is caused by excessive sweating combined with a large intake of water by mouth (salt is lost and fluid increased, thus reducing sodium concentration), excessive infusion of nonelectrolyte fluids, gastrointestinal suction plus water by mouth, and adrenal insufficiency, which causes large loss of electrolytes.

The symptoms of a sodium deficit are apprehension, abdominal cramps, diarrhea, and convulsions.

Dehydration results from loss of sodium and leads to peripheral circulatory failure. When sodium and water are lost from the plasma, the body attempts to replace them by a transfer of sodium and water from the interstitial fluid. Eventually the water will be drawn from the cells and circulation will fail; plasma volume will not be sustained.

Sodium excess may be present when the plasma sodium rises above 145 mEq/L. Its causes are excessive infusions of saline, diarrhea, insufficient water intake, diabetes mellitus, and tracheobronchitis (excess loss of water from lungs because of rapid breathing).

The symptoms of sodium excess are dry, sticky mucous membranes, oliguria, excitement, and convulsions.

Calcium

Calcium is an electrolyte constituent of the plasma present in a concentration of about 4.6–5.1 mg/dL ionized calcium.[4] Total calcium range is 8.9–10.3 mg/dL. Calcium serves several purposes. It plays an important role in formation and function of bones and teeth. As ionized calcium, it is involved in normal clotting of the blood and regulation of neuromuscular irritability.

The parathyroid glands control calcium metabolism. By acting on the kidneys and bones, PTH regulates the concentration of ionized calcium in the extracellular fluid. Impairment of this regulatory mechanism alters the calcium concentration. Hyperparathyroidism causes an elevation in the serum calcium level and a decrease in the serum phosphate level.

Calcium deficit may occur in patients with diarrhea or with problems in gastrointestinal absorption, in extensive infections of the subcutaneous tissue, and in burns. This deficiency can result in muscle tremors and cramps, in excessive irritability, and even in convulsions.

Calcium ionization is influenced by pH; it is decreased in alkalosis and increased in acidosis. With no loss of calcium, a patient in alkalosis may develop symptoms of calcium deficit: muscle cramps, tetany, and convulsions. This is due to the decreased ionization of calcium caused by the elevated pH.

A patient in acidosis may have a calcium deficit with no symptoms because the acid pH has caused an increased ionization of available calcium. Symptoms of calcium deficit may appear if acidosis is converted to alkalosis.

It is estimated that 98% of patients with *hypercalcemia*, or calcium excess, have one of the following three conditions: malignancy, hyperparathyroidism, or thiazide diuretic use.[4] Characteristics include muscular weakness, tiredness, lethargy, constipation, anorexia, polyuria, polydipsia, shortened QT interval on the electrocardiogram, and a serum calcium concentration greater than 10.5 mg/dL.

Other Electrolytes

The primary role of *magnesium* is in enzyme activity, contributing to the metabolism of both carbohydrates and proteins. Its serum concentration is 1.3 to 2.1 mEq/L.* A *magnesium deficit* is a common imbalance in critically ill patients. Deficits may also occur in less acutely ill patients, such as those experiencing withdrawal from alcohol and those receiving parenteral or enteral nutrition following a period of starvation. Neuromuscular irritability, disorientation, and mood changes are indicative of hypomagnesemia. *Hypermagnesemia* is generally uncommon, but it may be seen in patients with advanced renal failure. Magnesium is excreted by the kidneys; therefore, diminished renal function results in abnormal renal magnesium retention.[4]

Chloride, the chief anion of the extracellular fluid, has a plasma concentration of 97 to 110 mEq/L. A deficiency of chloride leads to a deficiency of potassium, and vice versa. There is also a loss of chloride with a loss of sodium, but because this loss can be compensated for by an increase in bicarbonate, the proportion will differ.[1]

Phosphate is the chief anion of the intracellular fluid; its normal level in plasma is 1.7 to 2.3 mEq/L.*

REFERENCES

1. Baxter Healthcare. (1977). *Fundamentals of body water and electrolytes* (pp. 5, 21). Deerfield, IL: Author.
2. Burgess, E. F. (1965). Fluids and electrolytes. *American Journal of Nursing, 65*, 90–95.
3. Crowell, C. W., & Staff of Educational Design, Inc., New York. (1967). Potassium imbalance. *American Journal of Nursing, 67*, 343.
4. Metheny, N. M. (1992). *Fluid and electrolyte balance* (pp. 4, 6, 8–11, 30–31, 88–92, 97, 104, 111, 112, 117). Philadelphia: J. B. Lippincott.
5. Metheny, N. M., & Snively, W. D., Jr. (1983). *Nurses' handbook of fluid balance* (4th ed., pp. 8, 9, 17, 51, 54, 68–81, 282). Philadelphia: J. B. Lippincott.

* Convert to mg/dL by multiplying by 1.2.

REVIEW QUESTIONS

1. Nonelectrolytes found in body fluid include which of the following?
   a. dextrose
   b. urea
   c. creatinine
   d. bicarbonate

2. Normal pH of the blood is:
   a. 6.35–6.45
   b. 6.75–7.25
   c. 7.35–7.45
   d. 7.45–7.65

3. Osmolality of normal blood plasma is:
   a. 210 mOsm/kg water
   b. 230 mOsm/kg water
   c. 270 mOsm/kg water
   d. 290 mOsm/kg water

4. Metabolic acidosis may be caused by which of the following?
   a. uncontrolled diabetes
   b. starvation
   c. renal disease
   d. hepatic disease

5. Which of the following controls distribution of water throughout the body?
   a. sodium
   b. potassium
   c. calcium
   d. phosphorus

6. Aldosterone is secreted by which of the following?
   a. adrenal glands
   b. hypothalamus
   c. thyroid gland
   d. pituitary gland

7. Normal ionized calcium concentration is:
   a. 2 mEq/L
   b. 3 mEq/L
   c. 5 mEq/L
   d. 6 mEq/L

8. The primary role of magnesium is:
   a. catalyst activity
   b. enzyme activity
   c. normal clotting
   d. neuromuscular activity

9. Normal plasma concentration of sodium is:
   a. 115–120 mEq/L
   b. 125–132 mEq/L
   c. 135–145 mEq/L
   d. 146–150 mEq/L

10. The homeostatic mechanism responsible for control of calcium metabolism is:
    a. parathyroid glands
    b. thyroid glands
    c. pituitary gland
    d. kidneys

_____

CHAPTER 18

Rationale of Fluid and Electrolyte Therapy

OBJECTIVES OF PARENTERAL THERAPY _____

Parenteral therapy has three main objectives: (1) to maintain daily body fluid requirements, (2) to restore previous body fluid losses, and (3) to replace present body fluid losses.

MAINTENANCE THERAPY _____

Maintenance therapy consists of providing all the nutrient needs of the patient: water, electrolytes, dextrose, vitamins, and protein. Of these needs, water is the most important. The body may survive for a prolonged period without vitamins, dextrose, and protein, but without water, dehydration and death occur.

Water

Water is needed by the body to replace the insensible loss that occurs with evaporation from the skin and evaporated moisture from the expired air. An average adult loses from 500 to 1000 mL water per 24 hours through insensible loss. The skin loss varies with the temperature and humidity.

Water must also be provided for kidney function; the amount needed depends on the amount of waste products to be excreted as well as the concentrating ability of the kidneys. Protein and salt increase the need for water.

Until 1925, parenteral fluids consisted solely of isotonic saline solutions. Because water is hypotonic and cannot be given IV, salt was added to attain isotonicity. If given IV, distilled water causes hemolysis; the distilled water is drawn into the blood cells because of the greater solute concentration, causing them to swell and burst. After 1925, glucose began to be used extensively to make water isotonic and to provide calories.

An individual's fluid requirements are based on age, height, weight, and amount of body fat. Because fat is water free, a large amount of body fat contains a relatively low amount of water; as body fat increases, water decreases in inverse proportion to body weight.[2] The normal fluid and electrolyte requirements based on body surface area have been found to be more constant than when expressed in terms of body weight. Many of

Sharon M. Weinstein: PLUMER'S PRINCIPLES & PRACTICE OF INTRAVENOUS THERAPY, FIFTH EDITION, © 1993 J. B. Lippincott Company

the essential physiologic processes such as heat loss, blood volume, organ size, and respiration have a direct relationship to the body surface area.[2] The fluid and electrolyte requirements are also proportionate to surface area, regardless of the the patient's age.[2] These requirements are based on square meters of body surface area and calculated for a 24-hour period. Nomograms are available for determining surface area (Figure 18-1).

Balanced solutions are available for maintenance. The average requirements of fluid and electrolytes are estimated for a healthy person and applied to the patient. The balanced solutions contain electrolytes in proportion to the daily needs of the patient, but not in excess of the body's tolerance, as long as adequate kidney function exists. When a

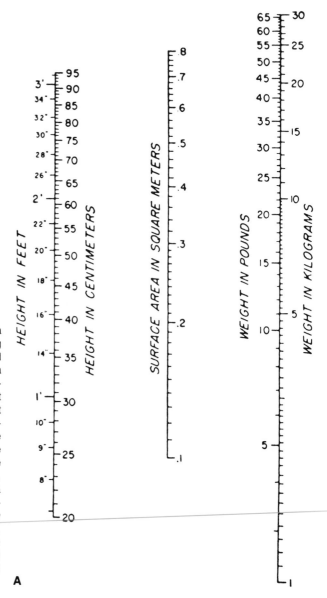

FIGURE 18-1 Body surface area nomograms for (**A**) infants and young children, and (**B**) older children and adults. To determine the surface area of the patient, draw a straight line between the point representing height on the left vertical scale to the point representing weight on the right vertical scale. The point at which the line intersects the middle vertical scale represents the patient's body surface area in square meters. (From Talbot, N. B., Sobel, E. H., McArthur, J. W., & Crawford, J. D. [1952, 1980]. *Functional endocrinology from birth through adolescence.* Cambridge, MA: Harvard University Press, © 1952, 1980 by the President and Fellows of Harvard College. Reprinted by permission.)

A

patient's water needs are provided by these maintenance solutions, the daily needs of sodium and potassium are also met. For maintenance, 1500 mL/m^2 body surface area is administered over a 24-hour period.[3]

Glucose

Glucose, a necessary nutrient in maintenance therapy, has important functions. Because it is converted into glycogen by the liver, it improves hepatic function. By supplying necessary calories for energy, it spares body protein and minimizes the development of

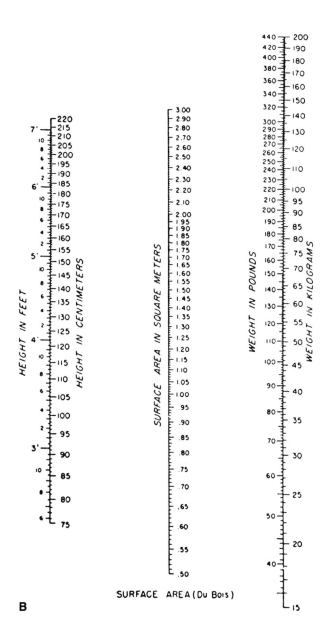

SURFACE AREA (Du Bois)

B

ketosis caused by the oxidation of fat stores for essential energy in the absence of added glucose.

The basic daily caloric requirement of a 70-kg adult at rest is about 1600 calories. However, the administration of 100 g glucose a day is helpful in minimizing the ketosis of starvation;[3] 100 g is contained in 2 L 5% dextrose in water or 1 L 10% dextrose in water.

Protein

Protein is another nutrient important to maintenance therapy. Although a patient may be adequately maintained on glucose, water, vitamins, and electrolytes for a limited time, protein may be required to replace normal protein losses over an extended period. It is necessary for cellular repair, wound healing, and synthesis of vitamins and some enzymes. The usual daily protein requirement for a healthy adult is 1 g/kg body weight.[2] Protein is available as amino acids; taken orally, it is broken down into amino acids before being absorbed into the blood.

Vitamins

Vitamins, although not nutrients in the true sense of the word, are necessary for the utilization of other nutrients. Vitamin C and the various B complex vitamins are the most frequently used in parenteral therapy. Because these vitamins are water soluble, they are not retained by the body but lost through urinary excretion. Because of this loss, larger amounts are required parenterally to ensure adequate maintenance than may be required when administered orally. Vitamin B complex vitamins play an important role in the metabolism of carbohydrates and in maintaining gastrointestinal function. Vitamin C promotes wound healing and is frequently used for the surgical patient.

Vitamins A and D are fat-soluble vitamins, better retained by the body and not generally required by the patient on maintenance therapy.

RESTORATION OF PREVIOUS LOSSES

Restoration of previous losses is essential when past maintenance has not been met—when the output has exceeded the intake. Severe dehydration may occur from failure to replace these losses. Therapy consists of replacing losses from previous deficits in addition to providing fluid and electrolytes for daily maintenance. Kidney status must be considered before electrolyte replacement and maintenance can be initiated; urinary suppression may result from decreased fluid volume or renal impairment. A hydrating solution such as 5% dextrose in 0.2% (34.2 mEq) sodium chloride is administered. Urinary flow will be restored if the retention is functional. The patient must be rehydrated rapidly to establish an adequate urinary output. Only after kidney function is proved adequate can large electrolyte losses be replaced. Potassium chloride must be used with considerable caution and is considered potentially dangerous if administered when renal function is impaired. A buildup of potassium, caused by the kidney's inability to excrete salts, can prove hazardous; arrhythmia and heart block can result from the effect of excess potassium on the heart muscle.

REPLACEMENT OF PRESENT LOSSES

Replacement of present losses of fluid and electrolytes is as necessary as daily mainte-nance and replacement of previous losses. The importance of accurate measurement of all intake and output cannot be underestimated as a means of calculating fluid loss. Fluid loss may also be estimated by determining loss of body weight; 1 L body water equals 1 kg, or 2.2 lb, body weight. An osmolality determination may indicate the water needs of the body. If necessary, a corrective blood urea nitrogen determination may be done in conjunction with the osmolality.

The type of replacement depends on the type of fluid being lost. A choice of appropriate replacement solutions is available. Excessive loss of gastric fluid must be replaced by solutions resembling the fluid lost, such as gastric replacement solu-tions. Excessive loss of intestinal fluid must be replaced by an intestinal replacement fluid. Examples of conditions that may result from current losses are alkalosis and acidosis.

Alkalosis

Alkalosis may occur from an excessive loss of gastric fluid, either by vomiting or suction. Gastric juices, with a pH of 1 to 3.5[3], are the most acid of the body secretions.[3] Excess loss of chloride causes an increase in the concentration of bicarbonate ions; total anions must always equal total cations. The patient's respiration becomes slow and shallow; the body attempts to correct alkalosis by retaining carbon dioxide. Because of the body's inability to ionize calcium in the presence of a high pH, muscular hyperactivity and tetany occur. The patient may become irritable, uncooperative, and disoriented.

Prompt recognition of symptoms is important for early treatment or for altering current treatment. Most alkalotic states secondary to gastric suction are corrected by sodium chloride and potassium chloride solutions. Special gastric replacement solutions are available. They contain ammonium chloride, which replaces the chloride without increasing the sodium. The hydrogen ions, liberated by urea in the conversion of ammonium chloride, correct alkalosis. These solutions, invaluable in certain conditions, can be potentially dangerous if given to patients with impaired liver or kidney function. Ammonia, metabolized by the liver, is converted into urea and hydrogen ion. If the liver fails to convert the ammonia to urea, ammonia retention and toxicity will result. Symptoms of ammonia toxicity include pallor, sweating, tetany, and coma; death may follow.

Acidosis

Acidosis may occur when the excessive fluid loss is alkaline, as are intestinal secretions, bile, and pancreatic juices. Intestinal secretions contain large amounts of bicarbonate ions; with the loss of these ions, the chloride ion concentration increases—and acidosis occurs. Symptoms include shortness of breath with rapid breathing (respiratory compen-sation to reduce carbon dioxide and correct acidosis). Weakness and coma occur. To replace lost alkaline secretions and correct acidosis, specific parenteral solutions contain-ing base salts, such as sodium lactate or sodium bicarbonate, are used.

ELECTROLYTE AND FLUID DISTURBANCES _____

Fluid and electrolyte imbalances occurring in the ill patient are serious, life-threatening complications. The correction of these imbalances is of vital concern to the patient's welfare. A discussion follows of a few of the most common clinical cases in which fluid disturbances contribute to serious complications, with emphasis on the physiologic changes accompanying these imbalances and the parenteral therapy necessary to correct them.

THE SURGICAL PATIENT _____

A knowledge of the endocrine response to stress helps the nurse better understand the imbalances and problems associated with them. It also contributes to safe and successful parenteral therapy. The nurse knows what to expect, is alert to the possible dangers of imbalances, and recognizes early symptoms.

Neuroendocrine Response

The neuroendocrine response stimulated by many anesthetic agents is further heightened by surgical stress. Apprehension, pain, and duration and severity of trauma give rise to surgical stress and contribute to an increased endocrine response during the first 2 to 5 days after surgery.

The stress reaction is normal and is nature's way of protecting the body from hypotension resulting from trauma and shock. Correction is often unnecessary and may, in fact, be harmful.

The two major endocrine homeostatic controls affected by stress are the pituitary gland and the adrenal gland (Figure 18-2). The posterior pituitary controls quantitative secretions of antidiuretic hormone (ADH). The anterior pituitary controls secretions of corticotropin, which stimulates the adrenal gland to increase mineralocorticoid secretions (aldosterone) and glucocorticoid secretions (hydrocortisone).[2] The adrenal medulla secretes vasopressors (epinephrine and norepinephrine) to help maintain the blood pressure.

A direct physiologic effect occurs when stress increases the secretions of these various hormones. When the posterior pituitary increases ADH secretions, antidiuresis is effected, thus helping maintain blood volume. When the anterior pituitary increases corticotropin secretions, the adrenal gland is stimulated to increase aldosterone and hydrocortisone secretion. These two adrenal hormones help maintain blood volume by causing the retention of sodium ions and chloride anions, thereby causing water retention, and promoting the excretion of potassium (loss of cellular potassium ions causes loss of cellular water into extracellular space, where it is retained by ADH to maintain blood volume).[2]

Hydrocortisone also promotes the catabolism of protein to provide necessary amino acids for healing and stimulates the conversion of protein and fat to glucose for metabolism during the stress period. This metabolic activity may elevate the blood sugar level, a finding that may mistakenly suggest diabetes mellitus. A drop in the eosinophil count and an elevated level of serum 17-hydroxycorticosteroid hormones indicate increased adrenal activity.[2]

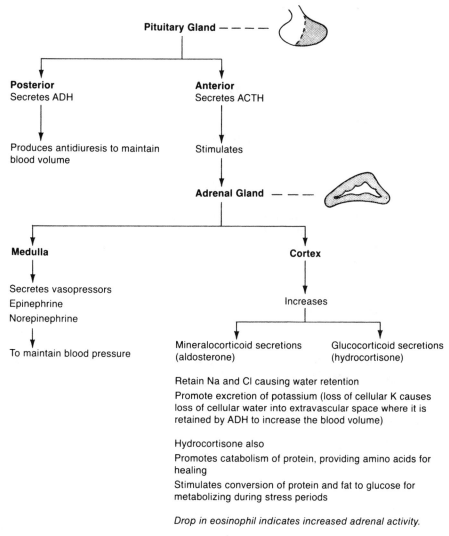

Pituitary Gland — — — —

Posterior
Secretes ADH

Produces antidiuresis to maintain blood volume

Anterior
Secretes ACTH

Stimulates

Adrenal Gland — — —

Medulla

Secretes vasopressors
Epinephrine
Norepinephrine

To maintain blood pressure

Cortex

Increases

Mineralocorticoid secretions (aldosterone)

Glucocorticoid secretions (hydrocortisone)

Retain Na and Cl causing water retention
Promote excretion of potassium (loss of cellular K causes loss of cellular water into extravascular space where it is retained by ADH to increase the blood volume)

Hydrocortisone also
Promotes catabolism of protein, providing amino acids for healing
Stimulates conversion of protein and fat to glucose for metabolizing during stress periods

Drop in eosinophil indicates increased adrenal activity.

FIGURE 18-2 Endocrine response to stress.

Fluid Needs

Accurate records of intake and output measurements are important for assessing fluid requirements and preventing serious fluid imbalances during the early postoperative period. The daily requirement of 1500 to 2000 mL varies with the patient's needs. Caution must be taken not to overhydrate the patient—the intake should be adequate but should not exceed the fluid losses.

We have seen how the adrenocortical secretions, increased by trauma and stress of surgery, cause some water and sodium retention. This retention may be severe enough to give a false picture of oliguria. Excessive quantities of nonelectrolyte solutions (such as 5% dextrose in water) administered at a time when antidiuresis is occurring may cause a serious fluid imbalance, hyponatremia.

Hyponatremia

In hyponatremia, the serum sodium concentration is less than normal. Water-yielding solutions, infused in excess of the body's tolerance, expand the extracellular compartment, lowering the electrolyte concentration. By osmosis, water invades the cells, with a resulting excess accumulation of intracellular fluid. Usually there is no edema because edema is the result of an excess accumulation of fluid in the extracellular compartment.[2]

Symptoms of water excess include confusion, hallucinations, delirium, weight gain, hyperventilation, muscular weakness, twitching, and convulsions. If these occur during the early postoperative stages, the nurse should suspect water excess. This is of particular concern in the young and the aged. Serious consequences, even death, can result.

Restricting the fluid intake may correct mild water excess, but for more severe cases, the administration of high concentrations of sodium chloride may be indicated. The electrolyte concentration of the plasma, increased by the concentrated saline, causes an increase in the osmotic pressure, drawing fluid from the cells for excretion by the kidneys.

Often parenteral therapy during the stress period consists of administering conservative amounts of 5% dextrose in water. Because some sodium retention results from the endocrine response to stress, caution is taken to avoid administration of excessive quantities of saline at a time when there is an interference in the elimination of salt. During this early period, the physician frequently gives 5% dextrose in quarter- or half-strength saline to avoid sodium excess.

Hypernatremia

In hypernatremia, the serum sodium concentration is higher than normal. This excess can cause expanded extracellular fluid volume or edema and possible disruption of cellular function (in potassium-depleted patients the sodium may replace the intracellular potassium).

Symptoms of sodium excess include flushed skin, elevation in temperature, dry and sticky mucous membranes, thirst, and a decreased or absent urinary output. Treatment consists of reducing the salt and water intake and promoting diuresis to eliminate the excess of salt and water from the plasma.

Nutrients

Carbohydrates

Carbohydrates provide an indispensable source of calories for the postoperative patient unable to receive oral sustenance. When carbohydrates are inadequate, the body will use its own fat to supply calories; the by-products are ketone bodies. These acid bodies neutralize bicarbonate and produce metabolic acidosis. The only by-products excreted in the metabolism of carbohydrates are water and carbon dioxide.

By providing calories for essential energy, carbohydrates also reduce catabolism of protein. During the stress response, the renal excretion of nitrogen (from the catabolism of protein) exceeds the intake. By reducing the protein breakdown, glucose helps prevent a negative nitrogen balance.

Carbohydrates do not provide adequate calories for the patient receiving prolonged therapy. One liter of 5% dextrose in water provides 170 calories. Many liters, a volume too great for most patients to tolerate, would be required to provide a patient with 1600 calories. Greater concentrations of glucose, 20% and 50%, may be administered to provide calories for patients unable to tolerate large volumes of fluid (*eg*, patients with renal insufficiency). The concentrated solutions must be administered slowly for glucose utilization to occur. Rapid administration results in diuresis; the concentrated glucose acts as a diuretic, drawing interstitial fluid into the plasma for excretion by the kidneys.

Alcohol

Alcohol solutions may be administered to the postoperative patient for nutritional and physiologic benefits. Nutritionally, the alcohol supplements calories provided by the glucose, 1 g ethyl alcohol yielding 6 to 8 calories.[3] Because alcohol is quickly and completely metabolized, it provides calories for essential energy, sparing fat and protein. Metabolized in preference to glucose, alcohol allows the infused glucose to be stored as glycogen.

Physiologically, alcohol produces a sedative effect, reducing pain; 200 to 300 mL of a 5% solution per hour produces sedation without intoxication in the average adult.[3] Alcohol also inhibits the secretion of ADH, promoting water excretion.

Solutions containing alcohol, particularly hypertonic solutions, can cause phlebitis. These solutions, if allowed to infiltrate, may cause tissue necrosis. The cannula should be carefully inserted within the lumen of the vessel and inspected frequently to detect any infiltration.

Protein

Patients who receive parenteral fluid therapy for a prolonged time require protein for cellular repair, wound healing, and growth. Stress states accompanying surgical procedures and trauma frequently result in protein deficiency.

During the stress period, increased secretions of glucocorticoids from the adrenal cortex cause protein breakdown and the conversion of protein and fat to glucose for energy. More urinary nitrogen is lost than normal. When nitrogen loss exceeds intake, the patient is said to be in a *negative balance*. This response to stress is normal. However, protein losses must be counteracted; preservation of body cell mass is essential. A depleted body cell mass can be restored only by hyperalimentation. Approximately 1 g/kg body weight is required by a healthy adult to replace normal protein loss.[3]

Because of the high ammonia level, extreme caution is required if administered to patients with hepatic insufficiency or emaciation. Organ-specific formulas have been developed for the patient with renal or hepatic disease.

Supplemental medications added to the solution may result in incompatibilities. Always check with the pharmacist before adding any medication to solutions.

Solutions, once opened, must be used immediately. Storing a partially used container of solution in the refrigerator for future use provides a culture medium for the growth of bacteria.

No solutions that are cloudy or that contain precipitate should be used.

Fat Emulsions

Fat emulsions provide a source of calories and essential fatty acids for metabolic processes. They provide a high caloric yield, 9 kcal/g as compared with 4 kcal/g from carbohydrates.

Potassium

Once the stress period is past, adrenal activity decreases and diuresis begins. At this time, usually after the second to the fifth postoperative day, potassium is given daily to prevent a deficit; potassium is not conserved by the body but is lost in the urine. Electrolyte maintenance fluids may be used or potassium may be added to parenteral solutions. When potassium is added to parenteral fluids, the container, bag, or bottle should be thoroughly shaken to mix and dilute the potassium. Potassium should *never* be added to a hanging container while the infusion is running; such action could result in a bolus injection of the drug. Rapid injection, which increases the drug concentration in the plasma, can result in trauma to the vessel wall and even in cardiac arrest. Potassium should never be given by IV push or bolus administration.

The status of the kidneys must be considered. If kidney function is inadequate, the patient must be rehydrated. During this infusion, the nurse must watch for diminished diuresis and notify the physician if antidiuresis occurs.

Usually 40 mEq/L is sufficient to replace normal potassium loss. It is usually infused over an 8-hour period. Premixed potassium-replacement solutions are available in a variety of strengths.

In extreme cases of hypokalemia, when the serum potassium concentration is less than 2.0 mEq/L, it may be necessary to infuse potassium at a much faster rate, not faster than 40 mEq/hr. When the serum K concentration reaches 2.5 mEq/L and ECG manifestations of hypokalemia diminish, the rate should be decreased to no more than 10 mEq/hr, using a solution that contains no more than 30 mEq/L.[4] Continuous monitoring by electrocardiography is required when high doses of potassium are infused. The solution containing potassium should be conspicuously labeled and must never be used when positive pressure is indicated—rapid infusion may result in cardiac arrest.

Potassium is irritating to the vein and may cause a great deal of pain, especially if infused into a vein where a previous venipuncture has been performed. Slowing the rate may decrease the pain.

Vitamins
Vitamins B complex and C are usually added to parenteral solutions if, after 2 or 3 days, the patient is unable to take fluids orally. Vitamin C is important in promoting healing in the surgical patient, and vitamin B complex aids carbohydrate metabolism.

Nursing Diagnoses
Nursing diagnoses for the postsurgical patient should address relevant fluid and electrolyte disturbances. Table 18-1 lists some possible nursing diagnoses for this patient.

THE BURNED PATIENT

The body mechanisms that regulate fluid and electrolyte balance are altered when severe burns occur. The changes during the first 48 hours must be recognized and dealt with. Fluid and electrolyte therapy sufficient to replace losses and maintain a status quo increase the patient's chances of survival. Awareness of these physiologic changes contributes to intelligent therapy and aids in the patient's recovery.

Fluid and Electrolyte Changes

Intravascular to Interstitial Fluid Shift
The shift from intravascular to interstitial fluid, followed by shock, begins immediately after the burn. This fluid shift represents the water, electrolyte, and protein lost through

TABLE 18-1
Examples of Nursing Diagnoses For a New Postoperative Patient After Abdominal Surgery

Nursing Diagnosis	Etiologic Factors	Defining Characteristics
FVD related to actual fluid loss and third-space fluid shift during surgical procedure	Vomiting after reaction to anesthesia GI suction Third-space fluid shift at surgical site	Postural tachycardia Postural hypotension initially; later, low BP in all positions Decreased skin turgor Decreased capillary refill time Oliguria (<30 mL/hr in adult) Weight change depends on cause (decreased if actual fluid loss, as in GI suction; usually increased if fluid loss is due to third-space shift, provided parenteral fluids are given in an attempt to correct hypovolemia)
Altered tissue perfusion (renal) related to hypotension during surgical procedure	Hypotensive effects of anesthesia Hypovolemia due to direct or indirect loss of fluid Hypovolemia due to inadequate parenteral fluid replacement	Oliguria or polyuria in presence of elevated serum creatinine
Alteration in sodium balance (hyponatremia) related to excessive ADH activity	Major surgery with its premedication, anesthesia, decreased blood volume, and postoperative pain results in increased ADH release (causing water retention with sodium dilution)	Serum sodium <135 mEq/L May be asymptomatic if Na >120 mEq/L Lethargy, confusion, nausea, vomiting, anorexia, abdominal cramps, muscular twitching
Alteration in acid–base balance (metabolic alkalosis) related to vomiting or gastric suction	Vomiting after reaction to anesthesia Gastric suction, particularly if patient is allowed to ingest ice chips freely	Tingling of fingers, toes, and circumoral region, due to decreased calcium ionization pH >7.45, bicarbonate above normal, chloride below normal
Altered nutrition (less than body requirements) related to negative nitrogen balance after surgical stress, and inadequate caloric intake	Catabolic response to stress of surgery Inability to tolerate oral feedings during first few postoperative days due to decreased GI motility, anorexia, nausea, and general discomfort Failure of health care providers to administer sufficient calories via the parenteral route	Weight loss of approximately 1/4 to 1/2 lb/day in adult (provided fluids are not abnormally retained) Perhaps a decrease in serum albumin, transferrin, and retinol binding protein levels (although delivery of a large volume of blood products or the long half-life of certain secretory proteins can interfere with correct interpretation)

BP, blood pressure; FVD, fluid volume deficit; GI, gastrointestinal.

(*From Metheny, N. M. [1992]. Fluid and electrolyte balance [2nd ed., p. 210]. Philadelphia: J. B. Lippincott.*)

the damaged capillaries, resulting in edema and a marked reduction in plasma volume. The severity of the shift depends on the degree and extent of the burn. In an adult with a 50% burn, the edema may exceed the total plasma volume of the patient. Parenteral fluids must be given immediately to replace the fluid loss and combat shock.

Dehydration

In the early phases of fluid shift from plasma to tissues, water and electrolytes are lost in larger quantities than is the protein (protein, because of its larger molecular size, does not readily pass through the capillary walls). The osmotic pressure, increased by the higher protein concentration of the plasma, draws fluid from the undamaged tissues and generalized tissue dehydration occurs.

A much more significant fluid loss occurs as exudate from the burned area, water in the form of vapor at the burned area, and blood lost through the damaged capillaries. These losses further contribute to dehydration and hypovolemia.

Decreased Urinary Output

Decreased urinary output occurs when the lowered blood volume causes a diminished renal blood flow. Increased endocrine secretions further contribute to the decreased urinary output; adrenocortical secretions cause sodium and water absorption; ADH causes increased water reabsorption by the kidneys.

In deep burns free hemoglobin, released by destruction of red blood cells, may produce renal damage.

Potassium Excess

In the early postburn period, when excessive amounts of potassium build up in the extracellular fluid, potassium excess occurs; cell destruction releases potassium and decreased renal flow obstructs normal excretion of potassium. Plasma potassium concentrations may rise to a dangerously high level. Because of the tendency to plasma potassium excess and the uncertainty of the extent of renal impairment in the burned patient, administration of potassium is contraindicated.

Sodium Deficit

When plasma is lost in edema and exudate, sodium, the chief electrolyte of the extracellular fluid, is lost with the plasma, and sodium deficit occurs. Further loss may occur as sodium moves into the cells to replace lost potassium.

Metabolic Acidosis

Acidosis develops within a few hours due to accumulation of fixed acids released from injured tissues.[2]

Fluid Needs

When moderate or severe burns occur, immediate fluid therapy is necessary to combat hypovolemic shock and prevent renal depression. A large-gauge indwelling venous catheter is inserted to ensure venous access during this critical period. Because the measurement of venous pressure is an important guide against overinfusion, a CVP line may be placed.

Solutions such as lactated Ringer's (LR), a balanced salt solution, is often used. It supplies salt and water and helps correct the metabolic acidosis associated with burns.

Hypertonic crystalloid solutions were introduced to decrease the fluid volume needed to correct burn shock and to minimize formation of edema. If used, they are prescribed during the first 24 hours of fluid therapy.[2] In general, they are prescribed after the first 24 hours of fluid therapy. Albumin is also frequently used. Non-protein colloids, including dextran and hetastarch, have molecular size and increased oncotic pressure to help maintain blood volume and cardiac output by pulling water from the interstitial space of nonburned tissue. Blood is generally not administered unless sufficient loss of blood has occurred from an associated injury. A nonelectrolyte solution, such as 5% dextrose in water, may be used to replace insensible water loss.

During the initial 24 hours, caution must be taken to avoid overzealous administration of water. During the early phase, water contributes little to the maintenance of normal cardiovascular function. Later, when fluid shifts back into the plasma, excess parenteral fluid can cause overburdened circulation and pulmonary edema. If smoke and heat damage have impaired lung function, the threat of pulmonary edema is further increased. Only enough fluid to maintain blood volume and urinary output is administered.

The shift from interstitial fluid to plasma begins on the second to third day after the burn and accounts for the large reduction in parenteral fluids. An increase in the urinary output should alert the nurse to the edema mobilization taking place and the need to decrease fluid therapy.

The "rule of nines" has been commonly used to estimate burned area (Table 18-2). The body's surface area is divided into areas equal to 9% or multiples of 9%. The portion of these areas that have sustained second- or third-degree burns is determined. The total represents the percentage of total body surface area burned. This method may be inaccurate in children, and hence, other charts are available for accurately determining percentage of body surface area burned.

Formulas

Fluid requirements for the first 24 hours range from 2 to 4 mL/kg body weight per percent of body surface area burned. Several factors must be considered, including age of the patient, size and depth of the burn, type of fluid, and complication factors such as inhalation injury, electrical burns, or multiple trauma.[2] Numerous formulas have been developed for this purpose (Table 18-3), but an ideal rate of infusion is one that maintains perfusion, as reflected by a urinary output of 0.5 mL/kg body weight per hour in the adult patient.

TABLE 18-2
"Rule of Nines" for Estimating Burned Body Area in Adults

Part of Body	Percentage of Body
Head and neck	9
Anterior trunk	18
Each arm	9
Posterior trunk	18
Genitalia	1
Each leg	18

TABLE 18-3
Formulas for Fluid Replacement/Resuscitation

	First 24 Hours			Second 24 Hours		
	Electrolyte	Colloid	Glucose in Water	Electrolyte	Colloid	Glucose in Water
Burn budget of F. D. Moore	1000–4000 mL lactated Ringer's solution and 1200 mL 0.5N saline	7.5% of body weight	1500–5000 mL	1000–4000 mL lactated Ringer's solution and 1200 mL 0.5N saline	2.5% of body weight	1500–5000 mL
Evans	Normal saline, 1 mL/kg/% burn	1.0 mL/kg/% burn	2000 mL	One half of first 24-hr requirement	One half of first 24-hr requirement	2000 mL
Brooke	Lactated Ringer's solution, 1.5 mL/kg/% burn	0.5 mL/kg/% burn	2000 mL	One half to three quarters of first 24-hr requirement	One half to three quarters of first 24-hr requirement	2000 mL
Parkland	Lactated Ringer's solution, 4 mL/kg/% burn				20%–60% of calculated plasma volume	
Hypertonic sodium solution	Volume to maintain urine output at 30 mL/hr (fluid contains 250 mEq Na/L)			One third of salt solution orally, up to 3500 mL limit		
Modified Brooke	Lactated Ringer's solution, 2 mL/kg/% burn				0.3–0.5 mL/kg/% burn	Goal: maintain adequate urinary output
Burnett Burn Center	Isotonic or hypertonic alkaline sodium solution/% burn/kg			D_5 ¼ NS maintenance	Colloid 0.5 mL/% burn/kg	D_5W (% burn) (TBSAm³)

TBSA: total body surface area.

(Hudak, C., Gallo, B., & Benz, J. [1990]. Critical care nursing [5th ed., p. 766]. Philadelphia: J. B. Lippincott, with permission.)

Assessment

Ongoing assessment of the patient is needed to allow tailoring of fluid replacement to individual needs. Monitoring parameters include urine volume, sensorium, vital signs, and central venous pressure.

Urine output is the best indicator of adequate fluid resuscitation. Adult output should be 30 to 50 mL/hr. Lack of urine output or a substantial decrease in volume may be attributed to inadequate fluid replacement, gastric dilation, or renal failure. Daily weights are a helpful tool for monitoring the burned patient. A weight gain of 15% to 20% may indicate fluid retention.

Adequacy of tissue perfusion is measured by assessing the patient's sensorium. Sensorium should remain normal with appropriate fluid replacement unless other factors, such as head injury, are present.

Vital signs should be monitored hourly in the burned patient. Blood pressure should remain at near normal values with consideration given to the patient's baseline pressure. Temperature may be elevated and tachycardia may be present. Rate and character of respirations should be evaluated. Peripheral pulses and capillary refill times should be monitored. Vasoconstriction of unburned skin is a compensatory response to help preserve normal blood flow in the hours immediately following a severe burn. Hence, unburned skin may be cool to the touch and appear pale at first.

Central venous and arterial pressure monitoring may be used to evaluate the effects of fluid replacement. Inadequate fluid replacement is evidenced by decreased urinary output, thirst, restlessness and disorientation, hypotension, and increased pulse rate. Circulatory overload may be indicated by elevated central venous pressure reading (15–20 cm), shortness of breath, and moist crackles.[2]

DIABETIC ACIDOSIS

Diabetic acidosis is an endocrine disorder causing complex fluid and electrolyte disturbances. It occurs when a lack of insulin prevents the metabolism of glucose, and essential calories are provided instead by the catabolism of fat and protein. Acidosis results from the accumulation of acid by-products. Knowledge of the physiologic changes in diabetic acidosis aids the nurse in early detection of imbalances and in an understanding of the treatment involved.

Physiologic Changes

Lack of insulin prevents cellular metabolism of glucose and its conversion into glycogen. Glucose accumulates in the bloodstream (*hyperglycemia*). When the blood sugar rises above 180 mg/100 mL, glucose spills over into the urine (*glycosuria*). The kidneys require 10 to 20 mL water to excrete 1 g glucose; water excretion increases (*polyuria*).

The body's fat and protein are used to provide necessary calories for energy. Ketone bodies, metabolic by-products, reduce plasma bicarbonate, and acidosis occurs.

Fluid and Electrolyte Disturbances

Dehydration
Dehydration results from excessive fluid and electrolyte losses. Cellular fluid deficit occurs when water is drawn from the cells by the hyperosmolality of the blood. Extracellular deficit occurs when (1) glycosuria increases the urinary output, (2) ketone bodies increase the load on the kidneys and the water to excrete them, (3) vomiting causes loss of fluid and electrolytes, (4) oral intake is reduced because of the patient's condition, and (5) hyperventilation is induced by the acidotic state.

Decreased Kidney Function

Dehydration lowers the blood volume, decreasing renal blood flow, and the kidneys produce less of the ammonia needed to maintain acid–base balance. Severe dehydration may lower the blood volume enough to cause circulatory shock and oliguria.

Ketosis

Ketosis is the excessive production of ketone bodies in the bloodstream. Ketone bodies are the end products of oxidation of fatty acids. Ketosis occurs when a lack of insulin results in excessive fatty acids being converted by the liver to ketones and the decreased utilization of ketones by the peripheral tissues. Electrolytes and ketone bodies, retained in high serum concentration, increase the acidosis; the increase in the number of hydrogen ions, from the retention of ketone bodies, may drop the blood pH to 7.25 and lower. The bicarbonate anions decrease to compensate for the increase in ketone anions and may drop the bicarbonate level to 12 mEq/L or less.[3]

Hyperglycemic Hyperosmolar Nonketotic Coma

Hyperglycemic hyperosmolar nonketotic (HHNK) coma is a syndrome that may develop in the middle-aged or elderly type II diabetic patient. This condition is often associated with the stress of cardiovascular disease, infection, or pharmacologic treatment with steroids or diuretics. It is also precipitated by too-rapid infusion of parenteral nutrition solution. Blood sugars may reach 4000 mg/dL but without the ketosis of diabetic ketoacidosis.[2] Fluid volume deficit is profound and may lead to death. Underlying factors contributing to development of diabetic ketoacidosis or HHNK coma are found in Table 18-4.

Signs and Symptoms of Diabetic Acidosis

The nurse should be familiar with the signs and symptoms that characterize diabetic acidosis. By recognizing impending diabetic acidosis, early treatment may be initiated and complications prevented.

1. *Hyperglycemia* occurs when a lack of insulin prevents glucose metabolism; glucose accumulates in the bloodstream.
2. *Glycosuria* occurs when the accumulation of glucose exceeds the renal tolerance and spills over into the urine.
3. *Polyuria*. Osmotic diuresis occurs when the heavy load of nonmetabolized glucose and the metabolic end products increase the osmolality of the blood, and the increased renal solute load requires more fluid for excretion.
4. *Thirst* is prompted by cellular dehydration arising from the osmotic effect produced by hyperglycemia.
5. *Weakness* and *tiredness* come from the inability of the body to use glucose and from a potassium deficit.
6. *Flushed face* results from the acid condition.
7. *Rapid deep breathing* is the body's defense against acidosis; expiration of large amounts of carbon dioxide reduces carbonic acid and increases the pH of the blood.
8. *Acetone breath* results from an increased accumulation of acetone bodies.

TABLE 18-4
Factors Contributing to Development of DKA* or HHNC* in Susceptible Persons

DKA	HHNC
Infections, illness	Chronic renal disease
Physiologic stresses (*eg*, trauma, surgery, myocardial infarction, dehydration, pregnancy)	Chronic cardiovascular disease
	Acute illness, infection
Psychological/emotional stress	Surgery, burns, trauma
	Hyperalimentation, tube feedings
Omission/reduction of insulin	Peritoneal dialysis
Failure of insulin delivery system (pump)	Mannitol therapy
	Pharmacologic agents
Excess alcohol intake	Chlorpromazine
	Cimetidine
	Diazoxide
	Diuretics (thiazide, thiazide-related, and loop diuretics)
	Glucocorticoids and immunosuppressive agents
	L-asparaginase
	Phenytoin
	Propanolol

* DKA = diabetic ketoacidosis; HHNK = hyperglycemic hyperosmolar nonketotic coma

(*From Metheny, N. M. [1992]. Fluid and electrolyte balance [2nd ed., p. 290] Philadelphia: J. B. Lippincott*)

9. *Nausea* and *vomiting* are caused by distention from atony of gastric muscles.

10. *Weight loss* accompanies an excess loss of fluid (1 L body water equals 2.2 lb, or 1 kg, body weight) and a lack of glucose metabolism.

11. *Low blood pressure* results from a severe fluid deficit.

12. *Oliguria* follows the decreased renal blood flow that results from a severe deficit in fluid volume.

Parenteral Therapy

Insulin is given to metabolize the excess glucose and combat diabetic acidosis. Because absorption is quickest by the bloodstream, insulin is administered IV. When given subcutaneously or intramuscularly, the slower rate of absorption of insulin may be further decreased by peripheral vascular collapse in the presence of shock. The dose of insulin, when administered by continuous infusion, is usually 4 to 8 U/hr.[3] Many types of infusion pumps are available to ensure accurate and continuous administration of medications.

Parenteral fluids are administered to increase the blood volume and restore kidney function. Early treatment of the hypotonic patient usually consists of the administration of sodium chloride (0.9% NaCl) to replace sodium and chloride losses and to expand the blood volume. Later, hypotonic fluids with sodium chloride may be used. Bicarbonate replacement may be necessary when severe acidosis is present.

Potassium administration is contraindicated in the early treatment of diabetic acidosis. During the later stages (10–24 hours after treatment), the plasma potassium level falls; improved renal function increases potassium excretion and, in anabolic states, as the glucose is converted into glycogen, a sudden shift of potassium from extracellular fluid to intracellular fluid further lowers the plasma potassium level. If the patient is hydrated, potassium should be administered when the plasma potassium concentration falls.

A severe potassium deficit may occur if symptoms are not recognized and early treatment begun. Symptoms include weak grip, irregular pulse, weak picking at the bedclothes, shallow respiration, and abdominal distention.

REFERENCES

1. Burgess, R. E. (1965). Fluid and electrolytes. *American Journal of Nursing*, 65, 90.
2. Metheny, N. M. (1992). *Fluid and electrolyte balance* (2nd ed., pp. 10, 56–58, 182, 223, 308, 311, 289–316). Philadelphia: J. B. Lippincott.
3. Metheny, N. M., & Snively, W. D., Jr. (1985). *Nurses' handbook of fluid balance* (4th ed., pp. 18, 19, 91, 147–154, 161, 185–192, 293–297). Philadelphia: J. B. Lippincott.
4. Dunagan, W., Ridner, M. (1989). *Manual of medical therapeutics* (26th ed.) Boston: Little, Brown and Co.

REVIEW QUESTIONS

1. Objectives of infusion therapy include which of the following?
   a. maintain daily requirements
   b. restore previous losses
   c. replace present losses
   d. restore future losses

2. Balanced solutions are used for:
   a. restoration of volume
   b. maintenance
   c. future losses
   d. fluid balance

3. Water-soluble vitamins not retained by the body include which of the following?
   a. vitamin C
   b. vitamin E
   c. B complex vitamins
   d. Vitamin B$_6$

4. Which electrolyte is considered potentially dangerous if administered to the patient with impaired renal function?
   a. sodium
   b. potassium
   c. phosphate
   d. calcium

5. One liter of body water equals how much body weight?
   a. 1 kg
   b. 2 kg
   c. 3 kg
   d. 4 kg

6. Blood volume is maintained by which of the following hormones?
   a. aldosterone
   b. cortisone
   c. hydrocortisone
   d. norepinephrine

7. Immediately following severe burns, what fluid shift occurs?
   a. interstitial to intravascular
   b. intravascular to interstitial
   c. plasma to tissues
   d. tissues to plasma

8. Rapid administration of 20% or 50% glucose promotes:
   a. diuresis
   b. dehydration
   c. hydration
   d. emesis

9. Decreased kidney function in diabetic acidosis is caused by:
   a. decreased renal blood flow caused by low blood pressure
   b. increased renal blood flow caused by low blood pressure
   c. increased renal blood flow caused by high blood pressure
   d. decreased renal blood flow caused by high blood pressure

10. What fluid shift occurs on the second to third day following a burn?
    a. interstitial to intravascular
    b. intravascular to interstitial
    c. plasma to tissue
    d. tissue to plasma

CHAPTER 19

Principles of Parenteral Fluid Administration

PARENTERAL FLUIDS

A knowledge of parenteral fluids is essential if the patient is to be protected from the rapid and critical changes in fluid and electrolyte balance caused by infusions.

Until the 1930s, IV fluids consisted of dextrose and saline; little was known about electrolyte therapy. Today, with more than 200 types of commercially prepared fluids available and with the great increase in their use, fluid and electrolyte disturbances are more common. With the increased administration of fluids in alternative care settings, nurses must know the chemical composition and the physical effects of the infusions they administer.

Nurses have a legal and professional responsibility to know the normal amount and both the desired and untoward effects of any IV infusion they administer. The type of fluid, the amount, and the rate of flow are determined only after the physician has carefully assessed the patient's clinical condition. Attention to detail and a comprehensive assessment of a patient's fluid and electrolyte status will ensure positive IV patient outcomes.

Definition of Intravenous Infusion

Today, methods of infusion have changed dramatically, and small-volume parenterals may be administered as a secondary infusate or in a volume-controlled reservoir for electronic drug delivery.

An infusion is usually regarded as an amount of fluid in excess of 100 mL designated for parenteral infusion, because the volume must be administered over a long period of time. However, when medications are administered by "piggyback" small volume parenterals (SVP) (50–100 mL), a shorter period (usually 30 minutes to 1 hour) may be required, whereas 150- to 200-mL volumes may require more than an hour.

Intravenous fluids are mistakenly referred to as *IV solutions*. The term *solution* is defined in the United States Pharmacopeia (USP) as liquid preparations that contain one or more soluble chemical substances usually dissolved in water. They are distinguished from injection, for example, because they are not intended for administration by infusion or injection.[11] They may vary widely in methods of preparation. The USP refers to

Sharon M. Weinstein: PLUMER'S PRINCIPLES & PRACTICE OF INTRAVENOUS THERAPY, FIFTH EDITION, © 1993 J. B. Lippincott Company

parenteral fluids as injections, and methods of preparation must follow standards for injection.

Official Requirements of Intravenous Fluids

Intravenous injections must meet the tests, standards, and all specifications of the USP applicable to injections. This includes quantitative and qualitative assays of infusions, including tests for pyrogens and sterility.

Particulate Matter

Each container must be carefully examined to detect cracks and the fluid examined for cloudiness or presence of particles. The final responsibility falls on the pharmacist and the nurse who administers the fluid. Tests to detect the presence of particulate matter and standards for an acceptable limit of particles have been established by the USP. A large-volume injection for single-dose infusion meets the requirements of the test if it contains not more than 50 particles per ml that are equal to or larger than 10.0 μm and not more than 5 particles per ml that are equal to or larger than 25.0 μm in effective linear dimension.[10]

pH

The pH indicates hydrogen ion concentration or free acid activity in solution.[7] All IV fluids must meet the pH requirements set forth by the USP. Most of these requirements call for a solution that is slightly acid, usually ranging in pH from 3.5 to 6.2.

Dextrose requires a slightly acid pH to yield a stable solution. Heat sterilization, used for all commercial solutions, contributes to the acidity.

It is important to know the pH of the commonly used IV fluids because it may affect the stability of an added drug and cause the drug to deteriorate. The acidity of dextrose solutions has been criticized for its corrosive effect on veins.

Tonicity

Parenteral fluids are classified according to the tonicity of the fluid in relation to the normal blood plasma. The osmolality of blood plasma is 290 mOsm/L. Fluid that approximates 290 mOsm/L is considered isotonic. Intravenous fluids with an osmolality significantly higher than 290 mOsm (+ 50 mOsm) are considered hypertonic, whereas those with an osmolality significantly lower than 290 mOsm (− 50 mOsm) are hypotonic.[2] Parenteral fluids generally range from approximately one-half isotonic (0.45% sodium chloride) to five to ten times isotonic (25% to 50% dextrose).

The tonicity of the fluid when infused into the circulation has a direct physical effect on the patient. It affects fluid and electrolyte metabolism and may result in disastrous clinical disturbances. Hypertonic fluids increase the osmotic pressure of the blood plasma, drawing fluid from the cells; excessive infusions of such fluid can cause cellular dehydration. Hypotonic fluids lower the osmotic pressure, causing fluid to invade the cells; when such fluid is infused beyond the patient's tolerance for water, water intoxication results. Isotonic fluids cause increased extracellular fluid volume, which can result in circulatory overload. By knowing the osmolality of the infusion and the physical effect it produces, the nurse is alerted to the potential fluid and electrolyte imbalances.

The choice of veins used for an infusion is affected by the tonicity of the fluid; hyperosmolar fluids must be infused through veins with a large blood volume to dilute the fluid and prevent trauma to the vessel.

The tonicity of the fluid affects the rate at which it can be infused; hypertonic dextrose infused rapidly may result in diuresis and dehydration.

Because of the direct and effective role osmolality plays in IV therapy, it is helpful for the nurse involved in the administration of IV fluids to be familiar with the terminology and subsequent calculations.

The osmotic pressure is proportional to the total number of particles in the fluid. The milliosmole is the unit that measures the particles or the osmotic pressure. By converting milliequivalents to milliosmoles, an approximate osmolality may be determined. A quick method for approximating the tonicity of IV injections follows.[13]

Fluids Containing Univalent Electrolytes

Each milliequivalent is approximately equal to a milliosmole because univalent electrolytes, when ionized, carry one charge per particle. Normal saline injection (0.9% sodium chloride) contains 154 mEq sodium and 154 mEq chloride per liter, making a total of 308 mEq/L, or approximately 308 mOsm/L.

Fluids Containing Divalent Electrolytes

Because each particle carries two charges when ionized, the milliequivalents per liter or the number of electrical charges per liter when divided by the charge per ion (2) will give the approximate number of particles or milliosmoles per liter. As an example, when 20 mEq magnesium sulfate is introduced into a liter of fluid, each particle ionized will carry two charges. By dividing 20 mEq or 20 charges by 2, an approximate 10 particles or 10 mOsm/L is reached for each component, or 20 mOsm/L total.

The osmolality of electrolytes in solution may be accurately computed but involves the use of the atomic weight and the concentration of the given electrolytes in milligrams per liter. The methods for accurately computing the osmolality of an electrolyte in solution and a whole electrolyte in solution follow.[10]

Osmolality of a Given Electrolyte in Solution

Formula: $\dfrac{\text{milligrams of electrolyte/L}}{(\text{atomic weight})(\text{valence})} = \text{milliosmoles/L}$

Example: 39 mg K/L

$$\frac{39}{39 \times 1} = 1 \text{ mOsm/L}$$

Example: 40 mg Ca/L

$$\frac{40}{40 \times 2} = \tfrac{1}{2} \text{ mOsm/L}$$

Osmolality of a Whole Electrolyte in Solution

The milliosmolar value of the whole electrolyte in solution is equal to the sum of the milliosmolar values of the separate ions. For example, determine the number of milliosmoles in 1 L of a 0.9% sodium chloride (NaCl) solution.

Formula (atomic) weight of NaCl = 58.5 g (58,500 mg)

1 millimole NaCl $\frac{1}{1000}$ formula weight = 58.5 mg

Assuming complete dissociation:

1 millimole NaCl = 2 m Osm of total particles *or*

each 58.5 mg of the whole electrolyte (NaCl) = 2 mOsm of total particles

To calculate the osmotic activity (expressed as milliosmoles) for 9000 mg (0.9% NaCl), use the following proportion:

$$\frac{58.5 \text{ mg (weight of 1 mOsm of whole electrolytes)}}{9000 \text{ mg (weight of whole electrolyte/L)}}$$

$$= \frac{2 \text{ mOsm (number of particles from whole electrolyte)}}{X \text{ (mOsm)}}$$

X = 307.7 mOsm

DEXTROSE IN WATER FLUIDS

When glucose occurs as a part of parenteral injections, it is usually referred to as *dextrose*, a designation by USP for glucose of requisite purity. Dextrose is available in concentrations of 2.5%, 5%, 10%, 20%, and 50% in water. To determine the osmolality or the caloric value of a dextrose solution, it is necessary to know the total number of grams or milligrams per liter. Because 1 mL water weighs 1 g, and 1 mL is 1% of 100 mL, milliliters, grams, and percentages can be used interchangeably when calculating solution strength. Thus, 5% dextrose in water equals 5 g dextrose in 100 mL equals 50 g dextrose in 1 L.

Calories

Hexoses (glucose or dextrose and fructose) do not yield 4 calories[15] per gram as do dietary carbohydrates (*eg*, starches). Each gram of hydrous or anhydrous dextrose provides approximately 3.4 or 3.85 calories, respectively. One liter of 5% glucose solution yields 170 calories; one liter of 10% glucose yields 340 calories[1] (See page 360).

Tonicity of 5% Dextrose in Water

Dextrose 5% in water is considered an isotonic solution because its tonicity approximates that of normal blood plasma, 290 mOsm/L. Because dextrose is a nonelectrolyte and the total number of particles in solution does not depend on ionization, the osmolality of dextrose solutions is determined differently from that of electrolyte solutions. One millimole (one formula weight in milligrams) of dextrose represents 1 mOsm (unit of osmotic pressure). One millimole of monohydrated glucose is 198 mg, and 1 L of 5% dextrose in water contains 50,000 mg. Thus:

$$\frac{50,000 \text{ mg}}{198 \text{ mg}} = 252 \text{ mOsm/L}$$

pH

The USP requirement for pH of dextrose solutions is 3.5 to 6.5. This broad pH range may at times contribute to an incompatibility in one bottle of dextrose and not in another when an additive is involved (see Chapter 22).

Metabolic Effects of Dextrose[12]

1. Dextrose provides calories for essential energy.

2. Because glucose is converted into glycogen by synthesis in the liver, it improves hepatic function.

3. It spares body protein (prevents unnecessary breakdown of protein tissue).

4. It prevents ketosis or excretion of organic acid, which frequently occurs when fat is burned by the body without an adequate supply of glucose.

5. When deposited intracellularly in the liver as glycogen, dextrose causes a shift of potassium from the extracellular to the intracellular fluid compartment. This effect is used in the treatment of hyperkalemia by infusing dextrose and insulin.

Indications for Use

Dehydration
Dextrose 2.5% in water and dextrose 5% in water provide immediate hydration to the dehydrated patient and often are used for hydrating the medical and surgical patient. Dextrose 5% in water is considered isotonic only in the bottle; once infused into the vascular system, the dextrose is rapidly metabolized, leaving the water. The water decreases the osmotic pressure of the blood plasma and invades the cells, providing immediately available water to dehydrated tissues.

Hypernatremia
If the patient is not in circulatory difficulty with extracellular expansion, 5% dextrose may be administered to decrease the concentration of sodium.

Vehicle for Administration of Drugs
Many of the drugs for IV use are added to infusions of 5% dextrose in water.

Nutrition
Concentrations of 20% and 50% dextrose in conjunction with electrolytes provide long-term nutrition. Insulin is frequently added to prevent overtaxing of the islet tissue of the pancreas.

Hyperkalemia
Infusions of dextrose in high concentration with insulin cause anabolism (buildup of body cells), which results in a shift of potassium from the extracellular to the intracellular compartment, thereby lowering the serum potassium concentration.

Dangers

Hypokalemia
Because the kidneys do not store potassium, prolonged fluid therapy with electrolyte-free fluids may result in hypokalemia. When cells are anabolized by the metabolism of glucose, a shift of potassium from extracellular to intracellular fluid may occur, resulting in hypokalemia.

Dehydration
Osmotic diuresis occurs when dextrose is infused at a rate faster than the patient's ability to metabolize it. A heavy load of nonmetabolized glucose increases the osmolality of the blood and acts as a diuretic; the increased solute load requires more fluid for excretion. A normal, healthy individual with a urinary specific gravity of 1.029 to 1.032 requires 15 mL water to excrete 1 g solute, whereas individuals with poor kidney function or low concentrating ability of the kidneys require much more water to excrete the same amount of solute.[8]

Hyperinsulinism
This condition may occur from a rapid infusion of hypertonic carbohydrate solutes. In response to a rise in blood sugar, extra insulin pours from the beta islet cells of the pancreas in its attempt to metabolize the infused carbohydrate. Termination of the infusion may leave excess insulin in the body, resulting in symptoms such as nervousness, sweating, and weakness caused by the severe hypoglycemia that may be induced. Frequently, after infusion of hypertonic dextrose, a small amount of isotonic dextrose is administered to cover the excess insulin.[8]

Water Intoxication
This imbalance results from an increase in the volume of the extracellular fluid from water alone. Prolonged infusions of isotonic or hypotonic dextrose in water may cause water intoxication. This condition is compounded by stress, which leads to inappropriate release of antidiuretic hormone (ADH) and fluid retention. The average adult can metabolize water at a rate of about 35 to 40 mL/kg per day, and the kidney can safely metabolize only about 2500 to 3000 mL/day in an average patient receiving IV therapy.[6] Under stress, the patient's ability to metabolize water is decreased.

Administration

Isotonic dextrose may be administered through a peripheral vein. Hyperosmolar fluids such as 50% dextrose in water should be infused into the superior vena cava through central venous access. Hypertonic dextrose administered through a peripheral vein with small blood volume may traumatize the vein and cause thrombophlebitis; infiltration can result in necrosis of the tissues.

Sodium-free dextrose injections should not be administered by hyperdomoclysis. Dextrose solutions, by attracting body electrolytes in the pooled area of infusions, may cause peripheral circulatory collapse and anuria in sodium-depleted patients.

Electrolyte-free dextrose injections should not be used in conjunction with blood infusions. Dextrose mixed with blood causes hemolysis of the red blood cells.

The amount of water required for hydration depends on the condition and the needs of the patient. The average adult patient requires 1500 to 2500 mL water each day. In patients with prolonged fever, the water requirement depends on the degree of temperature elevation. The 24-hour fluid requirement for a temperature between 101°F and 103°F increases by at least 500 mL; the requirement for a prolonged temperature above 103°F increases by at least 1000 mL.[4]

The rate of administration depends on the patient's condition and the purpose of therapy. When the infusion is used to supply calories, the rate must be slow enough to allow complete metabolism of the glucose (0.5 g/kg per hour in normal adults). The maximum rate should generally not exceed 0.8 g/kg per hour.[1] When the infusion is used to produce diuresis, the rate must be fast enough to prevent complete metabolism of the dextrose, thereby increasing the osmolality of the extracellular fluid.

ISOTONIC SODIUM CHLORIDE INFUSIONS

Sodium Chloride Injection (0.9%), USP (normal saline), contains 308 mOsm/L (sodium, 154 mEq/L; chloride, 154 mEq/L); has a pH between 4.5 and 7.0; and is usually supplied in volumes of 1000, 500, 250, and 100 mL. The term *normal* or *physiologic* is misleading because the chloride in normal saline is 154 mEq/L, compared to the normal plasma chloride value of 103 mEq/L, while the sodium is 154 mEq/L, or about 9% higher than the normal plasma value of 140 mEq/L. Because the other electrolytes present in plasma are lacking in normal saline, the isotonicity of the solution depends on the sodium and chloride ions, resulting in a higher concentration of these ions.[1]

Indications for Use

1. Extracellular fluid replacement when chloride loss has been relatively greater than or equal to sodium loss.

2. Treatment of metabolic alkalosis in the presence of fluid loss; the increase in chloride ions provided by the infusion causes a compensatory decrease in the number of bicarbonate ions.

3. Sodium depletion. When there is an extracellular fluid volume deficit accompanying the sodium deficit, an isotonic solution of sodium chloride is used to correct the deficit.[8]

4. Initiation and termination of blood transfusions. When 0.9% sodium chloride is used to precede a blood transfusion, the hemolysis of red blood cells, which occurs with dextrose in water, is avoided.

Dangers

0.9% Sodium chloride provides more sodium and chloride than the patient needs. Marked electrolyte imbalances have resulted from the almost exclusive use of normal saline. Untoward effects include the following:

Hypernatremia
An adult's dietary requirement for sodium is about 90 to 250 mEq/day, with a minimum requirement of 15 mEq and a maximum tolerance of 400 mEq.[3] When 3 L 0.9% sodium chloride or 5% dextrose in 0.9% sodium chloride is administered, the patient receives 462 mEq sodium (154 mEq/L × 3), a level that exceeds normal tolerance. Such an infusion at a time when sodium retention is occurring, as during stress, can result in hypernatremia.

The danger of hypernatremia is increased in the elderly, in patients with severe dehydration, and in patients with chronic glomerulonephritis; these patients require more water to excrete the salt than do patients with normal renal function. Isotonic saline does not provide water but requires most of its volume for the excretion of salt.

Acidosis

One liter of 0.9% sodium chloride contains one third more chloride than is present in the extracellular fluid. When infused in large quantities, the excess chloride ions cause a loss of bicarbonate ions and result in acidosis.

Hypokalemia

Infusion of saline increases potassium excretion and at the same time expands the volume of extracellular fluid, further decreasing the concentration of the extracellular potassium ion.

Circulatory Overload

Continuous infusions of isotonic fluids expand the extracellular compartment and lead to circulatory overload.

Requirements

In an average adult, the daily requirements of sodium chloride are met by infusing 1 L of 0.9% sodium chloride or 1–2 L of 4.5% sodium chloride, but the dosage depends on the patient's age, weight, clinical condition, and fluid and electrolyte and acid–base balance.[1]

ISOTONIC SALINE WITH DEXTROSE

Dextrose 5% in 0.9% Sodium Chloride

Dextrose 5% in 0.9% sodium chloride contains 252 mOsm dextrose (chloride, 154 mEq/L; sodium, 154 mEq/L); has a pH of 3.5 to 6.0; and is available in volumes of 1000, 500, 250, and 150 mL.

When normal saline is infused, the addition of 100 g dextrose prevents both the formation of ketone bodies and the increased demand for water the ketone bodies impose for renal excretion. The dextrose prevents catabolism and, consequently, loss of potassium and intracellular water.

Indications for Use
1. Temporary treatment of circulatory insufficiency and shock caused by hypovolemia in the immediate absence of a plasma expander.
2. Early treatment along with plasma or albumin for replacement of loss caused by burn.
3. Early treatment of acute adrenocortical insufficiency.

Dangers

The hazards are the same as those for normal saline (see preceding section).

Dextrose 10% in 0.9% Sodium Chloride

Dextrose 10% in 0.9% sodium chloride contains 504 mOsm/L dextrose (sodium, 154 mEq/L; chloride, 154 mEq/L), has a pH of 3.5 to 6.0, and is usually supplied in volumes of 1000 and 500 mL.

Indications for Use
This fluid is used as a nutrient and an electrolyte (sodium and chloride) replenisher.

Dangers
Hypernatremia, acidosis, and circulatory overload may result when normal saline is administered in excess of the patient's tolerance.

Administration
Dextrose 10% in 0.9% sodium chloride, because of its hypertonicity, must be administered IV, preferably through a vein of large diameter to dilute the fluid and reduce the risk of trauma to the vessel. Close observation and precautions are necessary to prevent infiltration and damage to the tissues.

HYPERTONIC SODIUM CHLORIDE INFUSIONS

These infusions include 3% sodium chloride (sodium, 513 mEq/L; chloride, 513 mEq/L) and 5% sodium chloride (sodium, 850 mEq/L; chloride, 850 mEq/L).

Indications for Use

Severe Dilutional Hyponatremia (Water Intoxication)
Hypertonic sodium chloride, on infusion, increases the osmotic pressure of the extracellular fluid, drawing water from the cells for excretion by the kidneys.

Severe Sodium Depletion
Infusions of hypertonic saline replenish sodium stores. An estimate of the sodium deficit can be made by taking the difference between the normal sodium concentration and the patient's current sodium concentration and multiplying it by 60% of the body weight in kilograms; sodium depletion is based on total body water and not on extracellular fluid.[9]

Administration

Hypertonic sodium chloride injection must be administered with great caution to prevent pulmonary edema. Frequent reevaluation of the clinical and electrolyte picture during administration is advised. A 3% or 5% solution of sodium chloride is used to correct the deficit if the fluid volume is normal or excessive; the amount of sodium administered depends on the sodium deficit in the plasma.[8]

Hypertonic saline solutions should be infused slowly (such as 200 mL over a minimum of 4 hours),[8] and the patient should be observed constantly. The fluid must be infused by vein, with great care to prevent infiltration and trauma to the tissues. Table 19-1 summarizes the important nursing considerations in the administration of hypertonic saline.

HYPOTONIC SODIUM CHLORIDE IN WATER

One-half hypotonic saline (0.45% saline containing sodium, 77 mEq/L, and chloride, 77 mEq/L) is used as an electrolyte replenisher. When there is a question regarding the amount of saline required, hypotonic saline is preferred over isotonic saline. In general, 0.45% sodium chloride is preferable to 0.9% sodium chloride.

TABLE 19-1
Summary of Important Nursing Considerations in Administration of Hypertonic Saline Solutions (3% and 5% NaCl)

1. Check the serum sodium level before administering these solutions and frequently thereafter.

2. Be aware that these solutions are dangerous and should be used only in critical situations in which the serum sodium is very low (such as less than 110 mEq/L) and neurologic symptoms are present.

3. Administer these solutions only in intensive care settings where the patient can be closely monitored. Watch for signs of pulmonary edema and worsening of neurologic signs. Use with great caution in patients with congestive heart failure or renal failure.

4. Be aware that only small volumes are needed (such as 5 mL or 6 mL/kg body weight of 5% NaCl) to elevate the serum sodium level by 10 mEq/L. For example, elevating the serum sodium level of a 70-kg patient from 110 to 120 mEq/L would require approximately 350 to 420 mL.

5. The serum sodium should not be raised more rapidly than 2 mEq/L/hr unless the clinical state of the patient indicates the need for more rapid treatment.

6. Use an electronic infusion device to administer the fluid; maintain close vigilance on the device as none is foolproof.

7. Be aware that the aim of therapy is not to elevate the serum sodium level to normal quickly; rather, it is to elevate it only enough to alleviate neurologic signs. It has been recommended that the serum concentration be raised no higher than 125 mEq/L with hypertonic saline.

8. Be aware that the physician may prescribe furosemide to promote water loss and prevent pulmonary edema. Urine should be saved as renal sodium and potassium losses may need to be measured to allow for replacement.

(From Metheny, N. M. [1992]. *Fluid and electrolyte balance* [2nd ed., p. 64]. Philadelphia: J. B. Lippincott.)

HYDRATING FLUIDS

Because solutions consisting of dextrose with hypotonic saline provide more water than is required for excretion of salt, they are useful as hydrating fluids. These solutions include 2.5% dextrose in 0.45% saline (dextrose, 126 mOsm/L, with sodium, 77 mEq/L, and chloride, 77 mEq/L), 5% dextrose in 0.45% saline (dextrose, 252 mOsm/L, with sodium, 77 mEq/L, and chloride, 77 mEq/L), and 5% dextrose in 0.2% saline (dextrose, 252 mOsm/L, with sodium, 34.2 mEq/L, and chloride, 34.2 mEq/L).

Indications for Use

1. Commonly called *initial hydrating solutions*, hypotonic saline dextrose infusions are used to assess the status of the kidneys before electrolyte replacement and maintenance are initiated.

2. Hydration of medical and surgical patients.

3. Promotion of diuresis in dehydrated patients.

Administration

To assess the status of the kidneys, the fluid is administered at the rate of 8 mL/m^2 body surface per minute for 45 minutes. The restoration of urinary flow shows that the kidneys have begun to function; the hydrating fluid may be replaced by more specifically needed electrolytes. If after 45 minutes the urinary flow is not restored, the rate of infusion is reduced to 2 mL/m^2 body surface per minute for another hour. If this does not produce diuresis, renal impairment is assumed.[8]

Initial hydrating fluids must be used cautiously in edematous patients with cardiac, renal, or hepatic disease. Once good renal function is obtained, appropriate electrolytes should be administered to prevent hypokalemia.

HYPOTONIC MULTIPLE-ELECTROLYTE FLUIDS

Hypotonic multiple-electrolyte fluids are patterned after the type devised by Butler. Butler, with his coworkers at the Massachusetts General Hospital, was the first to emphasize that basic water and electrolyte requirements are proportionate to the body surface area. Butler-type fluids are one third to one half as concentrated as plasma. They provide fluid to meet the patient's fluid volume requirement and in so doing provide cellular and extracellular electrolytes in quantities balanced between the minimal needs and the maximal tolerance of the patient. These fluids, because of their hypotonicity, provide water for urinary and metabolic needs and take advantage of the body's homeostatic mechanisms to retain the electrolytes and reject those not needed, thus maintaining water and electrolyte balance.[8]

Hypotonic fluids should contain 5% dextrose for its protein-sparing and anti-ketogenic effect.[5] The dextrose will increase the tonicity of the fluid in the container, but once infused the dextrose will be metabolized, leaving the water and salt. Whether the patient has received too much or too little water depends on the tonicity of the electrolyte and not the osmotic effect of dextrose.

A balanced solution of hypotonic electrolytes is ideal for routine maintenance. There are several modifications of the Butler-type fluids. Those containing 75 mEq total cation per liter are used for older infants, children, and adults.

Administration

A useful formula for maintenance water requirements, based on studies by Crawford, Butler, and Talbot, is: maintenance water equals 1600 mL/m^2 body surface area per day.[5] For obese or edematous patients, this should be calculated on ideal weight rather than actual weight. The water requirement must be patterned after the condition of the patient. When infection, trauma involving the brain, or stress lead to inappropriate release of ADH, maintenance requirements are less. Excessive fluid losses through urine, stool, expired air, and so forth require increased water. The rate of infusion is usually 3 mL/m^2 body surface per minute.

Dangers

Hyperkalemia
When renal function is impaired, IV potassium should be used cautiously. The nurse should be alert to signs of hyperkalemia. If such signs develop, the physician should be notified and the fluid replaced by more appropriate electrolytes.

Water Intoxication
The patient's tolerance limits for water can be exceeded. Care should be exercised in maintaining the prescribed flow rate and in ensuring that the patient receives the

prescribed volume of fluid. Water intoxication is more likely to occur when inappropriate release of ADH, in response to stress, causes water retention. These patients should be carefully watched to detect any early signs of an imbalance, so that a change in therapy can be initiated before the condition becomes precarious. Weighing the patient is the best way to monitor the status of water balance. Daily weights are extremely important in following the state of hydration in very ill patients.

ISOTONIC MULTIPLE-ELECTROLYTE FLUIDS

Many types of commercial replacement fluids are available. When severe vomiting, diarrhea, or diuresis result in a heavy loss of water and electrolytes, replacement therapy is necessary. Balanced fluids of isotonic electrolytes having an ionic composition similar to plasma are used.

Administration

Rapid initial replacement is seldom necessary. However, if impaired circulation and renal function of a severely dehydrated patient become evident and it is necessary to restore the patient's blood pressure quickly, 30 mL/kg of an isotonic fluid may be provided in the first hour or two.[5] Fluid overload must be prevented. Central venous pressure monitoring is especially helpful in the elderly patient and in patients with renal or cardiovascular disorders.

Extracellular replacement can generally be assumed to be complete after 48 hours of replacement therapy unless proved otherwise by clinical or laboratory evidence. To continue replacement fluids after deficits have been corrected may result in sodium excess leading to pulmonary edema or heart failure.[5] Patients receiving replacement therapy should be observed closely to detect any signs of circulatory overload.

Gastric replacement fluids provide the usual electrolytes lost by vomiting or gastric suction. They contain ammonium ions, which are metabolized in the liver to hydrogen ions and urea, replacing the hydrogen ion lost in gastric juices. They are useful in metabolic alkalosis caused by excessive ingestion of sodium bicarbonate. The usual adult dose is 500 to 2000 mL, and the rate should be consistent with the patient's clinical condition but not exceed 500 mL/hr.

Gastric replacement fluids are contraindicated in the presence of hepatic insufficiency or renal failure. They require the same precautions as any fluid containing potassium and should be avoided in patients with renal damage or Addison's disease. Also, the low pH causes incompatibilities with many additives.

Lactated Ringer's injection is considered safe in certain conditions. Because the electrolyte concentration closely resembles that of the extracellular fluid, it may be used to replace fluid loss from burns and fluid lost as bile and diarrhea. Lactated Ringer's injection has been useful in mild acidosis, the lactate ion being metabolized in the liver to bicarbonate.

Dangers

Three liters contains about 390 mEq sodium, which can quickly elevate the sodium level in a patient who is not deficient.[3] Lactated Ringer's injection is contraindicated in severe metabolic acidosis or alkalosis and in liver disease or anoxic states that influence lactate metabolism.

ALKALIZING FLUIDS

When anesthesia or disorders such as dehydration, shock, liver disease, starvation, and diabetes cause retention of chlorides, ketone bodies, or organic salts, or when excessive bicarbonate is lost, metabolic acidosis occurs. Treatment consists of infusion with an appropriate alkalizing fluid. These fluids include one-sixth molar isotonic sodium lactate (1.9%, with sodium, 167 mEq/L, and lactate ions, 167 mEq/L, and a pH of 6.0–7.3), one-sixth molar Sodium Bicarbonate Injection, USP (1.5%, with sodium, 178 mEq/L, and bicarbonate, 178 mEq/L, and a pH of 7.0–8.0), and hypertonic sodium bicarbonate injection (7.5% or 5%).

One-Sixth Molar Sodium Lactate

The lactate ion must be oxidized in the body to carbon dioxide before it can effect acid–base balance; the complete conversion of sodium lactate to bicarbonate requires about 1 to 2 hours.[1] Because oxidation is necessary to increase the bicarbonate concentration, sodium lactate is not used for patients suffering from oxygen lack, as in shock or congenital heart disease with persistent cyanosis. It is also contraindicated in liver disease because the lactate ions are improperly metabolized.

One-sixth molar sodium lactate is used when acidosis results from a sodium deficiency in such disorders as vomiting, starvation, uncontrolled diabetes mellitus, acute infections, and renal failure.[1]

The usual dose is 1 L of a one-sixth molar solution, but the dosage depends on the patient's condition and the serum sodium level. One-sixth molar infusion may be administered by venoclysis or hyperdermoclysis and usually at a rate not greater than 300 mL/hr.[1] The patient should be observed closely for any evidence of alkalosis.

Sodium Bicarbonate

Sodium Bicarbonate Injection, USP (1.5%, with sodium, 178 mEq/L, and bicarbonate, 178 mEq/L), is an isotonic solution that provides bicarbonate ions in conditions in which excess depletion has occurred. It is used for severe hyperpnea early in the treatment of severe acidosis until the signs of dyspnea and hyperpnea are relieved. The bicarbonate ion is released in the form of carbon dioxide through the lungs, leaving an excess of sodium cation behind to exert its electrolyte effect.[1] Recommendations and practice related to pharmacologic management of cardiopulmonary resuscitation (CPR) suggest a cautious use of sodium bicarbonate to manage acidosis.[8]

The usual dose is 500 mL in a 1.5% solution. The dosage depends on the patient's weight, condition, and carbon dioxide content. If the isotonic infusion is not available, it may be made by adding two 50-mL ampules containing 3.75 g each of sodium bicarbonate to 400 mL hypotonic saline. The fluid should be infused slowly intravenously. Rapid injection may induce cellular acidity and death. The patient should be watched for signs of hypocalcemic tetany, and calcium supplement should be administered if required; calcium does not ionize well in an alkaline medium. Extravasation of hypertonic sodium bicarbonate injections must be avoided.[1] Bicarbonate therapy should cease when the pH reaches 7.2.[9]

ACIDIFYING INFUSIONS

Normal saline (0.9% Sodium Chloride Injection, USP) is not usually listed among the acidifying infusions. However, because metabolic alkalosis is a condition associated with excess bicarbonate and loss of chloride, isotonic saline provides conservative treatment. When the chloride ions are infused, the bicarbonate decreases in compensation and the alkalosis is relieved.

Ammonium chloride, the usual acidifying agent, is available as isotonic 0.9% ammonium chloride injection (ammonium, 167 mEq/L; chloride, 167 mEq/L) and hypertonic 2.14% ammonium chloride injection (ammonium, 400 mEq/L; chloride, 400 mEq/L). The pH range is 4.0 to 6.0. Both concentrations are supplied in 1-L bottles.

Indications for Use

Ammonium chloride is used as an acidifying infusion in severe metabolic alkalosis caused by loss of gastric secretions, pyloric stenosis, or other causes. The ammonium ion is converted by the liver to hydrogen ion and to ammonia, which is excreted as urea.

Administration

The 2.14% ammonium chloride is usually used in the treatment of the adult patient; 0.9% ammonium chloride is used for children.[8]

The dosage depends on the condition of the patient and on an accurate chemical picture, including plasma carbon dioxide–combining power. Ammonium chloride must be infused at a very slow rate to enable the liver to metabolize the ammonium ion, not to exceed 5 m/L minute in adults.[1] Rapid injection can result in toxic effects, causing irregular breathing, bradycardia, and twitching.[1]

Precautions

Because its acidifying effect depends on the liver for conversion, ammonium chloride must not be administered to patients with severe hepatic disease or renal failure. It is contraindicated in any condition with a high ammonium level.

Contents of selected solutions and comments are found in Table 19-2.

EVALUATION OF WATER AND ELECTROLYTE BALANCE

A rational approach is necessary if the patient is to receive safe and successful IV therapy. In the past, emphasis was placed on the technical responsibility of the nurse in maintaining the infusion and in maintaining patent venous access. With the increase in the use of IV therapy, clinical disturbances in fluid and electrolyte metabolism are more common. Changes can occur quickly and in the absence of the physician. Today the nurse's responsibility consists of monitoring the fluid and electrolyte status of the patient as well as the progress of the infusion. Greater emphasis must be placed on the causes and effects of fluid and electrolyte abnormalities so that these imbalances may be anticipated and recognized before they become disastrous. The nurse should be familiar with the parameters used in evaluating fluid and electrolyte imbalances and in supplying fluid and electrolyte requirements.

TABLE 19-2
Contents of Selected Water and Electrolyte Solutions with Comments About Their Use

Solution	Comments

5% dextrose in water (D₅W):
  No electrolytes
  50 g of dextrose
	Supplies approximately 170 cal/L and free water to aid in renal excretion of solutes
	
	Should not be used in excessive volumes in patients with increased ADH activity or to replace fluids in hypovolemic patients

0.9% NaCl (isotonic saline):
  Na^+ 154 mEq/L
  Cl^- 154 mEq/L
	Not desirable as a routine maintenance solution because it provides only Na^+ and Cl^-, which are provided in excessive amounts

0.45% NaCl (½-strength saline):
  Na^+ 77 mEq/L
  Cl^- 77 mEq/L
	A hypotonic solution that provides Na^+, Cl^-, and free water Na^+ and Cl^- provided in fluid allows kidneys to select and retain needed amounts
	
	Free water desirable as aid to kidneys in elimination of solutes

0.33% NaCl (⅓-strength saline):
  Na^+ 56 mEq/L
  Cl^- 56 mEq/L
	A hypotonic solution that provides Na^+, Cl^-, and free water
	
	Often used to treat hypernatremia (because this solution contains a small amount of Na^+, it dilutes the plasma sodium while not allowing it to drop too rapidly.)

3% NaCl:
  Na^+ 513 mEq/L
  Cl^- 513 mEq/L
	Grossly hypertonic solutions used only to treat severe hyponatremia
	
	See Table 19-1 for summary of important nursing considerations in administration

5% NaCl:
  Na^+ 855 mEq/L
  Cl^- 855 mEq/L
	Dangerous solutions

Lactated Ringer's solution:
  Na^+ 130 mEq/L
  K^+ 4 mEq/L
  Ca^{++} 3 mEq/L
  Cl^- 109 mEq/L
  Lactate (metabolized to bicarbonate)
    28 mEq/L
	A roughly isotonic solution that contains multiple electrolytes in approximately the same concentrations as found in plasma (Note that this solution is lacking in Mg and PO₄.)
	
	Used in the treatment of hypovolemia, burns, and fluid lost as bile or diarrhea
	
	Useful in treating mild metabolic acidosis

Other isotonic multiple electrolyte solutions:
  Plasma-Lyte 148 (Baxter)
  Isolyte S (McGaw)
  Normosol R (Abbott)
    Na^+ 140 mEq/L
    K^+ 5 mEq/L
    Mg^{++} 3 mEq/L
    Cl^- 98 mEq/L
    HCO_3 50 mEq/L (or equivalent)
	Isotonic solution that can be used to replace extracellular fluid loss
	
	Because of relatively high bicarbonate content, can be used to correct mild acidosis

Hypotonic multiple electrolyte solutions:
  Plasma-Lyte 56 (Baxter)
  Normosol M (Abbott)
    Na^+ 40 mEq/L
    K^+ 13 mEq/L
    Mg^{++} 3 mEq/L
    Cl^- 40 mEq/L
    HCO_3 16 mEq/L (or equivalent)
	Hypotonic solution that supplies free water as well as electrolytes

(continued)

TABLE 19-2   *(Continued)*

Solution	Comments
Sodium lactate solution, $\frac{1}{6}$ M: Na⁺ 167 mEq/L Cl⁻ 167 mEq/L	A roughly isotonic solution used to correct severe metabolic acidosis (lactate is metabolized to bicarbonate in 1–2 hr by the liver.)
	Not used in patients with liver disease (lactate cannot be converted to bicarbonate in such individuals); also, not used in patients with oxygen lack (unable to adequately convert lactate to bicarbonate)
Sodium bicarbonate, 5%: Na⁺ 595 mEq/L Cl⁻ 595 mEq/L	A very hypertonic solution used to correct severe metabolic acidosis
	Should be cautiously administered at a slow rate, under careful volume control
	Should be administered only with extreme caution to salt-retaining patients (*eg,* those with cardiac, renal, or liver damage)
Ammonium chloride, 2.14%:	Acidifying solution used to correct severe metabolic alkalosis
	Due to high ammonium content, must be administered cautiously to patients with compromised hepatic function

(From Metheny, N. M. [1992]. *Fluid and electrolyte balance* [2nd ed., p. 173]. Philadelphia: J. B. Lippincott.)

Central Venous Pressure

Central venous pressure monitoring provides a simple, accurate, and valuable guide in detecting changes in blood volume and in assessing fluid requirements. It is particularly valuable in assessing the ability of the heart to tolerate the infusion. Many erroneous conclusions are drawn from false values recorded when the line is not properly responsive to right atrial pressures.

A normal venous pressure indicates an adequate circulatory blood volume.

An elevated venous pressure may mean an increase in circulatory volume and right heart pressure, with the possibility of circulatory overload. It may also indicate other problems such as a pulmonary embolus, myocardial infarction, or lack of digitalis. Determination of the hematocrit value will supplement clinical information.[6]

A low venous pressure, too low to measure, indicates that the patient has probably lost fluid or blood. One must not overlook the fact that fluid loss can result from drug-induced vasodilation,[8] or improper administration of IV fluids. If rapid infusion of dextrose exceeds the patient's tolerance, massive diuresis with dehydration and diminished circulatory volume may occur. The decreased venous blood return into the right atrium is reflected by a decrease in the central venous pressure.

Pulse

The pulse quality and rate provide valuable clinical information for assessing fluid and electrolyte changes in the patient. A high pulse pressure, bounding and not easily obliterated by pressure, indicates a high cardiac output caused by circulatory overload. A regular pulse, easily obliterated by pressure, indicates low cardiac output resulting from a lowered blood volume. A bounding, easily obliterated pressure signifies a drop in blood pressure with a wide pulse pressure, indicative of impending circulatory collapse. As the patient's condition deteriorates, the pulse will become rapid, weak, thready, and easily obliterated, signifying circulatory collapse.

Hand Veins

Examination of the hand veins provides a means of evaluating the plasma volume. The hand veins will usually empty in 3 to 5 seconds when the hand is elevated and will fill in the same length of time when the hand is lowered to a dependent position. Peripheral vein filling takes longer than 3 to 5 seconds in patients with sodium depletion and extracellular dehydration.[8] Slow emptying of the hand veins indicates overhydration and an excessive blood volume; slow filling indicates a low blood volume and often precedes hypotension. Hand veins that become engorged and clearly visible indicate an increase in the plasma volume secondary to an interstitial-to-vascular fluid shift or an increase in extracellular fluid volume.[8]

Neck Veins

Changes in fluid volume are reflected by changes in neck vein filling, provided the patient is not in heart failure. In the supine position, the patient's external jugular veins fill to the anterior border of the sternocleidomastoid muscle. Flat neck veins in the supine position indicate a decreased plasma volume.[8]

Weight

A sudden gain or loss in weight is a significant sign of a change in the fluid volume. A change in the volume of body fluid can be computed by weighing the patient daily at the same time of day, on the same scales, with the same amount of clothing. A loss or gain of 1 kg body weight reflects a loss or gain of 1 L body fluid. A rapid 2% loss of total body weight (TBW) indicates mild fluid volume deficit (FVD), and a rapid loss of 8% or more represents severe FVD. Conversely, weight gain occurs when total fluid intake exceeds total fluid output. A rapid 2% gain of; TBW indicates mild fluid volume excess (FVE); a 5% gain represents a moderate FVE; and 8% or greater indicates a severe FVE.[8]

Thirst

Thirst is an important symptom denoting a deficit in body fluid or, more specifically, cellular dehydration. This type of dehydration occurs when the extracellular fluid becomes hypertonic, either as a result of water deprivation or the infusion of hypertonic saline. The increase in osmotic pressure causes fluid to be drawn from the cells, resulting in cellular dehydration, the stimulus to thirst.

Normally, thirst governs the need for water but, in certain conditions, the lack of thirst may accompany dehydration. This is especially true in the aged, in whom thirst is not urgent. These patients may lose their thirst and as a result become severely dehydrated before the condition is recognized.

In the severely burned patient, the great thirst experienced may lead to ingestion of excess water and to a serious sodium deficit.

Intake and Output

Water intake and output should be carefully measured and recorded. Hourly urine output measurements may be particularly important. A urine output of 200 mL/hr indicates that too much water is being infused too rapidly. By regulating the urine output between 30 and 50 ml/hr the patient receives at least enough fluid for his kidneys to work efficiently.[6]

A decreased urinary output accompanies a decreased blood volume; changes in the arterial pressure and pressure in the glomeruli result in the oliguria or anuria of profound shock. The increase in urinary output accompanying an increase in blood volume is primarily caused by changes in arterial pressure and pressure in the glomeruli.[8] Output should include urine, vomitus, diarrhea, drainage from fistulas, and drainage from suction apparatus.[8]

Skin Turgor

Observing changes in skin turgor (elasticity) and texture is helpful in assessing the state of water balance. To test skin turgor, pinch the skin over the sternum, inner aspect of the thigh, or forehead in the adult or the medial aspects of the thigh or abdomen[8] in the child, and then release it; in the normal individual, the pinched skin will return to its original position. Skin that remains in a raised position for several seconds indicates a deficit in fluid volume.

A dry, leathery tongue may indicate a fluid volume deficit or mouth breathing. To differentiate between the two, the mucous membrane may be checked for moisture by running the finger between the gums and the cheek; dryness indicates a fluid volume deficit.

Tongue Turgor

Normally, the tongue has one longitudinal furrow. In the patient with fluid volume deficit, additional longitudinal furrows are present and the tongue is smaller because of the fluid loss. Not significantly affected by age, the tongue is a good parameter to measure in all age groups.

Edema

Edema reflects an increase in the extracellular fluid volume outside the circulating intravascular compartment. It depends on an imbalance or a disturbance in the exchange of water and electrolytes between the patient and the environment or the exchange of water and electrolytes between the compartments of the body. The fluid and electrolyte exchange between the body compartments may be affected by an alteration in the circulatory system, the lymphatic system, or the concentration of albumin in the serum; water and electrolytes escape from the circulation faster than they enter, and edema ensues. Edema may be generalized, as in congestive failure, localized, as with ascites, or peripheral.

By detecting edema early, a clinical imbalance may be corrected before the patient's condition deteriorates. Early peripheral edema may be detected by fingerprinting, a procedure in which the finger is rolled over the bony prominence of the sternum or tibia. As edema increases, pitting edema will occur and may be detected by pressure of the fingers on the subcutaneous tissue.

In generalized edema, such as that seen in cardiac failure, total extracellular water volume as well as interstitial edema increase. Symptoms such as venous engorgement, restlessness, dyspnea, cyanosis, and pulmonary rales indicate generalized edema.

Laboratory Values

Laboratory values, when used to supplement clinical observations, aid in forming diagnostic and therapeutic guidelines.

Electrolyte studies (serum sodium, potassium, chloride, bicarbonate, and pH) performed daily are important in assessing the fluid and electrolyte status of the patient receiving IV fluids. In patients with massive electrolyte losses, such studies may be required two or three times a day.

Blood cell count and *hematocrit* determinations are helpful in detecting hemoconcentration or hemodilution; hemoconcentration reflects a diminished plasma volume caused by dehydration, and hemodilution, an increased volume from overtreatment with water.

Measurement of *serum protein with the albumin–globulin ratio* helps in detecting a change in fluid volume; large quantities of parenteral fluid rapidly administered dilute and decrease the serum protein concentration. This determination is helpful when used to supplement clinical observation—otherwise it may be misleading and interpreted as showing actual depletion. A decrease in serum protein reduces the osmotic pressure of the extracellular compartment, causing some edema and loss of plasma volume.

Blood urea nitrogen should be measured frequently to evaluate kidney function, an important parameter in treating fluid and electrolyte imbalances.

CLINICAL DISTURBANCES OF WATER AND ELECTROLYTE METABOLISM

Most of the common clinical disturbances in water and electrolyte balance result from changes in the volume of total body water or in one or more of the fluid compartments of the body. Clinical disturbances in water and electrolyte metabolism have been classified into six types: isotonic, hypertonic, and hypotonic expansion and isotonic, hypertonic, and hypotonic contraction. These are discussed in the following pages and are summarized in Tables 19-3 and 19-4.

Isotonic Expansion

Isotonic expansion (circulatory overload) occurs when fluids of the same tonicity as plasma are infused into the vascular circulation. Because solutions isotonic to plasma do not affect the osmolality, there is no flow of water from the extracellular compartment to the intracellular compartment. The extracellular compartment expands in proportion to the fluid infused and is the only compartment affected. The increase in the volume of fluid dilutes the concentration of hemoglobin and lowers the hematocrit and total protein levels, but the serum sodium level remains the same.

Isotonic expansion is a critical complication of IV therapy. Patients who receive isotonic fluids around the clock are prime targets and should be observed closely for early signs of circulatory overload. 0.9% Sodium chloride or solutions containing balanced isotonic multiple electrolytes are used for preexisting or continuing fluid and electrolyte losses and are not the ideal fluids for maintenance therapy. The electrolyte isotonicity of these solutions causes expansion of the extracellular compartment and does not provide the extra water that balanced hypotonic solutions provide for the kidney to retain or secrete as needed.[3]

The early postoperative or posttrauma patient is susceptible to this critical complication. The increased endocrine response to stress during the first 2 to 5 days following surgery results in retention of sodium chloride and water.[8] When a patient under stress is receiving isotonic infusions, the nurse must anticipate and watch for signs of circulatory overload.

TABLE 19-3
Comparison of Three Types of Dehydration (Contraction)

	Isotonic	Hypertonic	Hypotonic
Cause	Loss of blood or isotonic fluid	Excess loss of water or insufficient intake	Loss of salt
Effect on fluid compartments	ECF volume ↓	ICF and ECF volume ↓	ICF volume ↑ ECF volume ↓
Clinical signs Weight	↓	↓	↓
Rate of H$_2$O excretion	↓	↓	↑
Rate of Na excretion	↓	↓	↓
Thirst	—	Early sign, due to cellular dehydration	—
Pulse rate	Regular, easily obliterated by pressure	Regular and normal in early stages	Increased, weak and thready, easily obliterated by pressure
Hand vein filling time (normal = 3–5 sec)	May ↑	May be normal	Normal to ↑
Behavior	—	Irritability, restlessness, possibly confusion	Possibly vomiting and cramps
Signs in late stages	Developing shock with pulse weak and thready	Skin turgor diminished; dry, furrowed tongue; death, possibly due to rise of osmotic pressure	Skin turgor may be diminished; thready pulse; possibly confusion and apathy; death from peripheral circulatory failure
Laboratory values Hematocrit	↑	↑	↑
Hemoglobin	↑	↑	↑
Total protein and albumin-globulin ratio	↑	↑	↑
Sodium concentration	—	↑	↓

ECF, extracellular fluid; ICF, intracellular fluid

Elderly patients receiving isotonic fluids must be carefully monitored because they have a lower tolerance to fluids and electrolytes. Because they are also likely to have some degree of cardiac and renal impairment, the ability of the kidneys to eliminate fluid is likely to be diminished. The status of these patients can change quickly.

In the patient who has had a craniotomy, large-volume isotonic infusions can increase the intracranial pressure and prove detrimental.

Patients who are potential candidates for isotonic expansion must be watched carefully and turned frequently to prevent fluid from settling in the lungs. Pulmonary edema can result from the cardiac and pulmonary side effects of IV therapy. The apices of the lungs which are high will tend to be fairly dry, but the bases of their lungs, posteriorly and inferiorly, can be fairly wet.[6] As a result, hypostatic pneumonia secondary to gravity may develop.

TABLE 19-4
Comparison of Three Types of Fluid Expansion

	Isotonic	Hypertonic	Hypotonic
Cause	Infusion of excess quantities of isotonic fluids	Infusion of excess quantities of hypertonic saline	Increased intake or infusion of water in excess of patient's tolerance
Effects on fluid compartments	ECF volume ↑	ECF volume ↑ ICF volume ↓	ECF and ICF volume ↑
Clinical signs			
Weight	↑	↑ depending on amount infused	↑
Rate of H_2O excretion	↑	↓	↑
Rate of Na excretion	↑	↑	↑
Thirst	—	Present	—
Pulse rate	Bounding, not easily obliterated by pressure	Full, bounding (significant)	May be regular and not easily obliterated by pressure
Hand vein emptying time (normal = 3–5 sec)	↑	↑	↑
Edema	May be present	Early, tibial edema; later, pitting edema; diminished skin turgor	Tibial edema with finger printing
Signs of intracranial pressure	—	—	Irritability, headache, confusion
Signs in late stages	Hoarseness, pulmonary edema, cyanosis, coughing, dyspnea	Water rales, pulmonary edema	Pulmonary edema
Other signs	—	Hoarseness (a frequent early sign)	Cramping of exercised muscles
Laboratory values			
Hematocrit	↓	↓	↓
Hemoglobin	↓	↓	↓
Total protein and albumin-globulin ratio	↓	↓	↓
Sodium concentration	—	↑	↓

ECF, extracellular fluid; ICF, intracellular fluid

Manifestations
The nurse who monitors IV infusions must be familiar with the early clinical manifestations that accompany isotonic expansion in order to recognize and prevent its development; mild pulmonary edema progressing to severe pulmonary edema is a late stage that must be prevented. Early clinical manifestations consist of: (1) weight gain; (2) increase in fluid intake over output; (3) a high pulse pressure, bounding and not easily obliterated, showing signs of high cardiac output; (4) increase in central venous pressure; (5) peripheral hand vein emptying time longer than normal 3 to 5 seconds when the hand is elevated from a dependent position; (6) peripheral edema, depending on the extent of

fluid expansion; and (7) hoarseness. If IV therapy is allowed to continue, isotonic expansion becomes more apparent and dangerous, with easily recognized signs: cyanosis, dyspnea, coughing, and neck vein engorgement.

Laboratory characteristics include a drop in the hematocrit value and reduced concentrations of hemoglobin and of total protein.

Treatment

Treatment for circulatory overload when detected early is relatively simple and consists of withholding all fluids until excess water and electrolytes have been eliminated by the body. After the condition is rectified, hypotonic maintenance fluids will provide the patient with fluid and a minimum daily requirement of electrolytes. The hypotonicity of the fluid allows the kidneys to maintain the needed amount and selectively retain or excrete the excess.

Isotonic Contraction

Isotonic contraction occurs when there is loss of fluid and electrolytes isotonic to the extracellular fluid, such as whole blood or large volumes of fluid from diarrhea or vomiting. The extracellular compartment contracts. Because the fluid lost is isotonic, the osmolality of the extracellular compartment remains unchanged and no movement of water occurs between the compartments; only the extracellular volume is affected.

Manifestations

Because of the loss of fluid, the hematocrit level and the concentrations of hemoglobin and total protein are increased. The serum sodium concentration does not change.

Clinical manifestations are: (1) weight loss; (2) negative fluid balance (a decrease in urinary output but a greater output than total fluid intake); (3) pulse regular in rate, easily obliterated by pressure, and, as the patient's condition deteriorates, becomes weak and thready; and (4) possible increase in peripheral hand filling time above the normal 3 to 5 seconds when the hand is moved from an elevated to a dependent position.

Treatment

Treatment consists of replacing the fluid loss with isotonic solutions containing balanced electrolytes.

Hypertonic Expansion

Hypertonic expansion occurs when the volume of body water is increased by the IV infusion of hypertonic saline. Sodium chloride 3% or 5% is used to replace a massive sodium loss or to remove excess accumulation of body fluids, but, if it is rapidly infused, hypertonic expansion can result. The saline increases the osmotic pressure of the extracellular compartment, causing water to be drawn from the intracellular compartment until both compartments are isosmotic. There is an increase in the volume of the extracellular compartment and a decrease in the volume of the cellular compartment. The osmolality of the extracellular fluid is higher than before the infusion but lower than the high level after the infusion because of the increased extracellular fluid volume.[1]

Caution must be used in the IV administration of hypertonic saline. Circulatory overload with hypernatremia can occur. An understanding of the reason for the infusion, the condition of the patient, the proper rate of administration, and the signs and symptoms of hypertonic expansion provides a basis for sound IV practice.

Manifestations

Clinical manifestations include a gain in body weight dependent on the volume infused. A small volume (500 mL) will not contribute to a significant weight gain.[13] An increased sodium load results in a decreased rate of water excretion; however, the abrupt increase in plasma volume may cause an increase in the rate of water excretion as the body attempts to excrete the excess salt and water. The degree of thirst will depend on the hypertonicity of the plasma and consequently the amount of cellular dehydration. Peripheral hand vein emptying time may be increased beyond the normal 5 seconds when the hand is elevated, but depends on the degree of expansion of the extracellular compartment. A bounding pulse is significant in detecting hypertonic expansion. The serum sodium concentration is increased. The hematocrit level and the concentrations of hemoglobin and total serum protein are decreased as a result of the expanded fluid volume in the extracellular compartment.

Treatment

Treatment consists of stopping the infusion to allow the kidneys to eliminate the overload of salt and water. If there are no cardiovascular side effects, 5% dextrose in water may be infused slowly to reduce the tonicity of the extracellular fluid and replace body water.

Hypertonic Contraction

Hypertonic contraction (hypertonic dehydration) occurs when there is a loss of water without a corresponding loss of salt. This condition occurs in patients who are unable to take sufficient fluid for a prolonged period or in patients with excess insensible water loss through the lungs and skin.

In the elderly, hypertonic dehydration is a common clinical disturbance; there is frequently a decrease in the thirst stimuli in response to hypertonicity of body fluids, and adequate intake of fluid is not met. In the unconscious or incontinent patient, frequency and excess urination may go undetected or may be recognized as a sign of good renal function. A loss of tubular ability to concentrate urine in the aged will result in a large urinary volume when an increased solute load is presented to the patient.[8] Elderly patients also have a diminished response to ADH. Large amounts of dilute urine may be lost, resulting in hypertonic dehydration.

To prevent fluid imbalance, the nurse must recognize that individuals differ widely in the water they require; patients whose kidneys do not concentrate well require more water than those whose kidneys concentrate well. The daily fluid requirement must be met.

In hypertonic contraction, the loss of water from the extracellular compartment results in an increase in the osmolality, causing water to flow from the cells to the extracellular compartment. Dehydration occurs as water leaves the cellular compartment to replace the plasma volume. Both compartments, the intracellular and the extracellular, are affected by the water loss; there is a decrease in volume and an increase in osmolality in both compartments. In contrast, in isotonic contraction only the extracellular compartment is affected and the contraction is more serious.

Because signs of hypertonic contraction are not obvious in the early stages, the nurse must anticipate such an imbalance and be alert to any changes.

Manifestations

Clinically, thirst is an early and reliable sign of hypertonic contraction but may be absent in the elderly, complicating early recognition of this imbalance. Weight loss occurs. Negative fluid balance (output greater than intake) is present. Hourly output measurements show a decrease in the rate of excretion of water. The pulse has a normal quality and is regular in the early stages of hypertonic contraction. The hand vein filling time may be within the normal limits; cellular fluid has partly replenished the plasma. Irritability, restlessness, and possibly confusion may be present. Skin turgor diminishes and is a sign of dehydration in the later stages. A dry mouth with a furrowed tongue indicates dehydration.

Laboratory studies show an increase in serum sodium concentration, hematocrit level, hemoglobin concentration, and total serum protein concentration.

Treatment

Treatment consists of hydrating the patient by administering a balanced hypotonic solution such as the Butler-type solutions; 2400 mL/m^2 body surface per day for moderate preexisting deficit and 3000 mL/m^2 body surface per day for severe preexisting deficit.[8] The usual rate for IV administration is 3 mL/m^2 body surface area. A therapeutic test for functional renal depression may be necessary before infusing water and electrolytes for maintenance.

Hypotonic Expansion

Hypotonic expansion (water intoxication, dilutional hyponatremia) occurs when the increase in the volume of body fluids is caused by water alone. Water expands the extracellular compartment, causing a decrease in the concentration. Water then diffuses into the cells until both compartments are isosmotic. Both the extracellular and the intracellular compartments are affected; the volume is increased and the concentration is decreased. The serum sodium concentration and the hematocrit, hemoglobin, and total serum protein levels are reduced.

Hypotonic expansion occurs in patients who are receiving large quantities of electrolyte-free water to replace excessive fluid and electrolytes lost from gastric suction, vomiting, diarrhea, or diuresis, or insensibly through the skin.

Patients receiving continuous infusion of 5% dextrose in water are particularly susceptible to water intoxication. This solution contains 252 mOsm dextrose per liter, making it an isotonic solution in the container. Once introduced into the circulation, the dextrose is quickly metabolized, leaving the water free to dilute and expand the extracellular compartment. With the decreased osmolality of the extracellular fluid, water diffuses into the cells and hypotonic expansion occurs.

The patient's tolerance to water can be exceeded by infusion of excess amounts of hypotonic fluids. The kidneys of the normal adult can metabolize water in amounts of 35 to 45 mL/kg per day, but the kidneys of the average patient can metabolize only 2500 to 3000 mL/day; above these volumes, abnormal accumulation of water occurs.[6]

Hypotonic expansion is more likely to occur during the early postoperative period, when retention of water is being affected by the response to stress, particularly in the elderly patient, in whom the response to stress is compounded by impairment in renal function. Small amounts of adjusted hypotonic saline (sodium, 90 mEq/L; chloride, 60 mEq/L; and lactate, 30 mEq/L) may be used in the early postoperative management of the aged.

Manifestations

When acute onset of behavioral changes, such as confusion, apathy, and disorientation, occurs in the elderly patient postoperatively, overhydration should be suspected. Central nervous system disturbances such as weakness, muscle twitching, and convulsions are seen, as are headaches, nausea, and vomiting.

Fluid intake is increased over fluid output. Weight gain is always present. Blood pressure usually is normal but may be elevated. Peripheral hand veins are usually full, and hand emptying time is increased beyond the normal 5 seconds when the hand is elevated from a dependent position. The pulse may be regular and not easily obliterated when pressure is applied.

Treatment

Treatment consists of withholding all fluids until the excess water is excreted. In severe hyponatremia, it may be necessary to administer small quantities of hypertonic saline to increase the osmotic pressure and the flow of water from the cells to the extracellular compartment for excretion by the kidneys. Hypertonic saline must be used cautiously and must not be administered to patients with congestive heart failure.

Hypotonic Contraction

Hypotonic contraction (hypotonic dehydration) occurs when fluids containing relatively more salt than water are lost from the body. This loss results in a decrease in the effective osmolality of the extracellular compartment. Water is drawn into the cells until osmotic equilibrium is established. Because of the invasion of water, the intracellular compartment is expanded and the extracellular compartment is contracted.

This imbalance may result from the loss of salt from any one of several sources: urine of patients receiving diuretics, fistula drainage, severe burns, vomitus, and sweat. The elderly are affected by the loss of small quantities of sodium.

Manifestations

Clinical manifestations include (1) weight loss; (2) negative fluid balance; (3) pulse rate increased, weak or thready, and easily obliterated; (4) increased hand filling time; and (5) decreased skin turgor.

Laboratory studies show a decrease in serum sodium concentration and an increase in hematocrit, hemoglobin, and total serum protein levels.

Treatment

Treatment of hypotonic contraction consists of replacing the fluids and electrolytes that have been lost. Because other electrolytes are usually lost along with the sodium loss, a balanced electrolyte solution may be administered.

REFERENCES

1. American Society of Hospital Pharmacists. (1992). Bethesda, MD: American Hospital Formulary Service, 1485, 1487, 1490, 1514, 1527–1529.
2. Burgess, R. E. (1965). Fluid and electrolytes. *American Journal of Nursing, 65,* 90.
3. Burns, W. (1972). Indications for IV therapy. In Health Care Worldwide. *Proceedings of Clinical Seminar* (pp. 7, 8, 12). San Francisco, 1968. North Chicago, IL, Abbott Laboratories.
4. Condon, R., & Nyhus, L. (Eds.). (1975). *Manual of surgical therapeutics* (3rd ed., p. 203). Boston: Little, Brown.

5. Drug and Therapeutic Information, Inc. (1970). Parenteral water and electrolyte solutions. *Medical Letter on Drugs and Therapeutics, 12*(19), 77.

6. Dudrick, S. J. (1971). Rational IV therapy. *American Journal of Hospital Pharmacy, 28,* 83–85.

7. Lebowitz, M. H., MaSuda, J. V., & Beckerman, J. H. (1971). The pH and acidity of intravenous infusion solutions. *Journal of the American Medical Association, 215,* 1937.

8. Metheny, N. M. (1992). *Fluid and electrolyte balance* (2nd ed., pp. 12–29, 169, 174, 273). Philadelphia: J. B. Lippincott.

9. Dunagan, W. & Ridner, M. (1989). *Manual of medical therapeutics* (26th ed., pp. 2, 65). Boston: Little, Brown & Co.

10. Stoklosa, M. J. (1974). *Pharmaceutical calcula-tions* (6th ed., pp. 236, 237). Philadelphia: Lea & Febiger.

11. United States Pharmacopeia. (1980). (20th ed., pp. 803, 1027). Easton, PA: Mack Publishing.

12. Vanatta, J., & Fogelman, M. (1988). *Moyer's fluid balance: A clinical manual* (4th ed., p. 45). Chicago: Year Book Medical Publishers.

13. Voda, A. M. (1970). Body water dynamics. *American Journal of Nursing, 70,* 2597, 2598, 2600–2601.

14. Weisberg, H. F. (1969). Parenteral fluid therapy in adults. In H. F. Conn (Ed.). *Current therapy* (p. 414). Philadelphia: W. B. Saunders.

15. Weisberg, H. F. (1964). Pitfalls in fluid and electrolyte therapy. *Journal of St. Barnabas Medical Center, 2,* 106.

REVIEW QUESTIONS

1. Fluids with the same tonicity as plasma are known as:
   a. isotonic
   b. hypotonic
   c. hypertonic
   d. base fluids

2. How many grams of dextrose are in 250 mL 20% dextrose in water?
   a. 25
   b. 50
   c. 75
   d. 100

3. How much water can the kidney safely metabolize in the average patient receiving IV therapy?
   a. 1500–1999 mL daily
   b. 2000–2499 mL daily
   c. 2500–2999 mL daily
   d. 3000–3500 mL daily

4. Hydrating fluids are used to:
   a. assess status of kidneys
   b. hydrate medical and surgical patients
   c. promote diuresis in dehydrated patients
   d. assess status of liver

5. What type of fluids are indicated when a retention of chlorides, ketone bodies, or organic salts occurs as in shock, liver disease, and starvation?
   a. alkalinizing fluids
   b. acetic fluids
   c. isotonic fluids
   d. hypertonic fluids

6. What fluid imbalance may result from continuous infusion of 5% dextrose in water?
   a. water intoxication
   b. dehydration
   c. hypertonic expansion
   d. peripheral edema

7. Loss of fluid and electrolytes of the same tonicity as plasma through vomiting, diarrhea, or loss of whole blood may result in:
   a. hypertonic contraction
   b. isotonic contraction
   c. hypotonic expansion
   d. hypertonic expansion

8. Which of the following sites is best used to assess skin turgor in the adult patient?
   a. skin over forehead or sternum
   b. skin over medial aspect of thigh
   c. skin over lateral aspect of thigh
   d. skin over abdomen

9. Which of the following parameters provide valuable information concerning fluid and electrolyte status?
   a. central venous pressure
   b. peripheral veins
   c. quality and rate of pulse
   d. laboratory values

10. Dextrose and hypotonic saline are considered hydrating fluids because:
    a. they provide more water than is required for excretion of salt
    b. the water they provide equals that needed for excretion of salt
    c. they minimize retention of salt
    d. they maximize retention of potassium in the cell

CHAPTER 20

Total Parenteral Nutrition

HISTORY

For centuries man has made attempts to feed patients via the IV route. When protein hydrolysates were developed in the 1930s, it became possible to provide IV amino acids to patients with a nonfunctioning gastrointestinal tract.[11,24] However, nutritive needs of the patient could not be met because the resultant hyperosmolar solution was too sclerosing to peripheral veins. Not until the discovery that central veins could be accessed successfully was it possible to give hypertonic solutions and actually "feed" the patient and provide hyperalimentation.[2,24]

Development of hyperalimentation began in the early 1960s in the Harrison Department of Surgical Research at the Hospital of the University of Pennsylvania. Stanley Dudrick devised a central venous system of feeding that resulted in the normal weight gain and growth of beagle puppies who were fed solely by vein.[10] Dudrick's animal experiments quickly led to human application; he successfully hyperalimented a severely ill infant who was unable to sustain herself with any type of gastrointestinal feeding due to small-bowel atresia.[29]

Dudrick's accomplishments led the way as this new therapy burgeoned during the 1970s, and clinicians realized its potential and its limitations. Hyperalimentation became a recognized specialty and nutritional support teams formed. In 1977, a multidisciplinary group of professionals was organized and the American Society for Parenteral and Enteral Nutrition (ASPEN) held its first Clinical Congress in Chicago.

The 1980s saw hyperalimentation evolve as a science, and this therapy of providing nutrients by vein in sufficient amounts to achieve anabolism became more commonly known as total parenteral nutrition (TPN) or parenteral nutrition (PN). Disease-specific formulas were developed to address the particular needs of patients with renal, cardiac, or hepatic disease and became commercially available. The rehabilitation of patients surviving catastrophic illnesses by maintenance on home TPN (HTPN) or home PN (HPN) led to the formation of support groups such as Life Line and the Oley Foundation (1983). Nutrition support research was enabled through the joint efforts of the Oley Foundation and ASPEN with annual reports of the Oasis Home Nutritional Support Patient Registry. Standards of care for TPN have been developed by the Intravenous Nurses Society (INS) and ASPEN (Appendices A and B).

Technology attempted to keep up with these new demands made by clinicians and patients alike as new-generation portable computerized pumps, semipermeable dressings, and three-in-one solutions were developed.

Sharon M. Weinstein: PLUMER'S PRINCIPLES & PRACTICE OF INTRAVENOUS THERAPY, FIFTH EDITION, © 1993 J. B. Lippincott Company

From this modest beginning, TPN has evolved into a sophisticated field of therapeutic intervention that has its own specialists and a large body of established knowledge. Research has proven TPN to be more beneficial in some disease states than others.[24] Indications and use in acquired immunodeficiency syndrome (AIDS), cancer, sepsis, and trauma needs further study. The role of amino acids such as arginine and glutamine; the indications for medium, short and/or long chain triglycerides; and the implications of antioxidants or "free radical scavengers,"[1] are just some areas where more research is needed.

INDICATIONS FOR PARENTERAL NUTRITION

A nutritional deficit often exists in hospitalized patients. This was illustrated in the classic studies by Blackburn and Bistrian, who found an incidence of 50% and 44% protein–calorie malnutrition in surgical and medical patients, respectively.[4,5]

Nurses are familiar with the isotonic IV fluid regimens prescribed for many patients—those awaiting surgery, those unable to eat postoperatively, those undergoing multiple days of testing that require NPO preparation, or those who are not eating well in the hospital for other reasons. The critical question should always be, "Does lack of nutritional support jeopardize the patient's well-being?" The answer, of course, depends on many variables, including the patient's nutritional status before disease or injury, the severity of the current illness or trauma, the patient's age, the degree of catabolism, and the anticipated length of time that the patient will be without gastrointestinal feeding.

The specific indications for nutritional support are as vast as the number of clinical conditions that prevent a patient from using the gastrointestinal tract for maintenance or achievement of anabolism. Some of the common indications for PN include gastrocutaneous fistulas; short-bowel syndrome; acute renal failure; trauma; large burns; inflammatory bowel disease; pancreatitis; prolonged ileus; large nitrogen losses from infected wounds, fistulas, or abscesses; respiratory failure; and sepsis (Table 20-1).

NUTRITIONAL ASSESSMENT

Ideally, nutritional assessment starts early in the admission. A screening process can be used to identify patients most at risk. This can be done in a variety of ways. Table 20-2 gives an example of how all patients at a cancer treatment center are screened for nutritional deficits. Patients identified as falling into the "B" (moderately) or "C" (severely) malnourished category would then automatically proceed to have a complete nutritional evaluation (Figure 20-1).

A nutritional assessment may include but is not limited to a complete history, including possible drug–nutrient interactions, anthropometric measurements, clinical and biochemical evaluation, level of immune competence, and the individual's nutrient requirements.

A complete history includes the medical, social, and dietary aspects. The medical history should include any acute or chronic diseases that may have an impact on nutrient intake or nutrient utilization and conditions that cause increased metabolic needs or increased fluid and electrolyte losses. The patient's weight (usual and current); patterns of alcohol, tobacco, and medication (prescription or over-the-counter) use; age; and level of activity are other factors to be addressed. Social factors that can influence nutrient

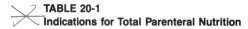

TABLE 20-1
Indications for Total Parenteral Nutrition

Primary therapy

Efficacy shown
 Short-gut syndrome
 Enterocutaneous fistula
 Renal failure due to acute tubular necrosis
 Hepatic failure (acute decompensation in the face of cirrhosis)
 Burns (when combined with aggressive enteral support)

Efficacy not shown
 Inflammatory bowel disease
 Anorexia nervosa

Supportive therapy

Efficacy shown
 Acute radiation enteritis
 Chemotherapy enteritis
 Perioperative support of the clearly malnourished patient

Efficacy not shown
 Chronic pancreatitis
 Perioperative support in "cardiac cachexia"
 Chronic protein loss from wounds or disease in excess of enteral
  repletion
 Prolonged respiratory support with ileus
 Cancer support
 Sepsis and trauma
 General perioperative support

---

intake are religion, income, substance abuse, and psychological or physical disabilities. A dietary history will reveal food allergies; intolerances; aversions; modifications (low sodium, low cholesterol); problems with chewing, taste, or appetite; and use of supplements (vitamins, minerals, meal replacement products).

Anthropometrics

Anthropometric measurements consist of simple, noninvasive, inexpensive techniques for obtaining body measurements used to evaluate a patient's nutritional status. Height and weight should be measured by the clinician because both decrease as adults age.[25] When obtaining the patient's weight, the level of hydration, accuracy of the scale, and consistency of serial measurements (same time, place, and attire) will contribute to the value of this measurement. Body frame size can be determined by wrist measurement or by elbow breadth.[14,21] In 1959, Metropolitan Life Insurance Company developed weight tables for adults based on sex, height, and frame size; these were updated in 1983 and are used to determine ideal weight and percent of ideal weight:

$$\% \text{ ideal body weight} = \frac{\text{Actual weight}}{\text{Ideal body weight}} \times 100$$

Although the percent of ideal body weight is important information and useful for patients on weight loss programs looking for goal weights, for ill and compromised

TABLE 20-2
Criteria for Identification of Malnourished Patients

	A*	B	C
Weight History			
Percent deviation from usual body weight (UBW)	85%–95%	75%–84%	<74%
and/or			
Percent involuntary weight loss	<5% over 1 mo	5% over 1 mo	>5%
	<7.5% over 3 mo	7.5% over 3 mo	>7.5%
	<10% over 6 mo	10% over 6 mo	>10%
Serum Albumin†	3.2–3.8	2.6–3.1	≤2.5
Transferrin	150–200 mg/dL	100–150 mg/dL	<100 mg/dL
and/or			
Prealbumin	10–15 mg/dL	5–10 mg/dL	<5 mg/dL

* The A B C classifications are primarily used to prioritize levels of care and to provide an initial basis for determining need for recommending parenteral or enteral nutrition.

Code A—mildly malnourished

Code B—moderately malnourished

Code C—severely malnourished

The above codes are determined during the initial nutrition screening. Other factors such as physical assessments, indirect calorimetry, body fat analysis, evaluation of food intake, feeding problems, etc., will have to be taken into consideration during the actual nutritional assessment.

† Normal values for serum albumin at this lab are 3.9–5.0 g/dL, which are higher than the universally accepted normal values of 3.5–5.0 g/dL. This arises from current laboratory methodology.

(Courtesy: Midwestern Regional Medical Center, Zion, IL.)

individuals it is more critical to assess percent of weight loss by comparing the patient's usual weight (before illness) to the current weight:

$$\% \text{ usual weight} = \frac{\text{Actual weight}}{\text{Usual weight}} \times 100$$

Calculating the degree of weight change also uses the patient's usual weight and the current weight:

$$\% \text{ weight change} = \frac{\text{Usual weight} - \text{Actual weight}}{\text{Usual weight}} \times 100$$

This is important because an individual may be 120% of ideal body weight but with the loss of 30 lb be identified as 78% of usual weight or moderately malnourished. Besides height and weight, skin-fold thickness, midarm muscle circumference, and arm muscle area are used to determine fat and skeletal muscle store (Table 20-3).

Clinical Evaluation

The clinical assessment is a physical examination provided by an experienced clinician looking for signs and symptoms that may indicate nutritional deficiencies. These include but are not limited to changes in hair, eyes, skin, nails, and systems evaluation (cardiac, gastrointestinal, respiratory, muscle skeletal, neurologic; Table 20-4).

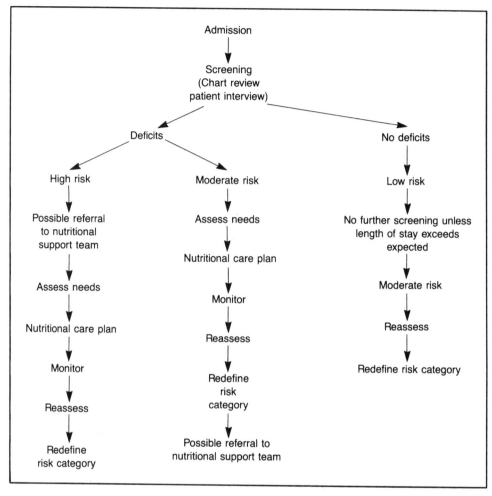

FIGURE 20-1 Nutritional screening. (Courtesy: Grant, DeHoog. Nutritional Assessment and Support, 1991.)

Biochemical Evaluation

Certain plasma proteins can be used to evaluate nutritional status because nutrient intake affects the synthesis of these visceral proteins. Serum albumin helps maintain oncotic pressure, and its values are affected by the patient's hydration status. The long half-life (20 days) of albumin makes it less valuable in monitoring acute nutrition changes. It is more useful in the initial screening process.[8] Serum transferrin is a more sensitive marker because its half-life is shorter (8–10 days).[12] Prealbumin is more sensitive yet with a half-life of 2 to 3 days, making it extremely sensitive to acute changes and giving a more accurate picture of visceral protein status.[3] Retinol-binding protein may not be as valuable in evaluating the visceral protein status because its half-life is so short (10–18 hours). Table 20-5 shows the normal values for these carrier proteins.

The creatinine height index (CHI) is also used to estimate the lean body mass. Creatinine is excreted in the urine each day in proportion to total body muscle. The actual

TABLE 20-3
Measurement of Mid-upper Arm Circumferences and Triceps Skin-Fold

These measurements allow for simple and quick assessment of nutritional status to identify muscle depletion and loss of caloric reserves.

	Standard	*90% Standard*	*80% Standard*	*70% Standard*	*60% Standard*
Arm Circumference (cm)					
Arm Circumference, Adults, Sexes Separate					
Male	29.3	26.3	23.4	20.5	17.6
Female	28.5	25.7	22.8	20.0	17.1
Muscle Circumference (cm)					
Muscle Circumference, Adults, Sexes Separate					
Male	25.3	22.8	20.2	17.7	15.2
Female	23.2	20.9	18.6	16.2	13.9
Triceps Skin-Fold (cm)					
Triceps Skin-Fold, Adults, Sexes Separate					
Male	12.5	11.3	10.0	8.8	7.5
Female	16.5	14.9	13.2	11.6	9.9

(Adapted from Jelliffe, D. B. [1966] *The assessment of the nutritional status of the community.* Geneva: World Health Organization)

daily creatinine excretion is compared to the expected daily loss of creatinine in an "idealized" normal individual of the same height:

$$\text{Creatinine height index (CHI)} = \frac{\text{Actual urinary creatinine}}{\text{Ideal urinary creatinine}} \times 100$$

Any loss of muscle tissue from malnutrition will be reflected in a reduction in creatinine excretion when compared to normal.[7] The patient's age, renal status, intake, and disease state may affect the results of this assessment parameter.[3]

A 24-hour urine for urine urea nitrogen (UUN) is obtained to determine nitrogen balance and is an objective method of evaluating the efficacy of the patient's nutritional prescription. For the patient to be in a positive nitrogen balance and an anabolic state, the amount of nitrogen taken by the patient (IV and PO) needs to be more than that excreted. A 24-hour urine collection is needed to measure the amount of urinary urea excreted. A factor of 4 g is added (2 g for fecal losses and 2 g for integumental losses) to measure total nitrogen excretion.

Nitrogen balance is then calculated by subtracting the amount of nitrogen lost from the amount of nitrogen given or taken by the patient:[7]

$$\text{Nitrogen balance} = \frac{\text{Protein intake}}{6.25} - (\text{Urinary urea nitrogen} + 4)$$

Cell-mediated immunity and total lymphocyte count (TLC) are measured to assess immune competency, an important component of host defense, and may be an indication

TABLE 20-4
Physical Assessment for Nutritional Deficiencies

I. Hair changes associated with protein–calorie malnutrition
   A. Lackluster
   B. Thinness, sparseness
   C. Pigmentation changes
   D. Easy pluckability (inspect comb, pillow, and bed for hair)

II. Lip changes
   A. Angular stomatitis
      1. Associated with deficiencies of one or more B vitamins
      2. Cracks, redness at corners of mouth
      3. May result in scars when healed
   B. Cheilosis
      1. Associated with riboflavin and niacin deficiency
      2. Vertical cracks in lips

III. Tongue changes
   A. Most changes associated with deficiencies of one or more B vitamins
   B. May change color (eg, become purplish red or beefy red)
   C. Fissures
   D. May be painful and hypersensitive, with burning
   E. Atrophy of taste buds; tongue may appear smooth and pale

IV. Skin changes
   A. Consider general characteristics of skin (dryness and flakiness may be associated with deficiency of vitamin A, essential fatty acids)
   B. Petechiae
      1. Hemorrhagic spots on skin at pressure points
      2. May occur in presence of liver disease or during anticoagulation
      3. Associated with deficiencies of vitamins C and K

(Adapted from Curtis, S. [1988]. Nutritional assessment. In C. Caldwell-Kennedy & P. Guenter [Eds.]. *Nutritional support nursing: Core curriculum.* Silver Spring, MD: American Society for Parenteral and Enteral Nutrition.)

of nutritional health.[3] The TLC indicates a patient's ability to fight infection and to maintain host integrity:

$$\text{Total lymphocyte count} = \frac{\% \text{ lymphocytes} \times \text{White cell count}}{100}$$

Delayed-type hypersensitivity (DTH) responses are assessed by measuring the response to intracutaneous administration of recall antigens (to which most people have had exposure) provoking a delayed cellular hypersensitivity response by a battery of antigens read at 24 and 48 hours. Plastic, disposable multiple test applicators are available, including tetanus toxoid, diphtheria toxoid, streptococcus, tuberculin Old, glycerin negative control, candida, trichophyton, and proteus. A positive reaction from any two of the skin test antigens is induration of 2 mm or greater. These results must be

TABLE 20-5 **Carrier Proteins**	**Normal Ranges**
Serum albumin	3.5–5.0 g/100 mL
	50%–65% of total protein
Serum transferrin (siderophillin)	250–300 mg/100 mL
Serum prealbumin	15.7–29.6 mg/mL
Serum retinol-binding protein	2.6–7.6 mg/100 mL

weighed with other findings in the nutritional assessment because nonnutritional factors can cause low TLCs and negative DTH responses.[28] Once the nutritional assessment data have been collected and evaluated, the optimal method for nutritional support must be selected. This decision process is depicted in Figure 20-2.

Three types of malnutrition have been identified:

1. *Maramus*—a gradual wasting of body fat and muscle and intact visceral protein stores. This patient is emaciated; maramus is often associated with chronic illness and starvation.

2. *Kwashiorkor* or *hypoalbuminemia*—loss of visceral protein stores in the presence of adequate fat and muscle. This patient may appear obese, and this condition is often associated with poor protein intake but adequate calorie intake.

3. *Mixed marasmus and hypoalbuminemia*—a combination of both fat loss and muscle wasting with depleted visceral protein stores.[9]

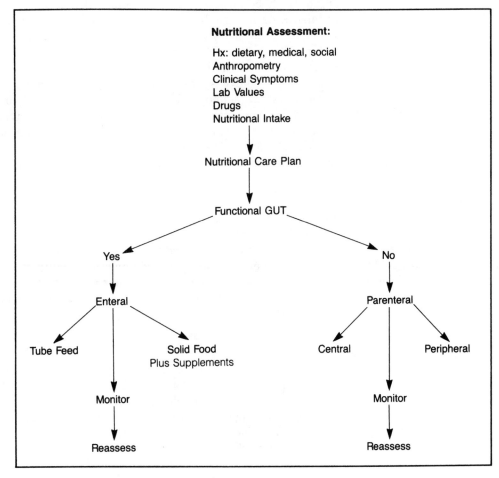

FIGURE 20-2 Nutritional support process. (Courtesy: Grant, DeHoog. Nutritional Assessment and Support, 1991.)

NUTRIENT REQUIREMENTS

The *basal metabolic rate* (BMR) is defined as the minimum amount of energy required by the body at rest in the fasting state needed to sustain life processes.[20] Age, sex, size, and stress affect the BMR. Two of the common methods of determining the BMR are by estimation and by measuring the resting energy expenditure (REE). The BMR is estimated by using the Harris-Benedict equation (Table 20-6) to arrive at the kilocalories needed per day (kcal/day). The REE can be obtained by indirect calorimetry. In hospitals, a mask or mouthpiece is placed on the patient for about 10 to 15 minutes and air exchange is measured. Additional calories are added to the BMR or REE to account for activity, weight gain, infection, and sepsis. A number of methods are available to calculate these extra needs[15,17] (see Table 20-6).

Solution Content

To supply protein-sparing, or "energy" calories, the solutions are admixed with large amounts of dextrose and final concentrations commonly range from 20% to 47% dextrose. If the proper calorie–nitrogen ratio is not provided, it is impossible to achieve positive nitrogen balance. As more has been learned about IV nutritional requirements, it has become clear that this ratio changes with different disease states and is not fixed for a particular patient but depends on changing clinical status. The currently accepted calorie–nitrogen ratio is 100 to 120 g non-protein calories per gram of nitrogen.[19]

The protein or nitrogen source is provided in the form of free amino acids directly into the circulation. These 22 amino acids are classified as essential (unable to be synthesized by the body) and nonessential (can be synthesized by the body) and are not stored in the body. Protein requirements are calculated individually for each patient. Each gram of protein yields 3.4 calories. The recommended daily allowance (RDA) is 18 g/kg body weight. Tables 20-7 and 20-8 list types of amino acid solutions available.

Dextrose

Dextrose is the carbohydrate source in TPN. Solution concentrations can vary from 2.5% to 70% (Table 20-9). Each gram of carbohydrate yields 3.4 kcal. The rate of glucose metabolism varies; it is recommended not to exceed 0.5 mg/kg per hour.[27] The demand for insulin increases proportionally with the amount of dextrose in the solution and coupled with stress of illness, infection, and so forth may cause a glucose intolerance requiring insulin administration. Replacing part of the dextrose calories with lipids can help alleviate this problem.

Lipids

Lipids are administered parenterally to prevent or treat essential fatty acid deficiency (EFAD) and to provide a concentrated calorie source because 1 g fat yields 9 kcal.

Essential fatty acid deficiency can be detected both biochemically and clinically. Biochemical lesions have been reported as early as 3 to 7 days following initiation of TPN, although clinical signs seem to take 3 to 4 weeks of dietary inadequacy before appearing. Biochemical lesions are diagnostic of EFAD and, thus, we now know that this deficiency state may exist in occult form for weeks before becoming clinically evident. Some clinical signs and symptoms of EFAD are dry or scaling skin, thinning hair, thrombocytopenia, and liver function abnormalities.

TABLE 20-6
Calculation of Nutrient Requirements

For the depleted patient, use the ideal body weight (IBW) to compute nutritional requirements. Use the current weight for patients at ideal weight or higher. Optimal weight gain during nutritional support is 0.5–1.0 kg (1.1–2.2 lb) per week. This can be achieved by giving additional 500 kcal/day in addition to calculated caloric requirements. Ideal body weight for height can be calculated by the following formulas:

> Ideal male weight = 50 kg (1st 5 ft) + 2.7 kg/inch over 5 ft
> Ideal female weight = 45.5 kg (1st 5 ft) + 1.8 kg/inch over 5 ft

Harris-Benedict

The Harris-Benedict formula has been found to be among the most useful and accurate for calculating basal energy requirements. The formula accounts for difference in age, current weight, height, and sex. An individual's basal energy expenditure (BEE) can be estimated by the following formula:

> Males: $66.5 + 13.8$ (wt) $+ 5.0$ (ht) $- 6.8$ (age)
> Females: $655.1 + 9.6$ (wt) $+ 1.8$ (ht) $- 4.7$ (age)

Jeejebhoy*

Jeejebhoy suggests an alternate method of estimating calories that will satisfy the needs of most patients.

Status	kcal/kg/IBW
Basal energy needs	25–30
Ambulatory with weight maintenance	30–35
Malnutrition with mild stress	40
Severe injuries and sepsis	50–60
Extensive burns	80

Long†

(BEE) formula:

$$BEE \times (AF) \times (IF)$$

AF (Activity Factor)		IF (Injury Factor)	
bedrest	1.2	minor surgery	1.2
ambulatory	1.3	skeletal trauma	1.35
		major sepsis	1.60
		severe burns	2.10

*From Jeejebhoy, K. (1976). Total parenteral nutrition. *Annals of the Royal College of Physicians and Surgeons of Canada, 9,* 287–300.

†From Long, C., (1979). Metabolic response to injury and illness: Estimation of energy and protein needs from indirect calorimetry and nitrogen balance. *Journal of Parenteral and Enteral Nutrition, 3,* 452–456.

Because EFAD is associated with decreased ability to heal wounds, adverse effects on red blood cell membranes, and a defect in prostaglandin synthesis, these disorders are ample reasons to be concerned with prevention of this deficiency state.

If fat is used as a major caloric source in TPN therapy, the amount of glucose in the system can be decreased and a peripheral vein approach to TPN becomes possible. Fat emulsions 10% provide 1.1 cal/mL, are isotonic, and therefore not sclerotic to

TABLE 20-7
Crystalline Amino Acid Profiles—The "Specialized Clinician" Concentration Files Comparison (Amino Acids Listed as a Percent of Total)

L-Amino Acids	Freamine 8.5% (No longer available)	Aminosyn 10%	Aminosyn II 10%	Freamine III 10%
Essential				
Isoleucine	6.9%	7.2%	6.6%	7.1%
Leucine	9.0%*	9.5%	10.0%	9.3%
Lysine + (free base)	9.0%*	7.2%†	10.5%	7.4%†
Methionine	5.2%	4.0%	1.7%	5.4%
Phenylalanine	5.6%	4.4%	3.0%	5.7%
Threonine	3.9%	5.2%	4.0%	4.1%
Tryptophan	1.5%	1.6%	2.0%	1.5%
Valine	6.5%	8.1%	5.0%	6.8%
Nonessential				
Alanine	7.0%	12.9%	9.9%	7.3%
Arginine (+)	3.6%	9.9%	10.2%	9.7%
Histidine (+)	2.8%	3.0%	3.0%	2.8%
Proline	11.1%	8.7%	7.2%	11.5%
Serine	5.8%	4.2%	5.3%	6.0%
Tyrosine	—	0.4%	2.2%‡	—
Glycine	21.1%	12.9%	5.0%	14.4%
Cysteine	<0.2%*	—	—	<0.2%*
Glutamic acid (−)	—	—	7.4%	—
Aspartic acid (−)	—	—	7.0%	—

* = Provided as the HCl salt

† = Provided as the acetate salt

‡ = Tyrosine concentration as tyrosine plus N-acetyl tyrosine

veins. The 20% lipid emulsions provide 2.2 cal/mL with an osmolarity of 333 mOsm/L, which makes them suitable for peripheral administration as well (Table 20-10).

Dosage and infusion rates depend on product concentration, the patient's age, and the stage of therapy. It is extremely important that the nurse be familiar with the manufacturer's current recommendations for use. Initial infusion rates are very slow for a limited period of time, and the patient is carefully observed for adverse reactions. To decrease the likelihood of adverse reaction, maximum daily dose should not be exceeded.

The patient's ability to eliminate infused fat from the circulation should be observed; lipemia must clear between daily infusions.

Administration of IV fat is contraindicated in patients with disturbances in normal fat metabolism such as pathologic hyperlipemia, lipoid nephrosis, or acute pancreatitis if accompanied by hyperlipemia.[30]

Lipid emulsions have been "piggybacked" into the dextrose and amino acid solution. However, it is now possible, with changes in compounding techniques, to mix all

Hepatamine 8%	Nephramine 5.4%	Novamine 8.5%	Travasol 8.5%	Travasol 10.0%	Trophamine 6%
11.3%	10.5%	4.9%	4.7%	6.0%	8.2%
13.6%	16.4%	6.9%	6.1%	7.3%	14.0%
7.6%	12.0%	7.8%†	5.7%*	5.8%*	8.2%†
1.3%	16.4%	4.9%	5.7%	4.0%	3.3%
1.3%	16.4%	6.9%	6.1%	5.6%	4.8%
5.6%	7.5%	4.9%	4.1%	4.2%	4.2%
0.8%	3.7%	1.6%	1.7%	1.8%	2.0%
10.5%	12.0%	6.4%	4.5%	5.8%	7.8%
9.6%	—	14.5%	20.7%	20.7%	5.3%
7.5%	—	9.8%	10.3%	11.5%	12.2%
3.0%	4.7%	5.8%	4.3%	4.8%	4.8%
10.0%	—	5.9%	4.1%	6.8%	6.8%
6.3%	—	3.9%	—	5.0%	3.8%
—	—	0.2%	0.4%	0.4%	2.3%
11.3%	—	6.9%	20.7%	10.3%	3.7%
<0.3%*	0.4%	0.4%	—	—	0.33%
—	—	4.9%	—	—	5.0%
—	—	2.9%	—	—	3.2%

(+) = Cationic amino acids

(−) = Anionic amino acid

(Reprinted with permission of Specialized Clinical Services, Tustin, CA)

three nutrients into one bag. This is referred to as "3:1, total nutrient admixture, or triple-mix" solution.

Vitamins

Vitamins are organic compounds essential for maintenance and growth that are not synthesized by the body.[18] There are two main groups: fat-soluble (A, D, E, K) and water-soluble vitamins (B complex, C). Vitamins are sensitive or become inactive with temperature changes and exposure to light. Therefore, they are added before administration and protected from direct light exposure.

There are commercially available vitamin admixtures. To meet the daily requirements set by the American Medical Association Nutrition Advisory Group, 10 mL of the mixture is added to the TPN solution.[22] However, because vitamin K is not included in the admixture, intramuscular injections may be given.

TABLE 20-8
Commercially Available Crystalline Amino Acid Groups Concentrations That Affect Acid/Base Balance (Amino Acid Groups as a Percent of the Total Amino Acids)

L-Amino Acids	Freamine 8.5% (No longer available)	Aminosyn 10%	Aminosyn II 10%	Freamine III 10%
Cationic amino acids	15.4%	20.1%	23.7%	19.9%
Anionic amino acids	—	—	14.4%	—
Serine/Glycine	26.9%	17.1%	10.3%	20.4%
Total sulfur containing amino acids	5.4%	4.0%	1.7%	5.6%
Acetate from lysine (mEq/L)	0	50	71.8	50.0
Acetate from acetic acid (mEq/L)	20.0	98.0	0	39.0
Total acetate (mEq/L)	20.0	148.0	71.8	89.0
Chloride (mEq/L)	45.0*	0	0.0	<3.0

* = As HCl from lysine HCl

† = From hydrochloric acid added as buffer

Minerals

Minerals can be divided into two basic groups: essential macronutrients (100 mg/day)—calcium, chloride, magnesium, phosphorus, potassium, sodium, sulfur; and essential trace elements or micronutrients (needed as few mg/day)—chromium, copper, fluoride, iodine, iron, manganese, molybdenum, zinc. These are given and adjusted based on laboratory values. These are also commercially available and may be given as admixtures or singly as the situation warrants.

PRODUCT HANDLING

Because nutritional support solutions cannot be sterilized terminally (they "caramelize" if autoclaved), they should be prepared in the pharmacy with stringent aseptic technique. The solutions should be mixed under a laminar flow hood by a pharmacist or trained technicians who are supervised by a clinical pharmacologist. The use of headgear, masks, and sterile gloves is desirable.

All additives should be placed in the dextrose–amino acids mixture at the time of initial mixing. Solution containers should be examined for integrity (bottles for cracks and bags for small punctures), and the solution should be inspected against a strong light to ascertain the presence of particulate matter or turbidity that could indicate bacterial contamination.

PATIENT MANAGEMENT

As mentioned earlier, TPN solutions are highly concentrated and contain large amounts of dextrose. These hypertonic solutions must be delivered into a wide-diameter blood vessel so that they may be rapidly diluted and not become sclerotic to the vein. Therefore,

Hepatamine 8%	Nephramine 5.4%	Novamine 8.5%	Travasol 8.5%	Travasol 10.0%	Trophamine 6%
12.1%	16.7%	23.4%	20.35%	22.1%	25.2%
—	—	7.8%	—	—	8.2%
17.6%	—	10.8%	20.7%	15.3%	7.5%
1.6%	16.8%	5.3%	5.7%	4.0%	3.3%
41.8	44.0	46.6	0	0	20.4
40.2	0	41.4	52.0	87.0	35.6
82.0	44.0	88.0	52.0	87.0	56.0
<3.0	<3.0	0	34.0*	40.0*	<3.0

(Reprinted with permission of Specialized Clinical Services, Tustin, CA)

the only veins acceptable for catheter tip location are the superior vena cava, the innominate vein, and the intrathoracic subclavian vein. The ideal location for the catheter tip is the middle of the superior vena cava.

Early attempts to administer TPN solutions often used the antecubital approach to the superior vena cava with polyvinylchloride catheters. These long catheters were frequently associated with painful thrombophlebitis, venous thrombosis, and sometimes, sepsis. Currently, however, antecubital catheters made of silicon elastomer are an acceptable alternative to the conventional subclavian or jugular catheter and are less thrombogenic than other materials.[13]

Subclavian or internal jugular percutaneous venipuncture remains the approach of choice for most clinicians. The external jugular vein is, however, usually too narrow to be easily cannulated. The addition of low-dose heparin sodium to the TPN solution has also been recommended to minimize the incidence of thrombosis.[16]

CATHETER INSERTION

Patient Considerations

Before the subclavian vein catheterization procedure is begun, the nurse should explain the procedure to the patient. Proper teaching beforehand tends to increase patient tolerance and markedly decrease the level of pain experienced during the procedure. In particular, the patient should be advised of the following aspects of the procedure:

1. The patient will be placed in the Trendelenburg (head-down) position to enable the vein to fill more readily.

2. The physician will be wearing a mask, gown, and gloves, and other personnel at the head of the bed will wear masks to prevent infection during the procedure.

TABLE 20-9
Dextrose Solution Concentrations

Dextrose Concentration (in %)	Calories/L	Calculated Osmolarity (mOsm/L)
2.5	85	126
5	170	250
7.7	260	390
10	340	505
11.5	390	580
20	680	1010
25	850	1330
30	1020	1515
38	1290	1920
40	1360	2020
50	1700	2525
60	2040	3030
70	2380	3530

(Source: American Hospital Formulary Service [1992]. American Society of Hospital Pharmacists)

3. The patient will be draped surgically, that is, small sterile towels will be placed around the area where the catheter will be inserted, and the patient's face will be turned away and loosely covered. Reassure the patient that he or she will be able to breathe normally and see clearly.

4. The physician will place a small towel roll along the vertebrae to hyperextend the neck and elevate the clavicles and support the head and shoulders.

5. The skin will be prepped with acetone, iodine, and alcohol.

6. The anesthetic will be administered a few minutes before the catheterization and may feel somewhat like a bee sting until it starts to work.

7. The search for the subclavian vein may produce unusual sensations, which may include pressure in the chest or pain.

When this teaching is done in a calm, matter-of-fact manner, it usually results in a less traumatic experience for the patient and, at the very least, one for which the patient was prepared. It is important to elicit feedback during the teaching so that the nurse can assess the patient's level of understanding and eliminate fears.

If the patient seems to be especially apprehensive, even after the preinsertion teaching has been done, administration of an analgesic or psychotropic medication should be considered.

Certain comfort measures can reduce the fear and isolation generated by an invasive procedure such as catheterization. The nurse should hold the patient's hand during the procedure. If the nurse has assembled the equipment in advance, he or she is free to support the patient while the physician places the catheter. The nurse should remember to maintain eye contact with the patient.

TABLE 20-10
Lipid Emulsions

Preparation Manufacturer	Intralipid® 10% Clintec	Intralipid® 20% Clintec	Liposyn® II 10% Abbott	Liposyn® II 20% Abbott
Concentration	10%	20%	10%	20%
Fat content g/100 mL				
Safflower oil	—	—	5	10
Soybean oil	10	20	5	10
Fatty acids (%)				
Linoleic acid	50%	50%	65.8%	68.8%
Oleic acid	26%	26%	17.7%	17.7%
Palmitic acid	10%	10%	8.8%	8.8%
Stearic acid	3.5%	3.5%	3.4%	3.4%
Linolenic acid	9%	9%	4.2%	4.2%
Egg phosphatides g/100 mL	1.2	1.2	up to 1.2	1.2
Glycerin g/100 mL	2.25	2.25	2.5	2.5
mOsm/L	260	260	276	258
pH	6–8.9	6–8.9	6–9	6–9
Calories/mL	1.1	2	1.1	2

Preparation Manufacturer	Liposyn® III 10% Abbott	Liposyn® III 20% Abbott	Nutrilipid® 10% McGaw	Nutrilipid® 20% McGaw
Concentration	10%	20%	10%	20%
Fat content g/100 mL				
Safflower oil	—	—	—	—
Soybean oil	10	20	10	20
Fatty acids (%)				
Linoleic acid	54.5%	54.5%	49%–60%	49%–60%
Oleic acid	22.4%	22.4%	21%–26%	21%–26%
Palmitic acid	10.5%	10.5%	9%–13%	9%–13%
Stearic acid	4.2%	4.2%	3%–5%	3%–5%
Linolenic acid	8.3%	8.3%	6%–9%	6%–9%
Egg phosphatides g/100 mL	up to 1.2	1.2	1.2	1.2
Glycerin g/100 mL	2.5	2.5	2.21	2.21
mOsm/L	284	292	280	315
pH	6–9	6–9	6–7.9	6–7.9
Calories/mL	1.1	2	1.1	2

(Source: American Hospital Formulary Service [1992]. American Society of Hospital Pharmacists)

It is the nurse's responsibility to take an active role in ensuring sterile technique, thereby protecting the patient. This means that if a glove becomes contaminated, the nurse should quickly give the physician a fresh pair. The nurse should take the initiative in maintaining asepsis.

Catheterization should be performed only by an experienced physician. The inside-the-needle catheter is placed in the standard method of subclavian venipuncture. When the needle is open to the air, before and during the threading of the catheter, the patient is asked to perform the Valsalva maneuver (forced expiration with a closed glottis). This maneuver is a precaution against possible air embolism and is easily accomplished by instructing the patient to "take a deep breath and hold it, bearing down and straining slightly." If the intubated patient is unable to do this, the nurse may produce the Valsalva maneuver by carefully maintaining inspiration with a manual resuscitation bag.

After the catheter is placed, one suture is placed at the catheter insertion site. This prevents in-and-out motion of the catheter, which could introduce skin organisms into the puncture wound, and also helps prevent accidental dislodging of the catheter. Because of the potential complications and discomfort associated with the procedure, repeated, unsuccessful attempts to catheterize a specific vessel are unjustified.

Immediate Postcatheterization Management

After the catheter has been sutured, the routine dressing is applied and a chest roentgenogram is taken immediately. Only isotonic solution should be infused at a slow keep-open rate (10–20 mL/hr) until the chest x-ray confirms central venous location. After it has been confirmed that the catheter tip is located in the superior vena cava or the innominate or intrathoracic subclavian vein, infusion of the initial TPN solution may be started.

It is unacceptable to have the catheter tip located in the heart, the inferior vena cava, or any extrathoracic vessel. Atrial rupture, valvular damage, myocardial irritability, and cardiac tamponade are some of the possible complications that have been reported when catheter tips are located in the heart. Although the inferior vena cava has a wide diameter, it is contraindicated for catheterization because it has been associated with catheter-induced thrombosis and occlusion. Extrathoracic veins are too narrow and will become sclerosed if used for TPN administration.

COMPLICATIONS

Complications are infrequent, but placement of a subclavian catheter can trigger serious events. Be particularly alert for signs of respiratory distress, pain, a slowly increasing hematoma, or any unexplainable symptom. Some of the possible complications following a subclavian puncture are listed in Figure 20-3.

Pneumothorax

Pleural puncture may occur inadvertently because of the anatomic proximity of the lung to the subclavian veins. Sharp chest pain or decreased breath sounds may be present, or the pneumothorax may be evident only radiographically. Treatment is based on symptoms. Sometimes a chest tube is indicated although smaller pneumothoraces often resolve spontaneously.

Hemothorax

The subclavian vein or adjacent vessels may be traumatized during venipuncture, possibly causing slow, constant bleeding into the thorax. This is particularly serious if the patient has a bleeding disorder. Symptoms and treatment are the same as those for pneumothorax.

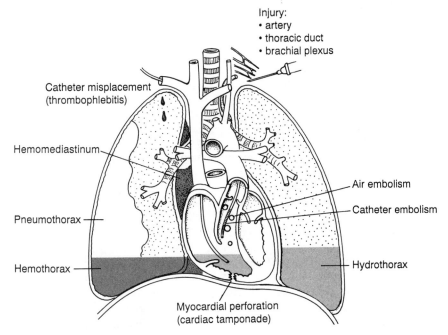

FIGURE 20-3 Complications of catheter insertion. (Adapted from Fisher, J. E. (1991). *Total parenteral nutrition* (2nd ed.). Permission granted by Fisher and Little, Brown & Co.)

Hydrothorax

The catheter may transect the vein and locate in the thorax, causing IV solutions to be infused directly into the chest. Symptoms and treatment for this complication are also like those for pneumothorax.

Inadvertent Arterial Puncture

It is possible to inadvertently enter an artery during attempted venipuncture. This is usually not a problem if the error is clinically observed and the patient treated immediately. Punctured arteries must receive direct pressure for at least 5 full minutes, timed by the clock, to stop bleeding. If the patient has a bleeding disorder or platelet abnormality, direct pressure must be applied for an even longer period. Therefore, one must be on the alert for a rapidly expanding hematoma, signs and symptoms of tracheal compression or respiratory distress, or a combination of these. If these symptoms occur, direct pressure must be placed on the arterial site and the physician must be called immediately.

Brachial Plexus Injury

A tingling sensation in the fingers, pain shooting down the arm, or paralysis of the arms may indicate brachial plexus injury. This is a rare complication of subclavian catheterization. The treatment is symptomatic and may not always resolve the injury. Physical therapy is indicated for paralysis.

Thoracic Duct Injury (Chylothorax)

The thoracic duct is enlarged in cirrhotic patients because of alterations in lymph flow and should be suspected when there is clear drainage from the insertion site. Therefore, it may be entered accidentally during catheter placement. A left-sided subclavian puncture should therefore be avoided in cirrhotic patients whenever possible.

Sheared Catheter with Distal Embolization

During the process of threading the catheter through the needle, the catheter should never be pulled back for redirection. The entire unit should be removed and a new catheter should be used. If the catheter is pulled back against the needle, it may shear off and embolize. In such cases, cardiac catheterization, with snaring of the catheter embolus under fluoroscopic control, may be necessary.

Air Embolism

Air embolism is a potential danger whenever the central venous system is open to the air. The exact amount of air necessary to cause death remains controversial. This reemphasizes the need for air embolism precautions during catheter placement. Signs and symptoms vary with the severity of the air embolism and may include dyspnea, apnea, hypoxia, disorientation, tachycardia, hypotension, or a precordial murmur. Severe neurologic deficits, including hemiplegia, aphasia, seizures, and coma, have reportedly been associated with air embolism. The pathophysiology of the neurologic deficit associated with air embolism is attributed to direct access of air into the cerebral circulation in most situations. Immediate treatment is aimed at preventing obstruction by air of the right ventricular outflow tract. The patient should be placed in the left lateral, head-dependent position, and direct intracardiac needle aspiration of air may be necessary.

Air embolism can also occur during IV administration set change either because of accidental disconnection of tubing junctions or through a tract left after catheter removal. Therefore, air embolism precautions during tubing change and catheter removal are essential, as is the proper securing of tubing junctions. Catheter removal should be followed immediately by placement of an occlusive dressing, such as ointment or petroleum jelly, gauze that is left on for at least 48 hours until the tract is totally healed. Rather than placing the patient in the Trendelenburg position, it is sufficient to have the patient flat in bed during these procedures. The Valsalva maneuver is always necessary, however.

Sepsis

Catheter-related sepsis remains the most dreaded complication of TPN therapy. In the early years of therapy, extraordinarily high rates of infection were reported. A number of studies followed, documenting acceptably low rates of sepsis correlated with careful adherence to aseptic technique and rigid implementation of therapy protocol.[23]

Catheter-related sepsis is caused predominantly by skin contaminants (from skin around the catheter entry area) and from the hands of health care personnel.[6,26] This is evident when those organisms most commonly cultured are identified as skin contaminants (Table 20-11). Bjornson and colleagues have demonstrated a relationship between a threshold number of organisms at the insertion site and colonization of the catheter.[6]

Clearly defining catheter-related sepsis has implications for nursing because the

TABLE 20-11
Catheter Sepsis Rate in Cancer Patients

Patient	Months on Catheterization	Episodes of Sepsis	Diagnosis	Organism	Catheter
DM	74	2	Ovarian	*Candida albicans* *Staphylococcus aureus*	Hickman
EC	14	1	Prostate	*Staphylococcus aureus*	Hickman
TL	20	1	Colon	*Staphylococcus aureus*	Port
HB	8	1	Carcinoid	*Staphylococcus epidermidis*	Hickman

(Reprinted with permission of Clinical Homecare, Ltd.)

sepsis is usually caused by organisms at the catheter insertion site that migrate along the catheter, rather than from in-line contamination.

Ideally, we want to be able to assess the effectiveness of care and prevent *avoidable* complications. Nurses are also primarily responsible for obtaining the updated data that provide more sensitive and accurate diagnostic indications of catheter-related sepsis. These data are partially derived from the results of semiquantitative cultures of catheter insertion sites and catheter tips.

Nutritional IV lines should be placed specifically for administration of TPN. Nurses should infuse TPN solutions only through a new catheter placed exclusively for this purpose. The nutritional IV system should not be used for central venous pressure monitoring, withdrawal of blood, "piggyback" infusions of medication, or IV bolus injection of drugs. Dual-lumen catheters have facilitated these goals of patient care.

Nurses have an important role in quality control because they are often first to witness an in-use violation, which renders the catheter unacceptable for TPN therapy. At some medical centers, a method of surveillance has been initiated that encourages staff nurses to call the nutrition support team and report any such violations.

Teaching programs should constantly remind staff that TPN patients are extremely susceptible to infection, especially fungal sepsis. This keeps the general level of staff awareness high.

The nurse should take certain steps when a TPN patient experiences a temperature elevation. All patients should have their temperature taken carefully every 6 hours. Any elevation in temperature should be a warning. Generally, a fever is considered to be a reading of 100°F (37.7°C) orally or 101°F (38.3°C) rectally. Certain drugs and disease states suppress the normal febrile response and affected patients must be assessed individually.

When an afebrile patient has a dramatic and unexpected temperature elevation, the entire IV system should be changed immediately, including the catheter. The system should be cultured to rule out solution contamination. A new container of TPN fluid should be hung through new tubing. If new TPN solution is unavailable, 10% dextrose in water, with insulin when appropriate, may be substituted to avoid rebound hypoglycemia. A complete "fever work-up," including a thorough history, physical examination, and culturing should be done. If no other source for the fever is obvious, the catheter should be removed and cultured. Immediate removal of the catheter is necessary because a dramatic, unabating temperature spike in a patient without an obvious reason for it could implicate the catheter and possibly result in septic shock if the source is not removed.

Typically, catheter sepsis presents as a low-grade fever for several days, progressing gradually to a high fever. Again, a complete fever work-up is necessary, although intervention varies with clinical findings and laboratory results. In all cases of suspected sepsis, the nurse should immediately notify the physician when fever presents and should participate in the thorough culturing necessary to determine the etiology of the fever. Thorough culturing includes urine, sputum, wound drainage, feces, blood, and invasive line sites. If possible, semiquantitative cultures of skin sites around catheter insertion sites and catheter tips should be done. Semiquantitative counts of organisms at the skin site or on the catheter tip yield important information that helps prevent the misinterpretation of "skin contamination, not catheter sepsis" when results are positive. For example, *Staphylococcus epidermidis* is a common skin contaminant of bacterial cultures, but it can also be a dangerous pathogen. If the skin site is growing abundant and unexpected numbers of this organism, infection is to be suspected. On the other hand, without the semiquantitative technique, results are merely qualitative, that is, positive or negative, and not especially useful as a diagnostic indicator.

Whether to continue therapy or remove the catheter is the physician's decision and varies with the patient's clinical status, culture results, and the nature of the offending organism. Some physicians now leave TPN catheters in when gram-negative bacteremia exists, treating the patient with the appropriate antibiotic. In an attempt to eradicate the septicemia before pulling the line, gram-positive bacteremia and fungemia require catheter removal and treatment as indicated before reinstitution of TPN therapy. Many TPN patients are compromised hosts and are particularly susceptible to fungal infection. Whenever this possibility exists, it is necessary to differentiate between colonization and deep tissue invasion, for example, of invasive candidiasis. Total parenteral nutrition should not be administered to a patient with deep tissue fungal invasion.

Misdirection

The chest radiograph taken after catheter insertion may show the catheter to be coiled, looped, in the opposite subclavian vein, in smaller vessels, or headed up into the jugular vein. All of these situations will require catheter repositioning. This is usually done by redirecting the catheter with a guidewire under fluoroscopy.

Arrhythmias

Various cardiac arrhythmias can be precipitated by the guidewire or the catheter, causing irritation to the myocardium. Repositioning the guidewire (during the insertion process) or repositioning the catheter after insertion will correct this problem.

Caval Perforation

This rare complication of central line placement may occur if the catheter erodes through the superior vena cava. Diagnosis is made when the chest radiography shows widening of the mediastinum and when there is no blood return from the line. Catheter removal will correct this potentially lethal complication if discovered early.

Metabolic Disturbances

The first principle of metabolic support in TPN therapy is the correct provision of all nutrients. Support solutions contain glucose, amino acids, electrolytes, minerals, vitamins, and trace elements. Intolerance to or insufficient amounts of any of these solution components can result in deficiency states or metabolic aberrations.

Be aware of the signs and symptoms that accompany fluid and electrolyte imbalance and vitamin and trace element deficiency and toxicity. Most commonly, however, metabolic complications of TPN therapy are associated with glucose imbalance.

In most adults, the maximum rate of glucose utilization is 0.8 to 1.0 g/kg body weight per hour. This means that some patients can tolerate constant IV infusion of the large glucose load found in hyperalimentation solutions without the assistance of exogenous insulin. As the highly concentrated glucose infusion is initiated, a pancreatic beta cell response occurs, creating the frequently found increased serum insulin levels. Initial infusions should begin slowly, usually at an approximate rate of 60 to 80 mL/hr for the average-weight adult. A gradual increase in flow rate, approximately 25 mL/hr per day, allows the pancreas to establish and maintain the increased insulin production necessary.

Glucose tolerance may, however, be compromised by sepsis, stress, shock, hepatic and renal failure, starvation, diabetes, pancreatic disease, and administration of some medications, particularly, certain steroids, diuretics, and tranquilizers. Age is another variable; the elderly and the very young are particularly susceptible to glucose intolerance. For these patients, administration of exogenous insulin often is necessary. Conversely, when the patient's illness induces a hypermetabolic state, and daily caloric utilization is accelerated, glucose tolerance may exceed 0.8 to 1.0 g/kg per hour (Table 20-12).

Urinary Glucose Measurement

Urine should be tested for sugar and acetone content every 6 hours around the clock. During the initial period of TPN, as glucose tolerance becomes established, glycosuria is not uncommon. Glycosuria should not be allowed to persist without clinical evaluation and treatment. Urinary sugar content greater than 2 + requires a serum glucose test to determine the exact concentration of sugar present. Because 4 + urinary sugar is an open-ended value, the serum glucose level should be measured immediately whenever this condition exists.

Treatment is directed to the cause of the glucose intolerance. Some patients require a reduction in initial infusion rates and then proceed to tolerance, which never requires exogenous insulin during therapy. Others require administration of insulin as needed.

Glycosuria may exist secondary to hypokalemia because potassium deficiency can cause glucose intolerance. This demonstrates the need for careful maintenance of the serum potassium level.

Certain drugs render a false positive result when the urinary glucose determinations are done by the copper reduction method (Clinitest). These drugs include the cephalosporins, vitamin C (in high doses), aspirin and other salicylates (in high doses), Aldomet (in high doses), Benemid, injectable tetracycline, Chloromycetin, and levodopa (in high doses).

To avoid false negative readings with the glucose oxidase method (Tes-Tape) of determining urinary glucose, the nurse should pay careful attention to a band of color

(text continues on page 370)

TABLE 20-12
Potential Metabolic Complications Associated with Total Parenteral Nutrition

Cause(s)	Prevention	Treatment
Hyperglycemia		
Carbohydrate intolerance → too rapid infusion of TPN	Urine S/A q8h	Decrease TPN rate or dextrose concentration of solution
Insulin resistance → stress, sepsis, diabetes	Accuchecks q6h	Add insulin to the solution and/or use sliding scale insulin coverage
	Be aware of meds that may cause glucose intolerance (ie, steroids)	Add lipids daily to prescription
	Start TPN infusion slowly	
Hypoglycemia		
Interruption of TPN infusion	Wean or slow down TPN infusion when stopping	Hang 10% D/W at same rate of TPN if unable to hang TPN
Excessive insulin administration	Hang 10% D/W at same rate of TPN if unable to hang TPN	Give IV glucose STAT. 50% dextrose may be needed. Maintain proper flow rate
	Maintain infusion rate; use an EID	
	Monitor urine/serum glucose levels	
Hyperglycemic Hyperosmolar Nonketotic coma		
Untreated glucose intolerance causes hyperosmolar diuresis, electrolyte imbalances, coma, death (40% mortality rate)	Appropriate glucose monitoring	Discontinue TPN insulin as needed
	Frequent chemistry profiles to assess electrolytes, osmolarity	Correct electrolyte imbalances
		Treat with hypotonic saline solution
Hyperkalemia		
Excessive potassium replacement	Monitor serum potassium	Stop or decrease potassium in solution
Renal disease—potassium cannot be excreted	Anticipate that a sodium deficiency may lead to hyperkalemia	Monitor pulse for changes (bradycardia)
Leakage of potassium from cells following severe trauma	Start TPN in stable patients	In severe hyperkalemia, dialysis may be necessary
	Accurate I/O to evaluate fluid balance	
Hypokalemia		
Excessive potassium losses (increase GI losses following diarrhea	Monitor serum potassium	Add potassium to TPN solution
Diuretic therapy	Anticipate potential potassium depletion with large GI losses	May need additional IVPB potassium run over 4–6 hr to correct severe deficiency
Large doses of insulin	Monitor I/O	Monitor pulse for tachycardia/arrythmia. Monitor for metabolic alkalosis (potassium loss may cause sodium retention)
	Be aware of drugs that cause excessive potassium loss	
	Be aware that patients severely malnourished are susceptible (refeeding syndrome)	
Hypernatremia		
Dehydration	Maintain I/O	Provide salt-free solution until corrected
Diarrhea	Monitor serum sodium	Provide enough free water to meet needs
Diabetes insipidus	Be aware of drugs that cause sodium retention (ie, steroids)	Treat or correct cause (ie, diarrhea)
Excessive replacement		

(continued)

TABLE 20-12   *(Continued)*

Cause(s)	*Prevention*	*Treatment*
Hyponatremia		
Diuretics	Accurate I/O	Give 3%–5% sodium chloride IV
GI loss (vomiting or fistula)	Urine specific gravity	Add sodium to TPN solution
Disease states (*ie*, renal failure/cirrhosis)	Accurate weights (to ensure fluid shifts)	Minimize GI loss (*ie*, vomiting if possible with medication)
Hyperphosphatemia		
Renal insufficiency	Accurate I/O	Low or no phosphate added
Excessive replacement	Specific gravity	Switch to renal failure formula
	Urine S/A help to access renal function	
Hypophosphatemia		
Insulin therapy	Monitor chemistry profile	Replace phosphate in TPN
Disease states Alcoholism Respiratory alkalosis Renal problems Severe diarrhea Malabsorption associated with low calcium and low magnesium levels	Be aware of potential disease states that cause low phosphate levels	Replace calcium as needed (repletion may cause calcium to drop)
Hypercalcemia		
Pancreatitis inactive/immobile patient excessive replacement	Monitor serum level Be aware of potential problems in immobile patient	Decrease calcium replacement in TPN
Hypocalcemia		
Vitamin D deficiency	Monitor serum levels	Replace by adding calcium to TPN, may require IVPB of calcium to correct severe deficiency; must also correct phosphate/magnesia to correct calcium
Insufficient replacement	Be aware of disease states, medications, malnutrition can cause hypophosphatemia	
Pancreatitis		
Hypomagnesia hypophosphatemia		
Metabolic acidosis		
Renal insufficiency	Monitor CO_2, potassium, sodium	Give bicarbonate
Diabetic ketoacidosis	To assess kidney function: accurate I/O, specific gravity, urine S/A	Monitor vital signs
Diarrhea		Decrease potassium in TPN solution to control diarrhea
Ureteral diversions		
Lactic acidosis (shock)		
Potassium excess		
Metabolic alkalosis		
Body fluid losses (vomiting)	Monitor serum, CO_2, potassium, chloride	Give ammonium chloride to replace chloride/potassium
Potassium deficit		Monitor vital signs
Chloride deficit		Control vomiting if possible

S/A, sugar/acetone; I/O, daily intake and output; GI, gastrointestinal; IVPB, IV piggyback

that might appear across a portion of the wet tape, even if the total wet surface has not changed color. The color of the band will demonstrate a true positive test in these cases. The glucose oxidase test may yield both false positive and false negative results when the patient is taking Pyridium; the Clinitest should be used for these patients.

Urinary sugar measurements are continued every 6 hours throughout therapy. A patient may become glucose intolerant at any time because of the previously mentioned conditions. Without this testing, hyperglycemia can exist undetected. Remember that glycosuria may be the first sign of sepsis. Serum glucose levels should be determined daily until the maintenance flow rate has been achieved. Thereafter, twice-weekly determinations should continue while the patient is receiving TPN. (See Chapter 26.)

Insulin Administration

When exogenous insulin is required, the dosage may be based on the urinary sugar level. This presupposes that the physician has determined the patient's renal threshold and knows the serum correlate for the particular level of glycosuria. Some forms of renal disease (*eg*, acute tubular necrosis) render urinary glucose measurements meaningless as an indicator of blood sugar concentration. A person with acute tubular necrosis can have, for instance, a blood sugar value greater than 1000 mg/100 mL and yield a negative urinary sugar test.

Regular insulin is usually added directly to the TPN solution. Amino acids in TPN are thought to bind a significant amount of the insulin. Patients have been benefitting from this method of IV insulin administration since the advent of TPN therapy. It is preferable to administer insulin through the solution because it provides a more constant serum insulin level than does periodic subcutaneous administration.

Flow Rates

The TPN solutions should be infused at a constant rate as ordered. Too-rapid infusion of these highly concentrated dextrose solutions can cause a hyperglycemic reaction or even hyperosmolar, nonketotic coma. The flow rate should not be adjusted to compensate for past increases or decreases in rate, but always should be reset to the rate ordered. The use of electronic infusion devices ensures accuracy.

When choosing the electronic infusion device, the nurse must be aware of the advantages and disadvantages that each device offers. It is particularly important to avoid pumps that are capable of generating high output pressure, which may result in a rupture of the IV system, thus creating the potential for air embolism and contamination.

Documentation

Accurate daily weights, measured at the same time of day, using the same scale, and with the patient wearing the same clothing, are important. Intake and output data should also be scrupulously recorded. Without this information, it is difficult for the physician to calculate and meet the nutritional needs of the patient.

Hypoglycemia

Hypoglycemia is chemically defined as a serum glucose level of less than 50 mg/100 mL. Many patients are asymptomatic at this level, and the disorder is identified only during routine blood chemistry studies. If patients complain of weakness, headache, chills, tingling in the extremities or mouth, cold and clammy skin, thirst, hunger, apprehension, or all of these, they may be manifesting initial signs of hypoglycemia. Other symptoms include diaphoresis, decreased levels of consciousness, and changes in vital signs. Hypoglycemia can progress to a seizure disorder if untreated.

Treatment depends on the cause. Hypoglycemia often occurs in the TPN patient whose glucose infusion has been abruptly decreased or terminated. After solution flow interruption, serum insulin levels remain elevated longer than serum glucose levels, and this can cause an insulin rebound phenomenon. If a catheter becomes kinked, the flow rate is decreased. If a patient unknowingly bends the IV tubing during position change, the flow rate will decrease and may even stop.

When a patient is transported to another area of the hospital (*eg*, for testing), it is important to ensure continuity of solution flow rate. Nursing personnel in the area of destination should be alerted so that they may become responsible for flow rate maintenance.

Hyperglycemia and Hyperosmolarity

When the body's ability to metabolize the glucose in TPN solutions is inadequate, hyperglycemia occurs. Initial glucose intolerance has already been discussed. However, unchecked, progressive glucose intolerance can lead to the life-threatening complication of hyperglycemic, hyperosmolar, nonketotic coma. Marked hyperglycemia and glycosuria may lead to an osmotic diuresis accompanied by dehydration, electrolyte imbalance, and a decreasing level of consciousness that can result in a comatose state, leading to death, if untreated. Reversal of this state requires immediate discontinuation of the TPN solution, aggressive fluid and electrolyte replacement, and correction of hyperglycemia by insulin administration and correction of acidosis with bicarbonates.

CARE AND MAINTENANCE

Dressing Change Procedures

Many procedural variations of catheter site care are equally effective and practical. The following procedure, based on the original method of JoAnn Grant and Stanley Dudrick, is still widely used.

A sterile dressing change kit is brought to the bedside and not opened until needed. Prepackaged kits are efficient because they eliminate collecting and preparing material in an unclean area and provide the correct equipment. If procedural instructions are enclosed in the kits, they provide the additional advantage of a teaching aid.

Method

Before the procedure is begun, the bedside table is cleansed with an antiseptic solution. The nurse then puts on a mask and washes his or her hands before beginning the dressing change. A mask should also be worn by the patient unless doing so will compromise the patient's respiratory function. The nurse wears sterile gloves and uses a sterile clamp to hold the solution-wet swabs.

First, the nurse scrubs the catheter insertion site with acetone, a defatting agent. Acetone should be applied repeatedly until the prepping sponges come away free of debris. The second prepping solution applied is tincture of iodine, used because of its antifungal and antibacterial properties. It is applied for 2 minutes, timed by a watch, and allowed to air dry before removal. Third, alcohol is applied continuously until all the iodine, which may cause irritation or burning if left on the skin, is removed. The alcohol should be allowed to air dry naturally without fanning or blotting.

The method of prepping used should emphasize the "clean-to-dirty" technique. The area should be prepared in concentric circles (Figure 20-4), beginning at the catheter insertion site and moving out to the periphery. A sponge that has touched the periphery should never be returned to the center. Careful attention must be given to cleaning the catheter and all its parts.

Topical antimicrobial ointment is applied to the catheter insertion site. The site is then covered with two small gauze sponges. The exposed skin is sprayed with tincture of benzoin, which toughens the skin and prevents breakdown of tissue, and allowed to dry. Some catheters are left in for a long time, but even with dressing changes every 48 hours, there will be little trouble with skin irritation if the skin has been carefully protected.

Gauze pads may be covered with transparent semipermeable dressings and treated as a tape-and-gauze application. TSM dressings are also frequently used.

Dressing material is handled so that the side touching the patient's skin is not touched by the nurse (Figure 20-5). The dressing is placed over the sponges in an air-occlusive manner, and the edges are sealed with tape.

A slit piece of tape may be placed up under the catheter hub to ensure occlusion of the dressing and to allow the nurse easy access to the hub when it is time to change the IV tubing.

Secure all junctions using junction-securement devices and tape securely (Figure 20-6).

Some useful hints about the dressing are as follows:

1. If the patient is sensitive to acetone as a defatting agent, alcohol may be substituted. Alcohol's value as a prepping agent is now under consideration.[21]

2. If the patient is iodine sensitive, povidone–iodine solution may be used. When povidone–iodine is applied, it should not be removed with alcohol because this can cause skin irritation. It should air dry and remain on the skin.

3. If tincture of benzoin irritates the patient's skin, or if it is contraindicated as it is with some of the newer dressing materials, try other adhesive sprays or skin prep materials.

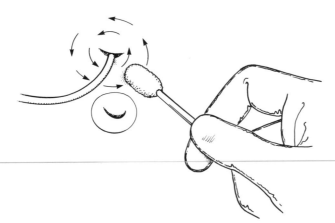

FIGURE 20-4 The area for catheter insertion is prepared in concentric circles.

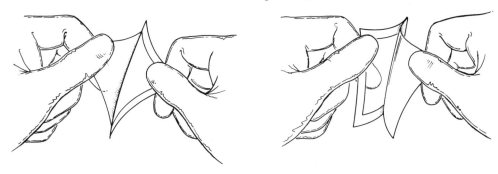

FIGURE 20-5 Handling dressing materials.

When the procedure is completed, the nurse documents it in the patient's chart. Any relevant condition is mentioned and the appropriate care plan is outlined. If erythema, edema, skin ulceration, or drainage exists, action must be taken immediately. If skin ulceration or purulent drainage is present, the physician should order appropriate cultures, and the catheter should be removed immediately.

Certification

Methods of "certifying" nurses to change TPN dressings are practiced nationwide. Preparation for certification entails witnessing a dressing change, reading the TPN literature, and attending an orientation session. The nurse then changes a dressing under the supervision of one of the nutrition support nurses or someone else who is authorized to certify. When the procedure has been performed satisfactorily, the nurse achieves certification. Some clinicians feel strongly that dressing changes should be done only by the nutritional support nurses. This is most desirable; when it is not possible, however, a method of certification may be helpful in ensuring rigidly controlled, standardized care.

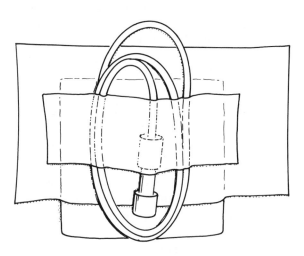

FIGURE 20-6 Completed dressing.

Intravenous Tubing and Filter Change

The IV tubing and filters should be changed every 24 hours according to INS Standards. It is most efficient to standardize the time of tubing, filter, and container changes for when the current day's supply expires and the next day's solutions have arrived in the clinical area. By changing the tubing and filter at the same time that the new container is hung, an additional break in the line is eliminated.

If a filter is used, its porosity should be 0.2 μm or less to effectively retain bacteria, fungi, and particulate matter. Many filters now available also have the ability to eliminate air. The method of filling the filter varies with different brands and is included on package instructions. Total nutrient admixture requires the use of a 1.2-μm filter.

There is *always* the risk of contamination when IV tubing is changed. Therefore, precautions must be taken. If the distal tip of the tubing has touched anything other than the inside of the catheter hub, it is contaminated and should be replaced. If changing the IV tubing is difficult, a small sterile sponge placed beneath the catheter hub will help to prevent accidental contamination of the IV tubing. This is an important step in maintaining asepsis.

During an IV tubing change, the patient should be lying flat in bed. When the catheter is open to the air, the patient should be instructed to perform the Valsalva maneuver. This maneuver enhances positive pressure of the central vessels, thereby decreasing the chance of accidental air embolism.

PREPARATION OF THE PATIENT FOR HOME PARENTERAL NUTRITION

Administration of HTPN may seem overwhelming to the patient and the family. The complexity of procedures may be difficult to handle. The amount of teaching done in the inpatient environment may be nominal because of precipitous discharge, changes in orders, or change in condition of the patient.

Home TPN may be administered as a continuous or cyclic infusion and as a standard formula with or without benefit of supplemental fat emulsion or as a triple-mix (3:1) solution. Regardless of the method chosen for a specific patient, the teaching program should be individualized for a patient's learning needs and homecare environment.

Patient teaching guides should be in place to facilitate the teaching process and to ensure confidence on the part of the patient and the family. At the minimum, teaching plans should encompass the following:

1. How to manage supplies (refrigeration, electricity, grounding requirements, battery power, emergency electronic infusion device replacement, reordering and maintaining inventory, disposal and safe handling)

2. How to prepare a work area (storage, work area, handwashing, principles of asepsis)

3. Catheter care (cap changing, clamping techniques, access of implanted devices, dressing changes, flushing techniques, problem solving and trouble shooting)

4. Administration of TPN and lipid emulsion (scheduling the infusion, handling electronic flow control devices and related equipment, rate changes, tapering, checking the solution, preparing additives, adding insulin or other drugs to the

solution, vitamin administration, connecting to the vascular device, disconnecting tubing from the catheter, method of delivering lipid emulsions)

5. Monitoring one's progress (patient drug information, knowledge of side effects and symptoms, recording of vital signs, accurate glucose determinations, urine sampling, intake and output). See Figure 20-7 for a sample home health record and guidelines for use.

6. Emergency interventions (problem solving for hypoglycemia, hyperglycemia, possible infection, overhydration)

The patient will have many questions, and answers should be provided before the patient leaves the inpatient setting.

Home Health Record

Guidelines For Patient TPN Home Health Record
This form will be available to the Home Health Nurse to help monitor patient's progress.

1. Patient's name.
2. Enter date daily.
3. Enter weight daily (same time).
4. Enter temperature reading twice a day.
5. Enter urine results (if appropriate) per physician's order.
6. Enter blood sugar value (if appropriate) per physician's order.
7. Enter amount of TPN infused.
8. Enter rate/amount of lipids infused.
9. Enter oral intake.
10. Enter urine output.
11. Enter other output.
12. Enter stool frequency/consistency.
13. Note dressing change by a check mark in the box. Indicate appearance of site by use of the key letter:
    C = clean/dry
    R = red
    D = drainage
    P = pain
    S = swelling
    L = loose
14. Enter information as noted in parentheses.
15. Enter any other situations/problems not addressed.
16. Save this record for Home Health Nurse.

A

Name:					
Date:					
Weight: _____lbs. _____kg.					
Temperature: a.m. p.m.					
Urine: A Sugar and acetone M P M					
Blood Sugar:					
Intake Rate/amount of TPN infused (cc's/24 hours)					
Lipids					
Albumin					
Antibiotics					
Oral fluid intake/24 hours (Total cc's)					
Output - Urine Other output (cc's) Type					
Stool frequency/ consistency L/F					
Dressing changed/site: C = clean/dry R = red D = drainage P = pain S = swelling L = loose					
General: (include problems, appetite, how you feel, foods eaten, supply problems, etc.)					

B

FIGURE 20-7 Home health record and guidelines for use for patient receiving TPN at home. (Courtesy: Midwestern Regional Medical Center, Zion, IL)

Arrangements for a home infusion provider should be determined as early as possible. Ideally, the home infusion nurse will visit the patient and family in the hospital to establish rapport, discuss learning needs, feelings, status, and the regimen ordered by the physician.

Standards of Practice for parenteral nutrition in the hospital also apply in the alternative care setting. Administration sets should be changed at 24-hour intervals. A 0.2-μm filter should be used unless 3:1 solution is being administered; then, a 1.2-μm filter is appropriate.

Infection is a common complication because the TPN solution is rich in nutrients, making it an excellent growth medium for microorganisms. The type of catheter may also influence the possibility of infection.

The patient should be taught to self-monitor for all signs and symptoms addressed in an inpatient clinical setting, including hyperglycemia and hypoglycemia. A patient receiving HTPN may be at risk for development of fluid overload. The patients should be taught to report edema, excessive weight gain, shortness of breath, and prominent neck veins.

The danger of possible air embolism is inherent. To prevent this complication, instruct the patient not to use scissors near the catheter; use only a soft-jaw clamp, tape all connections securely or use junction-securement devices, and keep an emergency repair kit in the home.

The patient should be familiar with the operation and maintenance of the electronic infusion device. A stationary pump will be used for ongoing infusion; a portable, ambulatory pump is preferred for cyclic therapy. The home infusion provider (see Chapter 26) should be available on a 24-hour basis for potential pump problems.

The benefits of HTPN clearly outweigh the risks, and patients today enjoy new freedoms and near-normal life-styles as a result of this added dimension to nutritional support therapy.

REFERENCES

1. Alexander, W. J., & Peck, M. D. (1991). Future considerations for nutrition. In J. E. Fischer (Ed.). *Total parenteral nutrition.* Boston: Little, Brown, p. 0294.

2. Aubanic, R. (1952). L'injection intraveineuse souse claviculaire. Advantage et technique. *Presse Medicale, 60,* 1456.

3. Barbul, A. (1991). Measurements of relevant nutrition data for determining efficacy of nutritional support. In J. E. Fisher (Ed.). *Total parenteral nutrition.* Boston: Little, Brown, pp. 153–164.

4. Bistrian, B. R., Blackburn, G. L., Vitale, J., & Cochran, D. (1976). Prevalence of malnutrition in general medical patients. *Journal of the American Medical Association, 235*(15), 1567.

5. Bistrian, B. R., Blackburn, G. L., Hallowell, E., & Heddle, R. (1974). Protein status of general surgical patients. *Journal of the American Medical Association, 230*(6), 858–860.

6. Bjornson, H. S., Colley, R., Bower, R. H., Doty, V. P., Schwartz-Fulton, J. T., & Fischer, J. E. (1982). Association between micro organism growth at catheter insertion site and colonization of the catheter in patients receiving TPN. *Surgery, 92,* 720.

7. Blackburn, G. L., Bistrian, B. R., Maini, B. S., Schlamm, H. T., & Smith, M. F. (1977). Nutritional and metabolic assessment of the hospitalized patient. *Journal of Parenteral and Enteral Nutrition, 1*(1), 11–22.

8. Church, J. M., & Hill, G. L. (1987). Assessing the efficacy of intravenous nutrition in general surgical patients: Dynamic nutritional assessment with plasma proteins. *Journal of Parenteral and Enteral Nutrition, 11,* 135.

9. Curtas, S. (1988). Nutritional assessment. In C. Kennedy-Caldwell & P. Guenter (Eds.). *Nutrition Support Nursing Core Curriculum* (2nd ed.), Silver Spring, MD: Aspen.

10. Dudrick, S. J. (1977). The genesis of intravenous hyperalimentation. *Journal Parenteral and Enteral Nutrition, 1,* 23.

11. Elman, R., & Weiner, D. O. (1939). Intravenous alimentation with special reference to protein (amino acid) metabolism. *Journal of the American Medical Association, 122,* 796.

12. Fletcher, J. P., Little, J. M., & Quest, P. K. (1987). A comparison of serum transferrin and serum prealbumin as nutritional parameters. *Journal of Parenteral and Enteral Nutrition, 11,* 144.

13. Flowers, J. F., Ryan, J. A., Jr., & Grough, J. (1991). Catheter related complications of total parenteral nutrition. In J. E. Fischer (Ed.). *Total parenteral nutrition.* Boston: Little, Brown, pp. 25–36.

14. Frisancho, A., & Flegel, P. (1983). Elbow breadth as a measure of frame size for US males and females. *American Journal of Clinical Nutrition, 37,* 311–314.

15. Hill, G. L. (1991). Nutritional assessment. In J. E. Fischer (Ed.). *Total parenteral nutrition.* Boston: Little, Brown, pp. 139–142.

16. Imperial, J., Bistrian, B. R., Bothe, A., Jr., Bern, M., & Blackburn, G. L. (1983). Limitation of central vein thrombosis in TPN by continuous infusion of low dose heparin. *Journal American College of Nutrition, 2,* 63.

17. Jeejeboy, K. (1976). Total parenteral nutrition. *Annals of the Royal College of Physicians and Surgeons of Canada, 9,* 287–300.

18. Kennedy-Caldwell, C. (1988). Substrate metabolism, vitamins. In C. Kennedy-Caldwell & P. Guenter (Eds.). *Nutrition Support Nursing Core Curriculum* (2nd ed., pp. 93–103), Silver Spring, MD: Aspen.

19. Kinney, J. M. (1991). Energy requirements for parenteral nutrition. In Fischer, J. E. (Ed.). *Total parenteral nutrition.* Boston: Little, Brown, pp. 181–187.

20. Knox, L. S. (1988). Nutritional requirements. In C. Kennedy-Caldwell & P. Guenter (Eds.). *Nutrition Support Nursing Core Curriculum* (2nd ed., p. 18), Silver Spring, MD: Aspen.

21. Lindner, P., & Lindner, D. (1991). How to assess degrees of fatness. In A. Grant & S. DeHoog. *Nutritional assessment and support* (1991, 4th ed.). Seattle: Grant and DeHoog.

22. Multivitamin preparations for parenteral use: A statement by the Nutrition Advisory Group. (1979). *Journal of Parenteral and Enteral Nutrition, 3,* 258.

23. Nelson, D. B., Kien, C. L., Mohr, B., Frank, S., & Davis, S. D. (1986). Dressing changes by specialized personnel reduce infection rates in patients receiving central venous parenteral nutrition. *Journal of Parenteral and Enteral Nutrition, 10,* 220.

24. Sax, H. C., Hasselgren, P-O. (1991). Indications. In J. E. Fischer (Ed.). *Total parenteral nutrition.* Boston: Little, Brown, p. 3.

25. Seltzer, F. (1983). Metropolitan height–weight tables. *Dietetic Currents, 10,* 17.

26. Sitzmann, J. V., Townsend, T. R., Siler, M. C., & Bartlett, J. G. (1985). Septic and technical complications of central venous catheterization: A prospective study of 200 consecutive patients. *Annals of Surgery, 202,* 766.

27. Torosian, M. H., & Daly, J. M. (1991). Solutions available. In J. E. Fischer (Ed.). *Total parenteral nutrition.* Boston: Little, Brown, pp. 13–15.

28. Twomey, P., Ziegler, D., & Rombleau, J. (1982). Utility of skin testing in nutritional assessment: A critical review. *Journal of Parenteral and Enteral Nutrition, 6,* 50.

29. Wilmore, D. W., & Dudrick, S. J. (1968). Growth and development of an infant receiving all nutrients exclusively by vein. *Journal of the American Medical Association, 203,* 860.

30. Wolfe, B. M., & Ney, D. M. (1986). Lipid metabolism in parenteral nutrition. In J. L. Rombeau & M. D. Caldwell (Eds.). *Parenteral nutrition,* Vol. 2. Philadelphia: W. B. Saunders.

REVIEW QUESTIONS

1. Which of the following porosity ratings is appropriate for use with total nutrient admixture solution?

   a. 0.2 μm

   b. 1.0 μm

   c. 1.2 μm

   d. 2.0 μm

2. Which of the following are fat-soluble vitamins?

   a. A, B, D, K

   b. A, C, E, K

   c. A, D, E, K

   d. A, B, C, D

3. Which of the following is indicative of marasmus?
   a. 120% IBW Albumin 2.4 Prealbumin = 13
   b. 120% IBW Albumin 3.9 Prealbumin = 25
   c. 80% IBW Albumin 2.4 Prealbumin = 13
   d. 80% IBW Albumin 3.8 Prealbumin = 25

4. A urinary urea nitrogen (UUN) is needed to for which of the following reasons?
   a. to determine kidney function
   b. to determine efficacy of nutritional support
   c. to determine protein calorie malnutrition
   d. to determine protein tolerance

5. Each gram of carbohydrate (CHO) yields how many kilocalories?
   a. 3.4
   b. 4
   c. 7
   d. 9

6. Each gram of fat yields how many kilocalories?
   a. 4.3
   b. 5
   c. 7
   d. 9

7. 10% lipid emulsion provides how many calories per mL?
   a. 1.0
   b. 1.1
   c. 2.0
   d. 2.2

8. The percentage of non-protein calories to fat should not exceed which of the following values?
   a. 50%
   b. 60%
   c. 65%
   d. 70%

9. A primary cause of catheter-related sepsis in the patient receiving TPN is which of the following?
   a. contaminated TPN solution
   b. skin contamination
   c. fibrin sheath formation
   d. infection from another source in the body

10. The non-protein calorie to nitrogen ratio most appropriate for the highly stressed patient is which of the following?
    a. 60 : 1
    b. 100 : 1
    c. 150 : 1
    d. 200 : 1

CHAPTER 21

Transfusion Therapy

During the past 5 years, many changes have occurred in transfusion therapy, partly because of the concentration on preventing transfusion-associated diseases. Transfusion therapy itself has taken a more definitive title, that of transfusion medicine. The understanding of acquired immunodeficiency syndrome (AIDS) is growing rapidly and brings new concerns to hospitals, patients, and staff, as well as the community. Medical and public education, changes in therapy and technology, and cost are paramount in transfusion medicine today. Various methods of autologous transfusion are being used to preserve the blood supply, decrease costs, and provide safer therapy to the patient.

Rules and regulations governing the procurement, storage, and administration of transfusion therapy have been established through national organizations and the Food and Drug Administration (FDA). Review of transfusion practice is also required by the Joint Commission on Accreditation of Healthcare Organizations (JCAHO). All staff working in this field should be knowledgeable and accountable for their practice.

Nurses administer transfusions in most hospitals and must acquire a greater knowledge base because patients will inquire about this integral part of their treatment. Administration of blood should be performed by competent, experienced, well-qualified personnel. Serious problems and complications that can lead to death and can result in litigation are associated with the administration of blood and its components. The IV nurse shares with the blood bank the responsibility for providing the safest transfusion therapy. Nurses must incorporate the fundamental principles of immunohematology into their daily nursing care; the indications, advantages, and disadvantages of a large variety of components; proper procedures for their safe administration; and the ability to recognize early symptoms of transfusion reactions and appropriate interventions. Being knowledgeable and maintaining the skills of administering blood and components will help decrease the risks in this important therapy.

The community has become more educated and, consequently, patients are questioning their treatment and clinical outcomes. Correct responses must be presented.

BASIC IMMUNOHEMATOLOGY

Immunohematology is the science that deals with antigens of the blood and their antibodies. An *antigen* is a substance capable of stimulating the production of an antibody and then reacting with that antibody in a specific way.

Sharon M. Weinstein: PLUMER'S PRINCIPLES & PRACTICE OF INTRAVENOUS THERAPY, FIFTH EDITION, © 1993 J. B. Lippincott Company

TABLE 21-1
ABO Classification of Human Blood

Group	Cell Antigens A	Cell Antigens B	Plasma Antibodies A	Plasma Antibodies B	% US Population
O	−	−	+	+	45
A	+	−	−	+	40
B	−	+	+	−	10
AB	+	+	−	−	5

The ABO system is the most important group of antigens for transfusion as well as transplantation. The synthesis of these antigens, which are located on the surface of red blood cells, is under the control of the A, B, and O genes. In the presence of the A gene, an individual makes A antigen and is classified as group A. Group B individuals have B antigens on their red blood cells, group AB individuals have both, and group O persons have neither (Table 21-1). These antigens are genetically inherited and determine the blood group of the individual.

The second most clinically important system for transfusion is the Rh system. About 85% of the Caucasian population has the D antigen on their red blood cells and are classified as D or Rh positive. The D antigen is lacking in the 15% of the population classified as Rh negative. Other common antigens in the system are C, E, c, and e.

About 50 other known blood group antigen systems containing about 500 antigens are known. Fortunately only a few systems, such as Kell, Duffy, and Kidd are commonly encountered.

Leukocytes also carry antigens on their surfaces. The most important group of these are human leukocyte antigens (HLA). Individuals who have been exposed to the red blood cells or leukocytes of other people through transfusion or pregnancy (maternal–fetal hemorrhage) may make antibodies to the foreign antigens carried on those cells.

An *antibody* is a protein in the plasma that reacts with a specific antigen. Antibodies are named for the antigen that stimulated their formation and with which they react. For example, an antibody against the D antigen formed after the transfusion of an Rh (D)-positive unit to a Rh (D)-negative recipient is called anti-D. Antibodies formed in response to exposure to foreign antigens are called *immune antibodies*. Some blood group antibodies are formed without exposure to allogenic red blood cells. The most important of these so-called naturally occurring antibodies are anti-A and anti-B. During the first few months of life, infants make IgM antibodies to whichever of the ABO antigens they lack. For example, a group A infant will make anti-B (see Table 21-1). It is these naturally occurring antibodies (the *isoagglutinins*) that can produce rapid hemolysis of red blood cells with the corresponding antigen that form the basis of ABO incompatibility.

MECHANISM OF IMMUNE RESPONSE

When a patient is transfused with allogenic blood bearing "foreign" (ie, non-self) antigens, the immune system may respond by producing antibodies. Phagocytic cells called macrophages play an important role in the defense system of the body. One of their roles in the immune response is to capture and process foreign antigens. It then "presents" the processed antigen to other members of the immune system, namely, the T and B lymphocytes. B cells, with help from T cells, begin to produce antibodies specific for the antigen presented to them by the macrophages. Stimulated by the appropriate foreign antigen, the B cell swells and changes its internal structure and differentiates into plasma cells to produce antibody.[16] Each plasma cell produces large quantities of antibody of the precise specificity and immunoglobulin class genetically programmed into the cell. The antibodies are secreted into a variety of body fluids, including the blood plasma.

The macrophages have also called on the T cells, which act as helpers or suppressors to B cell function. The intertwined relationship between T and B cells regulates the type and sensitivity of the immune response.

MECHANISM OF RED BLOOD CELL DESTRUCTION

Two mechanisms of red blood cell destruction are known: intravascular hemolysis and extravascular hemolysis. *Intravascular hemolysis* occurs within the vascular compartment. This mode of red blood cell destruction is the result of the sequential binding of antibody to a red blood cell with a foreign antigen on its surface. This antibody then fixes complement. If the entire complement cascade is triggered, a lytic complex is formed on the red blood cell membrane, which leads to rupture of the red cell, releasing hemoglobin into the intravascular compartment.

Antibodies that activate complement often agglutinate in vitro and can cause intravascular hemolysis in vivo. The most frequent cause of this type of red blood cell destruction is transfusion of ABO incompatible blood. Anti-A and anti-B are mostly IgM antibodies that are capable of engaging the complement and coagulation and kinin systems when they bind with their corresponding antigen. The consequences of this type of hemolysis are usually immediate and severe and are often fatal.

The other mechanism of red cell destruction, *extravascular hemolysis*, is more commonly seen as a result of incompatibilities in blood group systems other than the ABO system. Antibodies to these other blood group antigens are usually IgG. They bind to red blood cells with the corresponding antigen. Phagocytic cells of the reticuloendothelial system, particularly in the spleen, bind the IgG-coated red blood cells, ingest them, and destroy them extracellularly; hence the term, extravascular hemolysis. These IgG antibodies may also fix some amount of complement, but not enough to lyse the red blood cells. Instead, the complement-coated red blood cells are cleared from the circulation by the phagocytic cells of the liver, the Kupffer cells, and destroyed intracellularly. The consequences following extravascular hemolysis are not as severe as those of intravascular hemolysis but are recognizable by a drop in the hematocrit, an increase in the bilirubin level, and perhaps by the clinical signs of fever or malaise.

BLOOD GROUP SYSTEMS

The best known blood group system is the ABO system, which was discovered by Karl Landsteiner in 1901. Landsteiner described a classification of human blood based on agglutination reactions between the red blood cells and serum. The ABO system is the only system in which the reciprocal antibodies are consistently and predictably present in the sera of normal individuals whose red blood cells lack the corresponding antigen(s). The ABO system is the foundation of pretransfusion testing and compatibility.

In 1939, Levine and Stetson discovered the Rhesus (Rh) system, so called because of its relationship to the substance in the red blood cells of the Rhesus monkey. The Rh system is the second most important system in transfusion therapy. They found an antibody that agglutinated red blood cells in 85% of the individuals tested. The antigen causing the reaction is known as the Rh or D antigen. A person whose red blood cells have the D antigen is classified as Rh positive; lacking the D antigen, Rh negative. Because of the ease with which antibody D is made, grouping is done on all donors and recipients to ensure that D-negative recipients receive D-negative blood, except for reasonable qualifying circumstances. Rh-positive recipients may receive either Rh-positive or Rh-negative blood.

Antibodies to the Rh antigens are not present unless an individual has been exposed to Rh-positive red blood cells, either through transfusion or pregnancy. Individuals who develop Rh antibodies will have detectable levels for many years. If undetected, subsequent exposure may lead to a secondary immune response.

Occasionally, weak variants of the Rh D antigen are found, which are identified by special serologic tests. These individuals are termed weak D or Du positive, but are considered to be Rh positive both as donors and recipients.

Other blood group systems have been defined on the basis of reaction of cells with antibodies. Antibodies to antigens in the Kell, Duffy, Kidd, and Lewis systems are encountered frequently enough to be clinically important. Antibodies to the blood group antigens in most of the other systems are found so infrequently that they do not cause everyday problems. When present, these antibodies may produce hemolytic reactions. Once demonstrated, precautions must be taken to ensure that the patient receives compatible blood lacking the corresponding antigen. When difficulty arises in crossmatching or when a transfusion reaction occurs, these systems acquire special significance.

PRETRANSFUSION TESTING

The Donor

In addition to ABO and Rh group determination, a screen for unexpected antibodies, several other tests are performed on donor blood before it is released for patient use. Donor blood is tested for hepatitis B surface antigen (HBsAg), antibody to human T cell leukemia virus (anti-HTLV-I/II), antibody to hepatitis C virus and a serologic test for syphilis (STS). Antibody to hepatitis B core (anti-HBc) and alanine aminotransferase (ALT) testing are also performed, and no blood component is issued unless the test results are within established limits.

The Recipient

Tests performed on the intended transfusion recipient include ABO and Rh group determination and screen for unexpected antibodies. Before the administration of whole blood or red blood cell components, a major crossmatch (combining donor red blood cells and recipient serum or plasma) is performed to detect serologic incompatibility.

The American Association of Blood Banks (AABB) requires that if a patient has been transfused in the preceding 3 months with blood or a blood component containing red blood cells or has been pregnant within the preceding 3 months or if the history is uncertain or unavailable, the sample must be obtained from the patient within 3 days of the scheduled transfusion.[2] This requirement is made to rule out the possibility that a newly formed antibody is not missed.

In situations in which delay in provision of blood may jeopardize life, blood may be issued before completion of routine tests according to AABB standards.[2]

Recipients whose ABO group is not known must receive group O red blood cells.

Recipients whose ABO group has been determined by the transfusing facility, without reliance on previous record, may receive ABO group-specific whole blood or ABO group-compatible red blood cell components before other tests for compatibility have been completed.

Physicians must indicate in the record that the clinical condition is sufficiently urgent to release blood before compatibility testing is completed; the tag or label must conspicuously indicate that compatibility testing is not completed; and standard compatibility tests should be completed promptly.

ANTICOAGULANTS–PRESERVATIVES

Blood is routinely collected in plastic bags that contain one of two anticoagulant–preservatives. One of the anticoagulant–preservative systems currently used is citrate–phosphate–dextrose–adenine (CPDA-1). Blood collected in this anticoagulant–preservative may be stored for 35 days. The duration for storage is based on the standard that a minimum of 70% of the transfused red blood cells (stored for 35 days) must be present in the bloodstream of the recipient 24 hours after the transfusion. Providing a nutrient biochemical balance to red blood cells during storage is important to maintain viability and function of the components within the blood and to prevent physical changes. To minimize bacterial proliferation, specific temperatures must be maintained.

Each ingredient in the solution has a function. The phosphate acts as a buffer, slowing the drop in pH of the stored cells and improving viability. Sodium citrate, by combining with ionized calcium, inhibits clotting, thus serving as an anticoagulant. Dextrose (glucose) prolongs the life of the red blood cells by providing a nutrient source. Adenine is a substrate from which red blood cells can synthesize adenosine triphosphate (ATP). The red blood cell depends on ATP to maintain cell surface ion pumps.

A second group of anticoagulant–preservative systems is similar to CPDA-1. It differs, however, in that, once the platelet-rich plasma is removed from the unit, an additive solution containing saline, dextrose, and adenine is added to the packed red blood cells. This system permits storage for up to 42 days.

Additional solutions such as pyruvate and other compounds have been licensed and may be added to stored red blood cells nearing the end of their shelf-life. Called "rejuvenated" cells, these additives allow units to be stored even longer.

WHOLE BLOOD

Whole blood contains cells (red blood cells, white blood cells, and platelets), plasma (blood proteins, antibodies, water, and waste), and electrolytes.

Transfusions of whole blood are infrequent but may be indicated when an acute massive blood loss has occurred. Massive hemorrhage is usually defined as a patient

TABLE 21-2
ABO Compatibility for Whole Blood

Recipient	Donor
A	A
B	B
AB	AB
O	O

having more than 25% to 30% blood loss. Acute massive blood loss may result in hypovolemia and shock. The patient requires both oxygen-carrying capacity of the red blood cells and plasma for volume replacement. It is imperative to quickly restore the blood volume to improve oxygen delivery. Crystalloid and colloid solutions will only temporarily correct hypovolemia.

Whole blood, less than 4 to 5 days old, may be indicated for an exchange transfusion in a newborn.

Autologous transfusion, whereby the patient donates blood for himself, is frequently returned to the patient (donor) as a whole blood infusion.

Whole blood has many disadvantages. Patients must receive from their own blood group, which eliminates ABO compatibility between blood groups (Table 21-2).

With the continuous metabolic changes of red blood cells, definite changes take place in stored blood. The potassium leaks out of the cell and into the plasma. Studies have shown that the potassium level rises to approximately 21 mEq/L by day 21 after collection. Infusions of stored whole blood could potentially cause complications to patients with compromised cardiac status or in patients undergoing exchange transfusion. Another problem is the formation of microaggregates. As cells break down, this cellular debris may be detrimental to patients with lung disease, although physicians differ in opinion on the significance of microaggregates. Special filters are available and are designed to protect the infusion of this particulate matter.

Modified whole blood is prepared by removing the plasma, collecting the platelets and/or cryoprecipitate, and then returning the plasma back into the red blood cells. This product may be used for patients with hemorrhage and other clinical conditions when whole blood is warranted. Separate components may additionally be required.

Fresh whole blood, defined as being less than 24 hours old, has no valid indications. Although it contains viable platelets and other coagulation factors, a patient's deficit of these components should be specifically replaced with the component to correct the underlying problem.

Whole blood is stored at a temperature of 1°C (34°F) to 6°C (43°F) for 35 days, depending on anticoagulant–preservative.

The rate of administration for whole blood should be as rapid as necessary to correct and maintain hemodynamic status.

RED BLOOD CELL COMPONENTS

Packed Red Blood Cells

Packed red blood cells are prepared by removing approximately 225 to 250 mL of platelet-rich plasma from a unit of whole blood, either by centrifugation or sedimentation. This process packs the red blood cells and separates most of the platelet-rich plasma.

The red blood cell concentrate contains the same red blood cell mass as whole blood, 20% to 30% of the original plasma, and some leukocytes and platelets. Packed red blood cells generally have a hematocrit between 70% and 80%; thus, the viscosity of the unit is increased. One unit of packed red blood cells provides the same amount of oxygen-carrying red blood cells as a unit of whole blood.

The major indication for packed red blood cells is to restore or maintain oxygen-carrying capacity. Because of the reduced volume of the unit, the danger of circulatory overload is less—a definite advantage in patients with renal failure or congestive heart failure.

Because approximately two thirds of the plasma is removed, the patient is not subjected to infusions of additional potassium, citrate, or sodium.

Each unit of packed red blood cells is generally expected to raise the hematocrit 3% and the hemoglobin level 1 g/dL in the average 70-kg person. In infants, the hemoglobin level is expected to rise by 1 g/dL when administered at 3 mL/kg.

The expiration time of packed red blood cells is 35 to 42 days depending on the anticoagulant–preservative used.

Because most of the plasma is removed, thereby reducing the amount of anti-A or anti-B agglutinins (or both), group O may be given to other blood groups. In emergency situations, when time does not permit ABO determination, group O red blood cells may be given (Table 21-3).

Leukocyte-Poor Red Blood Cells

Leukocytes may be removed from red blood cells by several methods, including centrifugation, washing, or filtration. Filtration is the most effective, achieving a 2- to 3-log reduction in leukocytes, and is the method of choice.

Leukocyte-poor red blood cells are used to restore red blood cells to patients who have previously experienced two or more nonhemolytic febrile reactions and who may have developed antibodies against transfused leukocytes. These reactions may be extremely uncomfortable and may last for several hours. The component may also be considered for patients with diseases such as leukemia and aplastic anemia where it is anticipated that multiple transfusions will be administered. These patients are at risk of becoming refractory to platelet transfusions because of the formation of antibodies to leukocyte antigens, such as HLA antigens, which are also found on platelets. Patients who have a history of allergic transfusion reactions and are IgA deficient are also candidates for this component.

Leukocyte-poor red blood cells must be administered within 24 hours after preparation. Increasingly, special high-efficiency leukocyte removal filters are being used at the bedside.

TABLE 21-3
ABO Compatibility for Packed Red Blood Cells

Recipient	Donor
A	A or O
B	B or O
AB	AB, A, B, or O
O	O

The rate of infusion and ABO compatibility are the same as for packed red blood cells.

Frozen–Deglycerolized or Frozen–Stored Red Blood Cells

This component is prepared by freezing red blood cells with a cryoprotectant such as glycerol. The unit is thawed and washed before the transfusion.

Plasma is extracted from the whole blood. The red blood cells are then coated with glycerol. The red blood cells are frozen and stored at $-85°C$ until needed. After thawing, glycerol is removed by a variety of washing procedures. The component should be administered within 24 hours after the washing process occurs. The finished product contains less than 5% of the original donor platelets and leukocytes and has a hematocrit of approximately 80%.

Controversies exist as to the clinical importance and advantages or disadvantages for the use of this component. The major disadvantage is the substantial additional cost related to the process of preparing and storing the component and the cost of personnel involved. Therefore, the major clinical indication for using frozen deglycerolized red blood cells is to preserve blood from donors with rare blood groups. It is also useful to provide a plasma-free red blood cell component to patients who are sensitized to IgA or other plasma proteins. Because of the growing concerns over disease transmission, the increase in autologous donations may produce an increase in the number of units frozen if blood is donated more than 35 to 42 days before being needed.

The rate of infusion and ABO compatibility are the same as packed red blood cells.

Platelets

Platelets are available in two preparations: random donor concentrates made from units of whole blood and single donor concentrates obtained by plateletpheresis of a donor. Platelets contain factor III, a phospholipid that enhances the conversion of prothrombin to thrombin, which forms one of the most important steps in the coagulation process.[9]

Platelet transfusions are indicated for thrombocytopenia caused by uremia, massive loss of blood, chemotherapy, leukemia, and thrombotic thrombocytopenia purpura (TTP). The decision to transfuse platelets must be based on the clinical condition of the patient, the etiology of the thrombocytopenia, and the ability of the patient to produce platelets. Platelet transfusions should not be given on the basis of the number of red blood cells infused, but by the platelet count and signs and symptoms of hemorrhage. Platelets are not indicated for patients with thrombocytopenia secondary to TTP and idiopathic thrombocytopenic purpura (ITP).

Platelet concentrate prepared from whole blood contains a minimum of 5.5×10^{10} platelets in at least 75% of the units tested. Each unit contains about 40 to 70 mL and is expected to increase the platelet count by 5000 to $10,000/\mu L$ in a stabilized patient. Routinely, random donor platelets are transfused. Because of previous exposure to multiple transfusions of platelets, some patients become sensitized and develop platelet-specific and HLA antibodies. These patients are called refractory and are more likely to benefit from single donor platelets. Obtained by the process of plateletpheresis, these platelets may be produced from HLA-matched donors if necessary.[3]

Reactions to platelets may include disease transmission, graft-versus-host disease (GVHD), alloimmunization, febrile or allergic effects, and circulatory overload.

Platelet concentrates do not require crossmatching before infusion. Incompatibility between donor plasma and recipient red blood cells is usually clinically insignificant unless large numbers of platelet transfusions are required or if the patient is a small child. The rate of administration is 5 mL/min.

Specific leukocyte removal filters for platelets are available for effective leukocyte removal at the bedside.

Granulocytes

Granulocytes are obtained by the process of leukapheresis and are infrequently administered. Previously prescribed for gram-negative sepsis, new antibiotic regimens and improved management of infections have decreased the use of this component. Patients with chronic granulomatous disease or profound neutropenia may be candidates for granulocyte transfusion when it is expected that they will recover. These transfusions will only temporarily improve the patient's condition.

Granulocytes are stored at room temperature (20°–24°C; 68°–75°F) no more than 24 hours and preferably less than 6 hours. Because granulocytes are contaminated with donor red blood cells, they must be ABO compatible with the recipient's plasma.

Patients undergoing granulocyte transfusions are acutely ill and adverse effects are not uncommon. Febrile and pulmonary reactions may occur and cytomegalovirus (CMV) transmission is of particular concern.

Granulocytes are administered through a set containing the standard blood filter (80–170 μm) over a 4-hour period for adult and pediatric patients. Microaggregate filters should not be used.

PLASMA

Plasma is the liquid content remaining after the red blood cells have been removed from a unit of whole blood. It contains water, electrolytes, proteins (principally albumin), globulin, and coagulation factors.

Liquid Plasma

Single donor liquid plasma is stored at temperatures between 1°C (34°F) and 6°C (43°F) for no more than 26 days in citrate–phosphate–dextrose or 40 days in CPDA-1.[3]

Plasma plays an important role in the treatment of burns by supplying plasma proteins that are lost from the wound. Some of the clotting factor activity is lost during storage, limiting its use in patients with coagulation problems.

Under ordinary circumstances, single donor plasma should be compatible with the recipient's red blood cells. Because it lacks anti-A and anti-B agglutinins, AB plasma may be used for all ABO groups and in emergencies when the patient's blood group is unknown.

Fresh Frozen Plasma

Fresh frozen plasma (FFP) contains all the normal components of blood plasma including the clotting factors, in addition to 200 to 400 mg fibrinogen. It has a shelf life of 1 year when stored at a temperature of −18°C or lower. The plasma is separated from the cells and frozen within 8 hours of collection from the donor. The unit is kept frozen until the time of transfusion. It is then thawed in a water bath at 37°C (98.6°F) and optimally should be administered within 6 hours but no more than 24 hours after thawing to minimize the loss of the most labile clotting factors, factor V and factor VIII. To provide factors V and VIII, the component should be used within the first year of storage for treatment of coagulation disorders. After 12 months, FFP may be frozen for 4 more years provided it is relabeled "plasma" because it should not be used for correcting coagulation disorders. If cryoprecipitate has been removed from the plasma, the remaining unit must be labeled as such.

Fresh frozen plasma is beneficial to patients with demonstrated multiple coagulation deficiencies or inherited or acquired disorders. Because FFP is an isotonic volume expander, patients receiving multiple units should be monitored closely to prevent fluid overload. Fresh frozen plasma should never be used for volume expansion; this is more safely treated with crystalloid or colloid solutions. They are less expensive than FFP and lack the risk of transmitting disease. Fresh frozen plasma should not be used as a nutrient supplement.

The rate of administration may be 200 mL/hr (the approximate volume of each unit) or less if circulatory overload could be a potential complication. The pediatric rate of infusion should be about 1 to 2 mL/min. Although a crossmatch is not required, the component should be compatible with the recipient's red blood cells (Table 21-4).

Cryoprecipitate

Cryoprecipitate is a concentrate containing factor VIII (antihemophilic factor, AHF) extracted from cold-thawed plasma. It is the cold-insoluble portion of plasma after FFP has been thawed. It contains 80 to 120 U factor VIII, 40% to 70% of the plasma von Willebrand factor (vWF) and 150 to 250 mg fibrinogen in a 20- to 30-mL volume. The component is frozen at $-18°C$ for up to 12 months. It should be administered within 6 hours after thawing. Once thawed, the vWF and fibrinogen remain stable but factor VIII is labile.

In the past, this concentrate was predominately used to treat hemophilia and revolutionized the treatment of this sex-linked bleeding disorder. However, it is associated with the transmission of viral agents and should only be used for specific clinical conditions such as von Willebrand's disease. These patients have a platelet dysfunction and partial deficiency in the ratio of factor VIII to vWF and benefit from infusions of cryoprecipitate. It is the only component available to treat hypofibrinogenemia; previously available fibrinogen products have been withdrawn because of the increased risk of transmitting hepatitis.

For factor VIII replacement, repeated transfusions are required because the half-life of factor VIII is 8 to 12 hours in the circulation. Single units may be pooled into one

TABLE 21-4
ABO Compatibility for Fresh Frozen Plasma

Recipient	Donor
A	A or AB
B	B or AB
AB	AB
O	O, A, B, or AB

container and administered at a rate of 1 to 2 mL/min. Because cryoprecipitate contains few red blood cells, it should be administered under the same guidelines as plasma.

Plasma Derivatives

Normal Serum Albumin and Plasma Protein Fraction

Albumin comprises about 40% of the plasma protein and can be purified from raw plasma by several procedures. It replaces plasma in many clinical conditions. Albumin is available in two concentrations: 5% in 250 mL saline and 25% in 50 mL saline.

Albumin 5% is isotonic, being osmotically equivalent to an approximately equal volume of citrated plasma. It may be used to provide volume and colloid in the treatment of shock and burns. Initially after a burn, large volumes of crystalloid solution are needed to correct extracellular fluid losses because of fluid leakage into the intracellular compartment. Smaller amounts of colloid are required at this time. After 24 hours, large amounts of albumin are required to maintain intravascular volume and avoid hypoproteinemia, while smaller amounts of crystalloid are infused.

Albumin 25% is hypertonic and depends on additional fluids, either drawn from the tissues or administered separately for its maximal osmotic effect; 50 mL of 25% albumin is osmotically equivalent to 250 mL citrated plasma. It must be administered with caution because rapid infusion can result in circulatory overload or interstitial dehydration if administered to severely dehydrated patients without adequate amounts of supplemental fluid. It may be used for protein replacement in severe hypoalbuminemia and infused at a slow rate of 2 to 3 mL/min, adjusted to the patient's condition. Albumin may also be beneficial in newborns with hyperbilirubinemia because it will bind with additional bilirubin and reduce the complication of kernicterus.[14]

Administration of 5% and 25% albumin requires strict aseptic and antiseptic handling. Once the container is entered, it must be used immediately or discarded because albumin has no preservatives. Drugs should not be added to albumin nor should albumin be added to IV solutions. Albumin is a good culture medium and although bacterial contamination is rare, the product should be held, the lot number recorded, and the manufacturer and the FDA notified if reactions are suspected. More frequently, adverse reactions are caused by improper administration. Nursing plays an important role in assessing the patient's clinical condition, evaluating the patient, and ensuring proper rate of administration.

Both products have been heat treated to inactivate the hepatitis virus.

Plasma protein fraction (PPF) is not as highly purified as albumin and consists of 83% albumin and 17% alpha and beta globulins. It is used in a manner similar to albumin 5%. Neither albumin or PPF has any clotting factors and should not be considered "plasma substitutes."

There is no ABO or Rh matching for albumin or PPF.

Factor VIII Concentrate

Concentrates of factor VIII (AHF) are prepared from plasma by a variety of methods. Traditionally, plasma was fractionated by physiochemical techniques to provide factor VIII concentrates. Most recently, factor VIII has been extracted and purified from plasma using monoclonal antibodies to factor VIII. Clinical testing of a recombinant factor VIII is underway, and it should be marketed in the near future.[14] The newer techniques offer a higher activity of AHF and are less likely to transmit disease, but they are more costly. The levels vary, depending on the technique used to make the component but are usually too low to be useful for treating vWF disease. Various processes have been used to inactivate viruses to hepatitis and human immunodeficiency virus (HIV) in these preparations.

The clinical use of factor VIII concentrate is the treatment of hemophilia. The stability of the component allows patients to treat themselves at home and maintain a more normal life-style than they have in the past.

Once reconstituted, factor VIII concentrate should be administered immediately at a rate of 2 mL/min. Use of the administration set provided with the product is recommended.

No ABO or Rh matching is required.

Factor IX Concentrate

Factor IX concentrate is a commercially available lyophilized concentrated complex containing factor IX in addition to factors II, VII, IX, and X, which are vitamin K–dependent clotting factors synthesized in the liver. It is prepared by fractionation from large pools of human plasma. The product is treated by various methods to lower the incidence of transfusion-transmitted disease.

The clinical indication for factor IX concentrate is the prevention and control of bleeding in patients with hemophilia B, also known as Christmas disease. This disorder resembles hemophilia A. Patients have an abnormal gene that causes a defective synthesis of factor IX. Achieving therapeutic levels of factor IX with FFP would require infusion of large volumes. This product is the only concentrated available source for patients with this deficiency. Factor IX is also indicated for treating factor VII or X deficiencies and hemophilia A with factor VIII inhibitors.

The concentrate is provided with a sterile diluent. It should be reconstituted just before administration. The number of units of factor IX is printed on each vial.

The rate of administration is determined by the patient's condition and may be infused by drip or by push but should not exceed 10 mL/min.

Immune Globulin Intravenous

Immune globulin IV is prepared by cold fractionation from large pools of plasma. Currently six IV preparations are available. Most contain over 90% IgG antibodies and have an approximate half-life of 22 days.

The primary use of immune globulin IV is to supply sufficient amounts of IgG antibodies passively to patients who are unable to produce their own antibodies. Disease states most commonly requiring immune globulin are congenital agammaglobulinemia or severe combined immunodeficiencies. Because IV immune globulin preparations contain no preservatives, administration should begin promptly after the vial is opened or reconstituted. Dosage varies and depends on the patient's response and may be repeated every 3 to 4 weeks. It is recommended to use the infusion kit supplied with the product or transfer contents to a sterile vacuum bottle if one is not supplied. Rate of administration should also be determined by the manufacturer's guidelines.

Rh Immune Globulin

Rh immune globulin (RhIG) is a concentrate of IgG anti-D derived from plasma. It is administered by intramuscular injection to Rh-negative individuals to prevent Rh alloimmunization after being exposed to Rh-positive cells.

The Rh antibody produced by the Rh-negative mother of an Rh-positive infant is the cause of Rh hemolytic disease of the newborn (HDN). The preparation available, RhoGAM, should be administered within 72 hours after delivery and for other outcomes of pregnancy (abortion, miscarriage) or amniocentesis when a fetal–maternal hemorrhage could occur. Without RhIG protection, the mother has a 7% to 8% risk of developing anti-D. RhIG is also given antepartum at 28 weeks and again postpartum. This prophylaxis reduces the risk of immunization to about 1% to 0.1%.[3]

Mothers are not candidates for RhIG if the fetus is Rh negative or there is evidence of immunization to D not related to antepartum RhIG therapy.[2] Use of RhIG may be appropriate when an Rh-negative recipient receives Rh-positive red blood cells or components, such as platelets or granulocytes, which may contain sufficient cells to cause immunization.

One vial of RhoGAM is required for each 15 mL of Rh-positive red blood cells transfused.[3] Individual situations will dictate prophylaxis for red blood cell transfusions because the dose required is extremely large and causes discomfort.

Use of RhIG is not associated with viral transmission.[3]

BLOOD ADMINISTRATION

With the rapid advancement in transfusion therapy and more nurses being responsible for the administration of components, it is particularly important that they be well versed in every phase of the therapy. Nurses should not only be knowledgeable in the administration of components and monitoring patients during and after the transfusion, but also qualified to perform ABO and Rh certification of the components. The patient's safety depends on adherence to specific rules regarding safe administration. The transfusionist is responsible for the following:

1. Verifying the presence of a written physician's order for the transfusion
2. Verifying that documented informed consent has been obtained from the patient (if required by law or hospital policy)
3. Explaining the procedure to the patient
4. Verifying ABO and Rh compatibility between donor and recipient
5. Performing procedures relevant to patient–blood identification
6. Inspecting the unit before administration
7. Selecting and using proper technique and equipment
8. Observing the patient for 5 to 15 minutes at the beginning of the transfusion
9. Reminding the primary nurse to monitor the patient throughout the transfusion and for 1 hour after the transfusion
10. Documenting the transfusion appropriately

Issue and Transfer

Patient–blood identification is of paramount importance in preventing reactions from incompatible blood. The risk of identification errors is reduced by the use of triplicate requisitions or an on-line ordering system. Such requisitions, identifying the patient and indicating the amount and kind of blood and time needed, are sent to the blood bank with the blood sample.

The mode of transfer of blood components to the nursing unit depends on hospital policy. It may involve a pneumatic tube system, a messenger service, hospital personnel, or the individual who will administer the blood. One of the most common causes of hemolytic reaction is the accidental administration of incompatible blood from the wrong container to the patient. To prevent administration of incompatible blood, only 1 U should be transported by a person at a time.

Patient–Blood Identification

Absolute and positive identification of the donor blood and the patient must be made. All personnel handling the blood should be responsible for checking patient–blood identification. The nurse makes the final check and must decide whether to administer the blood or question it. *ABO and Rh compatibility identification* is made by comparing: (1) the patient's previous ABO and Rh determination with patient's and donor's ABO and Rh on the compatibility tag, and (2) the blood identification number on the blood container with the identification number on the blood tag and the blood unit itself.

Patient identification is made by checking the name and hospital identification number on the blood tag with the admitting sheet in the patient's clinical record. The patient then must identify himself or herself by complete name. Identity should never be made by addressing the patient by name and awaiting a response. Errors can occur from faulty response of medicated patients. Patients unable to respond should be identified by the primary or attending nurse. Hospital numbers on the identification bracelet must match hospital numbers on the tag to prevent errors in cases of similar names. Any discrepancy must be investigated and corrected before the blood is administered.

Blood must *never* be administered to a patient who has no identification bracelet.

Handling Blood

Gloves should be worn when handling any blood component. To prevent excessive warming, blood should be administered within 30 minutes of the time it leaves the bank. If blood is not maintained at 1°C (34°F) to 10°C (50°F) while outside the control of the blood bank, it cannot be reissued. Banked blood stored at 1°C (34°F) to 6°C (43°F) will exceed 10°C (50°F) in approximately 30 minutes at room temperature; blood that cannot be administered immediately should be returned to the blood bank within this time.

Blood should never be placed in nursing unit refrigerators because they are not controlled and contain no alarms to warn of temperature fluctuation.

If warmed blood is ordered, special blood-warming devices that maintain a controlled temperature should be used to warm the blood. Hot water and microwave ovens must never be used to heat blood.

Before administering the blood component, the expiration date should be noted to avoid infusion of an outdated component.

Sodium Chloride Injection, USP 0.9% (normal saline), may be used to initiate the infusion of red blood cells, whole blood, platelets, or leukocytes. Hypotonic or hypertonic solutions should not be used to dilute blood. Extreme hypotonicity causes water to invade the red blood cells until they burst, resulting in hemolysis. Hypertonic solutions dilute blood, resulting in reversal of this process with shrinkage of the red blood cells.

No medication or IV fluid (with the exception of 0.9% sodium chloride) should be added to blood or administered simultaneously through the same set.

Venipuncture

Peripheral veins with an adequate diameter should be used to ensure the flow of viscous components. The lower extremities are avoided in adults because thrombosis and blood pooling may occur. Areas of joint flexion should also be avoided.

The peripheral IV site should be checked frequently during the infusion for early detection of extravasation.

With the sophistication of IV therapy using centrally placed catheters, the infusion of blood components via percutaneous inserted central catheters and subclavian and tunnelled catheters or ports is acceptable.

Red blood cells and whole blood can usually be administered through an 18- or 20-gauge catheter, although smaller gauges may be used for other components. Often a 23-gauge catheter is used for pediatric patients. (See Chapter 25.)

Rate of Infusion

The rate of infusion is governed by the clinical condition of the patient and the viscosity of the component being infused. Infusions should be set at a slow rate for the first 15 minutes to avoid infusion of a large quantity of blood in case of an immediate reaction. Most patients can tolerate infusions of 1 U red blood cells in 1 to 1.5 hours. Patients in congestive heart failure or in danger of fluid overload require infusions given over a longer period of time, which should never exceed 4 hours.

External pressure devices and large-gauge catheters should be used when it is necessary to infuse blood rapidly. Administration of these transfusions should be the responsibility of the physician because certain risks may be involved.

Electronic infusion devices designed to administer blood and its components are frequently required for slow rates of infusion to pediatric and neonatal patients.

Blood Filters

A sterile pyrogen-free blood filter of 80 to 170 μm designed to remove debris, including clots, should be used for administration of most blood components. For best results, the entire surface area of the filter should be filled with the component because this provides an improved flow rate. A single filter may be used to infuse 2 to 4 U blood, although some institutions have a policy that a new filter is used with each component. Once the blood filter contains debris, it should be discarded. Continued use of such filters may result in bacterial contamination, a slowed rate of infusion, or hemolysis of the blood at room temperature.

Special leukocyte filters for red blood cells and platelets are available and are recommended to prevent febrile nonhemolytic reactions.

Microaggregate filters (20–40 μm) are designed to remove very small aggregates and fibrin. They may be useful in the setting of massive transfusions.

Filters are not required for the infusion of albumin or immune globulin.

Nursing Care

After initiation, the nurse/transfusionist should observe the patient for the initial 5 to 15 minutes of the infusion. Many of the fatal incompatible transfusion reactions produce symptoms early in the course of the infusion. Primary nurses also share a responsibility for safe transfusion administration. They must be familiar with the various transfusion reactions, be able to recognize adverse reactions, and know what procedures to follow.

If venous spasm occurs from the cold blood being infused, a warm pack applied to the vein through which the blood is being infused will relieve the spasm and increase the rate of flow.

Discontinuing the Transfusion

All data relevant to the transfusion should be recorded in the patient's clinical and transfusion records. Note the time the transfusion was complete, the volume of fluid infused, and the condition of the patient. Observation of the patient for 1 hour post-transfusion is recommended. Posttransfusion monitoring of laboratory values ensures that the clinical goal(s) was achieved.

Administration sets used to infuse blood components should be discarded within 24 hours after use. Bacterial growth may occur from the trapped proteins and debris contained in the set.

All transfusion-related equipment should be placed in biohazard waste receptacles. Follow institutional guidelines for observing universal precautions.

TRANSFUSION REACTIONS

Vast improvements in collection and storage methods, together with growing knowledge in the field of immunohematology, have increased the safety of transfusion therapy. However, an inherent risk still exists with every unit of transfused blood. Both the transfusionist and primary nurse should be aware of this fact and be alert to symptoms of untoward events. Reactions to administered blood cannot all be eliminated by ABO and Rh compatibility testing.

Whenever a transfusion reaction is suspected, the transfusion should be terminated and the IV kept open for possible therapeutic treatment. Vital signs should be taken, the physician should be notified, a blood sample of 10 mL should be sent to the blood bank with the blood container, and a transfusion reaction report completed (except for a simple allergic reaction). When a hemolytic reaction is suspected, urine should also be sent to the laboratory for urinalysis. Urinary output should be monitored and all urine saved and observed for hemoglobin or bilirubin.

Complete documentation of the reaction is important.

Transfusion reactions may be divided into two main classes: immediate and delayed. Both may be further divided into immunologic and nonimmunologic.

Immediate Effects

Immediate adverse effects of transfusion usually occur during or within 1 to 2 hours after the completion of an infusion. Therefore, closely monitor the patient during and after the transfusion to assess and identify signs and symptoms of impending reactions. Most immediate adverse effects are preventable and are caused by improper administration, failure to comply with standards, or lack of knowledge of the procedure or impact of the therapy.

The importance of thoroughly following written procedures and complying with policy are crucial for safe transfusion therapy.

Immunologic

The etiology of these adverse effects in the recipient are antigen–antibody reactions from red blood cells, leukocytes, or plasma proteins. They are usually produced by the body's response to foreign proteins.

Acute Hemolytic Reaction.   Acute hemolytic transfusion reactions occur when an antigen–antibody reaction occurs in the recipient caused by an incompatibility between the recipient's antibodies and the donor's red blood cells. Incompatibilities in the ABO blood group system are responsible for most of the deaths from acute hemolytic transfusion reactions.

The interaction of the isoagglutinins and ABO incompatible red blood cells activates the complement, kinin, and coagulation systems. The entire complement system is activated in the ABO mismatch, causing intravascular hemolysis. If the free hemoglobin released from the destruction of red blood cells is greater than the quantity that can combine with haptoglobin in the plasma, the excess hemoglobin filters through the glomerular membrane into the kidney tubules, and hemoglobinuria occurs.

The kinin system is activated by the antigen–antibody complex and produces bradykinin, which increases capillary permeability, dilates arterioles, and causes a fall in systemic blood pressure.

The coagulation system stimulates activation of the intrinsic clotting cascade, causing small clots in the circulation and may trigger disseminated intravascular coagulation (DIC), which in turn can cause formation of thrombi within the microvasculature.

Intravascular hemolytic reactions are often fatal. Investigation of fatal hemolytic transfusion reactions shows that the most common errors are misidentification—of the recipient sample sent to the blood blank, of the blood unit, or of the recipient.

Hemolytic transfusion reactions may be accompanied by chills, fever, flushing of face, burning sensation along the vein in which the blood is being infused, lumbar or flank pain, chest pain, frequent oozing of blood at the injection site and surgical areas, or shock. When reactions occur, the transfusion must be stopped at once and the vein kept open with 0.9% sodium chloride. When a Y blood tubing is used, a new setup (container of fluid and a new administration set) should be connected directly to the cannula. DO NOT OPEN THE FLOW TO THE NORMAL SALINE HANGING WITH THE Y BLOOD TUBING. To do so could result in the patient receiving additional incompatible blood cells contained in the Y tubing.

Vigorous treatment of hypotension and promotion of adequate renal blood flow are imperative. Therapy may consist of administration of volume, diuretics, and volume expanders to promote diuresis and to minimize renal damage. Urinary flow rates in adults should be maintained at or over 100 mL/hr for at least 18 to 24 hours.[3] Vasopressors, such as dopamine in low doses, dilate the renal vasculature while increasing cardiac output. Their use requires careful monitoring of the patient's urinary flow, cardiac output, and blood pressure. A diuretic agent such as furosemide is recommended to be given concurrently with adequate IV fluid replacement. The drug improves renal blood flow, thus minimizing the possibility of renal tubular ischemia and renal failure. Mannitol is infrequently used because, if ineffective, may cause hypervolemia and pulmonary edema.

The use of heparin therapy for the resulting DIC remains controversial and is dealt with after evaluating all consequences of the acute hemolytic reaction.

Prevention is the hallmark of therapy for this severe reaction. This reaction is preventable.

Febrile Nonhemolytic Reaction.   Febrile nonhemolytic reactions (FNR) are usually the result of antileukocyte antibodies in the recipient directed against the donor's white blood cells. Even though some leukocytes break down rapidly during storage, the membrane fragments are still capable of sensitizing patients in the same manner as intact leukocytes. Patients who have been sensitized by numerous transfusions or multiple pregnancies are more likely to develop FNH.

Febrile nonhemolytic reactions are defined as a rise in temperature of 1°C and usually occurs within 1 to 6 hours after the initiation of the transfusion. Febrile reactions may be accompanied by flushing of the face, palpitation, cough, tightness in the chest, increased pulse rate, or chills. As the name implies, no red blood cell hemolysis occurs. Antipyretics are used for treatment. When a patient experiences this reaction, there is a 1 in 8 chance that a similar reaction will occur with the next transfusion.[3] Documentation of the reaction is most important for possible prevention of future adverse effects.

Newly developed leukocyte removal filters are increasingly being used for filtration at the bedside. They are an efficient, effective, and convenient method of removing leukocytes and decreasing incidences of FNH. Deglycerolized red blood cells and washed red blood cells are also relatively depleted of leukocytes.

Anaphylactic Reactions.   Fortunately, anaphylactic reactions are rare. They may occur in patients who are IgA deficient and who have developed anti-IgA antibodies.

The two classic signs that an anaphylactic reaction is imminent are symptoms after only a few milliliters of blood or plasma has been infused and absence of fever. The reaction is characterized by coughing, respiratory distress, abdominal cramps, vascular instability, shock, and perhaps loss of consciousness. This medical emergency requires immediate resuscitation of the patient along with administration of epinephrine and steroids.

Prevention includes the use of autologous transfusions or obtaining units from donors who lack IgA. Reducing the plasma content of red blood cell and platelet transfusions may also be effective in reducing the severity of this reaction.

Urticaria.   These reactions are relatively uncommon and are based on a hypersensitivity response, probably to protein in donor plasma.

Urticarial reactions are usually mild and characterized by local erythema, hives, and itching. On occasion, fever may be present. The transfusion is usually interrupted and may be continued after the patient has responded to antihistamine therapy. If patients develop extensive urticaria or total body rash or fever, the transfusion may have to be discontinued. In these situations, washed or deglycerolized red blood cells may be indicated for future therapy.

Noncardiac Pulmonary Edema.   Although this reaction occurs infrequently, it can provoke severe symptoms. The usual etiology is a reaction between donor high titer antileukocyte antibodies and recipient leukocytes. The reaction can result in leukagglutination. The leukoagglutinins may become trapped in the pulmonary microvasculature. The reaction causes severe respiratory distress unassociated with circulatory overload and without evidence of cardiac failure. Chest radiography reveals bilateral pulmonary infiltrates consistent with pulmonary edema but without other evidence of left heart failure.

Clinical signs and symptoms other than respiratory distress include chills, fever, cyanosis, and hypotension. Treatment begins by discontinuing the transfusion and providing respiratory support measures. Once the donor has been implicated in such a reaction, that person's plasma should not be used for transfusion.

Nonimmunologic
Immediate nonimmunologic adverse effects are caused by external factors in the administration of blood; antigen–antibody reactions are absent.

Congestive Heart Failure.   Congestive heart failure may occur when blood or its components are infused too rapidly or given to a patient who has an increased plasma volume. The consequence is hypervolemia. Patients more prone to this adverse effect are the young and elderly and those with cardiac or renal disease.

Symptoms include a pounding headache, dyspnea, constriction of the chest, coughing, and cyanosis. The transfusion must be stopped and the patient placed in a sitting position. Rapid-acting diuretics and oxygen usually relieve the symptoms. If the condition is severe, a therapeutic phlebotomy may be indicated.

Prevention consists of frequent monitoring of those susceptible to congestive heart failure and the administration of concentrated components slowly.

This adverse effect is preventable.

Air Embolism.   This complication of transfusion therapy has been dramatically reduced with the use of plastic bags. It may result from faulty technique in changing equipment or plastic bags, careless use of Y-type administration sets, or air infused from one of the containers when fluid and blood are being pumped together. If air does enter the patient, acute cardiopulmonary insufficiency occurs.

Symptoms are the same as those for circulatory collapse: cyanosis, dyspnea, shock, and sometimes, cardiac arrest. The infusion should be stopped immediately and the patient turned on the left side, with the head down. This position traps air in the right atrium, preventing it from entering the pulmonary artery; the pulmonic valve is kept clear until the air can escape gradually. It may be necessary for the physician to aspirate the air with a transthoracic needle.

This adverse effect is preventable.

Citrate Toxicity.   Patients at risk of developing citrate toxicity or a calcium deficit are those who receive large quantities of citrated blood or have severely impaired liver function. The liver, unable to keep up with the rapid administration, cannot metabolize the citrate, which chelates calcium, reducing the ionized calcium concentration. Hypocalcemia may induce cardiac arrhythmia. This adverse effect may be encountered in the emergency room and operating room when large amounts of blood and components have been administered. Symptoms of hypocalcemia include tingling of the fingers, muscular cramps, convulsions, hypotension, and cardiac arrest.

Treatment consists of the administration of calcium chloride or calcium gluconate solution.

Hypothermia.   Hypothermia occurs commonly when large volumes of cold blood are infused rapidly.[13] Rapid infusions may cause chills, hypothermia, peripheral vasoconstriction, ventricular arrhythmias, and cardiac arrest. In many situations, warming blood to 35°C (95°F) with automatic blood warmers during rapid massive replacement prevents hypothermia. However, time does not always permit the setup of equipment. Many emergency rooms and trauma centers have dispensed with blood warmers and instead warm the IV solutions in special regulated warmers. In the emergency situation, the blood and IV fluid are infusing together; thus, the IV fluid warms the blood.[13]

This reaction is preventable.

Marked Fever with Shock.   Bacterial contamination of blood is the cause of this reaction and may occur at the time of donation or in component preparation. In addition to skin contaminants, cold-resistant gram-negative bacteria may contribute to this untoward event. Organisms such as *Pseudomonas* species, *Citrobacter freundii*, and *Escherichia coli* are potential causes. These organisms, capable of proliferating at refrigerator temperatures, release an endotoxin that initiates the reaction. It is potentially fatal when it occurs. Fortunately, it rarely does.

This complication can be prevented by inspecting the unit before administration. Observation of any discoloration of the blood or plasma or obvious clots should be reported.

Clinical manifestations of the reaction include high fever, flushing of the skin, "warm" shock, hemoglobinuria, renal failure, and DIC. These signs and symptoms are similar to those of an acute hemolytic reaction, so diagnosis must be made quickly. The transfusion should be discontinued; immediate therapy, including management of shock, steroids, and antibiotics, is required. Cultures obtained of the patient's blood, the suspected component, and all IV solutions will determine whether the bacteremia is caused by the blood or an IV-related infection.

This reaction is preventable.

Delayed Effects

These complications occur days, months, or years after the transfusion and usually are the result of alloimmunization or transmitted disease. To a great degree, prevention is unavoidable.

Immunologic
Delayed Hemolytic Reaction.   Delayed hemolytic reactions are caused by an immune antibody, produced by the body's response to a foreign antigen. These reactions are classified as primary and secondary. The primary or initial reaction is generally mild and may occur a week or more after the transfusion. Known as *primary alloimmunization*, it rarely produces symptoms and may be clinically insignificant. The degree of hemolysis depends on the quantity of antibody produced.

The secondary reaction occurs in a patient previously immunized by transfusion or pregnancy. These patients had formed a red blood cell alloantibody in the past, but the level of this alloantibody has become so low that it is serologically undetectable. On a later occasion, when donor red blood cells possessing the corresponding antigen are infused, they provoke the rapid increase in the specific antibody. The incompatible red blood cells survive until ample antibody is present to initiate a rejection response. The reaction is called secondary or *anamnestic (memory) response* and is caused by reexposure to the same antigen. These reactions are rarely caused by ABO incompatibility. A delayed hemolytic reaction is manifested by fever, mild jaundice, and an unexplained drop in the hemoglobin value. These coated cells are removed from the body by the reticuloendothelial system (extravascular hemolysis). A direct antiglobulin test may detect the antibody, but in a rapidly progressing delayed hemolytic reaction, this test may be negative.

Graft-versus-Host Disease. This is a very rare complication but presents severe complications and is often fatal. The usual cause is the transfer of immunocompetent T lymphocytes in blood components to a severely immunocompromised patient. The donor lymphocytes engraft and multiply in a severely immunodeficient recipient. These engrafted cells react against the foreign tissue of the host recipient, causing GVHD.[3]

Infusions of FFP or cryoprecipitate are largely acellular and do not cause the disease.

The onset of GVHD is usually 4 to 30 days after transfusion and begins with a high fever. Generalized erythroderma, anorexia, nausea and vomiting, and profuse diarrhea may follow. Bone marrow suppression and infection are the cause of death in 90% of patients dying from this disease.

Prevention is pretransfusion inactivation of lymphocytes by irradiating the blood component. Irradiation minimally affects red blood cells, platelets, and granulocytes.

Nonimmunologic

Hepatitis. Posttransfusion hepatitis (PTH) has been regarded as a complication of receiving blood since the 1940s and remains the most frequent adverse effect today.[15] It is predominantly transmitted by the hepatitis B virus (HBV) and the hepatitis C virus (HCV).

Hepatitis B virus accounts for less than 10% of PTH. The primary reasons for this low incidence are the elimination of paid donors and testing of all donors for the HBsAg. Increased donor scrutiny and the use of surrogate tests (ALT, HBcAB) to reduce PTH have also had an impact.

The average incubation period for HBV infection is 90 days with a range of 30 to 180 days. The length of the incubation period depends on the amount of HBV the patient is exposed to and the route of exposure.[3]

Hepatitis B can be transmitted directly by percutaneous inoculation of infectious serum or plasma by needle or transfusion of infectious blood. It can be indirectly transmitted by percutaneous introduction of infectious serum through minute skin cuts or abrasions, mucosal surfaces, or saliva or semen.[18]

Hepatitis B vaccine is advised for health care workers to actively immunize and eliminate the risk of acquiring infection by these routes. Health care workers who are at risk for exposure to blood and body fluids are advised to be vaccinated.

Manifested by elevated liver enzyme tests, anorexia, malaise, dark urine, fever, and jaundice, the disease usually resolves within 4 to 6 weeks.

Ninety percent of PTH is caused by neither type A nor type B hepatitis viruses and is designated as non-A, non-B (NANB) hepatitis. The predominant agent was recently identified and is HCV. Nearly 80% of NANB hepatitis is related to HCV. In 1990, a test for antibody to HCV was licensed by the FDA; the test is used to eliminate blood donors who have been exposed to HCV. Blood from donors is discarded if the test, an enzyme immunoassay (EIA), is repeatedly reactive. Because of the current sensitivity of the EIA, cases of HCV may be missed if the test is performed too early after the onset of acute hepatitis. This "window" period leads to false negative test results.

No licensed confirmatory test for HCV is available yet. Donors with elevated ALT concentrations and anti-HBc are also deferred because these surrogate tests seem to identify donors who have an increased likelihood of transmitting PTH. Antibody studies to anti-HBc appeared in some donors when HBsAg was negative. Potential donors who have the antibody will be deferred. The test may support another means of eliminating PTH.[10]

Modes of transmission appear to be similar to HBV and the majority of cases of HCV occur within 5 to 12 weeks after transfusion. The initial and acute illness is usually milder than HBV. Approximately 75% of patients are anicteric. Liver abnormalities persisting after 1 year indicate chronic hepatitis, and progression to cirrhosis in 20% of patients may occur.

Hepatitis from hepatitis A virus (HAV) is a rare cause of PTH largely because of the short time that viral particles remain in the circulation and the high prevalence of immunity in recipients of blood. Thus, its role in the etiology of PTH is infrequent and not significant.

The incidence of PTH has decreased over the past 10 years because of the screening of donors and the use of laboratory tests to identify at-risk donors.

Cytomegalovirus Infection.   Recognized to be present in blood and transmitted by transfusion, CMV poses little problem to most recipients. Patients predominately at risk of developing serious consequences of the infection are those who are immunocompetent; neonates; patients with malignancies who are immunosuppressed as a result of therapy of their disease; and transplant patients. The incidence of clinical disease doubles in these patients. Recently, CMV has gained additional attention because it appears to be a possible cofactor in patients with HIV infection.[6] Patients with HIV may have depression of cell-mediated immunity and be predisposed to opportunistic infections. Significant morbidity and mortality result.

Cytomegalovirus is in the herpes family and is transmitted by viable leukocytes in blood. The incubation period following transfusion is 3 to 8 weeks and 3 to 12 weeks following delivery.[18]

As a means to reduce CMV-related infection, CMV seronegative blood may be the best avenue of prevention. However, this special and limited product would only be available for selected patients.

Vaccines are available but not universally accepted as useful. The vaccine contains only one CMV strain and may have oncogenic potential; differences of opinion arise as to the danger of it causing virus activation.[4] Positive factors are that the vaccine stimulates cell-mediated immunity.

Malaria.   Eradicated in the United States and Canada, malaria is still prevalent in South and Central America, Africa, and Asia. The number of cases reported in the United States has increased because of immigrants and travelers. Although there is no practical laboratory test, diagnosis of the disease is made by identifying the organism on a blood smear. The patient may develop a high fever, which reflects lysis of the parasite from infected red blood cells and its release into the bloodstream.[14] Malaria parasite can be transmitted by blood transfusion.

New assays (indirect immunofluorescence and enzyme-linked immunoassays) are being used in Europe to qualify donors who are not infected but have a history of travel in malarial areas.[14]

Ater becoming symptomatic, taking antimalarial prophylaxis, or being in an endemic area, donors are deferred for 3 years. Immigrants, refugees, and citizens from endemic countries may be accepted as blood donors 3 years after departure from the area, if they are asymptomatic.[2]

Acquired Immunodeficiency Syndrome.   As early as 1983, those involved in transfusion medicine realized that a new disease was capable of being disseminated by transfusion.

Aggressive work began to safeguard the blood supply from AIDS. This infectious disease is caused by HIV. All units of blood in the United States and Europe have been tested for antibody to the virus (anti-HIV) since 1985 by enzyme-labeled immunosorbent assays (ELISA). When the ELISA is repeatedly reactive, a Western blot analysis is done as a confirmatory test. As of June 1992, all blood donors in the United States have to be screened for antibodies to both forms of HIV—HIV-1 and HIV-2. An additional confirmatory test, the recombinant DNA-derived HIV antigen-based immunoblot assay (RIBA-HIV 216) is being used by some agencies as a confirmatory test.[8]

The transmission of HIV has been and continues to be a focal point of discussion and research. It is transmitted by three primary routes: (1) sexual contact with an infected person, (2) parenteral exposure to infected blood or blood components (including needles shared among drug users), and (3) perinatally from an infected mother to her child.[11]

Clinical manifestations are weight loss, diarrhea, fever, lymphadenopathy, Kaposi's sarcoma, and opportunistic infections.

The HIV is a retrovirus that infects and kills CD4-positive lymphocytes (helper T cells), thereby destroying the immune system. It produces severe immunodeficiency and renders the individual vulnerable to opportunistic infections. The incubation period of the disease may exceed 7 years and the projection of the numbers of people in the United States infected with HIV was approximately 300,000 by the end of 1991.[14]

Although there has been a significant decrease in patients infected with AIDS by transfusions (1:225,000 per unit of blood transfused)[7] or about 2% of those transfused,[5] society is focused on this unfortunate consequence or adverse effect. Data on the disease reflect major geographic incidences. A decline in incidence of AIDS is not predicted at this time. Intense investigation to develop vaccines for active immunization is underway. Since the screening test became available, it is estimated that HIV transmission will occur in 1 of 40,000 to 1 of 250,000 U transfused.

To reduce the incidence of AIDS in transfusion therapy, the following measures are recommended: (1) the indications for the administration of blood components should be clear; (2) careful screening of donors and testing of donor units should be done; and (3) autologous transfusion should be used whenever possible.

Syphilis.   Serologic testing for syphilis is required by the FDA on all donor blood. Refrigerated blood storage has nearly eradicated the transmission of syphilis because temperatures of 4°C (39°F) have a spirocheticidal effect, thus eliminating treponemas after 72 hours.[3]

AUTOLOGOUS TRANSFUSIONS

All the techniques of autologous transfusion are accepted practice for appropriate candidates in a setting based on the patient's clinical condition.[12]

Autologous transfusion is the collection, filtration, and reinfusion of one's own blood; thus the donor and recipient are the same individual. The term autologous transfusion takes on several different meanings and methods—each applied to particular clinical conditions. They are predeposit donation (preoperative), hemodilution, intraoperative salvage, and postoperative blood salvage.

Autologous transfusion is an old practice that is making an impressive comeback.

The primary reasons for this change include advances made in technology, blood conservation, and the need to decrease the transmission of bloodborne diseases.

Predeposit (Preoperative) Donation

This technique is best used when a patient is planning an elective surgical procedure in which blood use is likely. The patient may plan periodic visits to a donor center for phlebotomies so that the patient's own red blood cells are stored for use later. By 1990, autologous transfusions accounted for as much as 5% of collected blood and, in some donor centers, as much as 20%.[17] As the public is becoming more aware of the hazards of disease transmission by transfusions, many patients will be more at ease knowing that they may receive their own blood through autologous transfusion programs.

Hemodilution (Perioperative)

In this procedure, 1 or 2 U of the patient's blood are collected and stored in the operating room until the end of the procedure. The patient receives infusions of a crystalloid or colloid solution to maintain plasma volume. Commonly done before cardiopulmonary bypass, hemodilution is limited by the patient's blood volume and hemodynamic considerations.[19] The hematocrit is reduced so patients with lung disease or hypo-oxygenation must be monitored closely. After the surgical procedure, the units of blood taken before surgery are infused back to the patient.[19]

Intraoperative Salvage

This method of autologous transfusion is gaining in acceptance and is being increasingly used. The technique involves aspirating blood from the operative site, washing the blood manually or using cell-washing machines, and reinfusing the blood back to the patient. The process may be performed completely in the operating room. It is most frequently used in cardiovascular, thoracic, orthopedic, neurologic, and hepatic surgery including transplants. The technique makes large volumes of blood immediately available when bleeding occurs in a clean operative procedure. The procedure is contraindicated in patients with malignancy or infection on the basis that reinfusion of cells may disseminate the tumor cells or infectious organism.

Sterile technique is mandated to avoid infectious agents from entering the system. Techniques vary with different equipment. Equipment and personnel costs can be high, but cost savings and improved medical care outweigh the disadvantages. Some programs are developed within hospitals; others may hire outside agencies to do "traveling" intraoperative autologous transfusions.

Postoperative Salvage

This technique involves collecting shed blood from patients following cardiac, trauma, orthopedic, and plastic surgery. Other clinical conditions may also be appropriate. The advantage of this technique is that it can be done for planned surgery or emergency operations and trauma. Blood collected through special equipment is collected, transfused, or discarded within 6 hours of initiating the collection and is not transfused to other patients. This technique is safe, simple, and cost effective. Combined with other methods of autologous transfusions described, the goal of avoiding homologous blood transfusions is closer.

Receiving one's own blood is the safest transfusion, and these modalities will be increasingly encouraged. Careful administration of autologous blood is still required. To avoid any errors, those administering the blood must verify all aspects of the component, including proper identification. Verification procedures should be identical to those for giving homologous transfusions.

In particular, IV nurses can play an important role in autologous transfusion and blood salvage techniques. Because of their skill, involvement, and knowledge of transfusions, their abilities translate well to these alternatives to conventional administration of homologous blood component therapy.

The goals of these programs are to conserve blood and prevent reactions, isoimmunization, and disease transmission. The success of these programs requires (1) availability of responsible staff 24 hours a day, especially if more than one machine is available; (2) preferably dedicated operators for each machine; (3) a quality improvement program; and (4) physician support and public awareness programs. The AABB endorses all modalities of blood conservation. All of these methods help in achieving the goals of autologous transfusions.

DIRECTED DONATIONS

Risk of transfusion-transmitted diseases has generated other programs whereby prospective patients may designate their own blood donors. Each donor enters the same process as any other, but the blood is labeled for a specific recipient provided screening tests are appropriate and the unit is compatible. If the blood is not compatible for the intended recipient, the donation is usually entered into the general supply.

The primary benefit of the program may be emotional because the patient feels more comfortable knowing the donors. This aspect is important and appreciated by patients and families. However, no data to date support the idea that the blood is safer than that from anonymous volunteer donors.[3]

REFERENCES

1. Alter, H. J., Tegtmeier, G. E., Jett, B. W., Ovan, S., Shih, J. W., Bayer, W. L., & Polito A. (1991). The use of recombinant immunoblot assay in the interpretation of anti-hepatitis C virus reactivity among prospectively followed patients, implicated donors, and random donors. *Transfusion, 31,* 771.

2. American Association of Blood Banks. (1991). *Standards for blood banks and transfusion services* (14th ed., pp. 8, 32, 37, 41). Arlington, VA: Author.

3. American Association of Blood Banks. (1990). *Technical manual* (10th ed., pp. 47, 62, 350, 369, 402, 419, 420, 426, 428, 446). Arlington, VA: Author.

4. Balfour, H. H. (1983). Cytomegalovirus disease: Can it be prevented? *Annals of Internal Medicine, 98,* 514–516.

5. Berkman, S. A., & Groopman, J. E. (1988). Transfusion—associated AIDS. *Transfusion Medical Review, 2,* 18–28.

6. Bhumbra, N. A., & Nankeruis, G. A. (1983). Cyto-

megalovirus infection. *Postgraduate Medicine, 73,* 62–68.

7. Petersen, L. R., Satten, G., Dodd, R. Y. et al. (1992). Current estimates of the infectious window period and risk of HIV infection from seronegative blood donations. In Program and abstracts of the Fifth National Forum on AIDS, Hepatitis and Other Blood-Borne Diseases, Atlanta, GA, March 30, 1992. Princeton, NJ: Symedco, 37.

8. Busch, M. P., Amad, Z. E., McHugh, T. M., Chien, D., & Polito, A. J. (1991). Reliable confirmation and quantitation of human immunodeficiency virus type I antibody using a recombinant-antigen immunoblot assay. *Transfusion, 31,* 129–136.

9. Guyton, A. C. (1986). *Textbook of medical physiology* (7th ed., pp. 76–77). Philadelphia: W. B. Saunders.

10. Hoofnagle, J. H. (1990). Posttransfusion hepatitis B. *Transfusion, 30,* 384.

11. Lifson, A. R. (1988). Do alternate modes for trans-

mission of human immunodeficiency virus exist? *Journal of the American Medical Association, 259,* 1353–1355.

12. Maffei, L. M., & Thurer, R. L. (1988). *Autologous blood transfusion: Current issues.* Arlington, VA: American Association of Blood Banks.

13. Pauley, S. Y. (1987). Massive hemorrhage in trauma. *Journal of the National Intravenous Therapy Association, 10,* 418.

14. Petz, L. D., & Swisher, S. N. (1989). *Clinical practice of transfusion medicine* (2nd ed., pp. 417, 653, 689, 696, 698, 702). New York: Churchill-Livingstone.

15. Sirchia, G., Giovanetti, A. M., Parravicini, A., Bellobuono, A., Mozzi, F., Pizzi, M. N., & Almini, D. (1991). Prospective evaluation of posttransfusion hepatitis. *Transfusion, 31,* 301.

16. Stroup, M., & Tracey, M. (1982). *Blood group antigens and antibodies* (pp. 29–30). Raritan, NJ: Ortho Diagnostics System.

17. Surgenor, D. M., Wallace, E. L., Hao, S. H. S., & Chapman, R. H. (1990). Collection and transfusion of blood in the United States. *New England Journal of Medicine, 322,* 1646–1651.

18. Thompson, J. M., McFarland, G. K., Hirsch, J. E., Tucker, S. M., Bewers, A. C. (1986). *Clinical nursing* (pp. 1544, 1550). St. Louis: C. V. Mosby.

19. Williamson, K. R., & Taswell, H. F. (1991). Intraoperative blood salvage: A review. *Transfusion, 31,* 662.

REVIEW QUESTIONS

1. The antigen in the ABO system that denotes one's blood group is located:
   a. on the red blood cell
   b. in the plasma
   c. in the serum
   d. on body tissue

2. Which of the following may stimulate a reaction?
   I. Antigen A combining with anti-A antibody
   II. Antigen AB combining with anti-AB antibody
   III. Antigen B combining with anti-A antibody
   IV. Antigen D combining with anti-D antibody
   a. I and II
   b. III and IV
   c. I, II, and IV
   d. all of the above

3. Which of the following indications is specific for the use of whole blood?
   a. acute blood loss
   b. surgical blood loss
   c. blood loss and coagulation disorders
   d. chronic anemia

4. Which of the following are autologous transfusions?
   I. perioperative
   II. preoperative
   III. intraoperative
   IV. postoperative
   a. I and II
   b. I, II, and III
   c. II, III, and IV
   d. all of the above

5. A patient, group O, may receive red blood cells from a donor who is:
   a. group A only
   b. group O only
   c. group A or O
   d. any group

6. A patient, group AB, may receive plasma from a donor who is:
   a. group A, AB, or O
   b. group AB or O
   c. group AB only
   d. any group

7. Intravascular hemolytic reactions are potentially caused by:
   a. ABO incompatibility
   b. Rh incompatibility
   c. ABO and Rh incompatibility
   d. none of the above

8. Which of the following is classified as a delayed transfusion reaction?
   a. febrile nonhemolytic
   b. citrate toxicity
   c. graft-versus-host disease
   d. allergic

9. A patient experiences the following signs and symptoms 1 hour after a unit of packed red blood cells has been infused: chills, increased pulse rate, fever, flushing of the face. Which of the following adverse reactions is suspected?
   a. citrate toxicity
   b. congestive heart failure
   c. febrile nonhemolytic reaction
   d. anaphylaxis

10. Treatment of choice for this reaction is:
   a. antipyretics
   b. therapeutic phlebotomy
   c. steroids
   d. IV calcium

PART V

Pharmacologic Applications of Intravenous Therapy

CHAPTER 22 _____

Drug Administration

ADVANTAGES _____

The vascular route for drug administration offers pronounced advantages, as follows:

1. Some drugs cannot be absorbed by any other route; the large molecular size of some drugs prevents absorption by the gastrointestinal route, whereas other drugs, unstable in the presence of gastric juices, are destroyed.
2. Certain drugs, because of their irritating properties, cause pain and trauma when given by the intramuscular or subcutaneous route and must be given IV.
3. The vascular system affords a method for providing rapid drug action.
4. The IV route offers better control over the rate of administration of drugs; prolonged action can be provided by administering a dilute infusion intermittently or over a prolonged period.
5. The vascular route affords a route of administration for the patient who cannot tolerate fluids and drugs by the gastrointestinal route.
6. Slow IV administration of a drug permits termination of the infusion if sensitivity occurs.

HAZARDS _____

Despite the advantages offered by the vascular route, certain hazards arise that are not found in other forms of drug therapy:

1. The possibility of incompatibilities when one or more drugs are added to the IV solution
2. Speed shock (a systemic reaction to a substance rapidly injected into the bloodstream)
3. Vascular irritations and subsequent hazards
4. Rapid onset of action, with inability to recall a drug once it has entered the bloodstream

Precipitation may occur when one or more drugs are added to parenteral solution.[9] It does not always occur at the time the solution is prepared, which increases the problem of

Sharon M. Weinstein: PLUMER'S PRINCIPLES & PRACTICE OF INTRAVENOUS THERAPY, FIFTH EDITION, © 1993 J. B. Lippincott Company

IV administration. Some drugs, stable for a limited time, degrade and may or may not precipitate as they become less therapeutically active. If administered IV, solutions containing insoluble matter carry the potential danger of embolism, myocardial damage, and effect on other organs such as the liver and the kidneys.

CLINICAL PHARMACOKINETICS

The pharmacokinetic basis of therapeutics requires the drug, route of administration, and frequency to achieve and maintain a proper drug concentration at the *receptor site* wherever it may occur within the body. If an insufficient amount of drug is present at this site, it may appear to be ineffective and therefore be discontinued. Conversely, the right drug may produce toxicity and be discarded simply because excessive amounts are present in the body. Awareness of drug pharmacokinetics is essential in reducing toxicity and potential excess drug dosages.

Therapeutic index is the margin between a drug's therapeutic and toxic concentrations at the receptor site.[5] Pharmacokinetic models describe and predict drug amounts and concentrations in various body fluids and the changes in these quantities over time. Factors influencing the pharmacokinetics of drugs may be found in Table 22-1.

Plasma concentration level (Cp) represents drug that is bound to plasma protein plus drug that is unbound or free. Two factors determine the degree of plasma protein binding. The first is the binding affinity of the drug for the plasma proteins; the second is the number of binding sites presently available or the concentration of plasma protein.[1] An acidic drug such as salicylate or phenytoin may be bound to albumin; a basic drug such as lidocaine or quinidine may be bound to serum globulins. Calculated plasma levels may assist the physician in evaluating effectiveness of therapy. Figure 22-1 notes concentration time curves following IV injection at three different rates.

The *compartment models* are essential for the IV nurse in understanding pharmacokinetic principles. The "one-compartment model" states that when a drug is introduced into the body, it is rapidly and homogeneously distributed throughout the entire space or compartment. Precise anatomic sites of drug distribution can only be determined by direct analysis of tissue concentrations, which is only possible in animal studies. The "two-compartment model" states that the first compartment is composed of blood volume and those organs or tissues that have a high blood flow. This compartment

TABLE 22-1
Factors Influencing the Pharmacokinetics of Drugs

Patient Characteristics	*Disease States*
Age	Liver disease
Sex	Renal disease
Body weight	Congestive heart failure
Body habits	Infection
Smoking habits	Fever
Alcohol consumption	Shock
Other coingested drugs	Severe burns

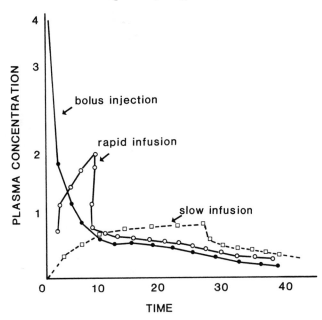

FIGURE 22-1 Concentration time curves following IV injection at three different rates.

equilibrates rapidly with administered drug, which is then distributed into the second compartment. Drug behavior in the body depends on both distribution and elimination.[1]

THERAPEUTIC DRUG MONITORING

The drug concentration level may be calculated after the initiation of a dosage regimen to ensure that it will produce the target concentration desired. It may also be measured periodically to ensure that it is still producing the desired target concentration or to determine if the therapeutic regimen is failing. Table 22-2 lists the types of patients needing therapeutic drug monitoring; ideal sampling times for various drug classes are listed in Table 22-3.[5]

Loading dose is the initial dose of drug ordered. Designed to produce an immediate target concentration, this is not always practical nor is it safe. An initial dose of lidocaine, calculated to achieve an average target concentration, may produce toxicity following administration as a bolus because it will reach high concentration in the heart and brain (toxic sites of action) before it is diluted by distribution elsewhere within the body.

TABLE 22-2
Patients Needing Therapeutic Drug Monitoring

Those on combination therapies

Those with renal dysfunction

Those with third-spacing

Those for whom therapeutic failure would prove catastrophic

Those who fail to respond to therapy despite appropriate dosing

TABLE 22-3
Ideal Sampling Times

Drug Classification	Sampling Time
Anticonvulsants	Predose
Antidepressants	Predose (lithium, 12 hr postdose)
Cardiovascular	Predose (propranolol, 6–10 hr postdose [Digoxin])
Antiasthmatics	Predose
Antibiotics	Predose and peak

Half-life is the time required for the plasma concentration of a drug or the total amount of drug in the body to decline by one half. Half-life of a drug depends on its volume of distribution (the distribution between the plasma and the various other fluids and tissues and the actual nature of distribution and clearance). During drug administration, it takes one half-life to reach 50% of steady state, two half-lives to reach 75%, three half-lives to reach 87.5%, and four half-lives to reach 93.75%. On discontinuation of a drug or after a drug dosage, it takes one half-life for the plasma concentration to fall to 50% of its initial level.[5]

INCOMPATIBILITIES

The number of possible drug combinations is overwhelming. Manufacturers provide an ever-increasing number of new drug products for the treatment of disease processes. Compounding of drugs for IV administration is generally performed by an IV admixture service as a component of a hospital-based or home infusion pharmacy. Today, admixture programs have expanded their service base, providing compounding service for extended care, ambulatory care, and any clinical setting in which infusion therapies are delivered.

All individuals responsible for mixing and compounding IV drugs must be alert to the hazards involved. Compatibility charts are provided through admixture services to alert the nursing professional to potential problems, particularly when additions to infusions in progress are made on a nursing unit or added in a patient's residence. Factors affecting the compatibility of drugs include order of mixing, quantity of the drug and solution, room temperature, and light. Incompatibilities are not always obvious to the naked eye; they may be classified as physical, chemical, or therapeutic.

Physical incompatibilities are those in which an undesirable change is physically observed (eg, sodium bicarbonate and calcium chloride forming an insoluble precipitate).[2,9]

Chemical changes are those occurring in the molecular structure or pharmacologic properties of a substance. They may or may not be physically observed (eg, penicillin and ascorbic acid lowering the pH).

Therapeutic incompatibilities are those in which an undesirable reaction results from the overlapping effects of two drugs given together or closely together (eg, penicillin and tetracycline inhibiting the bactericidal effect of penicillin).

CHEMICAL INTERACTIONS

The most common incompatibilities are the result of certain chemical reactions.[9]

1. *Hydrolysis* is the process in which water absorption causes decomposition of a compound. In preparing solutions of salt, the nurse should understand that certain salts, when placed in water, hydrolyze, forming a very strong acid and a weak base or a weak acid and a strong base. Because pH is a significant factor in the solubility of drugs, the increased acidity or alkalinity from hydrolysis of a salt may result in an incompatibility if another drug is added. *Example*: The acid salt sodium bicarbonate when placed in water hydrolyzes to form a strong alkali (sodium hydroxide) and a weak and unstable acid (carbonic acid). Many organic acids are known as weak acids because they ionize only slightly.[8]

2. *Reduction* is the process whereby one or more atoms gain electrons at the expense of some other part of the system.[8]

3. *Oxidation* is the corresponding loss of electrons occurring when reduction takes place. Antioxidants are often used as preservatives to prevent oxidation of a compound.[8]

4. *Double decomposition* is the chemical reaction in which ions of two compounds change places and two new compounds are thus formed.[8] A great many salts act by double decomposition to form other salts and probably represent the largest number of incompatibilities. *Example*: Calcium chloride is incompatible with sodium bicarbonate; the double decomposition results in the formation of the insoluble salt calcium carbonate.

pH AND ITS ROLE IN DRUG STABILITY

Because pH plays an important role in the solubility of drugs, it may be well to define it. pH is the symbol for the degree of concentration of hydrogen ions or the acidity of the solution. The weight of hydrogen ions in 1 L of pure water is 0.0000001 g, which is numerically equal to 10^{-7}. For convenience, the negative logarithm 7 is used. Because it is at this concentration that the hydrogen ions balance the hydroxyl ions, a pH of 7 is neutral. Each unit decrease in pH represents a tenfold increase in hydrogen ions.

It appears likely that the largest number of incompatibilities may be produced by changes in pH.[7] Precipitation occurs when a compound is insoluble in solution. The degree of solubility often varies with the pH. A drastic change in the pH of a drug when added to an IV solution suggests an incompatibility or a decrease in stability. Solutions of a high pH appear to be incompatible with solutions of a low pH and may form insoluble free acids or free bases. A chart denoting the pH of certain drugs and certain solutions to be used as a vehicle is helpful in warning of potential incompatibilities.

Factors Affecting Stability or pH

Many factors may affect the stability or pH of drugs:

1. *Parenteral solutions.* Some commonly prescribed drugs precipitate when added to IV solutions. Differences in the physical and chemical properties of each of these solutions may affect the stability of any drug introduced. A compound

soluble in one solution may precipitate in another. Sodium ampicillin deteriorates in acid solutions. This drug, when added to isotonic sodium chloride at a concentration of 30 mg/mL, loses less than 10% activity in 8 hours. However, when it is added to 5% dextrose in water, usually a more acid solution, its stability is reduced to a 4-hour period.

Another factor affecting the stability of drugs is the broad pH range (3.5–6.5) of dextrose solutions allowed by the United States Pharmacopeia (USP). A drug may be stable in one bottle of dextrose 5 percent in water and not in another.[2]

2. *Additional drugs.* One drug may be compatible in a solution, but a second additive may alter the established pH to such an extent as to make the drugs unstable.[6]

3. *Buffering agents in drugs.* An important consideration in the stability of drugs is the presence of buffers or antioxidants, which may cause two drugs, however compatible, to precipitate. For example, ascorbic acid, the buffering component of tetracycline, lowers the pH of the product and therefore may accelerate the decomposition of a drug susceptible to an acid environment.

4. *Preservatives in the diluent.* Sterile diluents for reconstitution of drugs are available with or without a bacteriostatic agent. The bacteriostatic agents usually consist of parabens or phenol preservatives. Certain drugs, including nitrofurantoin, amphotericin B, and erythromycin, are incompatible with these preservatives and should be reconstituted with sterile water for injection.

5. *Degree of dilution.* Solubility often varies with the volume of solution in which a drug is introduced. For example, tetracycline hydrochloride, mixed in a small volume of fluid, maintains its pH range over 24 hours. However, when added to a large volume (1 L), it degrades after 12 hours, becoming less therapeutically active.

6. *Period of time solution stands.* Decomposition of substances in solution is proportional to the length of time they stand. For example, sodium ampicillin with the high pH of 8 to 10 becomes unstable when maintained in an acid environment over a period of time.

7. *Order of mixing.* The order in which drugs are added to infusions often determines their compatibility.

8. *Light.* Light may provide energy for chemical reactions to occur. Therefore, certain drugs, such as amphotericin B and nitrofurantoin, once diluted must be protected from light.[6]

9. *Room temperature.* Heat also provides energy for reactions. After reconstitution or initial dilution, refrigeration prolongs the stability of many drugs.

VASCULAR IRRITATION

The hazards of IV therapy can be reduced by taking adequate precautions.

Vascular irritation is a significant hazard of drugs administered IV. Any irritation that inflames and roughens the endothelial cells of the venous wall allows platelets to adhere; a thrombus is formed. Thrombophlebitis is the result of the sterile inflammation. When a thrombus occurs, the inherent danger of embolism is always present.

If aseptic technique is not strictly followed, septic thrombophlebitis may result from bacteria introduced through the infusion cannula and trapped in the thrombus. This is much more serious because of the potential dangers of septicemia and acute bacterial endocarditis.

Preventive Measures

The following precautions must be observed to diminish the potential hazards of vascular irritation:

1. Veins with ample blood volume should be selected when infusing hypertonic solutions or solutions containing irritating compounds.
2. The cannula should be appreciably smaller than the lumen of the vein. A large cannula may occlude the lumen, obstructing the flow of blood; the solution then flows undiluted, irritating the wall of the vein.
3. The venipuncture should be performed at the distal end of the extremity to allow each successive puncture to be executed proximal to the previous. Hypertonic solutions, when allowed to flow through a traumatized vein, cause increased irritation and pain.
4. Veins in the lower extremities are susceptible to trauma and should be avoided.
5. Isotonic solutions should, when possible, follow hypertonic solutions to flush irritating substances from the veins.
6. The rate of infusion may contribute to the irritation. In a large vein, slow administration permits greater dilution of the drug with the circulating blood. In a small vein lacking ample circulating blood, a slow drip prolongs the irritation, increasing the inflammation.
7. Prolonged duration of an infusion increases the risk of phlebitis. After a 24-hour period the danger increases. Periodic inspection of the injection site to detect developing phlebitis is important. After 48 hours the injection site should be changed.
8. Precautions should be observed to avoid administering solutions containing particulate matter by:
   a. Proper reconstitution and dilution of additives
   b. Inspection of parenteral fluids before administration
   c. Use of freshly prepared solutions
   d. Use of a set with a filter when danger of precipitation exists
   e. Periodic inspection of solutions containing additives
   f. Avoidance of administration of cloudy solutions unless affirmed by the manufacturer

APPROVED DRUG LISTS

Lists of drugs approved for administration by nursing professionals in all clinical environments in which care is provided must be readily available. In the inpatient setting, the institution's pharmacy and therapeutics committee is the group that generally approves such lists. Intravenous nursing professionals are often members of this committee, and protocols are brought to this group for approval before a drug is added to the listing. The committee ideally provides a listing of approved drugs for administration by professional nurses, a listing of drugs approved for addition to infusions in progress, and a listing of investigational agents approved for administration.[3] In the alternative care environment, home health agencies and clinics should also develop lists that are subsequently approved by their medical directors before acceptance by the nursing community.

THE PHYSICIAN'S RESPONSIBILITY

A licensed physician writes and signs all orders for IV drugs and solutions. A complete order includes the drug or solution, route of administration, rate of administration in milliliters per hour, or the approximate length of time of administration of the infusion.

The physician also administers the drugs not on the approved drug list.

THE INTRAVENOUS NURSE'S RESPONSIBILITY

The IV nursing specialist is responsible for checking the physician's order for accuracy, completeness, and appropriateness. If a doubt exists regarding the compatibility or safety of an order, the physician should be consulted.

After checking for possible incompatibilities, determining the availability of appropriate venous access, and ascertaining possible drug sensitivities or allergic responses, the IV nurse initiates the infusion and adjusts the rate of flow consistent with the prescribed order. No coercion should be used on rational, adult patients. If the patient refuses the infusion, the physician should be advised.

The IV nurse observes the patient for some time following initial administration of drugs that may contribute to anaphylaxis. If the drug is being given for the first time in the monitored setting, documentation should indicate first-dose monitoring.

THE STAFF NURSE'S RESPONSIBILITY

The staff nurse is responsible for maintaining the infusion in progress and for monitoring patient response to treatment, possible side effects, rate of flow, and condition of site. In many inpatient settings, the staff nurse also hangs subsequent IV solutions, discontinues IV therapy, and documents IV care. Staff nurse responsibility for delivery of infusion therapy should be delineated by job description, responsibility, and training.

PREPARATION OF INTRAVENOUS SOLUTIONS AND ADDITIVES

Intravenous additives and solutions are best prepared in an IV additive station of the institution's pharmacy. Aseptic technique is best observed when a "clean room" approach is used. A laminar flow hood, proper illumination, and handwashing facilities are readily available in such a setting.

Admixing should be performed using aseptic technique. The IV policy and procedure addressing admixing should define potential hazards, compatibility, stability requirements, and the types of admixtures within the scope of practice. Safeguards should be implemented to protect personnel from potential health hazards associated with the admixing of medications.

Laminar flow is air flow in which the entire body of air within a confined area moves with uniform velocity along parallel flow lines.[2] Laminar flow hoods have a vital role in eliminating the hazard of airborne contamination of IV solutions and admixtures. Nurses should be familiar with the general operating guidelines of the hood. Vertical and horizontal hoods are available. Laminar flow hoods should be used within state and federal guidelines as well as the recommendations of the American Society of Hospital Pharmacists.

Extreme care in the preparation of solutions diminishes the risk associated with IV therapy.

1. *Aseptic technique is imperative.* Bacterial and fungal contamination of drug products and parenteral solutions must be avoided.
2. *Proper dilution of lyophilized drugs is essential.* Two special cautions to ensure complete solubility in the reconstitution of drugs must be observed.
   a. The specific diluent recommended by the manufacturer should be used.
   b. The drug should be initially diluted in the volume recommended.
3. *Introduction of extraneous particles into parenteral solutions must be avoided.* Fragments of rubber stoppers are frequently cut out by the needles used and accidentally injected into solutions. Large-bore (15-gauge) needles are practical for use in the nurses' station and appear to have fewer disadvantages than the smaller needles.
   a. Smaller needles may encourage particles that may be difficult to see on inspection.
   b. The small particles may be of a size capable of passing through the indwelling cannula.
   c. Filter aspiration needles, used when preparing admixtures, can remove particles.

A solution that on inspection contains fragments of rubber must be discarded.

Procedure in Compounding and Administering Parenteral Solutions

The following steps should be carried out in the preparation of solutions for infusion:

1. Inscribe order for drug additive directly from original order to medication label.
2. Substantiate drug orders with the drug product and the parenteral solution.
3. Inspect solution for extraneous particles.
4. Check drug product for:
   a. Expiration date—Outdated drugs should not be used because loss of potency or stability may have occurred.
   b. Method of administration
      (1) Intramuscular preparations are not usually used for IV administration; they may contain certain components such as anesthetics or preservatives not meant for administration by the vascular route.
      (2) Some are packaged in multiple-dose vials, which may contribute to contamination.
      (3) The dosage by the intramuscular route may not coincide with that for IV use.
5. With an accepted antiseptic, clean rubber injection site of both the drug product and the diluent.
6. Use sterile syringe and needle.
7. Reconstitute according to manufacturer's recommendation.

8. Check diluted drug for complete solubility before adding to parenteral solution.

9. After adding to solution, invert solution container to mix the additive completely.

10. Clearly and properly label solution container with:
    a. Name of patient
    b. Drug and dosage
    c. Date and time of compounding
    d. Expiration date
    e. Signature

11. As an added precaution to prevent errors, recheck label with used drug ampules before discarding ampules.

12. Inspect solution for precipitates; if any precipitates are present, discard the solution.

13. Substantiate identity of patient with solution prepared.

14. Perform venipuncture consistent with institutional policy and INS standards.[3]

15. Observe patient for a few minutes following the initial IV administration of any drug that may cause anaphylaxis.

16. Use added caution in administering any drug whose fast action could produce untoward reactions:
    a. Controlled-volume set
    b. Microdrip
    c. Electronic infusion device

17. Ensure first-dose delivery of drug in a clinically monitored environment.

General Safety Rules

The following safety rules for preparation and IV administration of drugs by nurses should be adhered to at all times:

1. Nurses will, on written order, prepare and administer only those solutions, medications, and combinations of drugs approved in writing by the Pharmacy and Therapeutics committee.

2. No IV infusion that is cloudy, discolored, or contains a precipitate should be given.

3. All IV infusions must be used or discarded within 24 hours of the time the container is opened.

4. Any question regarding chemical compatibility or the relative safety of any drug added to an IV infusion should be directed to the director of the pharmacy.

DRUG DELIVERY SYSTEMS

Manufacturers have kept pace with demands for improved drug delivery systems for use in all clinical settings in which infusion therapy is administered. Standard methods of drug delivery and terminology still apply.[10]

Intermittent infusion allows drugs to be administered on an intermittent basis through a slow keep-open infusion using a secondary container, single-dose additive, or multiple-dose admixture connected to a controlled-volume set. The intermittent infusion may also be given through a self-contained administration system such as an elastomeric pump. Intermittent infusions are often given through an *intermittent infusion device* (*heparin lock*) to conserve veins, allow freedom of motion between infusions, and provide a minimal amount of infusate for the patient whose intake may be restricted. Peripheral and central IV catheters are adaptable as intermittent infusion devices by the addition of a catheter plug or resealable adapter. Patency of these lines is maintained by administering an amount of flush solution sufficient to fill the internal diameter of the line in use. Dilute heparin solution (hence, heparin lock), is most often used. Saline solution may also be used, and the use of antibiotic flush in the immunocompromised patient is gaining support in the medical and nursing communities.

Intravenous push is the direct injection of a medication into the vein. It may be administered through the distal Y site of an administration set, through the intermittent infusion device, or via cannula. The terms "IV push" and "bolus" may be confusing. Drugs such as radiopaque dye used to visualize the cardiac chamber must be injected as a bolus (defined as a discrete mass). Most medications ordered as an IV push or bolus must be administered slowly, up to 30 minutes, depending on the drug itself. Rapid injection increases the drug concentration in the plasma, which may reach toxic proportions, flooding the organs rich in blood—the heart and the brain—and resulting in shock and cardiac arrest. The rate of administration, included with the order for the medication, can reduce any misconceptions and prevent the potential risk of a life-threatening reaction from too-rapid administration of the drug.

Because the IV push allows instant increased drug levels in the blood, it offers immediate relief to the patient. Nurses in many special care units are trained and authorized to administer specific IV pushes. In the past, the IV push was restricted to the intensive care unit, where the patient was monitored and where a potential crisis might arise requiring its immediate use in the absence of a physician. Today, nurses frequently administer IV push injections.

Many drugs, given as IV injections, can be potentially dangerous to the patient. The nurse must understand the action of the drug and assess the patient's condition before administering the medication.

Decreased tolerance to the drug can result from factors in the patient's condition[4] such as:

1. Decreased cardiac output
2. Reduced renal flow or poor glomerular filtration
3. Diminished urinary output
4. Pulmonary congestion
5. Systemic edema

Greater dilution of the drug and a longer injection time can prevent drug accumulation, reduce venous irritation caused by a low pH, and allow time to assess the patient's response and detect early reactions. Use of the manufacturer's recommended diluent is most important because different drugs require different diluents.

Reactions

Knowledge of the expected therapeutic effects of the medication, the recommended dosage range, the side effects, and the toxic symptoms is essential.

Side effects may be manifest as gastrointestinal distress including nausea, vomiting, and diarrhea; as allergic skin reactions; and as central nervous system dysfunction.[4]

Major reactions may consist of respiratory distress, anaphylaxis, cardiac arrhythmias, and convulsions.

Reactions must be detected and reported at once so that proper treatment can be administered.

Antidotes

Nurses who administer IV medications should have a knowledge of various antidotes and their use.

Emergency supplies of antidotes should be readily available. Many are available in prefilled syringes for emergency use. Sterile cartridge needle units, with accurately machine-measured doses, provide a closed-injection system ready for instant use.

Available antidotes may consist of:

1. Lidocaine hydrochloride (Xylocaine) for ventricular arrhythmias; useful in certain conditions of hyperactivity
2. Epinephrine (Adrenalin) for relief of hypersensitivity reactions, respiratory distress caused by bronchospasm, and cardiac arrest following anesthesia reaction
3. Diphenhydramine hydrochloride, USP (Benadryl) for allergic skin manifestations
4. Diazepam (Valium) for convulsions
5. Trimethobenzamide hydrochloride (Tigan), an antiemetic agent

Continuous administration is the term applied to medications mixed in a large volume of infusate and infused over a time period in excess of 2 hours.[12]

IMPORTANT CHECKPOINTS IN INTRAVENOUS DRUG ADMINISTRATION

The Drug

1. Understand the expected therapeutic effect of the medication.
2. Know the recommended dosage range and the length of time required for administration.
3. Understand the side effects and toxic symptoms that can occur.
4. Be knowledgeable in the use of the proper antidote and its location.

The Patient

1. Make positive identification of the patient. Do not rely on the patient's verbal identification of himself or herself.
2. Ascertain allergy history (food and drug).
3. Assess the patient's condition and be aware of any factors that can effect the drug action.
4. Know what medications the patient is receiving; be aware of therapeutic incompatibilities that may occur between any other medication the patient is receiving and the IV push medication.
5. Watch for the patient's response during and after the injection.

Preparation of the Medication

1. Check and recheck the order with the drug label.
2. Check the expiration dates of the drug and of the diluent.
3. Use the drug manufacturer's recommended diluent.
4. Clarify any questions or doubts with the patient's physician.

The Injection

1. Make sure that the cannula is within the lumen of the vessel.
2. Make sure that the drug is compatible with the IV solution if it is administered through a primary line. If incompatible, clamp the set and flush the injection port with compatible fluid. DO NOT USE STERILE WATER.
3. Ascertain the compatibility of the medication with heparin when a heparin lock is used. If incompatible, flush the lock with a compatible fluid before and after the IV injection.
4. Administer the medication at an evenly divided rate over the length of time recommended by the manufacturer, using a watch with a second hand.
5. Document the medication, time administered, dosage, time span for administration, any required flushing, the patient's response, and your initials.

Health Care Facility

Any institution that authorizes nurses to administer IV medications should provide:

1. Written policies for the IV injection of medications by nurses
2. A list of drugs with the recommended dosage range and rate of administration for each drug
3. A list of drugs that may be incompatible with IV injection medications
4. An educational agenda that includes information on the major reactions of the medications, their antidotes, their proper usage, nursing implications for use of drugs, and assessment and monitoring of patients

Drug delivery systems today provide a wealth of administration sets, delivery vehicles, and approaches to safe delivery of infusion therapies to patients. Each nursing professional *must* assume responsibility for becoming familiar with specific equipment used by the institution to provide safe drug therapy for all patients.

DRUG CALCULATIONS

An integral component of IV nursing practice is the ability to perform the mathematical calculations required to administer correct doses of medication and solution to patients. Accuracy in the administration of medications is a special concern when medications are administered IV.

Flow Rate Calculations

Flow rate calculations require the following base of information: amount of solution to be infused, duration of the administration, and drop factor of the set to be used. First, determine the amount of solution to be administered; then divide that number by the delivery time:

$$\frac{1000 \text{ mL}}{8 \text{ hr}} = 125 \text{ mL/hr}$$

Next, note the drop factor of the set being used. A macrodrip set takes 10, 15, or 20 drops to deliver 1 mL solution.

$$\frac{\text{No. drops/mL of set}}{60 \text{ (min in an hr)}} \times \text{total hourly volume} = \text{no. drops/min}$$

$$\frac{\text{mL/hr} \times \text{drop factor of set}}{60} = \text{drops/min}$$

For microdrip or pediatric systems, the equation is:

$$\frac{\text{mL/hr} \times \text{drop factor}}{60} = \text{drops/min}$$

Drug Dosage Calculations

Ratio and proportion or "desired over have" (D/H) may be easily applied to calculation of drug dosages for infusion therapy.[11] Rate of administration of IV drugs may be calculated in units per hour. For example, there are 12,500 U heparin sodium in 250 mL IV solution. The dose ordered is 800 U/hr.

$$\times = 250 \text{ divided by } 12,500$$
$$\times = 0.02$$

Then, calculate the rate of the prescribed dosage:

$$0.02 \text{ mL} \times 800 \text{ U} = 16 \text{ mL/hr}$$

In this example, you have 200 mg drug in 500 mL of 5% dextrose in water. You want to know the number of milligrams of drug your patient is receiving per hour. Determine the amount of drug per milliliter of solution by placing D/H or:

$$\frac{500}{20} = 25$$

$$\frac{200}{25} = 8 \text{ mg/hr}$$

Percent Solutions

The relationship between the amount of solute and the total quantity of solution is expressed as a percentage or ratio. Percentage strength of solution may be calculated in one of three ways:

1. Percent weight in weight (W/W)—the weight of the solute (drug) compared to the weight of the solution (g drug/100 g solution)
2. Percent weight in volume (W/V)—the weight of the solute compared to the volume of the total solution (g drug/100 mL solution)
3. Percent volume in volume (V/V)—the volume of the solute compared to the volume of the total solution (mL drug/100 mL solution)[11]

EXPIRATION DATES

Drug container expiration dates identify the date when a medication or product is no longer acceptable for use. Institutional policy and procedure should state that medications should not be administered beyond their expiration dates. Expiration dates should be verified by the nursing professional before drugs and infusates are given to patients.

ADMINISTRATION OF INVESTIGATIONAL DRUGS

State and federal regulations govern the administration of investigational agents. Signed informed consent is required before patients can participate in the investigation. An informed consent must be written by the investigator, approved by the institutional review board, signed by the subject, and witnessed. Before approval by the United States Food and Drug Administration (FDA), drug studies are conducted in four stages:

1. Phase I: Clinical Pharmacology and Therapeutics
   a. Evaluate drug safety.
   b. Determine an acceptable single drug dosage or levels of patient tolerance for acute multiple dosing.
2. Phase II: Initial Clinical Investigation for Therapeutic Effect
   a. Evaluate drug efficacy.
   b. Conduct a pilot study (Table 22-4).

TABLE 22-4
Types of Blinds in Pilot Studies of Investigational Drugs

Open label	No blind is used. Both investigator and patient know the identity of the drug.
Single blind	The patient is unaware of which treatment is being received, but the investigator has this information. In unusual cases, the investigator, not the patient, may be kept blind to the identity of the treatment.
Double blind	Neither the patient nor the investigator is aware of which treatment the patient is receiving. A double-blind design is generally considered to provide the most reliable data from a clinical study. This type of study is more complicated to initiate and conduct.
Combination	In part 1 of a study, one type may be used. In part 2 of the same study, another type may be used. A third part of the same study may use the same blind as part 1 or use an entirely different type of blind. The blind used may be changed during the course of the study according to certain criteria (eg, when inpatients are discharged, the double blind may be broken, and they may continue their treatment on open-label medication).

3. Phase III: Full-scale Evaluation of Treatment
    a. Evaluate the patient population for which drug is intended.
4. Phase IV: Postmarketing Surveillance
    a. Provide additional information about the efficacy or safety profile.

Policies and procedures should be developed pertaining to the administration of investigational agents, regardless of the clinical setting in which care is provided. Table 22-5 details factors to be considered for inclusion. Table 22-6 provides elements of informed consent.

TABLE 22-5
Factors to Consider as Criteria for Patient Inclusion*

Characteristics of Patient	Disease/Treatment	Environmental/Other
Sex	Disease evaluated	Patient recruitment
Age	Concomitant drugs	Patient cooperation
Weight	Previous drugs/nondrugs	Other drug studies
Education	Washout period of nonstudy drugs/	Participation in other study with
Race/ethnic	treatments	same drug
Social	History of diseases	Institutional status
Economic	Present clinical status	Environmental status
Pregnancy	Previous hospitalization	Occupation
Lactation		Geographic location
Use of:		Litigation
tobacco		Disability
caffeine		
alcohol		
drugs		
Diet		
Genetics		
Disabilities		
Hypersensitivity		
Other allergies		

*Also considered for exclusion

TABLE 22-6
Elements of Informed Consent

- Written by the investigator
- Approved by the institution's review board or ethics committee
- Signed by the subject (patient or volunteer) or authorized representative
- Witnessed

REFERENCES

1. American Hospital Formulary Service. (1992). Bethesda, MD: American Society of Hospital Pharmacists.
2. Edward, M. (1967). pH—an important factor in the compatibility of additives in intravenous therapy. *American Journal of Hospital Pharmacy, 24,* 442.
3. *Revised intravenous nursing standards of practice.* (1990). *Journal of Intravenous Nursing,* (Suppl.), S52–S53.
4. McGill, D. (1973). Giving IV push. *Nursing 73,* June, (3) 15–18.
5. Needham Clinical Laboratories (1983). *Therapeutic drug monitoring* (p. 11). Needham Heights, MA.
6. Pelissier, N. A., & Burgee, S. L. (1968). Guide to incompatibilities. *Lippincott's Hospital Pharmacy, 3,* 15.
7. Provost, G. E. (1966). Prescription compounding by nurses in hospitals. *American Journal of Hospital Pharmacy, 23,* 595.
8. Sackheim, G. L., Lehman, D. D., & Schultz, R. M. (1978). *Laboratory chemistry for the health sciences* (3rd ed., pp. 70, 71, 79). New York: Macmillan.
9. Webb, J. W. (1969). A pH pattern of IV additives. *American Journal of Hospital Pharmacy, 26,* 31–35.
10. Weinstein, S. M. (1992). Electronic drug delivery in the 1990s and beyond: A nursing perspective. *Pharmacy and Therapeutics, 17*(2), 228–231.
11. Weinstein, S. M. (1990). Math calculations for intravenous nurses. *Journal of Intravenous Nursing, 13*(4), 231–236.
12. Weinstein, S. M. (1991). *Nurses' handbook of intravenous medications* (pp. 605–606). Philadelphia: J. B. Lippincott.

REVIEW QUESTIONS

1. Chemical interactions that cause the most common incompatibilities include all of the following EXCEPT:
   a. hydrolysis
   b. decomposition
   c. reduction
   d. oxidation

2. The process that causes certain salts, when placed in water, to decompose, thereby altering the pH is known as:
   a. decomposition
   b. hydrolysis
   c. oxidation
   d. reduction

3. Factors that may affect the pH of drugs include all of the following EXCEPT:
   a. additional drugs
   b. buffering agents
   c. body temperature
   d. order/method of mixing

4. To diminish the potential hazards of vascular irritation, the nursing professional should do which of the following?
   a. avoid veins in lower extremities
   b. use a cannula smaller than the lumen of a vessel
   c. use the largest vein possible
   d. use the largest cannula possible

5. Which of the following are nursing responsibilities in the administration of drugs that potentially cause anaphylaxis?
   a. question patient regarding sensitivity
   b. observe patients following initial dose
   c. ensure administration of initial dose in a monitored environment
   d. have physician administer the drug

6. What special cautions should be observed to reduce the risk of particulate matter?
   a. dilute lyophilized drugs
   b. use filter as needed
   c. avoid use of powdered drugs
   d. observe before administration

7. Which of the following are advantages of IV administration?
   a. quicker drug action
   b. avoids reabsorption problems associated with gastrointestinal tract
   c. useful for patients without functioning gastrointestinal tract
   d. reduces trauma associated with intramuscular and subcutaneous delivery

8. Factors to be included as criteria for inclusion in a study are all of the following EXCEPT:
   a. sex
   b. age
   c. weight
   d. residence

9. Patients in need of therapeutic drug monitoring include those with:
   a. combination therapies
   b. renal dysfunction
   c. skin disorder
   d. third-spacing

10. Factors influencing the pharmacokinetics of drugs include all of the following EXCEPT:
    a. smoking
    b. alcohol
    c. habitus
    d. height

CHAPTER 23

Pain Management

ACUTE PAIN

Acute pain afflicts millions of patients worldwide. Effective control of acute pain is one of the most important issues in postoperative care today.[2] The following factors influence the incidence, intensity, and duration of pain experienced postoperatively:

- Site, nature, and duration of surgical procedure
- Type of incision
- Degree of intraoperative trauma
- Physiologic and psychological makeup of the patient
- Preoperative preparation
- Presence of complications
- Anesthetic management before, during, and after surgery
- Quality of postoperative care

Postoperative pain is more intense in those who have had upper abdominal, intrathoracic, renal, and lower abdominal surgery; extensive surgery of the spine; surgery of the major joints and large bones in the hand and foot; and other major surgical interventions. Traditionally, postoperative pain has been handled with potent opioids alone or in combination with nonopioid analgesics and other drugs. A major advance in the management of this type of pain has been the growth in the number of acute pain services in health care institutions nationwide. With the benefit of daily assessment of patients for the quality of analgesia and side effects, treatment is now provided by one of the following means:

- Systemic analgesics and adjuvant drugs (administered intramuscularly, IV, by continuous infusion, or as patient-controlled analgesia [PCA])
- Intraspinal opioids
- Regional analgesia
- Electrical analgesia through transcutaneous electrical stimulation or electroacupuncture
- Psychological analgesia in the form of hypnosis

Sharon M. Weinstein: PLUMER'S PRINCIPLES & PRACTICE OF INTRAVENOUS THERAPY, FIFTH EDITION, © 1993 J. B. Lippincott Company

Postoperative pain control influences one's ability to cough, deep breathe, and ambulate after major surgery. Much progress has been made in the field of postoperative pain management.

CHRONIC PAIN

Chronic pain, such as that associated with progressive cancer, long-term disability or illness, and chronic conditions has traditionally been more difficult to manage. The use of ambulatory therapy for the terminally ill patient has increased dramatically. Started during hospitalization or during a visit to a surgical center, continuous narcotic infusion is initiated slowly, and the drug dosage is increased consistent with a patient's clinical condition. An oncology patient who in the past would have been hospitalized for pain control is able to be safely maintained as an outpatient for an extensive time period.

NARCOTICS

Administration of spinal opiates has enhanced pain management and provided an alternative to narcotic administration by the intramuscular or oral route. Breakthrough pain may occur and should be treated during IV PCA by increasing the medication dose consistent with physician's orders. Breakthrough pain during intrathecal opiate administration should be supplemented with IV, intramuscular, or oral narcotic dosing. Breakthrough pain associated with epidural systems is discussed further in this chapter.

Side Effects

Side effects with spinal opiates include:

- Respiratory depression
- Somnolence
- Confusion

- Urinary retention
- Nausea
- Pruritus

Respiratory depression is the only serious side effect of spinal opiates and may be associated with somnolence or confusion. The IV nurse or pain specialist should assess the patient's mental status and count respiratory rate; some patients slow their breathing rate or breathe irregularly during normal sleep or at periods of rest. Apnea monitors have been used in some pain programs.

Presence of confusion or somnolence may indicate a significant level of narcotic in the brain and impending respiratory depression.

Urinary retention may be related to causes other than spinal narcotic administration, including surgery in the urinary tract system. Administration of Urecholine contracts the bladder and may help. Catheterization may also reverse retention.

Nausea may be reversed by narcotic antagonists, such as Nubain or Narcan. Nausea should be evaluated for possible relation to postsurgical ileus and the effects of general anesthetics.

Epidural morphine has been associated with a high incidence of pruritus when used for pain control in women after cesarean section. Epidural morphine has also been reported to be associated with reactivation of the herpes simplex virus labialis (HSVL) in these women.[1]

ACCESS FOR EPIDURAL PAIN MANAGEMENT

Epidural access may be achieved through the placement of a percutaneous epidural catheter, a fully implantable epidural access portal system, or a fully implantable drug infusion pump.[3,4,7]

Epidural Catheters

Epidural administration of pain medications offers analgesia, lower total drug use, fewer and lesser side effects, less sedation, earlier ambulation, and enhanced patient comfort. Initially, a small lumen, temporary catheter made of nylon or Teflon is placed. Long-term delivery is possible through the use of a long-term epidural catheter [average duration of use: 104 days; longest duration with the DuPen catheter[9] (Figure 23-1): 972 days and ongoing]. The epidural port can also be used.[6]

The Epidural Port

The epidural port consists of the portal and catheter and contains a 60-μm filter to remove large particulate matter. The catheter of the portal is positioned in the epidural space by percutaneous introduction, and a subcutaneous pocket is prepared for the portal over a bony prominence. The system is intended for repeated injection or infusion of preservative-free morphine sulfate into the epidural space.

THE EPIDURAL SPACE

Epi refers to the outside and *dura* refers to the covering of the spinal cord, enclosing the cerebrospinal fluid. This is, therefore, the part of the spinal canal outside the dura mater, enclosed by connective tissue covering the vertebrae and ligamentum flavum. Extending from the base of the skull to the coccyx, it ends at about S-1 in many patients (the spinal cord ends at about L-1). The regions and respective width may be found in Figure 23-2.

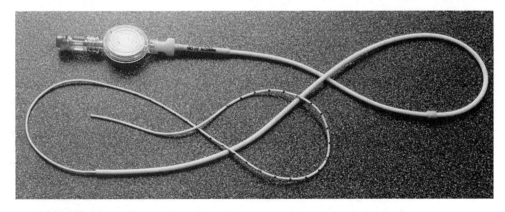

FIGURE 23-1 DuPen Epucath. (Courtesy: Davol, Inc., Subsidiary CR Bard Inc., Salt Lake City, UT)

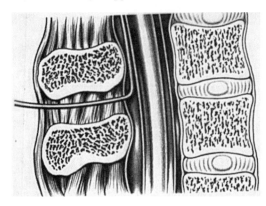

FIGURE 23-2   Close-up of L-1 epidural catheter placement.

This area is vascular; it supplies and drains blood from the vertebrae and spinal cord, and it is covered with spinal nerves. Filled with fatty tissue, blood vessels, lymphatics, and loose connective tissue, the epidural space has no "free" fluids. However, fluids injected into the epidural space spread in all directions between loose connective structures that occupy the space.

The intrathecal space is surrounded by the epidural space and separated from it by the dura mater. This space contains cerebral spinal fluid, which bathes the spinal cord.

Epidural pain management is the administration of narcotics into the epidural space to control one's pain. The advantage of administration of narcotics into this space is the ability to control pain with much lower volumes of narcotics. Potential candidates for epidural pain management should be evaluated for the following:

- Confirmed patient response to epidural medications
- Normal bleeding parameters
- Absence of active, untreated bacterial infection
- Acceptance of the therapy and understanding of potential side effects
- Adequate support systems to meet the patient's needs[5, 8, 10, 11]

CARE AND MANAGEMENT OF THE EPIDURAL CATHETER

Consistent with Intravenous Nursing Society (INS) Standards of Practice, the delivery of medications and maintenance and care of epidural catheters should be established in IV policies and procedures specific to the Nurse Practice Act. Policies and procedures for obtaining, delivering, administering, documenting, and discarding medication should be in accordance with state and federal regulations.

All medications administered by an epidural catheter should be preservative free. Alcohol is contraindicated for site preparation or when accessing the catheter because of the potential for migration of alcohol into the epidural space and possible resultant nerve damage. A 0.2-μm filter without surfactant should be used for medication administration. Before administration, the catheter should be aspirated to determine the absence of spinal fluid. Epidural catheters may be placed for short- or long-term use.

Mechanical problems may occur with the epidural catheter system, including leaking catheter hub, disconnected catheter, occluded catheter, or leaking at the skin site.

Bupivicaine Hydrochloride (Marcaine)

Combining a local anesthetic with epidural opiate may create more intense analgesia with an overall lower dose of narcotic agent. Intraspinal opiates block pain impulses within the spinal column at the level of the dorsal horn. Local anesthetics block nerve conduction at the nerve root level, thus preventing pain impulses from reaching the spinal cord. Side effects of high-dose bupivicaine hydrochloride include numbness, hypotension, urinary retention, and motor or sensory loss.

Epidural infusion is usually accomplished with administration of morphine sulfate (Infumorph) or fentanyl citrate. Patient-controlled analgesia is usually accomplished with administration of morphine sulfate, meperidine, or oxymorphone. Morphine is an opiate agonist that alters perception of pain at the spinal cord and in the higher levels of the central nervous system.

Aspiration of the Epidural Catheter

Indications for aspiration of the epidural catheter include inadequate pain control and oversedation. A normal effect is to visualize a small amount of blood-tinged or clear fluid flowing retrograde through the catheter into a 5- to 6-mL syringe. A blood-filled syringe is indicative of catheter migration into the intravascular space. Clear fluid in the syringe is indicative of catheter migration into the intrathecal space. In both cases, the infusion should be discontinued and the physician notified.

Flushing with Preservative-Free Saline

Flushing is performed to determine patency of the catheter; 3 mL preservative-free saline is instilled. If resistance is met, the connector to the epidural catheter should be loosened and a second attempt to flush should be made. If leaking occurs, the epidural catheter connector should be tightened.

Manipulating the Catheter Hub

If the catheter is disconnected and is lying open on the patient's bed *or* if it is leaking, the pump should be stopped and emergency interventions taken. If disconnected, the catheter should be cut 1/4 inch from its distal end with sterile scissors, and the connector should be replaced and tightened. If it is leaking at the hub, loosen the hub and remove the catheter from the hub. Reinsert the catheter as far as possible into the hub and tighten it. Take care not to overtighten the connection to prevent crimping the lumen. Restart the infusion pump and observe for leakage (Figure 23-3).

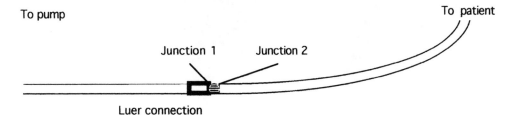

FIGURE 23-3 Epidural catheter and points at which damage may occur. 1 = Tighten catheter; 2 = Leak may occur.

Breakthrough Pain

Breakthrough pain with the epidural catheter is treated by administration of 2 to 4 mg morphine sulfate, IV, every 20 minutes as needed. If the patient is sensitive to morphine sulfate, 12.5 to 25 mg meperidine may be substituted, IV, every 20 minutes as needed.

Implanted Pumps

Advancements in medical technology have facilitated convenient alternatives to conventional methods of drug delivery. Systems such as the implanted pump (including pump, catheter, and optional access port) are implanted surgically and require periodic refilling. The pump weighs approximately 6 oz and stores and releases prescribed amounts of medication into the body (Figure 23-4). A computer programmer may be used by the physician or nurse during refill and checkup sessions to communicate with the pump and to set the prescription as ordered. The pump delivers a controlled amount of medication through a catheter to the area in the body where it will be most effective. These pumps are battery operated and generally last for 3 to 4 years. Potential risks include infection at the implant site, catheter plug or kinking, dislodgement, and leaking.

Patients should be cautioned to report redness, swelling, and pain near the incision and to avoid such activities as scuba diving, which would result in pump underinfusion and diminished drug effect. Diathermy and ultrasound treatments should be applied away from the pump site. Flow rates may be affected by atmospheric pressure, body temperature, blood pressure, and concentration and viscosity of the medication.

Possible complications include cessation of therapy caused by battery depletion, migration of the catheter access port, pocket seroma, rupture of the port connector at high injection pressures, complete or partial catheter occlusion, cerebrospinal fluid leak, and drug toxicity. The use of needles larger than 22 gauge may compromise the self-sealing properties of the septum. Huber-type needles are recommended to minimize

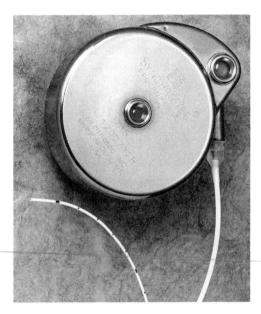

FIGURE 23-4 SynchroMed® Pump. (Courtesy: Medtronic, Minneapolis, MN)

septal damage. The IV nurse is cautioned to follow procedures for the use of implanted pumps, consistent with manufacturer's guidelines and institutional policy.

Patient Identification Card

When the pump is implanted, the surgeon should complete the patient registration and implantation record. The manufacturer will issue the patient a wallet-sized identification card containing information pertinent to the implanted pump. The physician should fill in the space provided for any medical emergency instructions. This card should be carried by the patient at all times.

Postimplantation Care

Patients should be monitored carefully after implantation to confirm proper pump performance, wound healing, and favorable response to therapy. The pump should not be used for the administration of drugs for several days after implantation to allow for adequate wound healing.

Patient Instructions

The patient should be instructed to:

1. Avoid traumatic physical activity to prevent tissue damage around the implant site.
2. Avoid long hot baths, saunas, and other activities that increase body temperature and result in increased drug flow.
3. Consult the physician during febrile illness to assess the effects of increased drug flow.
4. Consult the physician before air travel or change of residence to another geographic location. Adjustments in drug dosage may be required to compensate for an anticipated change in drug flow.
5. Avoid deep sea or scuba diving.
6. Report any unusual symptoms or complications relating to the specific drug therapy or the device.
7. Return at the prescribed time for pump refill.

Pump Refill Procedure

The pump will require refills at specific intervals, depending on the volume of the reservoir and the rate of administration.

The pump may be refilled as follows:

Equipment

Sterile fenestrated drape (1)

Sterile towel (1)

50-mL syringe with drug solution (1)

Sterile empty 50-mL syringe (1)

Sterile noncoring needle (1)

Sterile extension tubing with clamp (1)

Sterile gloves (1 pair)

Sterile 2 × 2 inch sponge (1)

Povidone–iodine swabs (3)

Heating pad (1)

Procedure

1. Warm 50-mL syringe with drug solution to 15° (59°F) to 35°C (95°F) with the heating pad.

2. Identify the outer perimeter of the pump by palpating the pump pocket. Locate pump septum.

3. Wash hands thoroughly and dry.

4. Using sterile technique, place all sterile items on opened sterile towel.

5. Put on sterile gloves.

6. Disinfect pump site with povidone–iodine. Use *three* separate preps. Start at the center of the pump and work outward beyond the periphery of the pump.

7. Place fenestrated drape over prepped pump site. Sterile template may be aligned over septum.

8. *Securely* connect *barrel* of empty 5-mL syringe and extension tubing to the noncoring needle. Close clamp.

9. Using a perpendicular angle, insert needle into center of septum.

10. Open clamp. Lower syringe barrel to below patient level and allow pump to empty.

11. Close clamp. Record returned volume, adding 1 mL for amount of drug remaining in extension tubing. Disconnect and discard syringe barrel.

12. *Securely* attach air-purged syringe with drug solution to extension tubing. Open clamp.

13. Using both hands, inject 5 mL solution into pump. Release pressure and allow drug to return to syringe. This test confirms proper needle placement. Continue to inject and check needle placement at 5-mL increments until syringe is emptied.

14. Pull needle out quickly and apply digital pressure with sterile sponge. If necessary, apply a sterile adhesive bandage.

PATIENT-CONTROLLED ANALGESIA

Patient-controlled analgesia allows the patient to control IV delivery of an analgesic and to maintain therapeutic serum levels of drug. The physician's order for PCA should include:

1. Loading dose, given IV push at initiation of therapy

2. Lock-out interval, during which the PCA device cannot be activated (usually 6–10 minutes)

3. Maintenance dose

4. Amount of drug patient will receive when the device is activated

5. Maximum amount the patient may receive within a given time frame

The PCA devices may have a pump with a call button or a wristband-type, disposable infuser. Factors to be considered in device selection include:

- Compatibility with currently used IV systems, poles
- Battery life
- Memory retention
- Display features
- Security features
- Safety features
- Commercial availability of prefilled syringes
- Delivery mode (PCA versus continuous infusion)

Ambulatory Infusion Pumps

A discussion of ambulatory infusion systems appropriate for pain management is contained in Chapter 12. Such devices have greatly enhanced our ability to manage acute, postoperative, and chronic pain in the hospital or alternative care setting. Units such as the CADD-PCA (Figure 23-5) are flexible; are programmable in milligrams or milliliters for use with a diversity of drugs and concentrations; are appropriate for subcutaneous, IV, and epidural delivery; are safe to use; are comfortable; and provide a total system of pain management and comprehensive support.

(text continues on page 438)

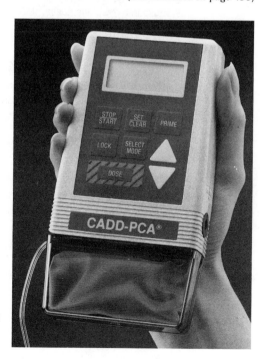

FIGURE 23-5 CADD-PCA® Ambulatory Infusion Pump. (Property of: Pharmacia Deltec, Inc., St. Paul, MN)

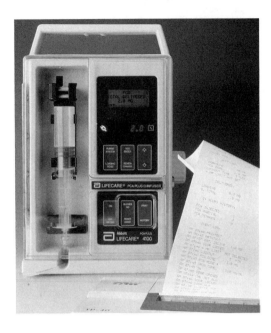

FIGURE 23-6 LifeCare PCA Plus II Infuser for pain management. (Courtesy: Abbott Laboratories, North Chicago, IL)

TABLE 23-1
Criteria and Rationale for RN Administration of Epidural Analgesia

Criteria	Rationale
Only postoperative patients would have epidural narcotics administered by RNs.	Chronic pain patients often require high doses that increase the risk of side effects.
Epidural medication would be limited to preservative-free morphine sulfate (MS).	The onset and duration of action of MS is well-known. Other medications would be administered by anesthesiologists.
RNs will only administer narcotics through epidural, not intrathecal, catheters.	There are greater risks of respiratory depression during intrathecal administration.
An apnea monitor would be used for the first 24 hr or longer until dosage has been stabilized.	Respiratory depression is most likely to occur within this time frame.
The anesthesiologist would be notified when: There is minimal or no pain relief following epidural administration. Clear or bloody fluid is aspirated from the catheter before injecting. Patient experiences pain on injection. Clear drainage is noted on the dressing.	These events indicate problems with the catheter.
Anesthesiologist will change the epidural dressing every 48 hr.	Epidural catheters are not sutured into place. The risk of dislodgement at time of dressing change is high.

(Reprinted from the *Oncology Nursing Forum* with permission from the Oncology Nursing Press, Inc. Camp-Sorrell, D., Fernandez, K., and Reardon, M. B. [1990]. Teaching oncology nurses about epidural catheters. *Oncology Nursing Forum,* *17*[5], 683–689.)

FIGURE 23-7 Patient care plan for postoperative pain control using epidural analgesia. Reprinted from the *Oncology Nursing Forum* with permission from Oncology Nursing Press, Inc. (Camp-Sorrell, D., Fernandez, K., & Reardon, M. B. [1990]. Teaching oncology nurses about epidural catheters. *Oncology Nursing Forum,* *17*[5], 683–689.)

Initials / In date	NURSING DIAGNOSIS/PATIENT PROBLEM DESIRED OUTCOME	ACTIONS/INTERVENTIONS SET & REVIEWED W/PATIENT/FAMILY [ ]YES [ ]NO	TARGET DATE	DATE OF DAILY REVIEW/INITIALS	RESOLUTION DATE EVALUATION
	1. Knowledge deficit related to the use of epidural analgesia for post-operative pain control. Patient demonstrates knowledge related to epidural catheter use for post-operative pain control and verbalizes understanding of need to report pain as soon as perceived	1. Describe the placement of the catheter, its use, who will administer pain medication and the use of an apnea monitor for immediate post-op period			
	2. Potential for injury due to catheter displacement (i e intrathecal space) Catheter will remain in epidural space or will be removed immediately if dislodged	1. RN will monitor: a The patency of the catheter b The condition of the dressing c Observe catheter site of intactness and hash marks indicating length d Negative aspiration before each medication adminstration			
	3 Potential for ineffective breathing pattern related to respiratory depression secondary to epidural analgesia Patient will exhibit effective breathing pattern: • respirations of six or greater, regular and non-labored	1 Maintain apnea monitor for first 24 hours or until a baseline dose is established to maintain patient comfort			

Initials	RN Signatures	Initials	RN Signatures

Primary Nurse

Social Worker:

Other

435

ini date	Initials	NURSING DIAGNOSIS/PATIENT PROBLEM DESIRED OUTCOME	ACTIONS/INTERVENTIONS SET & REVIEWED W/PATIENT/FAMILY [ ]YES [ ]NO	TARGET DATE	DATE OF DAILY REVIEW/INITIALS	RESOLUTION DATE EVALUATION
		3. Potential for ineffective breathing (Continued)	2 Have Naloxone (Narcan) 4mg available at all times while epidural narcotics are being used			
			3 Maintain IV access at all times while epidural catheter is in place			
			4 Monitor for signs of restlessness, miosis			
		4. Potential urinary retention related to atonic bladder from sacral analgesia Patient will demonstrate adequate urinary elimination.	1 If urinary catheter not in place, measure intake and output every four hours for first 24 hours and every eight hours thereafter			
		5. Potential for alteration in comfort related to displacement or dysfunction of the catheter. Patient will report adequate pain control	1 Use visual analog scale and Pain Flow Sheet to monitor patient comfort level every four hours			
			2 Administer medication as ordered or notify anesthesiologist of inadequate pain control. * Note: No other narcotics, tranquilizers or sedatives may be given unless ordered by anesthesiologist			

Initials	RN Signatures	Initials	RN Signatures

Primary Nurse:

Social Worker:

Other:

FIGURE 23-7 (Continued)

436

In date / Initials	NURSING DIAGNOSIS/PATIENT PROBLEM / DESIRED OUTCOME	ACTIONS/INTERVENTIONS SET & REVIEWED W/PATIENT/FAMILY [ ] YES [ ] NO	TARGET DATE	DATE OF DAILY REVIEW/INITIALS	RESOLUTION DATE / EVALUATION
	6. Potential for discomfort related to pruritis secondary to release of histamine from the morphine effect. :Patient will inform caregiver when itching begins. Patient will report relief of itching	1 Administer antipruritic as ordered by anesthesiologist PRN			
	7. Potential for hypotension related to vasomoter disturbance :Blood pressure will be maintained at adequate level	1 Monitor vital signs every four hours while epidural is in use 2 Maintain adequate intravenous or oral fluid intake 3 Elevate lower extremities 4 When getting OOB, allow patient to dangle at bedside first			
	8. Potential for injury related to infection secondary to epidural catheter. :Patient will remain infection-free as evidenced by absence of purulent drainage, redness or tenderness at catheter insertion site.	1 Monitor catheter insertion site every shift for redness, edema, drainage 2 Maintain strict sterile technique during preparation and administration of medications 3 Monitor temperature and WBC to detect possible infection.			

Initials	RN Signatures	Initials	RN Signatures

Primary Nurse

Social Worker:

Other

FIGURE 23-7 (Continued)

Epidural Catheter Checklist Medication Administration

Name: _____

Expectation: Performs epidural catheter care and the administration of medication safely.

	Date: _____		Date: _____	
	Yes	No	Yes	No
1. Checks physician order	____	____	____	____
2. Gathers supplies	____	____	____	____
3. Assesses patient	____	____	____	____
4. Maintains aseptic technique	____	____	____	____
5. Checks catheter placement	____	____	____	____
6. Administers medication	____	____	____	____
7. Documents procedure	____	____	____	____
8. Evaluates patient's response	____	____	____	____

Observer: _____   _____

The medication administration checklist is used to evaluate the clinical skills portion of the epidural catheter learning experience.

(Reprinted from the Oncology Nursing Forum *with permission from the Oncology Nursing Press, Inc. Camp-Sorrell, D., Fernandez, K., and Reardon, M. B. [1990]. Teaching oncology nurses about epidural catheters.* Oncology Nursing Forum, 17[5], 683–689.)

Stationary Infusion Devices

Abbott's LifeCare PCA Classic and PCA Plus II meet the needs of the sedentary patient receiving pain management. The Classic is a single-mode PCA device for low-cost PCA procedures. The Plus II has the ability to dose in micrograms or milligrams (Figure 23-6).

STAFF EDUCATION _____

Although information on the safe administration of epidural medication and monitoring of potential side effects is available, little has been written about preparing the registered professional nurse for administering and monitoring epidural analgesia. The initial step is to establish criteria and rationale on which the policy and procedure for administration of epidural analgesia would be based, as outlined in Table 23-1.

Development of a care plan illustrating potential side effects and appropriate nursing interventions is an essential component of the process. A sample care plan is detailed in Figure 23-7.

The clinical program should be intensive, and ideally, skills checklists may be used to identify criteria for assessing appropriate techniques. Sample checklists for medication administration and for discontinuing the catheter are shown.

Epidural Catheter Checklist Discontinuing Catheter

Name: _____

Expectation: Performs epidural catheter removal safely.

	Date: _____		Date: _____	
	Yes	No	Yes	No
1. Checks physician order	—	—	—	—
2. Gathers supplies	—	—	—	—
3. Assesses patient	—	—	—	—
4. Maintains sterile technique	—	—	—	—
5. Removes catheter slowly	—	—	—	—
6. Checks catheter tip	—	—	—	—
7. Cleanses insertion site	—	—	—	—
8. Applies dressing	—	—	—	—
9. Documents procedure	—	—	—	—
10. Evaluates patient's response	—	—	—	—

Observer: _____   _____

The discontinuing catheter checklist is part of the clinical skills evaluation.

(Reprinted from the Oncology Nursing Forum *with permission from the Oncology Nursing Press, Inc. Camp-Sorrell, D., Fernandez, K., and Reardon, M. B. [1990]. Teaching oncology nurses about epidural catheters.* Oncology Nursing Forum, 17[5], 683–689.)

DOCUMENTATION

Documentation should include the type of pain management provided, route of administration, methods used, IV or other access route, site care and maintenance, assessment of pain and degree of pain relief, and problems encountered in dealing with the particular type of access used. Flow sheets facilitate accuracy of documentation and provide a guideline for all areas of concern, including pain rating (intensity) and level of consciousness (Figure 23-8).

When PCA systems are implemented, the nurse records the date, time, medication, patient's name, room number, physician's name, and his or her name on an appropriate flow sheet. The continuous nature of the injection does not permit nursing to record the exact dosage administered on standard control sheets found in many health care institutions today. Many such facilities have developed individualized flow sheets specifically for PCA control (Figure 23-9).

The American Pain Society[6] has developed quality assurance standards for pain relief (Table 23-2).

(text continues on page 443)

PAIN ASSESSMENT FLOW SHEET

DATE:

MEDICATION ORDERED:

CONTINUOUS RATE:

PCA DOSE:

LOCKOUT:

CHECK ONE:

EPIDURAL: _____

INTRATHECAL: _____

IV-PCA: _____

(Addressograph Plate)

1 Hour Assessment

Date	Time	Sed. Scale	Respir. Rate	Med. Inf. As Ordrd. Tubing Secure

4-HOUR ASSESSMENT — Local Anesthetic

Pain Scale	B.P./ Pulse Lying	B.P./ Pulse Sitting	No Loss Of Sens. Lower Extrem.	Drsg. Dry Intact. No Edema S/S of Inf.

Checks Made Here - See Nurse's Notes:

Urinary Ret.	Pruritis	Break Through Pain	Catheter Checked For Placement	Drsg. Chg. (Kit Utied.)	Catheter Flushed 3cc NS.	Nausea Vomiting	Pulse Ox.	R.N.'s Initials

RN SIGNATURE / INITIALS:

N/V ECOG SCALE:
0 - No Nausea or Vomiting
1 - Nausea/Vomiting X 1/day
2 - Nausea/Vomiting Less Than X 6/day
3 - Vomiting X 6/day
4 - Dehydration - IV Therapy

PAIN SCALE:
0 - No Pain
1 - 2 - Discomfort
3 - 4 - Mild Pain
5 - 6 - Distress
7 - 8 - Severe Pain
9 - 10 - Excruciating Pain

SEDATION SCALE:
0 - No Sedation–Pt. Found Awake.
S - Normal Sleep–Easy To Awake.
1 - Mild Drowsy, Easy To Arouse.
2 - Moderate, Frequently Drowsy, Still Able To Arouse.
3 - Severely Somnolent, Unable To Arouse.

FIGURE 23-8 Pain assessment form. (Courtesy: Midwestern Regional Medical Center, Zion, IL)

PAIN ASSESSMENT ORDERS:

_____

_____

_____

_____

_____

_____

_____

_____

NURSE'S NOTES:

_____

_____

_____

_____

_____

_____

_____

_____

_____

_____

_____

_____

_____

_____

_____

_____

_____

_____

_____

_____

FIGURE 23-8   (_Continued_)

PATIENT-CONTROLLED ANALGESIA
Sample Flow Sheet

HOSPITAL I.D.   PATIENT I.D.

DATE_____   LOADING DOSE_____
MEDICATION——————   (IF APPLICABLE)

TIME	12MN	2A	4A	6A	8A	10A	12N	2P	4P	6P	8P	10P
DOSE VOLUME (ML)												
LOCK-OUT												
4 HR LIMIT (ML)												
# DOSE DEL.												
TOTAL VOL. DEL.												
SEDATION (1-5)												
PAIN (1-5)												
RESP. RATE												
NURSE'S SIG.												

ADMIN. SET
CHANGE

NEW PCA
UNIT

CONDITION
I.V. SITE

SCALES

SEDATION	PAIN
1 = WIDE AWAKE	1 = COMFORTABLE
2 = DROWSY	2 = IN MILD DISCOMFORT
3 = DOZING INTERMITTENTLY	3 = IN PAIN
4 = MOSTLY SLEEPING	4 = IN BAD PAIN
5 = ONLY AWAKENS WHEN AROUSED	5 = IN VERY BAD PAIN

FIGURE 23-9 Sample flow sheet for patient-controlled analgesia.

TABLE 23-2
American Pain Society Quality Assurance Pain Relief Standards

- Recognize and treat pain promptly.
  Chart and display pain and relief. (Process)
  Define pain and relief levels to initiate review. (Process)
  Survey patient satisfaction. (Outcome)
- Make information about analgesics readily available. (Process)
- Promise patients attentive analgesic care. (Process)
- Define explicit policies for use of advanced analgesic technologies. (Process)
- Monitor adherence to standards. (Process)

REFERENCES

1. Ackerman, W. E., Juneja, M. M., Kaczorowski, D. M., & Colclough, G. W. (1989). A comparison of the incidence of pruritus following epidural opioid administration in the parturient. *Canadian Journal of Anaesthesia*, 36(4), 388–391.
2. Bonica, J. J. (1990). Management of post-operative pain. In J. J. Bonica (Ed.). *The management of pain* (2nd ed., pp. 461–480). Philadelphia: Lea & Febiger.
3. Caballero, G. A., Ausman, R. K., & Himes, J. (1986). Epidural morphine by continuous infusion with an external pump for pain management in oncology patients. *American Surgeon*, 8(52), 402–405.
4. DuPen, S. L. (1987). A new permanent exteriorized epidural catheter for narcotic self-administration to control cancer pain. *Cancer*, 59, 986–993.
5. Hassenbusch, S. J., Pillay, P. K., Magdinec, M., Currie, K., Bay, J. W., Covington, E. C., Tomaszewski, M. Z. (1990). Constant infusion of morphine for intractable cancer pain using an implanted pump. *Journal of Neurosurgery*, 73(3), 405–409.
6. Max, M. (1990). American Pain Society quality assurance standards for relief of acute pain and cancer pain. In M. R. Bond, J. E. Charlton, & C. J. Woolf (Eds.). *Proceedings of the VI World Congress on Pain* (pp. 196–189). Amsterdam: Elsevier.
7. Paice, J. A. (1987). New delivery systems in pain management. *Nursing Clinics of North America*, 22(3), 715–726.
8. Patt, R. B. (1989). Interventional analgesia: Epidural and subarachnoid therapy. *American Journal of Hospice Care*, March/April, 11–14.
9. Product literature. Davol, Inc. Subsidiary of C. R. Bard, Inc., P.O. Box 8500, Cranston, RI ONC 60290–88810M.
10. Waldman, S. D. (1990). The role of spinal opioids in the management of cancer pain. *Journal of Pain and Symptom Management*, 5(3), 163–168.
11. Yablonski-Peretz, T., et al. (1985). Continuous epidural narcotic analgesia for intractable pain due to malignancy. *Journal of Surgical Oncology*, 29, 8–10.

REVIEW QUESTIONS

1. Pain management may be provided by which of the following?
   a. systemic analgesics
   b. continuous infusion
   c. intraspinal opioids
   d. regional analgesia

2. Breakthrough pain during IV PCA should be treated by:
   a. increasing medication dose consistent with physician's orders
   b. increasing medication dose consistent with nursing judgment
   c. oral narcotic dosing
   d. intramuscular dosing

3. Nausea may be reversed by narcotic antagonists, such as which of the following?
   a. Nubain
   b. Narcan
   c. Neupogen
   d. Naloxone

4. Epidural morphine has been associated with a high incidence of:
   a. pruritus
   b. pustule formation
   c. reactivation of HSVL
   d. confusion

5. Alcohol is contraindicated for site preparation or when accessing the catheter because of the potential for:
   a. migration into the epidural space
   b. possible nerve damage
   c. obliterating the catheter
   d. damage to the Silastic

6. Mechanical problems associated with the catheter include:
   a. occlusion
   b. disconnection
   c. leaking at hub
   d. leaking at site

7. Indications for aspiration of the epidural catheter include:
   a. adequate pain control
   b. inadequate sedation
   c. inadequate pain control
   d. oversedation

8. Clear fluid in the syringe following aspiration is an indication of:
   a. catheter patency
   b. catheter kinking
   c. catheter migration
   d. catheter damage

9. Quality assurance pain relief standards have been developed by which of the following?
   a. American Pain Society
   b. American Epidural Society
   c. American Association for Pain
   d. American Pain Control

10. Factors to be considered in device selection include:
   a. battery life
   b. memory retention
   c. display features
   d. safety features

CHAPTER 24 _____

Antineoplastic Therapy

Cancer chemotherapeutic agents present a unique challenge to the nurse responsible for their administration. Their history of being viewed as formidable substances with which to work is best overcome by the nurse interested in uniting highly refined IV skill with a keen awareness of how and why chemotherapy works. Successful nursing implementation of a chemotherapeutic regimen depends on a mutual understanding of the current goal of therapy (cure, control, or palliation); on the comprehensiveness of patient preparation and education; on the reliable knowledge and competence of the nurse caring for the patient with cancer; and, finally, on a healthy respect for these powerful chemicals themselves.

It is useful to know that oncology patients report their cancer experience as much more tolerable when they are cared for by nurses who are highly skilled in IV therapy. Thus, a unique opportunity awaits the professional who chooses to participate in this aspect of cancer care.

QUALIFICATIONS OF CLINICIANS _____

Credentialing

The privilege of administering antineoplastic agents must be preceded by extensive exposure to standardized educational preparation and practical experience. To provide consistently safe, high quality, and appropriate care to the patient, many centers currently mandate comprehensive training programs leading to credentialing in chemotherapy administration.

To provide a standardized framework for such credentialing, the Oncology Nursing Society (ONS) developed *Cancer Chemotherapy Guidelines*, a series of five modular professional education tools.[20,22,23] These guidelines provide structured recommendations for a combined theoretical and clinical curriculum, specific to acute, outpatient, or home care settings. Each module suggests a didactic core curriculum followed by a clinical practicum.

The didactic component includes basic information on the biology of cancer, pharmacology and principles of cancer chemotherapy, specific antineoplastic agents, the major principles governing the administration of chemotherapy, and patient assessment and management. This information is then applied during the clinical practicum, where

Sharon M. Weinstein: PLUMER'S PRINCIPLES & PRACTICE OF INTRAVENOUS THERAPY, FIFTH EDITION, © 1993 J. B. Lippincott Company

clinical skills are exercised and evaluated, before the nurse is considered qualified to administer chemotherapy safely and confidently.

The following sample course outline provides the major subjects that would be necessary to include in preparation for chemotherapy credentialing, whether it be to practice in a specific institution or to prepare for professional certification through the ONS.[20, 23, 32, 33]

I. Audiovisual component
  A. Historical overview of cancer chemotherapy
  B. Cell cycle
  C. Cellular kinetics
  D. Indications for use of antineoplastics
  E. Drug actions and classifications
  F. Drug development and investigative trials
  G. Therapeutic intent with combined modality therapy
  H. Side effects associated with cytotoxic agents
  I. Drug calculations, handling, preparation, storage, and disposal
  J. Normal dose ranges
  K. Drug administration techniques

II. Didactic component
  A. Individual facility policy statement and legal aspects
  B. Pharmacology of antineoplastics
  C. Drug calculation and reconstitution
  D. Drug administration principles and techniques
  E. Nursing management of side effects and common problems
  F. Patient and family education materials and teaching strategies
  G. Documentation
  H. Patient and family resources

III. Individual handout materials
  A. Nursing qualifications
  B. Policy and procedures
  C. List of approved drugs for administration by a nurse
  D. Samples of written patient education tools
  E. Nomogram to calculate body surface area
  F. Math test
  G. Pretest
  H. Class evaluation
  I. Bibliography
  J. Selected literature

IV. Clinical practicum
  A. Drug calculation
  B. Drug preparation and handling
  C. Drug storage and transport
  D. Drug administration techniques
  E. Management of complications
  F. Appropriate documentation
  G. Patient and family teaching and follow-up

The mechanics of delivering IV antineoplastic agents safely is only one aspect in caring for the cancer patient receiving cytotoxic agents. In addition, the nurse specializing in medical oncology needs a solid foundation of knowledge relevant to the specialty. Suggested areas for inclusion in basic oncology nursing education programs follow.

I. Pretherapy patient evaluation
   A. Performance status
   B. Nutritional status
   C. Hematologic assessment
   D. Psychosocial assessment
   E. Systems review
      1. Cardiac
      2. Renal
      3. Hepatic
      4. Pulmonary
      5. Gastrointestinal
   F. Diagnostic evaluation

II. Treatment selection
   A. Histology
   B. Location, size
   C. Prior therapy
   D. Therapeutic intent
      1. Cure
      2. Control
      3. Palliation
   E. Treatment type
      1. Primary
      2. Adjuvant
      3. Combined modality
   F. Drug calculation, scheduling, and dose modifications
   G. Treatment response

III. Principles of cancer chemotherapy
   A. Pharmacology
   B. Drug classifications
   C. Cellular kinetics
   D. Drug interactions
   E. Drug delivery (route, rate)

IV. Complications and toxicities
   A. Short-term
      1. Alopecia
      2. Gastrointestinal
      3. Bone marrow
      4. Allergic reactions
      5. Phlebitis and extravasation
      6. Psychosocial
   B. Long-term
      1. Genetic

        2. Oncogenetic
        3. Immunosuppressive
        4. Reproductive
        5. Psychosocial
    C. Specific organ toxicities
        1. Cardiac
        2. Renal
        3. Pulmonary
        4. Hepatic
        5. Gastrointestinal
        6. Neurologic
        7. Dermatologic
        8. Reproductive
V. Nursing care
    A. Early detection and prevention of complications
    B. Delivery of expert care
    C. Patient and family education
    D. Psychosocial support (newly diagnosed, remission, recurrence, terminal)
    E. Follow-up support needs

Remarkable progress in the field of cancer therapy relative to the use of antineoplastic agents as a major treatment modality poses a challenge to the clinician responsible for administration of these agents. Clinical investigation to discover new therapeutic methods of cytotoxic drug delivery is ongoing and vigorous in many cooperative groups. As a result, the nurse who chooses to maintain an expertise in this area is obliged to participate regularly in continuing education programs and to study current and related professional literature. The ONS recommends the development of an institutional mechanism for annually evaluating nursing knowledge and skill relative to chemotherapy administration and requires professional certification through reexamination every 4 years.[20]

LEGAL CONSIDERATIONS

Thorough understanding of legal implications as outlined in Chapter 2 is essential for the nurse who administers IV fluids and drugs. Additional legal considerations pertinent to cancer chemotherapy include:

1. The clinician should not administer cancer chemotherapy agents unless informed consent has been obtained. "If consent has not been obtained, the hospital or institution may be held liable if treatment is administered. Failure to obtain a patient's consent may constitute 'battery.' Battery may be defined as any physical contact of a patient without his permission."[6] Obtaining informed consent is the responsibility of a physician rather than a nurse in most states.[3]

2. The clinician should have in writing a clear statement of the lines of supervision.

3. The clinician should have defined what the standards of care are at the employing facility, what the scope of duty includes, and what "reasonable care" means in the particular area of practice.

4. The clinician should receive adequate training and supervision in IV fluid and drug administration before approaching the patient who is to receive chemotherapy. Written documentation of these qualifications in the clinician's personnel file is recommended.

5. A clinician should have completed the process of initial patient and family education regarding all medications that are part of the treatment regimen, including their side effects, with subsequent assertions of the patient's understanding and documentation of the same.

It is to the clinician's benefit to have defined in writing the scope of practice for each setting in which care is provided. The clinician should also explore the current medical liability insurance covering the practice. Some employers provide adequate coverage for care administered when the nurse is on duty. However, independent practitioners, instructors, or those working in physicians' offices may choose to obtain their own malpractice insurance. Unfortunately, as nurses assume greater responsibility in cancer chemotherapy administration, there may be an increased incidence of nurses involved in litigation proceedings. By taking care to ensure that the clinician is functioning within defined statutes, it is hoped that litigation can be avoided.[4, 14]

In addition to practice according to the care standards and policies and procedures of one's employer, the following organizations are resources for all nurses who are interested both in further defining the legal statutes that govern nursing practice and in national standards of IV and oncology nursing practice that pertain to the administration of chemotherapy:

- American Nurses Association
- Individual state departments of professional regulation (for data on state's Nurse Practice Act)
- Intravenous Nurses Society
- Oncology Nursing Society

Because the patient's clinical record contains the legally binding information used as evidence in litigation proceedings, thorough and appropriate nursing documentation is crucial. Miller has aptly described the essentials of adequate documentation, which include the time of significant incidence, a thorough and objective description of the care provided, a patient's state, and the exact nature of the physician's involvement.[17]

The expert nurse caring for the patient with cancer frequently practices at a level of autonomy that exceeds some other areas of nursing practice. Sometimes this allows for increased legal vulnerability. For instance, extensive telephone contact with oncology patients is common; the nurse is well-served by carefully working within the accepted scope of practice when responding to a patient's immediate needs. Also, the nurse is commonly the key clinician involved in clinical trials that call for take-home investigational drugs. It is unlawful for anyone other than a pharmacist or physician to dispense medication; thus, the packaging and delivery of investigational drugs is not a legal nursing function.

Finally, knowledge of common dosing and scheduling of cancer chemotherapy agents is undoubtedly the best protection for both nurse and patient from delivering an incorrect dosage of drug which, in the cases of some cancer chemotherapeutic agents, can be lethal.

PATIENT PARTICIPATION

Experience indicates that patient acceptance of and response to treatment are more favorable when they are actively involved in the therapy program. When administering cytotoxic agents, the nurse should involve the patient in all phases of care, even to the extent of actively soliciting the patient's assistance in assessing vein status. The wise clinician will listen to the patient who says, "The nurse tried three times to give me my medicine in that vein last week, and it didn't work." In addition to providing patients with a sense of control, the nurse is acknowledging a respect for the patient's knowledge of his or her body. The fact that patients frequently sense inner changes occurring in their bodies can be used to the clinician's advantage. Many patients can detect a coolness along the venous pathways as IV solutions are infused and can be assured that this is normal. Likewise, many patients can detect early extravasation before the therapist is able to do so. For this reason, the nurse should alert the patient to the signs of extravasation if vesicant agents are being infused and ask the patient to report them if they occur. These may include pain, burning, stinging, a feeling of tightness, tingling, numbness, or any other unusual sensation.

Several chemotherapy agents are associated with localized and generalized anaphylactic reactions, and, when reported early and treated properly, their course can be reversed or minimized. Patients are strongly encouraged to report symptoms of generalized tingling, chest pains or sensations, shortness of breath, or lightheadedness. The clinician should use sensitivity in imparting this information to the patient by assessing the patient's overall anxiety level before instruction.

In recommending that patients be encouraged to participate actively in the treatment program, the nurse creates the possibility that some patients may attempt to direct their care. Patient attempts at intimidation with statements such as, "This is the vein you must use today," or "I'll only give you one try, then you've got to go find someone else," should be anticipated. Undoubtedly, the patient doesn't realize how a remark like this can undermine a nurse's self-confidence. Several minutes spent explaining the rationale and process of vein selection to the patient may prevent a recurrence of the situation.

Once a working rapport has been established, the nurse will generally find that patient behavior shifts from this level of fear and anxiety to an almost implicit trust in the skill and judgment of the clinician with whom they are most familiar. This phenomenon of a patient's personal attachment to a particular chemotherapy nurse is a common observation that often begins before any chemotherapy is given, in the period of patient education. It is in the patient's best interest for the nurse to receive this exclusive partiality by encouraging a balanced relationship that disallows development of an unhealthy dependence from the outset. Patients are best served when directed toward their own inner resources and empowered to endure therapy without inordinate focus on "who's going to give me my treatment today."

PATIENT AND FAMILY EDUCATION

Nurses involved in the administration of chemotherapy have a tremendous opportunity to minimize treatment-related morbidity and thus, enhance their patients' quality of life. This opportunity is readily realized through the nurse's skill as a competent educator. Educating patients and their families or caregivers is as integral to the cancer treatment regimen as is vein selection for agent infusion.

The primary focus of this chapter deliberately places emphasis on the technical aspects of chemotherapy administration in the hope of satisfying the clinical needs of the IV nurse. At the same time, safe, skilled, efficient craftsmanship in antineoplastic agent delivery is only about half the vocation of contemporary IV therapy nursing professionalism; the more sensitive (and sometimes more influential) part of the art revolves around intuitive patient and family education, fashioned to address patient knowledge deficit. Some guidelines are presented. Brown and Hogan[3] proposed the following key considerations when tailoring a patient teaching plan.

1. The nurse must identify what patients and their families need and want to know about the disease, treatment, and measures to ameliorate their impact.
2. Mutually agreed on education goals must be established with the patient and the family. These should focus on patient and family needs, not on what the nurse intends to teach.
3. Educational methods and resources selected should be consistent with the patient's and family's learning needs and abilities.
4. Implementation of the educational program needs to consider how, when, and by whom the teaching will be done.
5. Evaluation of patient and family learning should be ongoing and focused, with goals established at the outset.
6. All components of the education process should be documented. An organized, systematic approach, such as a form in the medical record, is most efficient and effective.

Multiple psychosocial, emotional, and physiologic barriers are inherent in cancer patient education because of the nature of the disease and public perception of cancer and cancer therapy (Table 24-1).[24,30] The primary issue of nursing concern is whether the patient has received (which differs from having "been given") sufficient information to provide valid "informed consent."[3]

Including the patient's family in the educational process, providing patient-appropriate materials, and teaching in a physical environment that reduces anxiety are useful means to overcome some patient education barriers. Finally, many people need an opportunity to assimilate this important information over a period of time, and thus, require time between a teaching session and actual treatment.

Although it is imperative that patient education be an ongoing process, from the outset and for the duration of a patient's therapy, a natural division of three phases follows the evolution of the patient's experience. Table 24-2 summarizes the essential components of patient education.

Somerville[26] provides the following guidelines for the nurse who conducts oncology patient education. These are designed to evaluate the efficacy of the teaching content and technique by assessing the degree to which expected patient outcomes are achieved.

1. Patient demonstrates knowledge related to diagnosis and disease process.
   a. States the diagnosis and explains the disease process.
   b. Describes previous experience with cancer and cancer treatments.
   c. Acknowledges need for treatment.
   d. States alternatives to prescribed treatment.

TABLE 24-1
Examples of Potential Barriers to Successful Education of Patients Receiving Chemotherapy

Barrier Type	Examples
Emotional	Anxiety related to cancer diagnosis, anticipation of cancer therapy, cost issues
	Depression related to disease process and treatment
	Denial, used as coping mechanism
	External locus of control—learned helplessness and powerlessness
Physiological	Biochemical imbalances causing nausea and vomiting, fatigue, restlessness, irritability
	Altered consciousness caused by disease process and/or medications
Psychosocial	Cultural attitudes/beliefs/values that may yield unwillingness to learn ("My wife takes care of this kind of thing.")
	Refusal to claim ownership of self-care—attention to "self" perceived as "selfish" and culturally unacceptable
	Lack of inquisitiveness in effort to be seen as "good patient"
Functional	Compromised literacy level or language differences
	Being overwhelmed by new information (names of drugs, disease jargon, personnel names, schedules, etc.)
	Age, decreased retention or memory
Environmental	Busy, rushed, and distracting clinics
	Foreign, high technology, and threatening surroundings
	Close proximity to other patients can be restricting and depersonalizing

(Adapted from Somerville, E. T., Padilla, G. V., & Bulcavage, L. M. [1991]. Theories used in patient/health education. *Seminars in Oncology Nursing, 7*(2), 87–96; Villejo, L. & Meyers, C. [1991]. Brain function, learning styles, and cancer patient education. *Seminars in Oncology Nursing, 7*[2], 97–104.)

2. Patient demonstrates knowledge related to rationale for treatment with chemotherapy.
   a. Verbalizes need for chemotherapy.
   b. Verbalizes attitude toward and expectations about cancer treatment.
   c. States understanding of use of chemotherapy alone or in conjunction with other treatment modalities, if applicable.
   d. Identifies treatment protocol.
3. Patient demonstrates knowledge related to potential therapeutic effect of chemotherapy.
   a. States diagnosis and expected response to treatment.
   b. Identifies specific effect of treatment with chemotherapy drugs.
4. Patient demonstrates knowledge of treatment plan and schedule.
   a. Identifies drugs to be given.
   b. States frequency and duration of administration.
   c. Identifies studies and procedures that will be done before administration of chemotherapy.
   d. Identifies follow-up studies and procedures needed to evaluate treatment effect.

TABLE 24-2
Educational Essentials for Patients Receiving Chemotherapy

Common Goal to All Phases: To Lessen Patient's Knowledge Deficit Related to Chemotherapy

Phase	Goal	Nursing Actions
Pretreatment	To provide sufficient information to: Facilitate patient's ability to provide valid informed consent Provide nonthreatening environment conducive to learning and to accepting chemotherapy treatments confidently	Provide written, patient-appropriate educational materials containing specific chemotherapy agents before treatment is initiated; make allowances for extended learning period, if necessary
		Thoroughly discuss expectations of therapy
		Discuss anticipated procedure and administration technique, potential side effects, and planned interventions for symptom management
		Encourage patient involvement in decision-making regarding care and treatment plan
		Conduct patient teaching in a quiet, comfortable, and private environment
		Provide opportunity for patient and family to tour treatment area
		Provide opportunity to meet IV nurse assigned to case
		Provide nutritional counseling
		Provide opportunity for patient to express fears, concerns, and comprehension
		Emphasize variability and reversibility of side effects such as alopecia; offer patient assistance and alternatives
		Be absolutely honest with patient
Treatment	To provide sufficient information to: Enable patient to cope effectively with immediate effects of chemotherapy Achieve patient sense of participation in and control over care	Explain how chemotherapy works—cytotoxicity
		Instruct patient to report immediately any discomfort, pain, or burning during the administration of chemotherapy
		Review antiemetic schedule, foods to avoid, and hydration requirements
		Identify known side effects of each drug in use; instruct in precautions for thrombocytopenia—use of electric razors, nonabrasive toothbrush, ways to avoid constipation/Valsalva maneuver
		Review drug and food allergy history and record before first treatment—assess for multiple drug therapy complications—incompatibilities, and communicate to physician (*eg*, ASA-containing medications)
		Provide calender with schedule of treatments, appointments with physicians and labs, and expected time line for neutropenia/thrombocytopenia to occur
		Assist patient in energy conservation program and in setting realistic goals for work and social activities
		Discuss need for contraception and potential for infertility
		Discuss potential need for central venous access
		Instruct patient in oral hygiene and use of nonalcohol-based mouth rinses
		Encourage patient to bring written lists of questions to office/clinic visit, to avoid anxiety-related omission
Posttreatment (on-going)	To provide sufficient information to: Allow patient to demonstrate self-management, interventions to control side effects	Provide information regarding medical self-care in managing side effects of each drug treatment
		Explain reasons for follow-up studies to evaluate disease response
		Remind patient not to travel alone immediately after treatment (in most cases)

(continued)

TABLE 24-2 *(Continued)*

Phase	Goal	Nursing Actions
	Allow patient to function to maximum realistic potential	Instruct patient to report temperature >101.0°F (38°C), to report signs and symptoms of infection, increased bruising, blood in urine or stool, bleeding gums, rashes, fatigue, shortness of breath, sore throat, oral lesions, change in bowel habits, numbness or tingling in fingers or toes
		Stress importance of good personal hygiene; handwashing; and avoidance of rectal thermometers, enemas, and people with communicable diseases
		Encourage patient to call for assistance with any new or unusual medical developments and provide information on how to reach appropriate health care personnel 24 hr/day
		Confirm return appointments and assist with patient transport services, if needed or possible
		Phone patient after first and subsequent treatments, when problems are possible
		Solicit questions regarding response to treatment, patient concerns, comprehension, and self-care regimen
		Review and reinforce previous information related to diagnosis, disease, and treatment

(Prepared by M. M. McCluskey from McNally, J. C., Somerville, E. T., Miaskowski, C., & Rostad, M. [Eds.]. [1991]. *Guidelines for oncology nursing practice* [2nd ed.]. Philadelphia: W. B. Saunders; Groenwald, S. L., Frogge, M. H., Goodman, M. S., & Yarbro, C. H. [1990]. *Cancer nursing: Principles and practice* [2nd ed.]. Boston: Jones & Bartlett.)

5. Patient demonstrates knowledge of potential side effects of drugs.
   a. States mechanism of action of drugs.
   b. States reason for side effects.
   c. Identifies specific side effects that may occur with each drug.
   d. States self-management interventions to control side effects.
   e. States signs and symptoms to report to health care professionals.
   f. Identifies procedures for reporting signs and symptoms.
6. Patient demonstrates knowledge to manage treatment with chemotherapy.
   a. Maintains nutritional status to best of ability.
   b. Follows oral, body, and environmental hygiene measures.
   c. Maintains optimal rest and activity pattern.
   d. Uses safety precautions to prevent injury.
   e. Seeks and uses resources as necessary.
   f. Verbalizes reduced anxiety related to treatment with chemotherapy.
   g. States intention to comply with treatment plan.
7. Patient demonstrates knowledge relative to various access devices, if applicable.[26]

For further assistance with this important component of cancer chemotherapy administration, the reader is encouraged to refer to the comprehensive works of our oncology nursing colleagues who have thoroughly described nurses' responsibilities in ensuring patient and family understanding of the disease process, treatment, toxicities, and symptom management.[3, 11, 19, 25, 26]

DRUG PREPARATION, SAFE HANDLING, AND DISPOSAL

Administering cancer chemotherapy is not without the potential for occupational risks. Recommendations for safe handling of these agents must be followed to avoid clinician risks such as skin, mucous membrane, and eye irritation; lightheadedness; facial flushing; headache; nausea; and alopecia. These manifestations are said to be in direct relationship to time, amount, and method of exposure to specific classes of antineoplastics. Until more definitive studies are produced, prudent health care professionals will minimize potential health risks to themselves by following guidelines in antineoplastic policy and procedure development, as well as in drug preparation and handling.[3, 10, 20, 21, 29] Because of the teratogenic, mutagenic, and carcinogenic properties of antineoplastic agents, these guidelines should be followed strictly, especially by women who are planning pregnancy, who are pregnant, or who are breast-feeding (Table 24-3 and Figure 24-1).

The preceding discussion on safety issues as they apply to the administration of chemotherapy would be incomplete without the inclusion of the following concepts. Successful administration of chemotherapy demands seasoned and keen judgment on the part of the nurse, and because sound nursing judgment is based on scientific theory, to administer these agents in the absence of a clear understanding of why they are used and how they work is simply unsafe. Thus, expert technical skill aside, a basic understanding of the *indications for use* and the *mechanisms of action* is of pivotal value to the IV nurse and quality of patient care.

THE AGENTS

Indications for Use

Nitrogen mustard was the first modern chemical to be used as a therapeutic means to treat the uncontrolled cellular proliferation that characterizes cancer. This serendipitous discovery was the result of scientific observation that bone marrow depletion (hypoplasia) occurred in soldiers exposed to mustard gases during World War II. In the years immediately following, patients with leukemia and lymphomas were treated with nitrogen mustard and exhibited short-term but significant antitumor activity of this cytotoxic agent. The subsequent synthesis of various analogues to nitrogen mustard led to what is now the mainstay in the treatment of malignancies.[15]

Before these anticancer chemicals were discovered, surgery and radiotherapy were the primary techniques used for treating cancer. These modalities remain useful in treating localized tumors, which can either be surgically removed or destroyed by radiating the genetic material within the cancer cells.

Cancer, however, often is a systemic disease that requires systemic therapy. By its very nature of deviating from the normal attributes of cellular structure, function, and production, cancer has the characterizing ability to invade blood and lymph vessels and spread beyond the localized region of the primary disease site.[5] The ability of these aberrant cells to metastasize is the premise on which systemic anticancer therapy is based: chemotherapy is the primary systemic modality; immunotherapy is another systemic approach.

(*text continues on page 458*)

TABLE 24-3
Guidelines for Safe Handling and Disposal of Antineoplastic Agents

A. Drug Preparation
1. All antineoplastic drugs should be prepared by specially trained individuals in a centralized area to minimize interruptions and risk of contamination.
2. Drugs are prepared in a class II biologic safety cabinet (vertical laminar air-flow hood) with vents to the outside, if possible. The blower is left on 24 hr day, 7 days/wk. The hood is serviced regularly according to the manufacturer's recommendations.
3. Eating, drinking, smoking, and applying cosmetics in the drug preparation area are prohibited.
4. The work surface is covered with a plastic absorbent pad to minimize contamination. This pad is changed immediately in the event of contamination and at the completion of drug preparation each day or shift.
5. The prescribed drug is prepared using aseptic technique according to the physician's order, other pharmaceutic resources, or both.
6. Disposable surgical latex unpowdered gloves are used when handling the drugs. Gloves should be changed hourly or immediately if torn or punctured.
7. A disposable long-sleeved gown made of lint-free fabric with knitted cuffs and a closed front is worn during drug preparation.
8. A thermoplastic (Plexiglas) face shield or goggles and a powered air-purifying respirator should be used if a biologic safety cabinet is not available.
9. Because exposure can result when connecting and disconnecting IV tubing, when injecting the drug into the IV line, when removing air from the syringe or infusion line, and when leakage occurs at the tubing, syringe, or stopcock connection, priming of all IV tubing is carried out under the protection of the hood.
10. Other measures to guard against drug leakage during drug preparation include venting the vial and using large-bore needles, Luer lock fittings, and sterile gauze or sponge around the neck of the vial during needle withdrawal. Aerosolization may also be minimized by attaching an aerosol protection device (CytoGuard, Bristol-Myers) to the vial of drug before adding the diluent.
11. Once reconstituted, the drug is labeled according to institutional policies and procedures; the label should include the drug's vesicant properties and antineoplastic drug warning.
12. Antineoplastic drugs are transported in an impervious packing material and are marked with a distinctive warning label.
13. Personnel responsible for drug transport are knowledgeable of procedures to be followed in the event of drug spillage.

B. Drug Administration
1. Chemotherapeutic agents are administered by registered professional nurses who have been specially trained and designated as qualified according to specific institutional policies and procedures.
2. Before administering the drugs, the nurse ensures that informed consent has been given and clarifies any misconceptions the patient might have regarding the drugs and their side effects.
3. Appropriate laboratory results are evaluated and found to be within acceptable levels (eg, complete blood count, renal and liver function).
4. Measures to minimize side effects of the drugs are carried out before drug administration (eg, hydration, antiemetics and antianxiety agents, and patient comfort).
5. An appropriate route for drug administration is ensured according to the physician's order.
6. Personal protective equipment is worn, including disposable latex surgical gloves and a disposable gown made of a lint-free, low-permeability fabric with a closed front, long sleeves, and elastic or knit closed cuffs (optional).
7. The work surface is protected with a disposable absorbent pad.
8. The drug or drugs are administered according to established institutional policies and procedures.
9. Documentation of drug administration, including any adverse reaction, is made in the patient's medical record.
10. A mechanism for identification of patients receiving antineoplastic agents is established for the 48-hr period following drug dispensing.
11. Disposable surgical unpowdered latex gloves and a disposable gown are worn when handling body secretions such as blood, vomitus, or excreta from patients who received chemotherapy drugs within the previous 48 hr.
12. In the event of accidental exposure, remove contaminated gloves or gown immediately and discard according to official procedures.
13. Wash the contaminated skin with soap and water.
14. Flood an eye that is accidentally exposed to chemotherapy with water or isotonic eye wash for at least 5 min.
15. Obtain a medical evaluation as soon as possible after exposure and document the incident according to institutional policies and procedures.

(continued)

TABLE 24-3 *(Continued)*

C. Drug Disposal
1. Regardless of the setting (hospital, ambulatory care, or home), all equipment and unused drugs are treated as hazardous and disposed of according to the institution's policies and procedures.
2. All contaminated equipment including needles are disposed of intact to prevent aerosolization, leaks, and spills.
3. All contaminated materials used in drug preparation are disposed of in a leak-proof, puncture-proof container with a distinctive warning label and are placed in a sealable 4-mil polyethylene or 2-mil polypropylene bag with appropriate labeling.
4. Linen contaminated with bodily secretions of patients who have received chemotherapy within the previous 48 hr is placed in a specially marked laundry bag, which is then placed in an impervious bag that is marked with a distinctive warning label.
5. In the event of a spill, personnel should don double surgical latex unpowdered gloves; eye protection; and a disposable gown made of a lint-free, low-permeability fabric with a closed front, long sleeves, and elastic or knit closed cuffs.
6. Small amounts of liquids are cleaned up with gauze pads, whereas larger spills (>5 mL) are cleaned up with absorbent pads.
7. Small amounts of solids or spills involving powder are cleaned up with damp cloths or absorbent gauze pads.
8. The spill area is cleaned three times with a detergent followed by clean water.
9. Broken glassware and disposable contaminated materials are placed in a leak-proof, puncture-proof container and then placed in a sealable 4-mil polyethylene or 2-mil polypropylene bag and marked with a distinctive warning label.
10. Contaminated reusable items are washed by specially trained personnel wearing double surgical unpowdered latex gloves.
11. The spill should be documented according to established institutional policies and procedures.

(From Goodman, M. S. [1991]. Delivery of cancer chemotherapy. In S. B. Baird [Ed.]. *Cancer nursing: A comprehensive textbook* [p. 294]. Philadelphia: W. B. Saunders.)

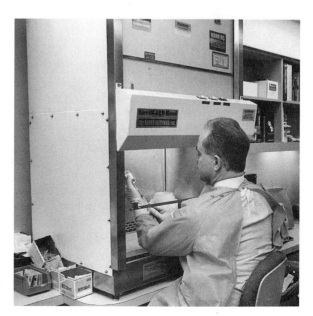

FIGURE 24-1 An oncologic pharmacist prepares the drug, using aseptic technique, in a class II biologic safety cabinet (vertical laminar air-flow hood).

Mechanisms of Action

Chemotherapy controls cancer by using chemical agents, which are cytotoxic, to kill rapidly dividing cells. The ultimate purpose of their use is to destroy as many cancer cells as possible with minimal impact on healthy cells.[27] As seen in Table 24-4, the use of chemotherapy is responsible for cure in about 12% of human cancers and has significant effect on improved survival in another 40% to 50%. The remaining cancers are less responsive to chemotherapy as a "curative modality."[5] Another legitimate role of chemotherapy is palliative treatment for patients with advanced or incurable disease. Even when there is no real hope of complete cure, cancer cells often remain somewhat sensitive to chemotherapies and can be controlled. Agents are introduced to control pain caused by tumor pressure, to ease fluid obstruction, and to "quiet" hypercalcemia and other organic processes.

The agents are grouped according to their specific effect on cancer cell chemistry and on the phase of the cell cycle in which they interfere. The cell cycle refers to the time required for a single cell to reproduce itself.[11] Chemotherapeutic agents fall into two categories. *Cell cycle phase-specific agents* are active only during a particular point in the cell replication cycle; *cell cycle phase-nonspecific agents* are active at any point in that cycle. Regardless of the specific or nonspecific timing and location of drug impact, the basic mechanism of all cancer chemotherapeutic agents is similar—they inhibit DNA synthesis. This, in turn, disables cell reproduction; the cell then dies.[25]

Chemotherapy is further categorized into five major groups: alkylating agents, antimetabolites, plant alkaloids, antitumor antibiotics, and hormones. Within each of these categories are found multiple agents of various toxicities, all relating to their antineoplastic properties.

One can make sense of the predictable toxicities when keeping in mind the property that lends activity to all of the agents, the destruction of rapidly dividing cells. It follows that the cell lines of host tissues that are normally rapidly dividing—such as bone marrow, hair follicles, and gastrointestinal mucosa—exhibit the toxic side effects so frequently seen, such as cytopenias, alopecia, and mucositis.

This relationship is demonstrated in Figure 24-2, which illustrates the special burden of systemic therapy not associated with surgery and radiotherapy. Toxicities associated with systemic chemotherapy are linked to patient-related factors such as type of malignancy, patient age, performance status, and level of health before and during therapy.[5]

Table 24-5 provides a quick reference for the IV nurse needing basic preparation, handling, and administration information in abbreviated form. The table includes the most frequently seen toxicities, which appear according to organ systems (*eg*, hematologic, dermatologic, gastrointestinal, genitourinary, hepatic, and neurologic). Comprehensive tables have been published and should be used for more detailed information on indications for use, routes of delivery, pharmacokinetics, and dosing, which vary extensively as new protocols indicate the use of new combinations of existing drugs.[5–7,11]

Rationale for Combined Modality Therapy

Although any one of the cancer treatment modalities may be used alone, often they are used in combination with one another. Chemotherapy is frequently used as an adjuvant treatment to assist in curing or controlling disseminated disease. Combining the available

TABLE 24-4
Classification of Tumors According to General Sensitivity to Chemotherapy

Tumors Responsive to Chemotherapy

Tumors Curable in Advanced Stages by Chemotherapy

Choriocarcinoma

Acute lymphocytic leukemia (in children and adults)

Hodgkin's disease

Diffuse large cell lymphoma

Lymphoblastic lymphoma (in children and adults)

Follicular mixed lymphoma

Testicular cancer

Acute myelogenous leukemia

Wilms' tumor

Burkitt's lymphoma

Embryonal rhabdomyosarcoma

Ewing's sarcoma

Peripheral neuroepithelioma

Neuroblastoma

Small cell cancer of the lung

Ovarian cancer

Tumors Curable in the Adjuvant Setting by Chemotherapy

Breast cancer

Osteogenic sarcoma

Soft tissue sarcoma

Colorectal cancer

Tumors Responsive in Advanced States but not yet Curable by Chemotherapy

Bladder cancer

Chronic myelogenous leukemia

Chronic lymphocytic leukemia

Hairy cell leukemia

Multiple myeloma

Follicular small-cleaved cell lymphoma

Gastric carcinoma

Cervical carcinoma

Soft tissue sarcoma

Head and neck cancer

Endometrial cancer

Adrenocortical carcinoma

Medulloblastoma

Polycythemia rubra vera

Prostate cancer

Glioblastoma multiforme

Insulinoma

Breast cancer

Carcinoid tumors

Tumors Poorly Responsive in Advanced Stages to Chemotherapy

Osteogenic sarcoma

Pancreatic cancer

Renal cancer

Thyroid cancer

Carcinoma of the vulva or penis

Colorectal cancer

Non-small cell lung cancer

Melanoma

Hepatocellular carcinoma

(From DeVita, V. T. [1989]. Principles and practice of cancer chemotherapy. In V. T. DeVita, S. Hellman, & S. A. Rosenberg [Eds.] *Cancer: Principles and practice of oncology* [p. 297]. Philadelphia: J. B. Lippincott. Used with permission.)

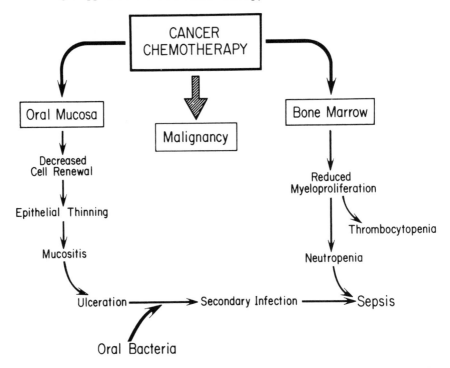

FIGURE 24-2   Effects of systemic cancer chemotherapy on the oral, basal, and epithelial cells and on the bone marrow stem cells. (From Sonis, S. T. [1989]. Oral complications of cancer therapy. In V. T. DeVita, S. Hellman, & S. A. Rosenberg [Eds.]. *Cancer: Principles and practice of oncology* [3rd ed., p. 2146]. Philadelphia: J. B. Lippincott. Used with permission.)

modalities is done in an attempt to optimize cancer cell kill, while minimizing their associated toxicities.[11]

With the exception of oral alkylating agents used for chronic leukemias, single-agent chemotherapy regimens are almost unheard of in contemporary medicine.[16] Simultaneous multiple-agent use capitalizes on synergistic drug actions on the cell cycle to maximize antitumor effects. Combining the agents also modifies dose-limiting toxicities.

Table 24-6 provides a list of common combinations of cytotoxic agents.[18] The IV nurse should be familiar with these combinations to answer patients' questions regarding the specific cytotoxic effects for which they should be prepared in relation to each of their drugs. The most illustrative and classic example of combination chemotherapy is the MOPP regimen (mechlorethamine [Mustargen], vincristine [Oncovin], procarbazine, and prednisone) used to treat Hodgkin's disease.[11]

The specific and fixed sequence in which the drugs are given yields specific and predictable toxicities. Figure 24-3 illustrates this regimen's depleting effect on bone marrow, which results in neutropenia, known as the nadir.[3,11]

Combining cytotoxic agents, then further combining them with one or more additional types of therapy, potentially provides the greatest collective benefit of each modal-

(*text continues on page 471*)

TABLE 24-5
Quick Reference to Commonly Administered Parenteral Chemotherapeutic Agents

Drug	Amt/Vial	Diluent	Final Concentration	Usual Dose	Usual Administration Technique	Comments and Major Toxicities
Asparaginase Enzyme Nonchemotherapeutic agent	10,000 IU	5 mL SWI 2 mL SWI	2000 IU/mL 5000 IU/mL	15–25,000 U/m² as a single dose	IVP slowly over 30 min IVPB (D5W, NS) in up to 1000 mL. IM	Acute liver dysfunction. Nausea and vomiting common and may be severe; Hypersensitivity rxns; Depression, lethargy, and drowsiness
Bleomycin Antitumor Antibiotic	15 U	7.75 mL NS	2 U/mL	10–20 U/m² qwk or twice weekly IM, IV or SQ. Constant infusions over 3–7 days at 20 U/m²/day.	IVP, IM or SQ. IVPB (rare)	Pulmonary fibrosis; Hypersensitivity rxns, fever and chills (premedicate with Tylenol); Skin rxns common (especially pruritic erythema); Reversible alopecia; Mucositis, stomatitis, and mild nausea and vomiting
Carboplatin Platinum complex	450 mg 150 mg 50 mg	45 mL SWI 15 mL SWI 5 mL SWI	10 mg/mL	360–400 mg/m² q4wk	IV infusion ONLY (D5W,NS) May dilute to as low as 0.5 mg/mL	Leukopenia and thrombocytopenia nadir at day 21; recovery by day 28–30; Nausea and vomiting (less severe than with Cisplatin); Increase in serum creatinine and BUN; DO NOT USE ALUMINUM NEEDLES
BCNU (carmustine) Alkylating agent	100 mg	3 mL of provided diluent. Then 27 mL SWI.	3.3 mg/mL	150–200 mg/m² q6wk	IVPB ONLY (D5W, NS) Infuse in 100–250 mL of fluid over 1–2 hr	Delayed leukopenia 4–5 wks after administration, with nadir lasting 1–2 wks; Thrombocytopenia with nadir 4–5 wks after administration lasting 1–2 wks; Nausea and vomiting common occurring 2–6 hr after administration and lasting 4–24 hr; Painful venous irritation during administration. Dose-related pulmonary fibrosis; Dose-related renal failure
Cisplatin Platinum complex	50 mg AQ	Already in solution	1mg/mL	20–40 mg/m² day × 3–5	IV infusion ONLY (D5W, NS)	Nausea and vomiting— often severe starting

(continued)

TABLE 24-5 *(Continued)*

Drug	Amt/Vial	Diluent	Final Concentration	Usual Dose	Usual Administration Technique	Comments and Major Toxicities
	100 mg AQ			days q 3–4 wks	250–1000 mL Infuse over 1–8 hr Ensure adequate hydration	about 1 hr after treatment and lasting 24 hr
				20–120 mg/m² given as a single dose q 3–4 wk		Nephrotoxicity is dose related
						Ototoxicity with tinnitus and/or hearing loss is dose dependent
						Moderate leukopenia and thrombocytopenia with a nadir on day 18–23 and recovery by day 39
						Alopecia and electrolyte imbalances
						PROTECT FROM LIGHT.
						USE 5-μM FILTER FOR SOLNS CONTAINING MANNITOL.
						DO NOT USE ALUMINUM NEEDLES
Cyclophosphamide (Cytoxan) Alkylating agent	1000 mg 500 mg	50 mL SWI 25 mL SWI	20 mg/mL	500–1500 mg/ m² q 3–4 wks	IVP over 5–10 min. (usually doses <750 mg).	Acute hemorrhagic cystitis in poorly hydrated individuals at doses of 1–2 g/m².
					IVPB (D5W, D5NS) infuse in 100–150 mL over 15–30 min	FORCE FLUIDS Leukopenia with a nadir of 8–14 days and recovery in 18–25 days; nausea and vomiting with an onset within 4–6 hr after treatment and lasting 8–10 hr
						Alopecia in 50% occurring approx. 3 wk after treatment
						Medium to low risk of pulmonary toxicity
						Cardiac necrosis with high dose
						Nail and skin hyperpigmentation
						Nasal stuffiness during administration
						Testicular atrophy and amenorrhea
Cytarabine (ARA-C) Antimetabolite	1000 mg 500 mg	10 mL SWI 10 mL SWI	100 mg/mL 50 mg/mL	100–150 mg/m² IV or SQ for 5–10 days	IVP (low dose) over 1–2 min IVPB (D5W, NS) in up to 1000 mL fluid for high-dose therapy	Leukopenia and thrombocytopenia with a nadir in 5–7 days
				20–30 mg/m² intrathecally		Nausea and vomiting dose related
				High dose: 3 g/m² q12hr for 6 days		Medium to low risk of pulmonary toxicity

(continued)

TABLE 24-5 *(Continued)*

Drug	Amt/Vial	Diluent	Final Concentration	Usual Dose	Usual Administration Technique	Comments and Major Toxicities
						Stomatitis and diarrhea
						Lethargy and keratoconjunctivitis with high doses (use dexamethasone eye drops)
						Alopecia (occasional)
						Cerebellar toxicity
DTIC (dacarbazine) Alkylating agent	200 mg 100 mg	19.7 mL SWI 9.9 mL SWI	10 mg/mL	75–125 mg/m²/ day for 10 days repeated q 4 wk	IVP over 1 min IVPB (D5W, NS) in up to 250 mL	Leukopenia and thrombocytopenia with a nadir at 21–25 days
				50–250 mg/m²/ day for 5 days repeated q 3 wk	Infuse over 30 min	Severe nausea and vomiting common. Occurs 1–3 hr after treatment usually lasting up to 12 hr
				650–1450 mg/ m² as a single dose q 3–4 wk		Anorexia
						Flulike symptoms with high doses
						Alopecia and facial flushing
						IRRITANT: avoid extravasation. Local pain at injection site. Slow rate of infusion to decrease pain from venous spasm.
						PROTECT FROM LIGHT
Dactinomycin Antitumor Antibiotic Vesicant	0.5 mg	1.1 mL SWI	0.5 mg/mL	*Adults* 1–2 mg/m² q 3 wk or 0.25 mg/m² day × 5 days q 3–4 wk	IVP slowly over 2–3 min IVPB (D5W, NS) in 50–100 mL over 20–30 min	Leukopenia and thrombocytopenia occurring in 7–10 days with nadir at approx. 3 weeks
				Children 0.25–0.5 mg/m² day × 5 days. Not to exceed 0.5 mg/day		Nausea and vomiting common and severe occurring immediately or a few hours after treatment lasting 4–20 hr—may be prolonged
						Erythema, hyperpigmentation and alopecia
						Stomatitis, dysphagia, proctitis and diarrhea
						Skin irritation or even necrosis in previously irradiated areas ("radiation recall")
Daunorubicin (Cerubidine) Antitumor Antibiotic	20 mg	4 mL SWI	5 mg/mL	30–60 mg/m²/ day for 2–3 days q 3–4 wks	IVP slowly over 2–3 min Continuous infusion	Leukopenia with nadir between 1–2 wk, recovery in 2–3 wk
						Thrombocytopenia less

(continued)

TABLE 24-5 *(Continued)*

Drug	Amt/Vial	Diluent	Final Concentration	Usual Dose	Usual Administration Technique	Comments and Major Toxicities
Vesicant					IVPB (D5W, NS) in 50–100 mL to infuse over 20–30 min	significant with nadir at 4–15 days and recovery in 2–3 wk
						Nausea and vomiting commonly occurring 1 hr after dose and lasting for several hours
						Diarrhea and stomatitis
						Rash, alopecia totalis
						Cumulative cardiotoxicity at max. lifetime dose of 500–600 mg/m² (aggravated by concurrent radiation)
						Fever
						Red urine—advise patient
						PROTECT FROM LIGHT
Doxorubicin (Adriamycin) Antitumor Antibiotic Vesicant	200 mg MDV	Already in solution	2 mg/mL	60–75 mg/m² as a bolus injection of a continuous infusion over 2–4 days q 3–4 wk 30 mg/m² daily for 3 days q 3–4 wk	IVP slowly over 20–30 min IVPB (D5W, NS) in 50–100 mL over 20–30 min Continuous infusion over 24–96 hr via IV fluid or EID	Leukopenia and thrombocytopenia with a nadir at 10–14 days and recovery in 21 days
						Alopecia (usually complete), hyperpigmentation of nailbeds and dermal creases
						Nausea and vomiting, sometimes severe, anorexia, stomatitis—especially with daily × 3 schedule
						Radiation recall: irritation of previously irradiated areas
						Arrhythmias and ECG changes
						CHF due to cardiomyopathy related to total cumulative dose (risk greater at doses above 550 mg/m²
						May enhance cyclophosphamide cystitis
						Advise patient of red discoloration of urine occurring up to 24 hrs after administration
						"Adria" flare may occur: erythematous streak up the vein

(continued)

TABLE 24-5 (Continued)

Drug	Amt/Vial	Diluent	Final Concentration	Usual Dose	Usual Administration Technique	Comments and Major Toxicities
Etoposide (VP-16) Plant alkaloid	100 mg	Already in solution	20 mg/mL	50–100 mg/m²/ day × 5 days	IVPB (D5W, NS) ONLY in 250 mL over at least 30 min to 1 hr	Incompatible with heparin and 5-FU PROTECT FROM LIGHT Leukopenia (dose-related), primarily granulocytopenia; nadirs within 7–14 days and recovery within 20 days. Thrombocytopenia uncommon. Alopecia: mild and reversible Nausea and vomiting: mild; anorexia in 10%–13% Hyperbilirubinemia and increased transaminase levels more common with high dose protocols Peripheral neuropathy TRANSIENT HYPOTENSION ASSOCIATED WITH RAPID ADMINISTRATION: INFUSE OVER 30 MIN TO 1 HR Discontinue infusion if hypersensitivity/bronchospasm occurs.
Fluorouracil (5-FU) Antimetabolite	500 mg	Already in solution	50 mg/mL	300–450 mg/m²/ day IVP × 5 days q 28 days 300–750 mg/m² IVP weekly or every other week 1000 mg/m² infused over 24 hr × 4–5 days	IVP at any convenient rate Continuous infusion (D5W, NS) CADD pumps over 5 days Intraocular 1 mg/0.1 mL in preservative-free NS	Leukopenia nadir at 9–14 days, with recovery in 21–25 days. Thrombocytopenia nadir at 7–14 days with recovery by approx. day 30. Both are dose limiting and less common with continuous infusion. Dermatitis, nail changes, hyperpigmentation, alopecia and chemical phlebitis with long term infusion (see Figure 24-12). Nausea, vomiting, and anorexia. Diarrhea (may be severe) can be dose limiting. Stomatitis is more common with 5-day infusion.

(continued)

TABLE 24-5 *(Continued)*

Drug	Amt/Vial	Diluent	Final Concentration	Usual Dose	Usual Administration Technique	Comments and Major Toxicities
						Pharyngitis
						Cerebellar ataxia and headache
						PROTECT FROM LIGHT
Idarubicin (Idamycin) Antitumor Antibiotic Vesicant	10 mg 5 mg	10 mL NS 5 mL NS	1 mg/mL	12 mg/m² /day for 3 days	IVP over 10 to 15 min	Myelosupression, dose limiting
				8–15 mg/m² as a single dose q 3 wk sometimes used	IVPB (D5W, NS) in any convenient volume	Nausea, vomiting, diarrhea, and stomatitis
						Alopecia, extravasation reactions, and rash
						Transient arrhythmias, decreased LVEF, and CHF
						PROTECT FROM LIGHT
	1 gm 3 gm 200 mg	20 mL SWI 60 mL SWI Already in solution	50 mg/mL 100 mg/mL	1–1.2 g/m² over 5 consecutive days q 3–4 wk	IVPB ONLY (D5W, NS, D5NS) in 250–1000 mL over 30 min or more	Leukopenia, thrombocytopenia (dose limiting); anemia
				Higher doses have been given over 2–3 days	IVP over 5 min. IVPB (D5W, NS) 50–100 mL over any convenient time	Nausea, vomiting, anorexia, constipation, and diarrhea
						Alopecia, rash, and urticaria
				20% of Ifosphamide dose given just before 4 and 8 hr after Ifosphamide		Increased ALT, AST, and hyperbilirubinemia
						Hemorrhagic cystitis and hematuria. Encourage ample fluids: HYDRATION OF >2 L/DAY TO MAINTAIN URINARY OUTPUT AND FREQUENT VOIDING. USE OF MESNA RECOMMENDED.
Ifosphamide (Ifex) Alkylating agent Mesna						Somnolence, lethargy, disorientation, confusion, dizziness, and malaise
						Chemical thrombophlebitis
Uroprotective agent (nonchemotherapeutic agent)						MESNA: Nausea, vomiting, diarrhea, abdominal pain, and altered taste
						Rash and uticaria
						Lethargy, headache, joint or limb pain, fatigue
Leucovorin, Calcium Tetrahydrofolic acid derivative Nonchemotherapeutic agent	350 mg 50 mg	17.5 mL SWI 5 mL SWI	20 mg/mL 10 mg/mL	Methotrexate rescue: 10–25 mg/m² q 6 hr × 6–8 doses	IVP at any convenient rate IM PO IVPB (D5W, NS) 50–250 mL over 15 min	Rare hypersensitivity reactions
				To potentiate the effect of 5 FU: 20–500 mg/ m²/dose		

(continued)

TABLE 24-5 *(Continued)*

Drug	Amt/Vial	Diluent	Final Concentration	Usual Dose	Usual Administration Technique	Comments and Major Toxicities
Mechlorethamine (Nitro Mustard) Alkylating agent Vesicant	10 mg	10 mL SWI	1 mg/mL	Hodgkin's disease: 6 mg/m² on days 1 and 8 of a monthly cycle (MOPP regimen) Up to 0.4 mg/kg as a single agent monthly	IVP over 1–3 min into the tubing of a rapidly running IV	Leukopenia and thrombocytopenia within 24 hr, with a nadir at 6–8 days to 3 wk Severe nausea and vomiting beginning 1–3 hr after treatment and lasting approx. 8 hr. Diarrhea Discoloration of infused vein and phlebitis Alopecia and stomatitis Vesicant: use of the antidote sodium thiosulfate is indicated if extravasation occurs Advise patient of metallic taste Amenorrhea and impaired spermatogenesis Mechlorethamine is incompatible with other antineoplastic agents and IV fluids due to its instability.
Methotrexate Antimetabolite	200 mg 50 mg 1 g	Already in solution preserv. free 19.4 mL SWI	25 mg/mL 50 mg/mL	Solid tumors: 20–40 mg/m² every 1–2 wk Leukemias and lymphomas: 200–500 mg/m² every 2–4 wk Intrathecal: Usually 12 mg in preservative-free NS	IVP (<100 mg) at any convenient rate IVPB (D5W, NS) in up to 500 mL over 30 min to 1 hr Intrathecally IM	Leukopenia and thrombocytopenia with high dose Stomatitis, sore throat, and pruritis with high dose Diarrhea can be severe with melana. Hematemesis Nausea and vomiting uncommon with low-dose therapy Renal dysfunction with high dose. Hepatic dysfunction more likely in patients receiving long-term continuous or daily treatment. Encephalopathy with multiple intrathecal doses. Confusion, ataxia, tremors, irritability, seizures, and coma Hypersensitivity rxns associated with fever, chills, and rash

(continued)

TABLE 24-5 *(Continued)*

Drug	Amt/Vial	Diluent	Final Concentration	Usual Dose	Usual Administration Technique	Comments and Major Toxicities
						Skin erythema, depigmentation or hyperpigmentation, alopecia, and photosensitivity
						Doses >80 mg/wk should be accompanied by leucovorin rescue (see under leucovorin)
Mitomycin C Antitumor Antibiotic Vesicant	20 mg 5 mg	50 mL SWI 10 mL SWI	0.5 mg/mL	10–20 mg/m² q 6–8 wk	IVP over 1–5 min IVPB (D5W, NS) in up to 250 mL over 30 min	Leukopenia and thrombocytopenia: delayed, cumulative, and dose limiting; anemia. Leukopenia nadir at day 25, recovery by day 32–39. Thrombocytopenia nadir at day 28, recovery by day 42–49
						Stomatitis, alopecia, dermatitis, and pruritis
						Nausea, vomiting, anorexia, and diarrhea
						Hepatomegaly and liver failure
						Parasthesias, fatigue, lethargy, weakness, and blurred vision
						Interstitial pneumonitis. Discontinue drug if acute bronchospasm occurs.
						Nephrotoxicity with high doses (>50 mg/m²)
						Pain on injection and phlebitis
Mitoxantrone Antitumor Antibiotic	20 mg 25 mg 30 mg	Already in solution	2 mg/mL	10–12 mg/m²/ day × 5 days for induction therapy for ANLL Other: 12 mg/m² q 3–4 wk	IVP has been used (over 3 min. or more), but IVPB preferred route IVPB (D5W, NS) in at least 50 mL over not <3 min	Leukopenia and thrombocytopenia nadirs at 10–12 days, with recovery on day 21
						Alopecia (mild), pruritis, and dry skin
						Nausea, vomiting, diarrhea, and stomatitis (mild)
						Cumulative cardiomyopathy (CHF), arrhythmias, and chest pain (occasional)
						Hypersensitivity rxns may include hypotension, uticaria, and rash

(continued)

TABLE 24-5 *(Continued)*

Drug	Amt/Vial	Diluent	Final Concentration	Usual Dose	Usual Administration Technique	Comments and Major Toxicities
						Advise patient of blue/green discoloration of urine, stool, and sclerae for 24–48 hr after treatment.
						May also discolor veins
						Fever, conjunctivitis, phlebitis, and amenorrhea
Streptozocin Antitumor Antibiotic Nitrosourea	1000 mg	9.5 mL NS	100 mg/mL	500–1000 mg/m²/day × 5 days q 3–4 wk 1–1.5 g/m² weekly	IVP over 15 min or more IVPB (D5W, NS) in up to 250 mL over 1–2 hr Continuous infusion × 5 days	Anemia (common). Leukopenia and thrombocytopenia (rarely dose limiting). Eosinophilia
						Nausea and vomiting common and occasionally severe; anorexia, diarrhea, and abdominal cramps
						Nephrotoxicity common (dose related) with proteinuria
						Vein irritation during administration: slow infusion to minimize pain
						Transient increases in ALT, AST, alk phos, and LDH.
						Glucose intolerance and glycosuria
Thiotepa Alkylating agent	15 mg	1.5 mL SWI	10 mg/mL	Nontransplant: 12–16 µg/m² q 1–4 wk Transplant: 900 mg/m² Intrathecal: 1–10 mg/m² q 1–2 wk Bladder instillation: 30–60 mg q 1–4 wk Intracavitary: 0.6–0.8 mg/kg through the same tubing used to remove fluid from the cavity	IVPB (D5W, NS) in 50–100 mL over 10 min Bladder instillation: in 50 mL NS	Thrombocytopenia (more prominent) and leukopenia with nadirs at 14 days and recovery after 2–4 wk. Anemia
						Alopecia (rare with low dose)
						Hypersensitivity rxns include hives, rash, and pruritis
						Nausea, vomiting, anorexia, and stomatitis dose dependent
						Headache, dizziness, and weakness of lower extremities
						Paresthesias associated with intrathecal administration
						Azoospermia and amenorrhea
						Pain at site of injection

(continued)

TABLE 24-5 *(Continued)*

Drug	Amt/Vial	Diluent	Final Concentration	Usual Dose	Usual Administration Technique	Comments and Major Toxicities
Vinblastine (Velban) Plant alkaloid Vesicant	10 mg	10 mL NS	1 mg/mL	6–10 mg/m² q 2–4 wk	IVP over 1 min IVPB not recommended, but stable in NS at a concentration of 20 mg/mL Continuous infusions have been given over 96 hr or longer through a central venous catheter	Marked leukopenia with early nadirs. Thrombocytopenia and anemia Alopecia. Skin and soft tissue damage if extravasated (treat with SQ injections of hyaluronidase and application of heat to disperse drug). Rash and photosensitivity Nausea, vomiting, and constipation; abdominal pain, anorexia, diarrhea, and stomatitis Peripheral neuropathy, myalgias, headache, seizures, depression, dizziness, and malaise Acute bronchospasm more common when administered with Mitomycin C Severe jaw pain Phlebitis and vein discoloration Azoospermia and amenorrhea
Vincristine (Oncovin) Plant alkaloid Vesicant	1 mg	Already in solution	1 mg/mL	0.5–1.4 mg/m² q1–4 wk Usually the maximum dose is 2 mg	IVP over 1 min Occasionally given as a continuous infusion (D5W, NS) over 96 hr via a central line	Leukopenia (mild and rare), thrombocytopenia (rare) Alopecia; skin and soft tissue damage if extravasated (use SQ hyaluronidase and application of heat to disperse drug); rash Nausea, vomiting (rare); constipation (place patient on bowel regimen). Abdominal pain, anorexia, and diarrhea New labeling requirements must specify "for IV use only" (intrathecal administration is fatal) Peripheral neuropathy, parasthesias, constipation, paralytic ileus, and myalgias

(continued)

TABLE 24-5 *(Continued)*

Drug	Amt/Vial	Diluent	Final Concentration	Usual Dose	Usual Administration Technique	Comments and Major Toxicities
						Acute bronchospasm more common when administered with Mitomycin C
						Severe jaw pain

ALT, alanine aminotransferase; ANLL, acute nonlymphocytic leukemia; AST, aspartate aminotransferase; alk phos, alkaline phosphatase; BUN, blood urea nitrogen; CHF, congestive heart failure; ECG , electrocardiographic; IVP, intravenous push; IVPB, intravenous piggyback; LDH, lactate dehydrogenase; LVEF, left ventricular ejection fraction; MDV, multiple-dose vial; NS, normal saline; rxn(s), reaction(s); SQ, subcutaneous; SWI, sterile water for injection.

(Prepared by Christopher Charlton, RPh, and M. M. McCluskey, RN, OCN, CRNI, St. Joseph Hospital, Chicago IL. [1992]. From: Dorr, R., & Fritz, W. [1980]. *Cancer chemotherapy handbook*. New York: Elsevier; Hubbard, S. M., Seipp, C. A., & Duffy, P. L. [1992]. Administration of cancer treatments: Practical guide for physicians and oncology nurses. In V. T. DeVita, S. Hellman, & S. A. Rosenberg [Eds.]. *Cancer: Principles and practice of oncology* [3rd ed., pp. 2371–2375]. Philadelphia: J. B. Lippincott; ECOG drug information sheets [1992]. [4th ed.]. Madison, WI: Eastern Cooperative Oncology Group.)

ity and thus the greatest likelihood of cure. When using a combination of modalities for either cure or significant control, the patient may experience significant toxicity. However, most patients report (especially when cured) that the toxicities caused by the treatment were worthwhile.[5]

Goodman rightfully places importance on the impact of a nurse's positive attitude when offering data about chemotherapy toxicities and likely side effects, offsetting it by stressing the dramatic potential benefits of treatment, to foster hope for patients and families.[9]

ROUTES AND MODES OF ADMINISTRATION

Pretreatment Assessment

During the pretreatment period before drug administration, two critical nursing functions are performed—patient education and patient assessment.[20] Proper pretreatment evaluation can have tremendous impact on the efficacy of the nurse's plan of care and on the patient's chemotherapy experience itself. Answers to the following questions should be ascertained by the nurse preparing the patient for chemotherapy, with patient support and data.

1. Does the patient sufficiently understand the instruction given to provide fully informed consent?

2. Is the patient receiving chemotherapy for the first time? If not, is the record complete regarding previous chemotherapy experience (physical and emotional response, experience with and management of side effects)?

3. Has patient's and family's ability to manage at home been assessed? Is patient familiar with resources available to assist with chemotherapy sequelae?

4. Is patient's physical history clear to the nurse administering treatment? Have all

TABLE 24-6
Anticancer Drug Combinations

ABVD	Doxorubicin + bleomycin + vinblastine + dacarbazine
CHOP	Cyclophosphamide + doxorubicin + vincristine + prednisone
CMF	Cyclophosphamide + methotrexate + fluorouracil
COPP	Cyclophosphamide + vincristine + procarbazine + prednisone
CVP	Cyclophosphamide + vincristine + prednisone
CY–VA–DIC	Cyclophosphamide + vincristine + doxorubicin + dacarbazine
FAC	Fluorouracil + doxorubicin + cyclophosphamide
FAM	Fluorouracil + doxorubicin + mitomycin
MOPP	Mechlorethamine + vincristine + procarbazine + prednisone
MPL + PRED	Melphalan + prednisone
MTX + MP + CTX	Methotrexate + mercaptopurine + cyclophosphamide
VAC	Vincristine + dactinomycin + cyclophosphamide
VBP	Vinblastine + bleomycin + cisplatin
VP–L–Asparaginase	Vincristine + prednisone + asparaginase

(From National Cancer Institute. [1990]. *Chemotherapy and you—A guide to self-help during treatment.* Bethesda, MD: U.S. Department of Health and Human Services. Used with permission.)

compromised organ systems been considered in dose determination/calculation (especially liver and kidneys, which must metabolize and clear the agents)?

5. Is the patient ready for therapy? Has the patient mobilized available coping mechanisms to sustain the experience?

6. Is patient prepared for potential hair loss?

7. Has an antiemetic regimen, both medical and dietary (in clinic, in home), been explained and initiated?

8. Does the patient have special hydration and electrolyte replacement needs? If so, are they ordered appropriately? Does patient understand need to continue fluid after chemotherapy. Will patient be able to take in and retain adequate fluids posttreatment?

9. Have laboratory values been obtained within the last 48 hours? Are they within normal limits (*eg*, complete blood counts, platelets, blood urea nitrogen, creatinine, liver function studies)?

10. Does the nurse have the therapy protocol or the written and signed physician order that clearly specifies patient name, drug name(s), dosage per square meter of body surface area, total dose, and rate/frequency/route of administration?

11. Is the patient as physically comfortable as possible and in a position where the nurse call-light is immediately available?

12. Are all necessary treatment supplies (*eg*, safe handling equipment, IV therapy materials, and hazardous waste containment) easily reachable? Is the environment lighted adequately to facilitate patient observation and for venipuncture purposes? Is environment conducive to privacy, especially in the event of emesis? (See Figure 24-4.)

13. Is the nurse prepared for anaphylaxis or extravasation? Is proper equipment for

MOPP/ABV ± D Administration Schedule and Corresponding White Blood Cell Count Nadirs

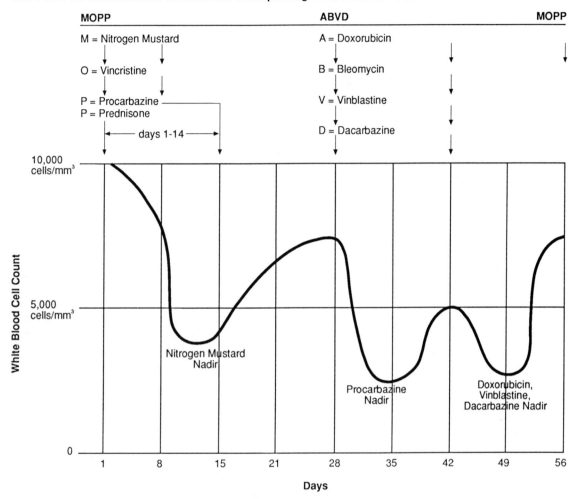

FIGURE 24-3 MOPP/ABV ±D administration schedule and corresponding white blood cell count nadirs. (From Goodman, M. S. [1986]. *Cancer: Chemotherapy and care* [p. 16]. Evansville, IN: Bristol-Myers. Used with permission.)

these emergencies readily available? (See Tables 24-7 and 24-8.) Are the necessary professionals immediately available in the event of patient emergency?

14. Does the patient have adequate venous access?

Resolution of these areas is necessary to prepare the patient to receive conventional chemotherapy adequately. Individual patients often require extended pretreatment evaluations for special needs, such as those who are exceptionally anxious, who have poor family or social support, or who are to receive investigational antineoplastic drugs. When chemotherapeutic protocol changes, any or all of these steps must be repeated or modified to update and educate the patient on new drug regimen.

When the nurse and the patient have combined their resources to satisfy these questions, chemotherapy administration may begin.

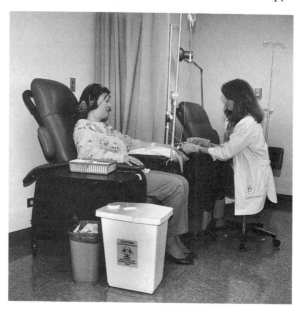

FIGURE 24-4 An environment conducive to successful chemotherapy administration is well lit and contains the necessary equipment, including adjustable infusion chair with arm rests, easily reached IV therapy equipment and materials, biohazardous waste container, safe handling materials, emesis basin, sphygmomanometer, emergency and extravasation equipment, and available nurse-call system.

Systemic Drug Delivery

Chemotherapy is delivered through a variety of routes; most common routes are oral and IV.[25] Antineoplastic agents are given orally if they can be absorbed and tolerated by the gastrointestinal tract. Most agents do not meet these criteria, however. Thus, the IV route is customary.

Successful IV drug administration requires careful vein selection and venipuncture. Vein selection depends on the purpose and length of infusion and on the vesicant or irritant properties of the drugs. Peripheral veins may be used for bolus or short-term infusion; central venous access is preferred for patients who require long-term infusions or who are at risk of extravasation caused by vein fragility or inaccessibility.

For peripheral venous access, patients should be positioned comfortably in a chair with extended arm rests, with hand and arm stabilization. Before venipuncture, the nurse schedules ample and unhurried time to assess both arms and hands to avoid areas of sclerosis, thrombosis, hematoma, or phlebitis (Figure 24-5). The examination of both arms also gives the nurse the baseline reference should changes occur during treatment.

If veins are obscure, moderately warm moist compresses may be applied to patient's hands and forearms. Clothing can be loosened to allow full view of the IV site. Watches and tight jewelry should be removed if they constrict the venous pathway or impede the smooth flow of drugs along the venous network.

Vascular irritation associated with IV administration of chemotherapy agents and phlebitis often can be minimized if arms are alternated from treatment to treatment. Alternating arm IV sites allows time for healing. Documentation should specify which arm was used for each treatment. If not informed of this procedure, and if treated by various nurses, a patient unwittingly may choose to have all treatment in one arm for personal preference, increasing the potential for phlebitis.

At all times, nurses should be vigilant in observing sterile venipuncture techniques, universal precautions, and safe handling of chemotherapeutic agents. Oncology patients

TABLE 24-7
Emergency Drugs and Equipment

Drugs	Strength	Volume
Epinephrine 1:1000 (1 mg/mL)	1:10,000	10 mL
Anhydrous theophylline	400 mg	100 mL
Diphenhydramine	50 mg	1 mL
Hydrocortisone	2 mL	100 mL
Dopamine (200 mg)	800 μg	250 mL
Levarterenol bitartrate	2 mg	500 mL
Sodium bicarbonate	8.4%	50 mEq/50 mL
Furosemide	40 mg	4 mL
Diazepam	10 mg	2 mL
Lidocaine	100 mg	5 mL
Naloxone hydrochloride	0.1–0.4 mg	5 mL
Nitroglycerine (sublingual)	0.15 mg	

Equipment

Suction machine with catheters

Oxygen tank with nasal and face mask

Ambu bag with adult–child face mask

Syringes and needles

Standard resuscitation equipment

*Check daily and restock as necessary.

(From Goodman, M. S. [1991]. Delivery of cancer chemotherapy. In S. B. Baird [Ed.]. *Cancer nursing: A comprehensive textbook* [p. 295]. Philadelphia: W. B. Saunders. Used with permission.)

on cytotoxic agents often are leukopenic as a result of treatment, and therefore, are more susceptible to a direct route for systemic contamination. Thus, aseptic technique must be strictly followed.

Venipunctures can be performed using the most distal veins first, moving proximally with successive administrations (from hand to forearm).[28] If a forearm venipuncture is unsuccessful, or if blood drawing was performed and a successful site then established in the hand of the same arm, the possibility exists that the drugs can leak out of the previous site and into the surrounding tissues. In the case of a vesicant, necrosis could result.

The large veins along the distal forearm (cephalic, median, and basilic veins) are easily accessible and may provide safe and convenient venipuncture sites. Using these larger veins diminishes the risk of chemical phlebitis caused by the caustic properties of many agents, especially when they are given as a bolus (IV push).[13] This area is also preferred because, in the event of extravasation, there is a greater area of soft tissue (than over the hand, for instance) that may be more easily grafted, thereby avoiding functional impairment.[9]

Frequently, IV solutions contain admixtures, which may be incompatible with cytotoxic drugs, such as the combination of doxorubicin and heparin sodium, which results in an obvious precipitate. Also, the possibility exists that venous irritation and phlebitis may result.

TABLE 24-8
Extravasation Kit: Items and Quantities

Needles	18 gauge (2)
	25 gauge (2)
	filter needle (1)
Tape	1 inch paper
Telfa pads	4 × 4 in (4)
Sterile gauze dressing	4 × 4 in (2)
Alcohol wipes	(4)
Syringes	Tuberculin
	3 mL
	5 mL
	10 mL
	20 mL
Local anesthetic	Ethyl chloride
Diluent	Sterile saline: 10 mL (1) preservative-free
	Sterile water: 10 mL (1)
Steroid cream	1% topical lotion (optional)
Antidotes	10% sodium thiosulfate (10 mL)
	Hydrocortisone solution (100-mg vial)
	Dexamethasone: 4 mg/mL
	Hyaluronidase (150 U) (in refrigerator)
	Dimethyl sulfoxide (50%–100%) topical
Latex gloves	
Hot pack	
Cold pack	
Policy and procedure for extravasation management	
Extravasation record	

Restock kit after each use. Kit should be available wherever vesicant drugs are being administered.

(From Goodman, M. S. [1991]. Delivery of cancer chemotherapy. In S. B. Baird [Ed.]. *Cancer nursing: A comprehensive textbook* [p. 295]. Philadelphia: W. B. Saunders. Used with permission.)

The use of preexisting IV sites is not recommended for vesicant chemotherapy administration. If the existing IV line is the only site available for nonvesicants, these precautions must be observed:

1. The dressing should be completely removed and vein patency ensured before treatment.

2. The tubing must be changed before and after chemotherapy if the IV contains admixtures.

3. A flush of approximately 50 to 100 mL IV fluids must be infused before and after

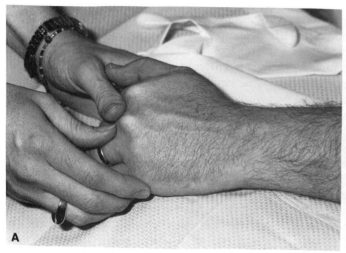
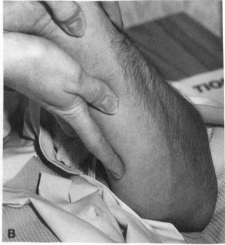

FIGURE 24-5 **(A)** Thorough examination of the hands and arms is performed before vein cannulation to avoid the use of phlebitic, bruised, inflamed, or sclerotic areas. **(B)** One useful and often overlooked peripheral site is the basilic vein on the medial aspect of the forearm.

treatment. (The nurse must ascertain that the additional fluid volume is allowable with patients who are on volume restriction.)

When establishing new IV lines, areas of joint flexion such as the wrist and antecubital fossa also should be avoided. The chosen vein should feel smooth and resilient, not hard or cordlike.[13] Several factors contraindicate use of the antecubital fossa.

1. Important anatomic structures, like median nerves and brachial arteries, are located in this area. If extensive tissue necrosis occurs in this area, amputation is a potential complication. At a minimum, extensive tissue necrosis could require long, expensive and psychologically traumatic reconstructive efforts.

2. Prolonged infusions restrict arm mobility because elbow function is limited during infusion.

3. Veins in the antecubital fossa traditionally are used for blood specimens. Repetitive needle insertions and infusions of chemotherapeutic agents could fibrose this area, precluding successful blood sampling.

4. Early subcutaneous infiltration is often more difficult to visualize because of the amount of subcutaneous fat and tissue present in this area.[17]

Despite the nurse's degree of technical competence, occasionally a nurse may have difficulty locating a vein. An arbitrary limit of three unsuccessive venipunctures is suggested before the nurse seeks assistance from a coworker. Repetitive venipunctures increase anxiety levels of both patient and nurse, which may decrease the of successful vein cannulation.

An arm with impaired circulation should not be used for the ve otoxic ag the lower extremities. Stagnant or sluggish blood flow ing the ge potentiate a local reaction and delay the agent from

Impaired circulation can exist in the extremities with an invading neoplasm, existing phlebitis, varicosities, the side of a mastectomy with axillary node dissection, an immobilized fracture, extensive hematomas, or inflamed areas.

Most chemotherapy regimens can be administered on an outpatient basis. When treating an outpatient peripherally, a stainless steel winged infusion needle is preferred. Often nurses are forced to cannulate veins in elusive areas, such as between the knuckles, or the cephalic vein as it arches over the bones on the radial wrist. Because of the position of these veins, the nurse may choose to tape the tubing securely, rather than the needle wings, to the skin, so as to not dislodge the needle.

It is important to understand that the short bevel of the needle may be dislodged from the vein with some IV push medications. So, the wings of the small scalp-vein needle should be secured to the skin whenever possible, with a short strip of tape. When securing the needle to the skin, the tape should be applied so that the needle insertion site and the immediate surrounding area are visible for inspection. A common site of extravasation is just above the needle insertion site. If obscured, subtle infiltration evidence may go unnoticed. Tubing should be taped independently and looped so that blood return can be seen when checked during administration. After needle placement has been secured, the remainder of the IV set should be arranged so that it will remain intact and functional in the event of sudden movement, such as vomiting.

Before cytotoxic drugs are administered, the vein's patency must be tested with IV fluid flush solutions. If fragile veins burst or if the needle has perforated the wall of the vein, conventional IV fluids can be absorbed without damage to surrounding tissues. Infusion of flush solution is exceedingly important before administering cytotoxic agents through a heparin lock or a permanent central venous catheter to avoid drug incompatibilities. At least 10 mL IV fluid should be used between drugs to avoid inopportune chemical interactions. Likewise, after all chemotherapy agents have been administered, approximately 50 mL IV fluid should be infused as a final flush to clear the line and vein.

Apply slow, even pressure when giving drugs by IV push. If resistance is encountered, the drug infusion can be stopped and the cause sought. If the bevel of the needle is against the wall of the vein, a careful repositioning may resolve the problem. Small-gauge needles offer more resistance. If the clinician applies great force, the patient may experience pain or venous spasm. In addition, a fast and forceful infusion of push medications can cause some patients to experience nausea and exaggerated hypersensitivity sensations (eg, nasal congestion with Cytoxan). To avoid these problems, chemotherapy should be delivered using even "push" pressure while maintaining constant supervision of administration process.

Figure 24-6 illustrates the standard procedure for drug delivery via the scalp vein, which uses either the two-syringe technique or a side port of a freely flowing IV line. Short-term chemotherapy may also be given by the conventional mini-infusion (piggyback) method. Regardless of the administration method, needle stability and adequate blood return must be checked every 1 to 2 mL, when injecting a vesicant. If any doubt exists regarding vein patency, it is urgent to immediately discontinue drug administration; resume the drug is a nonvesicant, a new cannulation site should be established to resume treatment; if the drug is a vesicant, the site should be treated as an extravasation.

After therapy treatment, the clinician removes the cannula, using a dry sterile sponge; then applies pressure to the site with the extremity elevated until bleeding stops; and dressing to the site. With thrombocytopenia being a common result of

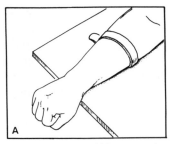

Apply tourniquet to mid-forearm, palpate radial pulse and loosen tourniquet if pulse cannot be felt. Have patient open and close fist for venous distention.

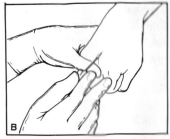

Cleanse injection area and hold patient's hand, using thumb to keep skin taut and anchor vein. Place needle in line with vein, bevel up, about one-half inch below proposed entry site.

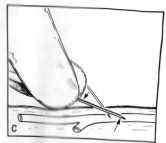

Insert needle through skin and tissue at 45° angle, relocate vein, decrease needle angle slightly and slowly enter vein with a downward then upward motion.

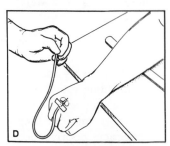

Remove tourniquet and tape scalp vein tubing.

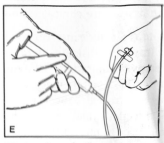

Attach syringe of saline, aspirate to remove air and irrigate.

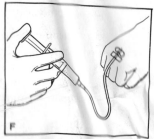

Remove saline syringe, attach chemotherapy syringe and inject slowly, checking for blood return and swelling.

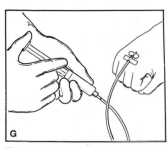

Flush catheter with saline solution.

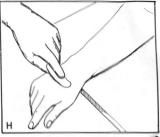

Remove needle, apply pressure to prevent bleeding and apply Bac

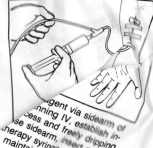

agent via sidearm of running IV, establish access and freely dripping use sidearm, insert needle therapy syringe and administer, maintaining even pressure

drugs. (From Goodman, M. S. Used with permission.)

FIGURE 24-6 Venipuncture and periph
[1986]. *Cancer: Chemotherapy a*

eous tissues can occur. The resulting
may preclude future use of that site until
nst handling heavy items with the
nous vasculature, who require long-te
ceive vesicant agents for a prolonged tim

chemoth
hemator
healed.
arm or
Pa
mother

require a venous access device.[10,25] Venous access devices can be for either long- or short-term use and can be tunnelled, nontunnelled, or implanted subcutaneously. They can be percutaneously inserted, either centrally or peripherally, eventually to dwell in the superior vena cava or above the junction of the right atrium.[8] They have become state of the art in chemotherapy administration because of the ease of placement, convenience, and safety they afford. Elimination of the anxiety of peripheral venipuncture can enhance patient serenity and comfort dramatically.

Other advantages include:

1. The patient's peripheral venous system is preserved.

2. The device can be used also for blood and nutritional products, antibiotics, analgesics, antiemetics, and cytotoxic agents, singly or in tandem.

3. Home infusions of vesicants and multiple drug therapies that once were safe and prudent only in acute care clinical settings are possible.

Potential disadvantages include insertion and maintenance costs, thrombus formation that might follow improper or inadequate irrigation, infection or sepsis, air embolism, and catheter severing or migration. Before discharge, the patients and family need meticulous training on device maintenance techniques, including take-home written instructions. If improperly instructed, patients may experience catheter occlusions caused by inadequate irrigation, infections (may require device removal) from poor aseptic technique, or air embolism caused by line mismanagement (connections poorly taped, clamps mishandled). These devices offer enormous quality-of-life advantages, but require more than the ordinary level of patient involvement, responsibility, and maintenance activities. Table 24-9 shows the various devices that provide long-term venous access.

Selection of venous access devices depends on frequency of access need, longevity of treatment, mode of administration, venous integrity, and patient preference.[25] Criteria for patient assessment are featured in Table 24-10. Common placement sites appear in Figure 24-7. These devices primarily are used for IV therapy, but also can be placed intra-arterially for organ profusion or intraperitoneally for "belly baths."[9,16]

The development of venous access devices implanted in a subcutaneous pocket offers an alternative to conventional central venous lines. Advantages include reduced infection and external catheter care requirements, and diminished risk of drug infiltration and necrosis from irritating drugs as compared to peripheral administration.[7] Various manufacturers have produced implantable devices; an example appears in Figure 24-8. To ensure continuous infusions of vesicant drugs (such as Adriamycin, Mitomycin, or Oncovin) administered through implanted devices because of the potential risk for vesicant resulting in extravasation. Proper needle placement should be ensured every 8 hours, which would require hospitalization if a continuous infusion is necessary through these devices. This is not the case with Hickman, an in-dwelling Silastic central venous catheter, such as Hickman, Broviac devices.

These are so simple and reliable that there is real risk of nurse complacency with these devices. Individual manufacturer recommendations for catheter volumes, lumen followed strictly because specific diameters, and flow rates vary from model to model. When complications occur, flushing. They are rare and (usually) avoidable if normal precautions are observed for chemotherapy administration.

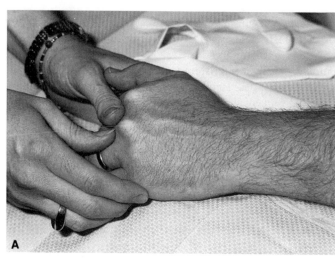
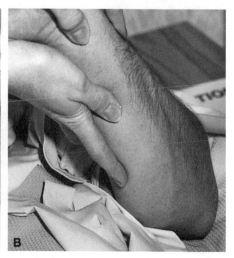

FIGURE 24-5 (**A**) Thorough examination of the hands and arms is performed before vein cannulation to avoid the use of phlebitic, bruised, inflamed, or sclerotic areas. (**B**) One useful and often overlooked peripheral site is the basilic vein on the medial aspect of the forearm.

treatment. (The nurse must ascertain that the additional fluid volume is allowable with patients who are on volume restriction.)

When establishing new IV lines, areas of joint flexion such as the wrist and antecubital fossa also should be avoided. The chosen vein should feel smooth and resilient, not hard or cordlike.[13] Several factors contraindicate use of the antecubital fossa.

1. Important anatomic structures, like median nerves and brachial arteries, are located in this area. If extensive tissue necrosis occurs in this area, amputation is a potential complication. At a minimum, extensive tissue necrosis could require long, expensive and psychologically traumatic reconstructive efforts.

2. Prolonged infusions restrict arm mobility because elbow function is limited during infusion.

3. Veins in the antecubital fossa traditionally are used for blood specimens. Repetitive needle insertions and infusions of chemotherapeutic agents could fibrose this area, precluding successful blood sampling.

4. Early subcutaneous infiltration is often more difficult to visualize because of the amount of subcutaneous fat and tissue present in this area.[17]

Despite the nurse's degree of technical competence, occasionally the nurse may have difficulty locating a vein. An arbitrary limit of three unsuccessful venipunctures is suggested before the nurse seeks assistance from a coworker. Repetitive venipunctures increase anxiety levels of both patient and nurse, which may decrease the chance of successful vein cannulation.

An arm with impaired circulation should not be used for cytotoxic agents nor should the lower extremities. Stagnant or sluggish blood flow through the venous system can potentiate a local reaction and delay the agent from reaching the general circulation.

Impaired circulation can exist in the extremities with an invading neoplasm, existing phlebitis, varicosities, the side of a mastectomy with axillary node dissection, an immobilized fracture, extensive hematomas, or inflamed areas.

Most chemotherapy regimens can be administered on an outpatient basis. When treating an outpatient peripherally, a stainless steel winged infusion needle is preferred. Often nurses are forced to cannulate veins in elusive areas, such as between the knuckles, or the cephalic vein as it arches over the bones on the radial wrist. Because of the position of these veins, the nurse may choose to tape the tubing securely, rather than the needle wings, to the skin, so as to not dislodge the needle.

It is important to understand that the short bevel of the needle may be dislodged from the vein with some IV push medications. So, the wings of the small scalp-vein needle should be secured to the skin whenever possible, with a short strip of tape. When securing the needle to the skin, the tape should be applied so that the needle insertion site and the immediate surrounding area are visible for inspection. A common site of extravasation is just above the needle insertion site. If obscured, subtle infiltration evidence may go unnoticed. Tubing should be taped independently and looped so that blood return can be seen when checked during administration. After needle placement has been secured, the remainder of the IV set should be arranged so that it will remain intact and functional in the event of sudden movement, such as vomiting.

Before cytotoxic drugs are administered, the vein's patency must be tested with IV fluid flush solutions. If fragile veins burst or if the needle has perforated the wall of the vein, conventional IV fluids can be absorbed without damage to surrounding tissues. Infusion of flush solution is exceedingly important before administering cytotoxic agents through a heparin lock or a permanent central venous catheter to avoid drug incompatibilities. At least 10 mL IV fluid should be used between drugs to avoid inopportune chemical interactions. Likewise, after all chemotherapy agents have been administered, approximately 50 mL IV fluid should be infused as a final flush to clear the line and vein.

Apply slow, even pressure when giving drugs by IV push. If resistance is encountered, the drug infusion can be stopped and the cause sought. If the bevel of the needle is against the wall of the vein, a careful repositioning may resolve the problem. Small-gauge needles offer more resistance. If the clinician applies great force, the patient may experience pain or venous spasm. In addition, a fast and forceful infusion of push medications can cause some patients to experience nausea and exaggerated hypersensitivity sensations (eg, nasal congestion with Cytoxan). To avoid these problems, chemotherapy should be delivered using even "push" pressure while maintaining constant supervision of administration process.

Figure 24-6 illustrates the standard procedure for drug delivery via the scalp vein, which uses either the two-syringe technique or a side port of a freely flowing IV line. Short-term chemotherapy may also be given by the conventional mini-infusion (piggyback) method. Regardless of the administration method, needle stability and adequate blood return must be checked every 1 to 2 mL, when injecting a vesicant. If any doubt exists regarding vein patency, it is urgent to immediately discontinue drug administration. If the drug is a nonvesicant, a new cannulation site should be established to resume the treatment; if the drug is a vesicant, the site should be treated as an extravasation.

After chemotherapy treatment, the clinician removes the cannula, using a dry sterile sponge; applies pressure to the site with the extremity elevated until bleeding stops; and then applies a dressing to the site. With thrombocytopenia being a common result of

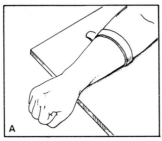

A

Apply tourniquet to mid-forearm, palpate radial pulse and loosen tourniquet if pulse cannot be felt. Have patient open and close fist for venous distention.

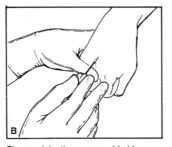

B

Cleanse injection area and hold patient's hand, using thumb to keep skin taut and anchor vein. Place needle in line with vein, bevel up, about one-half inch below proposed entry site.

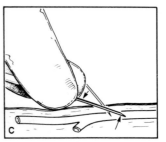

C

Insert needle through skin and tissue at 45° angle, relocate vein, decrease needle angle slightly and slowly enter vein with a downward then upward motion.

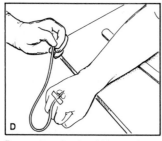

D

Remove tourniquet and tape scalp vein tubing.

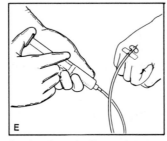

E

Attach syringe of saline, aspirate to remove air and irrigate.

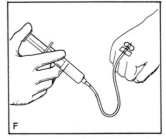

F

Remove saline syringe, attach chemotherapy syringe and inject slowly, checking for blood return and swelling.

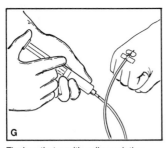

G

Flush catheter with saline solution.

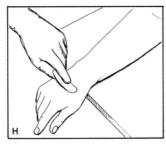

H

Remove needle, apply pressure to prevent bleeding and apply Band-Aid.

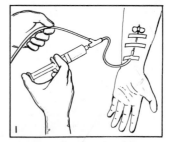

I

If administering agent via sidearm of continuously running IV, establish intravenous access and freely dripping fluid. Cleanse sidearm, insert needle of chemotherapy syringe and administer drug, maintaining even pressure.

FIGURE 24-6   Venipuncture and peripheral administration of chemotherapeutic drugs. (From Goodman, M. S. [1986]. *Cancer: Chemotherapy and care* [p. 21]. Evansville, IN: Bristol-Myers. Used with permission.)

chemotherapy, blood leakage into the subcutaneous tissues can occur. The resulting hematoma may be painful and unsightly and may preclude future use of that site until healed. Also, patients should be cautioned against handling heavy items with the treated arm or hand.

Patients with impaired peripheral venous vasculature, who require long-term chemotherapy infusion, or who are to receive vesicant agents for a prolonged time, may require a venous access device.[10, 25] Venous access devices can be for either long- or short-term use and can be tunnelled, nontunnelled, or implanted subcutaneously. They can be percutaneously inserted, either centrally or peripherally, eventually to dwell in the superior vena cava or above the junction of the right atrium.[8] They have become state of the art in chemotherapy administration because of the ease of placement, convenience, and safety they afford. Elimination of the anxiety of peripheral venipuncture can enhance patient serenity and comfort dramatically.

Other advantages include:

1. The patient's peripheral venous system is preserved.
2. The device can be used also for blood and nutritional products, antibiotics, analgesics, antiemetics, and cytotoxic agents, singly or in tandem.
3. Home infusions of vesicants and multiple drug therapies that once were safe and prudent only in acute care clinical settings are possible.

Potential disadvantages include insertion and maintenance costs, thrombus formation that might follow improper or inadequate irrigation, infection or sepsis, air embolism, and catheter severing or migration. Before discharge, the patients and family need meticulous training on device maintenance techniques, including take-home written instructions. If improperly instructed, patients may experience catheter occlusions caused by inadequate irrigation, infections (may require device removal) from poor aseptic technique, or air embolism caused by line mismanagement (connections poorly taped, clamps mishandled). These devices offer enormous quality-of-life advantages, but require more than the ordinary level of patient involvement, responsibility, and maintenance activities. Table 24-9 shows the various devices that provide long-term venous access.

Selection of venous access devices depends on frequency of access need, longevity of treatment, mode of administration, venous integrity, and patient preference.[25] Criteria for patient assessment are featured in Table 24-10. Common placement sites appear in Figure 24-7. These devices primarily are used for IV therapy, but also can be placed intra-arterially for organ profusion or intraperitoneally for "belly baths."[9, 16]

The development of venous access devices implanted in a subcutaneous pocket offers an alternative to conventional central venous lines. Advantages include reduced infection risk, no external catheter care requirements, and diminished risk of drug infiltration and vein sclerosis from irritating drugs as compared to peripheral administration.[7] Various manufacturers have produced implantable devices; an example appears in Figure 24-8.

Long-term infusions of vesicant drugs (such as Adriamycin, Mitomycin, or Oncovin) are not administered through implanted devices because of the potential risk for needle dislodgement, resulting in extravasation. Proper needle placement should be ensured and documented every 8 hours, which would require hospitalization if a continuous infusion of vesicants is necessary through these devices. This is not the case with vesicant drugs infused through an in-dwelling Silastic central venous catheter, such as Hickman, Broviac, or Groshong devices.

Venous access devices are so simple and reliable that there is real risk of nurse complacency in treating patients with these devices. Individual manufacturer recommendations for care and maintenance should be followed strictly because specific diameters, volumes, lumen size, and clamping procedures vary from model to model. When complications occur, they are severe, often life-threatening. They are rare and (usually) avoidable if normal professional standards and practices are observed for chemotherapy administration.

TABLE 24-9
Types of Venous Access Devices and Indications for Their Use

Silastic Atrial Catheters

Frequent venous access required for blood sampling, blood products, therapy, etc.

Bone marrow transplant recipient

Patient with leukemia

Single bolus injections of chemotherapy

TPN and antibiotic therapy

Short- or long-term chemotherapy infusions (vesicant or nonvesicant)

Inpatient/outpatient chemotherapy infusion

Significant other or patient capable of caring for device

Small-Gauge Central Venous Catheters

Short-term infusion chemotherapy (2–3 mo)

Short-term infusion of vesicant chemotherapy

Inpatient/outpatient infusion therapy

Single bolus injections of chemotherapy

Frequent venous access needed for chemotherapy

Infrequent blood sampling via peripheral vein

Brief life expectancy

Significant other or patient capable of caring for device

Implanted Ports

Infrequent venous access required

Single bolus injections of chemotherapy

Inpatient/outpatient infusion of nonvesicant chemotherapeutic agents

Short- or long-term chemotherapy

Used for TPN, blood transfusions, fluid replacement, or antibiotics

Infrequent blood sampling required

Patient physically unable to care for VAD

A young child: frequent venous access not required

Cosmesis/patient preference

TPN, total parenteral nutrition; VAD, venous access device.

(Adapted from Goodman, M. S., & Wickham, R. [1984]. Venous access devices: An overview. *Oncology Nursing Forum, 11*[5], 16–23.)

Infusion Systems

Venous access devices provide another key benefit to the patient who requires continuous or intermittent chemotherapy: the ability to be treated at home. The use of external ambulatory infusion systems to deliver antineoplastics reduces the patient's need to be hospitalized, reduces total cost, and allows patient autonomy within familiar home surroundings.

External ambulatory infusion systems may or may not be mechanical, but all are self-powered in that they are independent of household electrical power. The systems generally are lightweight, reusable, and battery powered and infuse either through a

TABLE 24-10
Patient Assessment Criteria for a Vascular Access Device

Criteria
Frequency of venous access
Longevity of treatment
Mode of administration
Venous integrity
Patient preference

Low Priority	High Priority
Infrequent venous access	Frequent venous access
Short-term therapy	Long-term indefinite treatment period
Intermittent single injections	Continuous infusion chemotherapy
Administration of nonvesicant/ nonirritating drugs	Home infusion of chemotherapy
No previous IV therapy	Administration of vesicant/irritating drugs
Both extremities available	Venous thrombosis/sclerosis due to previous IV therapy
Venous access with two or fewer venipunctures	Venous access limited to one extremity
Patient does not prefer VAD	Prior tissue damage due to extravasation
	Multiple (>2) venipunctures to secure venous access
	Patient prefers VAD

VAD, Vascular access device.
(From Goodman, M. S., & Wickham, R. [1984]. Venous access devices: An overview. *Oncology Nursing Forum, 11*[5], 16–23.)

piston-valve (Autosyringe) or peristaltic mechanism (CADD; Figure 24-9). The disposable Travenol Infuser, on the other hand, exerts positive pressure as a balloon containing the drug deflates into the venous access device at a rate determined by balloon pressure. All these systems can be set for the rate of volume administration. Mechanically powered pumps have alarm systems that detect backpressure, which occurs with occlusion or infiltration. These pumps also detect air in the line; the alarm sounds when the fluid reservoir is empty.

[Any list published here of available products and technologies in ambulatory infusion systems could be obsolete within weeks of publication. Intravenous clinicians are better served with a suggestion to keep abreast of manufacturer-provided instructional materials, patient education information, and trouble-shooting support services of the devices currently favored in one's own clinical setting.]

The nurse must be fully familiar with system operation to educate the patient and family in the areas of early detection of complications, including line occlusion, thrombo-

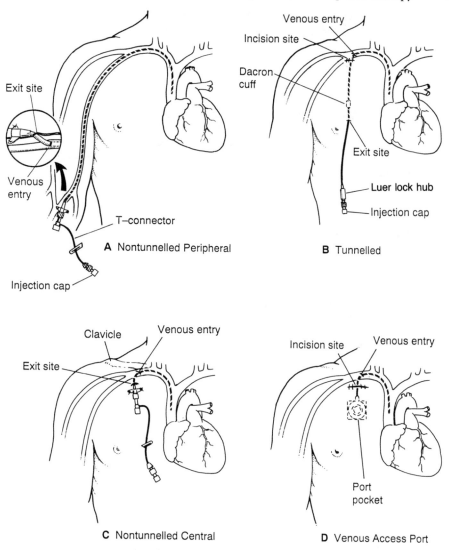

FIGURE 24-7 Common sites for long-term venous access devices. (From Wickham, R. [1987]. Techniques for long-term venous access. In Fifth National Conference on Cancer Nursing Proceedings, [p. 10]. Atlanta: American Cancer Society. Used with permission.)

sis, infiltration or extravasation, and system failure. The ONS has developed course contents and clinical practicum recommendations for nursing education and practice, which the nurse may find helpful in preparing patients to succeed with these systems.[22]

The factors to consider when recommending the use of an ambulatory infusion system are:

1. Level of patient and family understanding of pump function, alarm, features; level of patient and family compliance, reliability, dexterity, and comfort with devices; eyesight keen enough to see pump function clearly

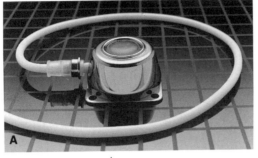

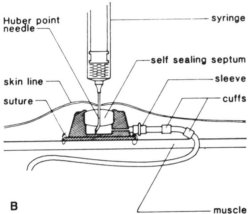

FIGURE 24-8 **(A)** PORT-A-CATH® Implantable Access System (Property of Pharmacia Deltec, Inc., St. Paul, MN) **(B)** A subcutaneously implanted port with Huber point needle penetrating the skin and the injection septum. (From Hubbard, S. M., Seipp, C. A., & Duffy, P. L. [1989]. Administration of cancer treatments: Practical guides for physicians and oncology nurses. In V. T. DeVita, S. Hellman, & S. A. Rosenberg [Eds.]. *Cancer: Principles and practice of oncology* [3rd ed., p. 2382]. Philadelphia: J. B. Lippincott. Used with permission.)

2. Proximity to health care provider, 24 hours a day, in the event of pump failure or occlusion

3. Drug regimen that matches device capacities and features

4. Insurance coverage of unit rental or purchase cost

Infusion systems can be attached by belt or shoulder straps for ease of patient movement. Mechanical systems generally require hands-on programming and reprogramming, requiring an on-site nurse visit when changes are needed.

The same is true for replenishing of fluid and drug reservoirs. Promised for the near-term future are astounding developments to ease ambulatory infusions, such as a system that allows pump reprogramming both by computer and over telephone lines, and without hands-on human intervention.

Regional Drug Delivery

Although chemotherapy is most commonly administered systemically by the IV route, some tumors respond better when locally exposed to antineoplastic agents. As a result, alternative methods of drug administration have been established to deliver high local concentrations of chemotherapeutic agents into a body cavity or into the organ site of the tumor. These drugs are given directly into the area of known malignancy, such as intraperitoneal, to treat malignant ascites or metastatic seeding of peritoneum from ovarian carcinoma; intravesical to treat bladder cancer; intrathecal or intraventricular for cancers known to have invaded the central nervous system; intrapleural for malignant

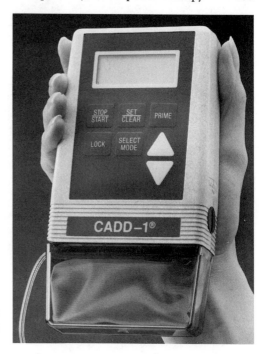

FIGURE 24-9 CADD-I Ambulatory Infusion pump, model 5100 HFX. (Property of: Pharmacia Deltec, Inc., St. Paul, MN)

effusions and sclerosing purposes; topical for early malignancies of the integumentary; or intra-arterial for the regional delivery of chemotherapy into the liver through the hepatic artery.[12]

Another advantage of the regional delivery of these infusions is that they can "bathe" the affected body cavity or organ without imposing toxic effects to the whole system.

The most likely alternative route of chemotherapy administration that may involve the IV nurse is the intra-arterial infusion that uses a totally implanted infusion pump (Figure 24-10). This route generally is used to treat primary hepatic tumors or hepatic metastasis of colorectal, stomach, esophageal, pancreatic, breast, lung, or malignant melanoma.[28] Intra-arterial infusion is also used to treat large amounts of localized disease in primary head and neck tumors, brain tumors, and widespread metastatic disease in the pelvis by giving large drug concentrations through the arteries that supply these areas.[3]

The most commonly used totally implantable drug delivery system is the Infusaid Pump. The Food and Drug Administration (FDA) has approved its use commercially for 5-FU, methotrexate, floxuridine (FUDR), heparin, morphine sulfate, insulin, and some aminoglycosides. The pump is powered by a volatile fluorocarbon vapor pressure, using a system of bellows, the exertion of which forces the fluid out of the drug chamber at a specified rate. This vapor pressure is influenced by changes in body temperature, atmospheric pressure, and drug viscosity. Because the pump's flow rate increases by roughly 10% for each degree centigrade increase in body temperature, patients must comply with the requirement to report fever, so that the scheduled pump refill may be adjusted, if necessary.

Also, because infection and thrombosis are the most common complications of

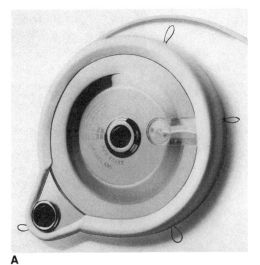

A

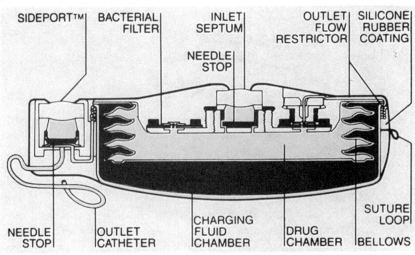

| SIDEPORT™ | BACTERIAL FILTER | INLET SEPTUM | OUTLET FLOW RESTRICTOR | SILICONE RUBBER COATING |

NEEDLE STOP

| NEEDLE STOP | OUTLET CATHETER | CHARGING FLUID CHAMBER | DRUG CHAMBER | SUTURE LOOP / BELLOWS |

B

FIGURE 24-10 **(A)** Infusaid Pump for chemotherapy administration. **(B)** Internal components of Infusaid Pump. (Courtesy: Intermedics Infusaid, Inc., Norwood, MA)

arterial infusion, patients also must report pain, changes in temperature of the skin over the pump, color, sensation, or fluid leakage.[13]

The pump is filled with the chemotherapy agent (in its active form) or saline to perfuse the area constantly. The device is refilled by percutaneous injection, approximately every 1 to 2 weeks.[10] The side port of the device may be used for direct intra-arterial access. The nurse must be entirely knowledgeable of the techniques and risks of this route of drug delivery before attempting administration and must strictly adhere to device manufacturer data and institutional policy and procedure for accessing and filling these pumps.

These devices also serve as effective pain management by infusing low-dose narcotics by intrathecal or subcutaneous modes of delivery.

Intrathecal therapy is another alternative route of cancer chemotherapy that might involve the IV nurse. This method may use a cerebrospinal access device, such as the Ommaya reservoir, subcutaneously implanted, to avoid repeated lumbar punctures in treating meningial carcinomatosis, the infiltration of the leptomeninges of the brain by cancer. The reservoir provides access to the cerebrospinal fluid through a burr hole in the skull (Figure 24-11).

Hubbard and coworkers[13] described the nursing procedure for use and maintenance of these devices as follows:

> First, the reservoir is pumped several times, to fill the device with spinal fluid. Then, the skin is prepared and the reservoir is obliquely punctured, using sterile technique, with a 25–27 gauge scalp-vein needle. Enough spinal fluid is removed for laboratory studies and to keep exchanges isovolumetric. A chemotherapeutic agent is then injected slowly into the reservoir through the scalp-vein needle, which is then flushed with Elliott's B solution. After the needle is removed, the reservoir is pumped to distribute the drugs into the intraventricular space. Preservative-free morphine sulfate also can be administered into an Ommaya reservoir to achieve prolonged periods of pain relief.

CONTROVERSIAL ISSUES

Some elements of chemotherapy administration policy and procedure have earned unanimous consensus. Others are handled in various ways, depending on personal experience, opinion, and talent. Until further investigation results in definitive direction, some controversy will remain in a few areas of chemotherapy theory and practice. Some examples follow.

The Oncology Nursing Society acknowledges that there are issues considered controversial among practicing clinicians. Below are several of those issues needing further investigative studies. An attempt is made to address the issues without being judgmental. Current researchers have yet to agree on a method of approach for these issues.

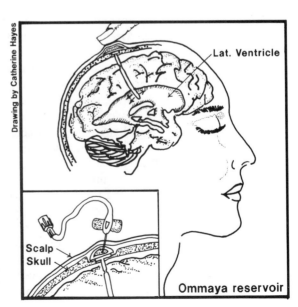

FIGURE 24-11 Cerebrospinal fluid reservoir (Ommaya type) facilitates repeated intraventricular administration.

A. Use of the antecubital fossa for administering chemotherapeutic agents
  1. Favoring the use of the antecubital fossa
     a. Larger veins permit more rapid infusion/administration of drugs.
     b. Larger veins permit potentially irritating chemotherapeutic agents to reach the general circulation sooner with less irritation to smaller veins.
  2. Avoiding the use of the antecubital fossa
     a. Arm mobility is restricted with a needle in place.
     b. The risk of extravasation is increased because of patient mobility (*eg*, coughing, vomiting).
     c. Infiltration could cause extensive reconstruction efforts to be necessary, with limited arm use during the healing process, resulting in increased morbidity and decreased function.
     d. Because of the subcutaneous tissues, early infiltration is more difficult to assess.
     e. Many chemotherapeutic agents are thought to cause venous thrombosis. Blood is usually drawn from the antecubital fossa. Fibrosed veins would make blood drawing more difficult.

B. Needle size
  1. Favoring the use of a larger gauge (*eg*, 19- and 21-gauge scalp-vein needles)
     a. Potentially irritating chemotherapeutic agents can reach the general circulation sooner, with less irritating effect on the peripheral veins.
     b. Drug administration time is decreased, which reduces the patient's exposure to a potentially stressful environment.
  2. Favoring the use of a smaller gauge (*eg*, 23- and 25-gauge scalp-vein needles)
     a. Smaller gauge needles are less likely to puncture the wall of a small vein.
     b. Scar tissue may be formed with needle insertion; small-gauge needles cause less scar tissue formation.
     c. Less pain may be experienced by the patient during the insertion of a smaller gauge needle.
     d. Increased blood flow around a smaller bore needle increases dilution of the chemotherapeutic agent.
     e. Mechanical phlebitis may be minimized with a smaller bore needle.
     f. Potential episodes of nausea and vomiting may be decreased by slow infusion of the chemotherapeutic agents.

C. Methods of drug sequencing
  1. Favoring the administration of vesicants first
     a. Vascular integrity decreases over time.
     b. The vein is most stable and less irritated at the initiation of the treatment.
     c. The initial assessment of vein patency is most accurate.
     d. The patient's awareness of symptomatic changes becomes less accurate over time.
  2. Favoring the administration of vesicants last
     a. Vesicants are irritating and may increase vein fragility.
     b. Venous spasm can occur at the beginning of IV push or bolus therapy, which the patient may report as painful; the nurse must decide if the complaint is spasm or infiltration.

D. Side arm versus direct push administration
  1. Favoring side arm administration

      a. Freely running IV lines allow for maximal dilution of drugs that could be potentially irritating.

      b. Can more readily interrupt the administration of the drug while maintaining venous access.

  2. Favoring direct push administration

      a. Integrity of the vein can be more easily assessed and the early signs of extravasation noted more easily.[20]

COMPLICATIONS

Despite the skill of the nurse and the use of appropriate administration techniques, patients will occasionally experience problems unique to the administration of cytotoxic agents.

Venous Fragility

Elderly, poorly nourished, and debilitated patients are often predisposed to having fragile veins. The unskilled nurse may unknowingly cause painful and unsightly hematomas that prevent future use of veins until healing occurs. If a patient has fragile veins, the nurse should attempt to cannulate the vein without the use of a tourniquet because tourniquet distention and rapid engorgement may cause the wall of the vein to rupture when the tourniquet is released. A second nurse may apply gentle hand pressure above the venipuncture site to effect distention. Other alternatives that can be used to distend veins include applying moderate heat or having the patient pump or clench the fist. Gravity flow may be maximized by having the patient dangle the hand and arm. Light tapping of the site with the nurse's finger may also be used to effect venous distention without the use of a tourniquet.

    With all maneuvers, patients with fragile veins should be approached cautiously, with adequate time being allowed by the therapist to effect an adequate venipuncture at the first attempt.

Localized Acute Allergic Reactions

Reactions should be anticipated in any patient receiving IV cytotoxic agents. Localized allergic reactions, commonly called "flare," often are associated with the administration of doxorubicin hydrochloride.[31] The first appearance may be that of erythema along the venous pathways. Blotchiness, hivelike urticaria, or the rapid appearance of welts may also occur as the first sign noted. The patient may complain of itching, stinging, or an increased sensation of heat in the area. Some feel that the reaction is caused by an intercellular release of histamines, which increases cell membrane permeability. Increased cellular permeability may permit drug leakage into the subcutaneous tissues.[31] Other possibilities include drug interactions or contaminants or a molecular extravasation through the vascular endothelium.

    Preventive measures include additionally diluting the chemotherapy agent either by adding the drug to 100 to 200 mL solution or by administering the drug piggyback.* A

---

* Piggyback refers to a method of infusion through the sidearm of the IV tubing while additional diluent is infusing.

chart similar to Table 24-5 may assist the nurse unfamiliar with rates and methods of administering cytotoxic agents.

Should a localized allergic reaction occur, many practitioners feel that, to prevent chemical cellulitis, the drug should be discontinued and a new venipuncture site established. Before removing the IV needle, the administration of additional fluid not containing drugs should be infused in an attempt to resolve the erythematous reaction. The medications listed below are suggested to treat localized sensitivity reactions. All require a physician's order before their administration.

Hydrocortisone sodium succinate (Solu-Cortef). Slow IV push, 25 to 50 mg, antiinflammatory agent

Benadryl. IV push, 25 to 50 mg, antihistamine

Venous Spasm

Several cytotoxic agents are associated with complaints of severe pain or spasm along the venous pathway. Carmustine (BiCNU) is diluted with absolute alcohol, which may be the offending agent. The breakdown products from photodegradation of dacarbazine (DTIC) may be responsible for the acute local burning associated with the use of this drug.

Mechlorethamine hydrochloride (Mustargen) can also cause pain, especially in patients who have received chemotherapy over extended periods. Although the administration of these agents should alert the therapist to the possible occurrence of this problem, it should be mentioned that *any* agent is capable of causing venous pain in the patient at any time. In addition, venous spasm or pain can also occur if a small-gauge needle is used and the treatment is administered by forceful pushing on the plunger of the syringe. Measures suggested for alleviating venous pain or spasm include:

1. Slowing the drug infusion rate.
2. Additionally diluting the drug.
3. Applying either warm or cool compresses to the arm during infusion. Unfortunately, the use of either warm or cool maneuvers at this time is empirically decided. Some patients will respond to one approach and some to the other. The nurse is reminded to take care that second-degree burns do not occur with temperature alteration maneuvers.
4. Administering Xylocaine 1%—0.25 mL (3 mL total), as needed. A physician's order and an allergy history should be obtained before administering the drug.

Chemical phlebitis is a risk associated with the administration of most IV cancer chemotherapy agents. With many treatment programs involving the combination of two or more cytotoxic agents, the risk is increased. Early phlebitis can be associated with pain, erythema, occasional limb edema, and a sensation of warmth in the affected extremity. As the acute symptom subsides, the venous pathways may retain a dark bluish to brown discoloration for some time. Often associated with this are complaints from the patient of restricted arm use. Acute phlebitis reactions can interfere with the patient's routine daily living activities and interrupt usual sleep patterns. Noninvestigational drugs frequently associated with causing phlebitis are:

Actinomycin D	Cisplatin
Carmustine	Dacarbazine

Daunorubicin	Streptozotocin
Doxorubicin hydrochloride	Vinblastine
Mechlorethamine hydrochloride	Vincristine
Mitomycin C	

Extreme caution should be taken by the nurse to prevent the occurrence of phlebitis. Should phlebitic reactions occur in both arms, IV chemotherapy treatment may need to be discontinued pending resolution of the problem. Inability to aggressively treat progressive disease with IV cytotoxic agents may jeopardize the patient's chances for long-term disease control. When possible, nonsclerosing agents in the same drug category are substituted for the offending agent. Occasionally a patient will display phlebitic reactions to any IV drug administered.

In addition to the preventive measures suggested in Chapter 22 (section on vascular irritation) to diminish the possible occurrence of phlebitis, the nurse may elect to adopt the following measures:

1. Administer hydrocortisone sodium succinate (Solu-Cortef), 25 to 50 mg, slow IV push. It is empirically suggested that half the total dose be administered pretreatment after ascertaining vein patency and the remaining half after the final flush has been administered and just before the needle is removed. A physician's order is necessary before this drug can be administered.

2. Additionally dilute the agent. Reducing the drug concentration may lessen the occurrence of phlebitis.

Unfortunately, some patients will develop phlebitis despite the most cautious effort of the nurse to prevent its occurrence. Repetitive needle insertions necessary for blood sampling and the administration of multiple IV chemotherapy agents increase the possibility that phlebitis and thrombosis will occur. Therapeutic measures that may be indicated once phlebitis has occurred include:

1. Elevation of the affected extremity
2. Application of topical heat
3. Administration of systemic analgesics (with a physician's order)

Ideally, the venous status should be assessed before the patient receives any chemotherapy treatments. If the veins are deep and difficult to visualize or palpate with tourniquet distention, or if the peripheral veins are extremely small, central venous options should be considered as an alternative to repeated peripheral attempts with each chemotherapy treatment.

Generalized Anaphylactic Reaction

The clinician should be prepared for the occurrence of an anaphylactic reaction at any time, with any drug, in any patient. Before initiating treatment, the nurse should understand the facility's policy for the administration of cytotoxic agents. Knowledge of the procedure for initiating emergency care and awareness of the location of an emergency cart are essential for the clinician who administers cytotoxic agents. For example, some hospital policies state that the nurse may not administer cancer chemotherapy agents without a physician being present. In addition, many institutions do not permit nurses to administer investigational drugs until their safety has been established and approval has been granted by the pharmacy and therapeutics committee. The rationale for this practice is that investigational drugs do not have the years of accumulated experience available with commercial drugs. Because documented clinical experience is lacking, many policy makers feel that unknown side effects cannot adequately be assessed and managed by nurses.

In anticipating the possibility of anaphylaxis, the nurse should continuously monitor the patient for signs of flushing, shaking, sudden agitation or anxiety, nausea, vomiting, urticaria, hypotension, generalized pruritus, throbbing in the ears, palpitation, paresthesias, or any respiratory distress (wheezing, coughing, shortness of breath, or an asthma-type reaction). If undetected, a generalized anaphylactic reaction can cause convulsions and cardiopulmonary arrest.

Before initiating therapy, the nurse should position the patient so that the reclining position can easily be managed if necessary (see Figure 24-4). The nurse will find it most difficult to treat an anaphylactic reaction if the patient is seated at a table without a bed nearby. In addition, an emergency cart with the appropriate medications should be readily available as well as the stethoscope and sphygmomanometer (see Table 24-7).

Some facilities initiate a "standing order" sheet for each patient signed at treatment initiation by the responsible physician. This valuable timesaving procedure permits the clinician to initiate emergency treatment until physician assistance arrives.

The nurse should also obtain a baseline blood pressure reading before treatment. If the patient is normally hypotensive, establishing a normal blood pressure reading will be useful if symptoms of shock occur. Also, the baseline reference point of the patient's mental status should be assessed. The presence of metastatic brain disease or other mental alterations, if not noted early, can be misleading for the therapist who is attempting to determine if early symptoms of anaphylaxis are being manifested (*eg*, agitation, ing to determine if early symptoms of anaphylaxis are being manifested (*eg*, agitation, anxiety, speech disorders, and mental confusion).

Regardless of whether a patient displays a mild reaction such as generalized pruritus or sustains a complete cardiovascular collapse, the nurse should be prepared to:

1. Recline the patient safely and quickly.
2. Administer basic cardiopulmonary resuscitative measures.
3. Maintain a patent IV line for emergency drug administration.
4. Provide reassurance to the patient.
5. Administer appropriate drugs, as ordered.
6. Monitor the patient until the reaction subsides.

Prevention of anaphylaxis is a goal with the administration of all cancer chemotherapeutic agents. The nurse should be aware of the agents known to cause anaphylaxis and be prepared to administer those agents as recommended in the product brochure.

1. *Bleomycin sulfate (Blenoxane).* The package insert recommends treating patients with 2 U or less with the first two doses.
2. *Cisplatin (Platinol).* No specific recommendations for dose attenuation or length of time of administration. Suggestions for symptom management are listed in the product brochure.

3. *Asparaginase (Elspar).* Desensitization should be performed before administering the first dose of Elspar on initiation of therapy to positive reactors and on retreatment of any patient in whom therapy is deemed necessary after carefully weighing the increased risk of hypersensitivity reactions.

In addition, an allergy history should be obtained and charted even though it is presumed to have been done by the physician. Precautionary measures to use when potential anaphylactic reactions are possible might include:

1. Test dosing
2. Antihistaminic, steroidal, and/or anti-inflammatory/antipyretic pretreatment
3. Uninterrupted dosing to prevent a significant buildup of reactive antibodies[6]

Extravasation

The treatment of local infiltrations of cancer chemotherapy agents is controversial. No treatments have well-documented efficacy.[6] Controlled clinical trials are undoubtedly lacking in this area because of the low number of accruable patients treated by skilled clinicians and because of the ethical issues associated with a control or no-treatment arm. It is often difficult, in fact, to ascertain that an infiltration actually has occurred. Table 24-11 outlines the venous reactions nurses may observe as compared to actual extravasations. No trained nurse would knowingly permit an infiltration of sclerosing agents to continue to the point of being frankly obvious. Therefore, justifications of studies involving patients have been ethically and morally difficult to defend. Because of the particularly morbid effect of doxorubicin hydrochloride (Adriamycin) on tissues, the majority of studies on extravasation have been conducted using this drug.

The consequences to the patient of extensive tissue necrosis are numerous (Figure 24-12). Areas to be considered include the following:

1. *Pain.* Extensive necrotic areas frequently require narcotics for pain control.
2. *Physical defect.* Patients may be unable to work for indefinite periods. If full range of motion is required in patient's employment, for example, permanent functional compromise will carry severe quality-of-life implications. If they are employed in areas where public exposure is great, the cosmetic defect may have a severe emotional impact (see Figure 24-12).
3. *Cost.* In many instances, patients bear the financial responsibility for the lengthy and numerous hospitalizations and extensive plastic surgery procedures that may be necessary. If patients are debilitated, additional time may be required and secondary medical problems may occur.
4. *Disease control.* Valuable time may be lost if patients are unable to continue medical treatments to control the disease process. Myelosuppression from previous chemotherapy treatments may cause a necrosed area to become secondarily infected, thus lengthening the interval before which chemotherapy treatments can be reinitiated.
5. *Time.* Patients who are employed or attend school may be unable to do so until healing occurs. The inability to sustain oneself financially may be an additional hardship for the entire family.

TABLE 24-11
Nursing Assessment of Extravasation versus Other Reactions

Assessment Parameter	Extravasation		Irritation of the Vein	Flare Reaction
	Immediate Manifestations of Extravasation	Delayed Manifestations of Extravasation		
Pain	Severe pain or burning lasting min or hr, eventually subsiding; usually occurs while the drug is being given and around needle site	48 hr	Aching and tightness along the vein	No pain
Redness	Blotchy redness around needle site, not always present at time of extravasation	Later occurrence	The full length of the vein may be reddened or darkened	Immediate blotches or streaks along vein, usually subsides within 30 min with or without treatment.
Ulceration	Develops insidiously, usually 48–96 hr later	Later occurrence	Not usually	Not usually
Swelling	Severe swelling usually occurs immediately	48 hr	Not likely	Not likely; wheals may appear along vein line
Blood return	Inability to obtain blood return; presence–rate	Good blood return during drug administration	Usually	Usually
Other	Change in the quality of infusion	Local tingling, sensory deficits	—	Urticaria

(From Oncology Nursing Society. [1992]. *Cancer chemotherapy guidelines: Module V, Recommendations for the management of vesicant extravasation, hypersensitivity and anaphylaxis.* Pittsburgh.)

6. *Psychological impact.* The five points above emphasize that this is a difficult time for the patient. Communication between the health care team and patient may be strained because of the therapist's own feelings of guilt.

Prevention

Undoubtedly, years of experience in administering cytotoxic agents will perfect the clinician's technique. However, despite the skill of the health care team, extravasation of tissue-sclerosing agents can occur. This statement is underscored in an effort to allay the inevitable anxiety experienced by nurses who administer cytotoxic agents. The emphasis should be on the perfection of IV techniques, anticipating and planning for the possibility of extravasation and detecting and treating *early* suspected infiltration. Although there is no guarantee that extravasation will not occur, there is reasonable assurance that the extent of involvement will be minimized by the services of an astute clinician. Prevention is the most effective strategy to avoid extravasation. Details of the strategies are outlined in Table 24-12.

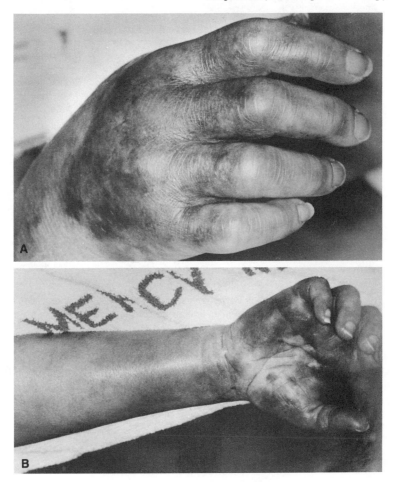

FIGURE 24-12 Extravasation of vesicant agents.

Patient Education
The patient must be informed of the possible consequences when cancer chemotherapy agents are being administered. Informed consent is a necessity. Knowledge of the possibility of extravasation constitutes an essential part of informed consent. Of course, such information should be conveyed in a sensitive manner so as to allay unnecessary fears. Naturally, the unconscious or irrational patient should not have cytotoxic agents infused without a nurse being in constant attendance. The rational and cooperative patient may report stinging, burning, pain at the cannula insertion site, or any unusual sensation. It should be emphasized, however, that extravasation can occur in the absence of these reported symptoms.

General Precautions
In administering cytotoxic agents, the clinician should understand and adhere to the following eight guidelines:

(text continues on page 500)

TABLE 24-12
Extravasation of Vesicant Antineoplastic Agents: Preventive Strategies

Risk Factor	Preventive Strategy	Rationale
Skill of the Practitioner	Chemotherapy administration only done by registered nurses who are specifically trained and supervised.	Procedures for management of extravasation vary according to the drug infiltrated.
		Certain drugs (streptozocin or BCNU) may cause a burning sensation during infusion, which is normal. However, it is abnormal and indicative of a problem if burning occurs during infusion of drugs such as doxorubicin and mitomycin.
	No attempts by practitioner to do procedures beyond his or her expertise.	
	Practitioners are skillful in venipuncture.	Procedures change rapidly. Techniques need to be learned and mastered before assuming responsibility for administration of chemotherapy.
	Practitioners are knowledgeable of the signs and symptoms of extravasation and drug therapy.	
	Practice is based on institutional policies and procedures that are routinely updated to meet the changing standards and methods of practice.	The definition of customary care in the community helps dictate standard of practice.
Condition of the Veins Small fragile veins	Use conventional methods for venous distention such as heat and percussion.	Risk of vesicant drug seepage exists with repeated venipuncture.
Access limited owing to axillary surgery, vein thrombosis, prior extravasation	Assess all available arm veins. Assess veins in a methodical fashion, taking time to select the most appropriate vein.	Multiple vein injections lead to thrombosis and limited availability.
Long-term drug therapy Multiple vein punctures	If practitioners do not feel confident in their ability to cannulate a person's veins successfully, they should seek the assistance of a colleague.	
	After attempting one or two injections without success, the practitioner should seek the assistance of a colleague before trying again.	
	A patient who consistently needs two or more attempts to secure venous access should be considered a candidate for a VAD.	Before the advent of vascular access devices (VADs), multiple venous injections to administer a drug might have been accepted as the only method of drug administration. This is no longer the case. Instead, treatment should be delayed until a VAD can be placed.
	The time to place a VAD is before an extravasation, not after.	
		Most VADs can be used immediately or within 24–48 hr, so delay in drug therapy is not usually an issue.
Drug Administration Technique	Vesicant agents are never given as continuous infusions into a peripheral vein.	The risk of infiltration of a vesicant from a peripheral vein infusion is great owing to the following: Blood return is not assessed frequently.

(continued)

TABLE 24-12   (Continued)

Risk Factor	Preventive Strategy	Rationale
		The longer the infusion, the greater the possibility of needle dislodgment.
		The patient can move the extremity, which could dislodge the IV cannula.
		Even a small amount of vesicant can cause tissue damage.
		Infiltration can be subtle and difficult to detect until a large volume has infiltrated.
		The patient may be sedated from an antiemetic and be unable to report sensations associated with extravasation.
	If peripheral line is on a controlled infusion pump, disconnect pump before injection of chemotherapy.	The pump forces drug into the tissues.
	When a vesicant is to be given as a continuous infusion, the drug should be infused via an external based central venous catheter whenever possible.	When an implanted port already exists, the patient is taught to check the needle three times a day to ensure placement during continuous infusion of a vesicant.
		The incidence of vesicant drug extravasation from ports used for continuous infusion is well documented and presents a risk to be avoided, if possible.
	Vesicant agents are most commonly administered using the two-syringe technique or through the side port of a free-flowing peripheral intravenous line.	The two-syringe technique allows for proper assessment of blood flow and resistance in the vein.
		A scalp-vein needle causes minimal vein irritation.
	Two-Syringe Technique Select an appropriate vein.	
	Begin a new IV line using a scalp vein needle (25 or 23 gauge).	
	Access vein using a single approach.	A subtle leak can be caused by accidentally piercing the vein before accessing it; avoid searching for a vein with repeated approaches.
	Flush line with 8–10 mL saline. Assess for brisk, full blood return and any evidence of infiltration. Check for swelling at the site, redness or pain, and lack of blood return.	
	Once access is ensured, switch to syringe of chemotherapy.	
	Dilute drugs according to the package insert.	Increasing the dilution increases the time it takes to administer the drug, thus increasing risk of infiltration.
	Inject drugs slowly and with minimal resistance.	The speed of the injection is determined by the resistance in the vein. Resis-

(continued)

TABLE 24-12 *(Continued)*

Risk Factor	Preventive Strategy	Rationale
	Assess for blood return every 1–2 mL infusion.	tance will vary depending on the size of the needle used.
	Flush with 3–5 mL of saline between each drug and 8–10 mL at the completion of the infusion of the drug or drugs.	
	Side-arm Technique Ensure proper venous access site. The IV fluid should be additive free.	The main rationale for the side-arm technique is the added dilution of the drug by the continuous drip of the IV fluid.
	Cannula used to access the vein should be at least a 20 gauge to ensure an adequate blood return and fluid flow.	Common pitfalls Not using a large enough cannula for a brisk infusion of infusate.
	Secure cannula but do not obstruct entrance site.	Vesicant backs up into IV line.
	Pinch off tubing and assess for blood return.	IV line has to be pinched off to inject vesicant, which defeats the purpose.
	Test the vein with 50–100 mL to ensure an adequate and swift drip of infusion.	Clinician tends to take eyes off of the site of drug infusion to watch fluid drip more than with two-syringe technique.
	With IV fluid continuing to drip, slowly inject vesicant into IV line.	
	Do not allow vesicant to flow backward.	
	Do not pinch off tubing except to assess for blood return.	
	Assess for blood return every 1–2 mL injection.	
	Flush scalp-vein needle with saline at the completion of injection.	
Order of Vesicant Drug Administration (*Note*: Sequencing is probably unimportant. The most critical issue is adequately testing the vein with saline [8–10 mL] before administering any drug [vesicant or nonvesicant]).	Give vesicant first.	Vascular integrity decreases over time.
		Practitioner's assessment skills are most acute initially.
		Patient may be more sedated from antiemetic and less able to report changes in sensation at infusion site as time goes on.
	Give vesicant between two nonvesicants.	Chemotherapy is irritating to the veins. Nonvesicants are presumed to be less irritating than vesicants.
	Give vesicant last.	Because venous spasm occurs early during the injection, it is less likely to be confused with pain of extravasation if vesicant is given last.
		It is assumed that because the vein tolerated the nonvesicants, it will also tolerate the vesicant.

(continued)

TABLE 24-12 *(Continued)*

Risk Factor	Preventive Strategy	Rationale
Site of Venous Access: Choosing the Best Vein	VADs, including tunneled catheters, implanted ports, and nontunneled central venous catheters, are indicated when patients have small, frail veins and are in need of long-term indefinite chemotherapy, continuous infusion of vesicant drugs, or both.	VADs are important options for patients with poor venous access.
	Although a VAD is a good way to prevent extravasation, it is not indicated just because someone is receiving a vesicant drug.	Externally based catheters are ideal for continuous infusion of vesicant chemotherapeutic agents because the risk of extravasation is very minimal.
	Peripheral access is optimal in the large veins of the forearm, especially the posterior basilic vein. After these, the metacarpal veins of the dorsum of the hand are easy to access and stabilize. The veins over the wrist are risky because of potential damage to tendons and nerves should extravasation occur.	Expert technique and a knowledgeable clinician are the most cost effective and safe means of administering vesicant drugs.
	Note: A large straight vein over the dorsum of the hand is preferable to a smaller vein of the forearm.	Veins in the forearm are large and adequately supporting by surrounding tissue. Adequate tissue exists around veins to provide coverage and promote healing should a problem occur.
	The antecubital fossa is to be avoided for vesicant drug administration.	The area is dense with tendons and nerves. Seepage of a vesicant can be subtle and go unnoticed. Damage here can result in loss of structure and function.
	If the antecubital fossa appears to be the only vein available for access, the patient needs an access device.	
	Hold chemotherapy—insert VAD.	Risking extravasation and subsequent tissue damage is not worth the temptation to give "just one more treatment" before considering other options.
		There is no evidence that delaying chemotherapy for 24 hr in selected cases is detrimental to the overall outcome.
	Avoid administering chemotherapy in lower extremities.	Risk for thrombosis is increased when chemotherapy is given in lower extremities.
Using a Preexisting IV Line	Do not use a preexisting peripheral intravenous line if any of the following are true: The IV cannula was placed more than 12 hr earlier. The site is reddened, swollen, or sore, or there is evidence of infiltration. The site is over or around the wrist. Evidence of blood return is sluggish or absent. The IV fluid runs erratically and the IV seems positional.	It is unreasonable to disregard the potential for a perfectly adequate venous access line because it was not started by the person administering the vesicant drug. Our ability to assess the vein and evidence of blood return should be adequate to ensure the practitioner of an adequate and safe venous access.

(continued)

TABLE 24-12 *(Continued)*

Risk Factor	Preventive Strategy	Rationale
	If the IV fluid runs freely; the blood return is brisk and consistent; and the site is without redness, pain, or swelling, then there is no reason to inflict unnecessary pain by injecting the patient again.	
	Prior dressings must be carefully removed over the cannula insertion site to fully visualize the vein during injection of the vesicant agent.	Dressings and tape can severely impede both visually and tactilely an assessment for an extravasation.

(From Goodman, M. S. [1991]. Delivery of cancer chemotherapy. In S. B. Baird [Ed.]. *Cancer nursing: A comprehensive textbook* [pp. 300–302]. Philadelphia: W. B. Saunders. Used with permission.)

1. *Anticipate the possibility of extravasation.* Before initiating treatment, the clinician should know which agents are capable of producing tissue necrosis (see Table 24-5).

    A conveniently posted chart listing vesicant agents and their recommended antidotes should be available (Table 24-13). In addition, the antidotes should be readily available for administration. Several studies suggest that delay in adminis-

TABLE 24-13
Recommended Antidotes for Vesicant/Irritant Drugs

Chemotherapeutic Agent	Antidote		Antidote Preparation
	Pharmacologic	Nonpharmacologic	
Mechlorethamine Nitrogen Mustard, (Mustargen)	Isotonic sodium thiosulfate	Cold compresses	Mix 4 mL 10% Na thiosulfate with 6 mL sterile H$_2$O for injection. (1/6 molar solution results). If using Na thiosulfate 25% mix 1.6 mL with 8.4 mL sterile H$_2$O for 1/6 molar solution.
Vincristine (Oncovin)	Hyalouronidase (Wydase)	Warm compresses	Mix with 1 mL NaCl (150 U/mL)
Vinblastine (Velban)			
Vindesine (Eldisine)			
Teniposide (VH-26)			
Etoposide (VP-16)			
Cisplatin (Platinol)	Isotonic sodium thiosulfate		Mix 4 mL of 10% Na thiosulfate with 6 mL sterile H$_2$0 for injection. (1/6 molar solution results).
Note: (large extravasations of concentrated solutions produce tissue necrosis)			If using Na thiosulfate 25% mix 1.6 mL with 8.4 mL sterile H$_2$O for 1/6 molar solution.

SQ, subcutaneous.

(From Oncology Nursing Society [1992]. *Cancer chemotherapy guidelines: Module V, Recommendations for the management of vesicant extravasation, hypersensitivity and anaphylaxis.* Pittsburgh.)

tering antidotes may increase the severity of local tissue reaction. The policy for the application of heat or cooling as used by the nurse's facility should be understood (Table 24-14). If standing orders are available, they should be signed by the individual physician and placed in the chart. Planning ahead can often minimize the severity of damage to the subcutaneous tissues.

2. *When in doubt, stop the infusion of the chemotherapy agent.* If there is any doubt in the nurse's mind that the cancer chemotherapy agent is not infusing properly, then the drug should *immediately* be discontinued. There is general agreement that the greater the amount of extravasation into the subcutaneous tissues, the more severe is the local tissue destruction. If veins are at a minimum, the therapist may elect to replace the drug with normal saline and infuse sufficient quantities while watching for signs of extravasation.

3. *Infuse at least 5 to 10 mL normal saline before cytotoxic agents are administered to ascertain vein patency.* Only when the clinician is sure beyond a doubt that the solution is infusing into the vein and not into the subcutaneous tissues should cytotoxic agents be administered. Additional infusion of normal saline may be necessary to satisfy the therapist. Once again, if there is any doubt about needle placement at any time during the drug infusion, normal saline should be infused or the venipuncture site changed.

4. *The nurse should be aware of a slow leak or insidious infiltration.* If the needle punctures the posterior wall of the vein, chemotherapy agents could leak into the

Method of Administration	Comments	References	
		Humans	Animals
1. Inject 1–4 mL (1/6 molar) through existing IV line cannula.	1. Na thiosulfate neutralizes mechlorethamine	26 33	34
2. Administer 1 mL for each mg extravasated.	2. Initiate treatment immediately.		
3. Inject SQ if needle removed.	3. Avoid multiple injections of antidote. Irrigate area with single injection as effectively as possible.		
1. Inject 1–4 mL through existing IV line cannula.	1. Enhances absorption and dispersion of the extravasated drug.	35 36	11 37
2. Administer 1 mL for each mL extravasated.	2. Warm compresses increase systemic absorption of the drug.		38 39
3. Inject SQ if needle removed.			
1. Inject 1–4 mL (1/6 molar) though existing IV line cannula.	1. Inactivates Cisplatin on contact.	40	42
2. Administer 1 mL for each mL extravasated.	2. Treatment not recommended unless a large amount of a highly concentrated solution is extravasated.	41	39
3. Inject SQ if needle removed.			

TABLE 24-14
Rationale for Use of Heat and Cooling for Extravasations

I. Heat
   A. The desired effect is to:
      1. Increase blood supply and increase the dispersion of the enzyme hyaluronidase (Wydase) into the subcutaneous tissues.
      2. Promote healing after the first 24 hr by increasing blood supply.
      3. Enhance the absorption of the vesicant agent (theoretic effect of vasodilation).
   B. Opponents of the use of heat feel that vesicant agents injure the cells' metabolic mechanisms. Heat increases metabolic demands and therefore may decrease cellular destruction.*

II. Cooling
   A. The desired effect is to:
      1. Decrease the blood supply and decrease the absorption of drugs into the subcutaneous tissues.
      2. Constrict peripheral veins which decrease blood supply to the area and thereby minimize localized pain.
      3. Decrease the absorption and diffusion of the vesicant agent, thereby resulting in local tissue "pooling" (theoretic effect of vasoconstriction).
   B. Proponents of the use of a cooling maneuver feel that it decreases many enzymatic reactions and decreases the destructive effect of released white cell components (*eg*, lysozymes). Cooling also slows cellular metabolic rates and may improve survival of marginally injured tissues.*

(*Personal communication*: V. Hentz, M.D., Plastic Surgery, Stanford University Medical Center, Stanford, California. In S. A. Miller [1980]. *Oncology Nursing Forum*, 7[4], pp. 8–16. Reprinted with permission.)

deep subcutaneous tissues. If small-gauge needles are used and if a large amount of subcutaneous fat is present, this infiltration could remain unnoticed for some time. This reemphasizes the need to initially assess the venipuncture site and immediate surrounding skin for comparison. Some nurses outline the suspected area of infiltration with a pen and watch for the outlined area to change in dimension while infusing normal saline.

5. *The nurse should be available to monitor the flow rate and check the blood flow frequently.*[†] When administering drugs by IV push,[†] the nurse should pull back on the plunger of the syringe approximately every 3 to 4 mL to note blood backflow. Although a good blood return does not guarantee that extravasation has not occurred, any change in blood backflow should be investigated. Repositioning of the needle may be necessary if the bevel is against the wall of the vein. Infiltration is the most frequently seen complication in IV therapy. Thus frequent observation (every 2–3 minutes), especially when vesicant agents are being infused, is necessary. Nurses who work on inpatient units, with additional patients to care for, frequently are not permitted the time to return to a patient's room every 2 to 3 minutes to monitor chemotherapy infusions. For that reason, many facilities have written policies that infused vesicant agents are not permitted unless the nurse is in constant attendance and are never to be infused using a mechanical infusion system.[23]

6. *A replacement nurse should have a thorough orientation.* Patients appreciate the security of knowing that a replacement nurse is qualified to assume their care

† Push refers to an injection directly into the vein through the tubing of a needle.

when their regular nurse leaves. Introducing the patient to a replacement nurse is a courtesy often forgotten but greatly appreciated by the patient. The replacement nurse should take the time to examine the IV site, check for vein patency, and review the chemotherapy drugs and rate of infusion. Both nurses should feel comfortable with the transition, and it should be accomplished in an unhurried atmosphere. The replacement nurse does not have a baseline pretreatment reference point for comparison and, if the IV site has not been examined closely with the nurse who initiated the procedure, uncertainties can later occur.

7. *A patient should not be permitted to leave the treatment area when vesicant agents are being infused.* Hospitalized patients frequently have diagnostic studies and therapies scheduled when chemotherapy is being administered. When patients are gone from the unit for extended periods and when physical maneuvering is expected, the possibility for needle dislodgement exists. In general, the larger the volume of drug extravasated, the greater the degree of tissue necrosis. Knowing this, the nurse should be cautioned against sending the patient away from his or her close supervision. If it is absolutely essential that the patient leave the treatment area, the cytotoxic agents should either be temporarily discontinued and normal saline substituted pending the patient's return, or the nurse should accompany the patient to supervise the drug infusion.

    The last general precaution should be kept foremost in the therapist's mind.

8. *If there is ever any doubt that the cytotoxic agent may not be infusing properly, it should be discontinued and a new site established.* This may seem difficult to defend in patients with a scarcity of veins for whom venipuncture is difficult and painful. However, when vesicant agents are being administered, there should be no hesitancy in restarting the IV if doubt exists to the vein's patency.

Treatment

It was mentioned previously that many early infiltrations are difficult to detect. A point bearing reemphasis is that if extravasation is *suspected* when vesicants are being administered, it should be treated as a *presumed* extravasation. General guidelines to follow when vesicants have extravasated are outlined in Tables 24-14 and 24-15. Recommended antidotes are found in Table 24-13.[23] At this time, clinicians are not in agreement as to the best method of managing suspected infiltrations.

Documentation

The nurse should be informed that for medicolegal purposes and to facilitate memory recall, documentation should be completed as soon after the extravasation as possible. Potential litigation often does not reach the courts until several years after the incident. Although the therapist is permitted to review the medical documents, the situation will more readily be recalled if charting is complete and recorded in detail at the time of the incident. Documentation should include:

1. Facility's nurses' notes to include:
   a. Date
   b. Time
   c. Type of venous access (needle type and size)
   d. Insertion site
   e. Number of venipuncture attempts and location

TABLE 24-15
Suggested Guidelines for the Treatment of Extravasation Associated with Vesicant Agents

Procedure	Rationale
1. Stop the infusion.	1. To prevent further drug leakage into the subcutaneous tissues.
2. Aspirate back remaining drug in the needle and tubing by drawing back on the syringe.	2. To remove any residual drug.
3. Superimpose normal saline.	3. To dilute the extravasated agent.
4. Administer by IV push suggested antidotes (physician's order needed). (See Table 24-13.)	4. To intentionally extravasate the antidote via the same route as the extravasated drug.
5. Remove the needle.	5. To facilitate step 6. The site can no longer be used as an IV route.
6. Administer suggested antidotes (see Table 24-13) SQ with multiple punctures into the suspected extravasation site.	6. Direct infiltration of the antidote into area of greatest concentration.
7. Elevate extremity.	7. To minimize swelling.
8. Apply heat or cooling pack.	8. See Table 24-14.
9. Apply topical antidotes.	9. To minimize surface (skin) inflammatory and erythematous reactions.
10. Obtain a plastic surgery consult.	10. Early plastic surgery intervention with wound débridement is mentioned by several authors when doxorubicin HCl has extravasated. When doxorubicin was initially introduced clinically, the necrotic ulcers from extravasation were followed without débridement. The ulcers showed no tendency to heal spontaneously. It is believed that doxorubicin attaches to the DNA molecule and causes cell death. It is thought that the drug is then released to attach to adjacent living cells with further cellular destruction. Early excision is advised to stop this progression.
11. Document in writing in official patient record.	11. To enhance later recall and for medicolegal purposes.
12. Call the patient.	12. To follow symptomatology and ensure that appropriate interventions are initiated.

SQ, subcutaneous.

  f. Drug(s)
  g. Drug sequence
  h. Drug administration techniques
  i. Approximate amount of drug extravasated or suspected of extravasating
  j. Patient complaints and statement
  k. Nursing management of extravasation
  l. Photo documentation (as per institution policy)

STANFORD UNIVERSITY HOSPITAL and CLINICS
Stanford Medical Center
Stanford, California 94305

CHEMOTHERAPY DRUG EXTRAVASATION RECORD

______ Diagnosis ______ Drug and/or Drug Regimen

Home Phone No. ______

DATE: ______

Route of Administration
____I.V. Push
____Piggyback
____In Dilution amt. & sol.
____I.M. (location)
____Sub. Q. (location)
____Flush only
____Other

Needle Size
____Scalp Vein Butterfly
____#25
____#23
____#21
____#19
____Other

Condition of Veins
____Soft, Pliable
____Fragile, thin-walled
____Thready
____Hard, Knotty
____Other (Specify)

Injection Site

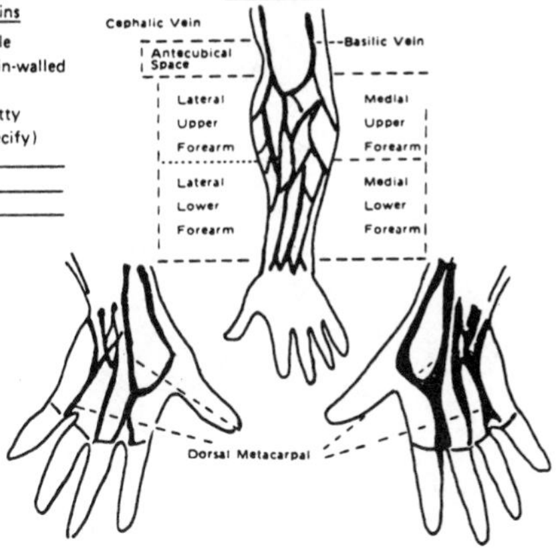

Sequence of Drugs
1st drug ______
Amt/Name/Method of Flus

Approx. amt. Infiltrate

Concentration:

Doctor Notified:
____Time of extravasation.
____Time M.D. called
____Time Responded

Appearance of Infiltration Site:
Describe:

Agents and Amt. Used
____SoluCortef 25 mg. (I.V. Push)
____Xylocaine 1% (I.V. Push)
____Wydase (S.Q.)
____Decadron LA
____Na Bicarb. (I.V. Push)
____Na Bicarb. (S.Q.)
____Na Thiosulfate (I.V. push/S.Q.)
____Other

Color and Dimension of Infiltration Site:
Describe:

Nursing Assessment/Patient Comments:

Plan and Follow-up (Use reverse side if necessary):

Signature and Date

FIGURE 24-13 Extravasation record used at Stanford University Hospital and Clinic. (From Miller, S. A. [1980]. *Oncology Nursing Forum, 7*[4], pp. 8–16. Used with permission.)

m. Appearance of site
n. Physician notification
o. Plastic surgery consultation/notification, if indicated
p. Follow-up instruction given to patient
q. Date of return visit
r. Nurse's signature[23]

2. Extravasation record (Figure 24-13)
3. Incident report

Successful administration of cancer chemotherapy is a multidimensional combination of skill and science, of clinician competence and professional discernment, of a fully prepared and participatory patient and a talented and sensitive clinician—with the willingness to learn all that one can learn to facilitate and deliver optimal care to the person sustaining the cancer experience, while realizing that this experience is a personal and individual one, always.

REFERENCES

1. Bender, C. M. (1987). Chemotherapy. In C. R. Ziegfeld (Ed.). *Core curriculum for oncology nursing* (pp. 225–235). Philadelphia: W. B. Saunders.
2. Bingham, E. (1985). Hazards to health workers from antineoplastic drugs. *New England Journal of Medicine, 313,* 1220–1221.
3. Brown, J. K., & Hogan, C. M. (1990). Chemotherapy. In S. L. Groenwald, M. H. Frogge, M. S. Goodman, & C. H. Yarbro (Eds.). *Cancer nursing: Principles and practice* (2nd ed., pp. 230–273). Boston: Jones & Bartlett.
4. Crudi, C., & Larkin, M. (1984). *Core curriculum for intravenous nursing.* Philadelphia: J. B. Lippincott.
5. DeVita, V. T., Hellman, S., & Rosenberg, S. A. (Eds.). (1989). *Cancer: Principles and practice of oncology* (3rd ed.). Philadelphia: J. B. Lippincott.
6. Dorr, R. T. (1980). *Cancer chemotherapy handbook.* New York: Elsevier.
7. Fischer, D. S., & Knobf, M. T. (1989). *The cancer chemotherapy handbook* (3rd ed.). Chicago: Year Book Medical Publishers.
8. Goodman, M. S., & Wickham, R. (1984). Venous access devices: An overview. *Oncology Nursing Forum, 11*(5), 16–23.
9. Goodman, M. S. (1986). *Cancer: Chemotherapy and care.* Evansville, IN: Bristol Laboratories.
10. Goodman, M. S. (1991). Delivery of cancer chemotherapy. In S. B. Baird (Ed.). *Cancer nursing: A comprehensive textbook* (pp. 291–320). Philadelphia: W. B. Saunders.
11. Guy, J. L. (1991). Medical oncology—the agents. In S. B. Baird (Ed.). *Cancer nursing: A comprehensive textbook* (pp. 266–290). Philadelphia: W. B. Saunders.
12. Holleb, A. I. (1991). *American Cancer Society textbook of clinical oncology.* Atlanta: American Cancer Society.
13. Hubbard, S. M., Seipp, C. A., & Duffy, P. L. (1989). Administration of cancer treatments: Practical guide for physicians and oncology nurses. In V. T. DeVita, S. Hellman, & S. A. Rosenberg (Eds.). *Cancer: Principles and practice of oncology* (3rd ed., pp. 2369–2402). Philadelphia: J. B. Lippincott.
14. *Revised intravenous nursing standards of practice.* (1990). Journal of Intravenous Nursing. (Suppl.).
15. Johnson, B. L., & Gross, J. (Eds.). (1985). *Handbook of oncology nursing.* New York: John Wiley & Sons.
16. Lokich, J. J. (1987). *Cancer chemotherapy by infusion.* Chicago: Precept Press.
17. Miller, S. A. (1980). Legal implications for the nurse involved in cancer chemotherapy administration. In R. T. Dorr & W. L. Fritz (Eds.). *Cancer chemotherapy handbook* (pp. 743–754). New York: Elsevier.
18. National Cancer Institute. (1990). *Chemotherapy and you—A guide to self-help during treatment.* Bethesda, MD: U.S. Department of Health and Human Services.
19. Oncology Nursing Society & American Nurses Association. (1987). *Standards of oncology nursing practice.* Kansas City: American Nurses Association.
20. Oncology Nursing Society. (1988). *Cancer chemotherapy guidelines: Modules I–IV.* Pittsburgh:
21. Oncology Nursing Society. (1989). *Safe handling of cytotoxic drugs: Independent study module.* Pittsburgh:
22. Oncology Nursing Society. (1989, I & II). (1990, III). *Access device guidelines, recommendations for nursing education and practice. Module I, catheters; Module II, implanted ports and reservoirs; Module III, pumps (infusion systems).* Pittsburgh:
23. Oncology Nursing Society. (1992). *Cancer chemotherapy guidelines: Module V, recommendations for the management of vesicant extravasation, hypersensitivity and anaphylaxis.* Pittsburgh:
24. Padilla, G. V., & Bulcavage, L. M. (1991). Theories used in patient/health education. *Seminars in Oncology Nursing, 7*(2), 87–96.
25. Petersen, J. (1991). Chemotherapy. In S. B. Baird (Ed.). *A cancer sourcebook for nurses* (6th ed., pp. 73–83). Atlanta: American Cancer Society.
26. Somerville, E. T. (1991). Knowledge deficit related to chemotherapy. In J. C. McNally, E. T. Somerville, C. Miaskowski, & M. Rostad (Eds.). *Guidelines for oncology nursing practice* (2nd ed., pp. 57–61). Philadelphia: W. B. Saunders.
27. Suddarth, D. S. (Ed.). (1991). *Lippincott manual of nursing practice.* Philadelphia: J. B. Lippincott.
28. Tennenbaum, L. (1989). *Cancer chemotherapy: A reference guide.* Philadelphia: W. B. Saunders.
29. U.S. Department of Labor, Office of Occupational Medicine, Occupational Safety and Health Administration. (1986). *Work practice guidelines for personnel dealing with cytotoxic (antineoplastic) drugs.* (Publ. No. 8.1.1). Washington, DC:
30. Villejo, L., & Meyers, C. (1991). Brain function, learning styles, and cancer patient education. *Seminars in Oncology Nursing, 7*(2), 97–104.
31. Vogelzang, N. (1979). Adriamycin flare: A skin reaction resembling extravasation. *Cancer Treatment Reports, 63,* 2067–2069.
32. Welch-McCaffery, D. (1985). Rationale, development and evaluation of a chemotherapy certification course for nurses. *Cancer Nursing, 8,* 255–262.
33. Ziegfeld, C. R. (Ed.). (1987). *Core curriculum for oncology nursing.* Philadelphia: W. B. Saunders.

REVIEW QUESTIONS

1. Which of the following is NOT a goal of cancer chemotherapy?
   a. cure
   b. control
   c. palliation
   d. surgery

2. Which of the following actions may prevent anaphylactic reactions during administration of antineoplastic agents?
   a. obtain an allergy history
   b. have an emergency cart available
   c. obtain and record baseline vital signs
   d. establish baseline mentation assessment

3. Which of the following statements concerning extravasation is true?
   a. may occur in presence of a blood return
   b. never occurs in presence of blood return
   c. may be prevented by using central veins
   d. never occurs with peripherally inserted central catheters

4. If a second venipuncture site is needed and the patient's other arm may not be used, the second site should be located:
   a. distal to the original
   b. proximal to the original
   c. in the lower extremity
   d. in a central line

5. All of the following drugs are established vesicants EXCEPT:
   a. dactinomycin
   b. daunorubicin hydrochloride
   c. doxorubicin
   d. dacarbazine

6. All of the following elements of documentation of extravasation are essential EXCEPT:
   a. number of attempts at venipuncture
   b. date and time of treatment
   c. antineoplastic agents and their sequence
   d. approximate quantity of drug extravasated (or suspected of extravasation)

7. Knowledge of which of the following areas is essential to effectively administer antineoplastic therapy?
   a. clinical pharmacology
   b. safe drug calculations
   c. proper disposal
   d. preparation and handling

8. Which of the following is NOT a barrier to a patient's thorough understanding of cancer treatment with antineoplastic therapy?
   a. anxiety
   b. compromised literacy
   c. denial
   d. familiar environment

9. Which of the following precautions should NOT be taken when preparing and handling IV antineoplastic agents?
   a. wear protective equipment, consistent with OSHA guidelines
   b. prepare drug in class II biologic safety cabinet
   c. label all syringes and containers
   d. clip all needles carefully

10. All of the following factors should be considered before establishing a venipuncture site on a patient receiving antineoplastic agents EXCEPT:
    a. avoid areas of impaired lymphatic drainage
    b. drug sequencing
    c. baseline reference points of vital signs and mental status is required
    d. patient education

PART VI

Special Applications of Intravenous Therapy

CHAPTER 25

Pediatric Intravenous Therapy

This chapter focuses on features of IV therapy unique in dealing with pediatric patients. A major subdivision between neonatal and general pediatrics is outlined because these two groups have vastly different IV requirements. In this chapter, patient monitoring, including equipment, procedures, and techniques will be discussed for each type of IV therapy. Nursing responsibilities for each therapy will also be highlighted.

PRELIMINARY CONSIDERATIONS

How do the needs of a pediatric patient differ from those of an adult? Body circumference of the adult alters relatively little from the onset of adulthood through the remainder of life, whereas body circumference of a child must accommodate more than a threefold increase in length and approximately a 20-fold increase in weight between birth and adolescence.[2] Thus, the stress levels and basal metabolic rates of a child are exceedingly higher than those for an adult. A more subtle area of concern is the child's developmental needs, which require patience, education, and understanding from the IV nurse. A full comprehension of the child's developmental stage according to age enables the health care team to provide appropriate, nonthreatening care. Furthermore, understanding the child's developmental stage enhances the ability of the staff to recognize that needs of children vary markedly, not only by stress levels but by growth and developmental levels.

Some common reasons for IV therapy in the pediatric patient include:

1. *Maintenance of fluid and electrolyte balance.* The younger the child the greater the risk not only of fluid and electrolyte imbalance, but also of fluid overload and congestive heart failure. Rehydration of a child with diarrhea may seem routine, but complexities can arise even in a child who requires fluid for rehydration when experiencing respiratory distress, altered electrolyte balance, or other complications. In this situation, manipulations according to actual fluid restriction are made.

2. *Antibiotic therapy.* The most common pediatric disease requiring antibiotic therapy is sepsis. Even before a child who displays the symptoms of sepsis (*ie,* increased heart rate, irritability, temperature spikes) is actually diagnosed, prophylactic IV antibiotics are routinely administered while a complete sepsis work-up is in progress (*eg,* urine cultures, throat cultures, blood cultures, wound

Sharon M. Weinstein: PLUMER'S PRINCIPLES & PRACTICE OF INTRAVENOUS THERAPY, FIFTH EDITION, © 1993 J. B. Lippincott Company

cultures, and so forth). If the sepsis work-up reveals a positive blood culture, the IV antibiotics are continued for a complete 10-day course of therapy. If the sepsis work-up is negative, the prophylactic IV antibiotics are discontinued. Antibiotic therapy is also used for treatment of cystic fibrosis, meningitis, osteomyelitis, and many other indications.

3. *Medication therapy.* In addition to antibiotics, many medications used in adults are also used in children. These include drugs such as aminophylline; insulin; cimetidine (Tagamet); ranitidine (Zantac); electrolytes; anticonvulsants and sedatives; vasoactive drugs such as dopamine (Intropin), isoproterenol (Isuprel), and nitroprusside (Nipride); immunosuppressant agents such as cyclosporine (Sandimmune); and a host of other IV medications. In many cases, drugs have not yet been approved for pediatric IV administration, but are used based on ongoing and published research studies, experience in adults, and the emergency status of the child. For this reason, children are often referred to as "therapeutic orphans," indicating a lack of information regarding interaction between a medication and the body processes of the child.[4] Emergency medications and fluids for respiratory and cardiac arrest may be administered by the intraosseous (IO) route (discussed later in this chapter) versus the IV route if IV access cannot be obtained.

4. *Anticancer drugs.* Most chemotherapy or anticancer drugs required for treating childhood cancers use the IV route because of efficacious absorption. There are many more IV protocols designed for the child with cancer compared to the adult, primarily because most childhood cancers are unique to children (*eg,* Wilms' tumor, neuroblastoma, and retinoblastoma). Precision in regulating the specific IV chemotherapy along with monitoring IV clearance is crucial in this group because of the incremental risk of fluid overload, electrolyte imbalances, and chemotherapy side effects.

5. *Nutritional support.* Administration of IV nutrition begins by peripheral or central line. These nutrients provide calories essential to meet the demands of the growing child. A section on this important form of IV therapy follows later in this chapter.

6. *Transfusion therapy.* Blood components most often used in children include packed red blood cells, platelets, and fresh frozen plasma. These products are administered in milliliters per kilogram; dosages are based on the volume limits of the child and the desired therapeutic outcome. In addition, components derived from a unit of plasma may be administered to children with special needs, as in the use of cryoprecipitate for treatment of hemophilia A and coagulation factor concentrates for treatment of factor deficiencies. Gamma globulin therapy expanded because of the availability of IV IgG versus intramuscular gamma globulin. This product is approved for treatment of immunodeficiencies and idiopathic thrombocytopenic purpura (ITP) and is being studied as a means of heightening the immune response in many other adult and pediatric disorders, such as acquired immunodeficiency syndrome (AIDS), neonatal sepsis, and cystic fibrosis.[15] A procedure unique to the neonatal population is exchange transfusion, where blood volume is gradually removed and replaced to correct such conditions as hemolytic disease of the newborn (HDN). Although transfusion

therapy is covered fully in Chapter 21, an overview of the therapeutics unique to pediatric patients will be discussed in this chapter.

Two of the main considerations in administration of IV therapy to children are emotional preparation of the child and initiation of IV access. The next several sections will look at these topics in detail, including special nursing considerations for treating pediatric patients. Specific IV therapeutic modalities will be described, following emotional considerations and peripheral and central IV access.

EMOTIONAL CONSIDERATIONS

What other considerations are essential to maintain the highest caliber of care in children? Even though children of varied ages and intellectual capacities all receive similar IV therapies, pre- and post-IV therapy education must be given, taking these variables into account. A child's capacity for understanding the significance of IV therapy, including the importance of not manipulating the IV site, usually occurs between the ages of 3½ to 5 years, depending on the individual child. Explanations of all procedures must be given to both the child and the parent.

Nursing assessments should include developmental level of the child, influence of the disease process and IV therapy on the child's psyche and body image, previous experience with venipuncture, and desire of parents or parental figures to be present during IV initiation. The presence of parents during a painful or invasive procedure is controversial and needs to be evaluated on a case-by-case basis. Parents may provide emotional support and represent security during an actual procedure, but should not be used to restrain a child, unless no other assistance is available (*ie*, home care). If a parent chooses to not accompany a child into the treatment room for the IV insertion, this decision should be honored by the IV nurse and parents should not be made to feel guilty; provision of comfort and praise after an IV insert provides an ideal means of parental involvement after the procedure is completed.

Establishing Trust

To gain insight into the problems of establishing trust, the practitioner should recognize the child's viewpoint. A thought-provoking question for practitioners is, "How can I expect the child to totally trust me when I am about to hurt him or her by performing a venipuncture?" Usually it is best to tell the child that the venipuncture will hurt but only for a short time. Define the term *time* not by minutes—young children will not understand this—but by comparison to other procedures, for example, "The actual IV puncture takes about the same time as it takes me to take your temperature, get you a glass of orange juice, or for you to finish your dinner." Inform the child that even though this therapy may be painful initially, it should make him or her feel better like before the illness. *Always be honest* with a child.

Specifically, do not promise a certain number of IV attempts or "only one stick," because a child will lose trust if several attempts are necessary. Give the child the opportunity to cry, providing as much privacy as possible. If old enough, let the child participate in the therapy; a child's ability to rip tape, open alcohol swabs, and hold tubing may provide tasks and distraction, particularly in the school-age group. Fear of needles may be assuaged by telling a child that once the IV is in place, the needle is no longer there, and only a small "straw" is in the vein. This theory can be reinforced during play therapy.

Play Therapy

Play therapy, consisting of practicing IV therapy on a doll, is an ideal teaching strategy that allows emotional preparation through acting out. It may not, however, always be practical because of the urgency of IV therapy or the availability of dolls. When it is pragmatic, nurses certainly can participate in this form of play therapy for teaching purposes, or they may seek such assistance from the child-life workers.

Use of Restraints

In younger children, especially those in the toddler group, great care must be taken to protect the IV site. In general, restraints are seldom used at children's medical centers because it is not only very confining but also creates a sense of frustration and mistrust in the child. Only on a rare occasion, with an extremely uncooperative child or a child who may injure himself or remove the IV, may restraints be used.

An armboard usually serves as an adequate restraint (Figure 25-1) and can be taped to the treatment table to provide passive restraint during IV insertion.

Establishing Rapport

Another important aspect of IV therapy is establishing rapport with the family and child through good communication. Communication differs with all age groups according to the child's intellectual level. Adolescents, in particular, require a great deal of individual attention and allowance for their independent nature versus their dependent situation. Adolescents feel grown up and desire the opportunity to assess their disease status; they deserve the opportunity to participate in the decision-making aspect of their care. Adolescents are easily hurt when criticized. They feel that they are grown up but lack the

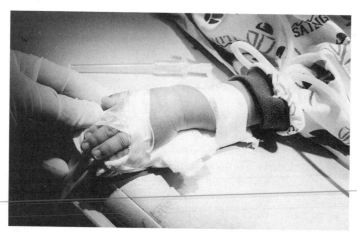

FIGURE 25-1   An armboard is used to support the area of the IV site and provide light restraint during IV insertion.

experience and knowledge of the adult. Therefore, educational techniques practiced with adolescents should encompass a commonsense approach, permitting each adolescent an opportunity to deal with IV therapy to the best of his or her ability. Overexpectation and performance pressure from the IV practitioner can result in emotional conflicts and depression in this age group.

PREPARATION FOR VENIPUNCTURE

From infancy to adolescence, children go through different developmental stages, and pre- and post-IV care should be geared toward these stages, including preparation for the procedure, IV site protection, and mobility and safety needs. Infants are provided with comfort, such as a pacifier during IV insert, and observed for aspiration if feeding occurred just before the procedure. Toddlers and preschool-age children are prepared immediately before the IV start in simple, positive terms, such as "We are going to start the IV now." School-age children can be prepared slightly in advance, afforded with privacy and small tasks, and allowed to cry, but hold still. Adolescents can be prepared well in advance and encouraged to make decisions regarding their care, such as having an IV restarted later in the day so they can go out on pass from the hospital for several hours, and participating in self-care, such as monitoring for IV site complications, maintaining intake and output with supervision, even setting up home total parenteral nutrition (TPN), or accessing an implanted port. The teenage population may test caregivers and express the need for independence by not always being compliant with therapy, so monitoring and encouragement are still needed, and planning a schedule with the teenager may be beneficial.

Care must be taken to assess each child individually, not just according to age or physiologic development. In some cases, children have disease processes that cause reduction in growth, such as in children with renal disease. Psychological age and ability must be considered when looking at the emotional needs of a child.

PERIPHERAL AND CENTRAL INTRAVENOUS ACCESS

Let us now analyze sites appropriate for IV therapy, from peripheral to central locations. Depending on the child's age, a site for administering IV drugs is typically more difficult to find than in an adult. Both hydration status and previous IV therapy may be used as predictors of difficulties in obtaining an intact venous access. In the child, the site selected for IV therapy should involve minimal risk and allow maximum efficiency and safety.[9]

When selecting the optimal site for IV therapy, certain basic strategies should be followed. An excellent site in the neonate and infant is the head because the scalp has an abundant supply of superficial veins (Figure 25-2). The bilateral superficial temporal veins just in front of the pinna of the ear or the metopic vein, which runs down the middle of the forehead, are generally easy to find and involve minimal patient risk.

Scalp veins are readily available until about 12 to 18 months of age, when hair follicles mature and superficial layers of skin thicken, making venous access difficult. When inserting an IV in the scalp, one must be aware of artery location, because it is difficult to distinguish veins from arteries in this area. Inadvertent arterial puncture reveals bright red blood, pulsation, and blanching of skin caused by arteriospasm when the IV device is flushed.[14] The IV device should be removed and pressure held on the site

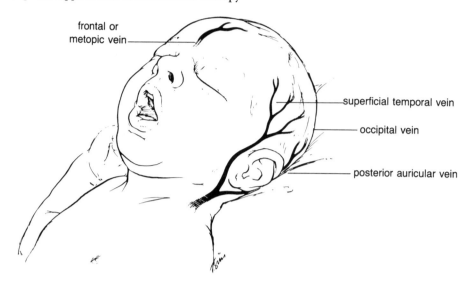

frontal or metopic vein

superficial temporal vein

occipital vein

posterior auricular vein

FIGURE 25-2 Sites for scalp vein infusions.

until bleeding stops. Use of an "arterial" IV could result in damage to the artery and the area to which oxygenated blood is delivered. The scalp as an IV site can also be distressing to parents, who may believe that the IV is in the brain. If the head must be shaved, shave or clip the smallest area possible, saving this hair for the parents as the child's first haircut, thus alleviating some distress at the use of this site.[14] Scalp IVs can restrict mobility and be easily dislodged; with the advent of small IV catheters for peripheral access, scalp veins are no longer the first choice for IV access in babies.

Other favorable peripheral IV sites include the hand, forearm, upper arm, foot, and antecubital fossa, moving from distal to proximal locations. Some unusual sites such as axilla, abdomen, and popliteal area have also been used when chronically ill infants and children exhibit greatly diminished peripheral venous access from long use (Table 25-1). Foot veins are used up to walking age and occasionally in older children where other usual sites are not available, such as in burn or multiple trauma patients. Depending on the regulations of the State Board of Nursing and institutional policy, external jugular and femoral veins are used for IV access and obtaining blood samples, although these last two sites are usually reserved for IV access by a physician or surgeon.

Peripheral Intravenous Devices

Before and during the 1970s, the device of choice for pediatric IV access was the winged infusion needle. This device was used for short-term IV therapy and withdrawal of blood samples for laboratory analysis. In the late 1970s, 22-gauge catheter-over-needle devices made of plastic, then Teflon, became available and could be used for longer lasting IV access in pediatric patients.[2] Winged infusion needles are still used for blood sampling in many pediatric institutions because the vacuum withdrawal method of blood sampling used in adults is often too aggressive for tiny pediatric veins.

Catheter-over-needle device design has advanced to include thin-wall cannulas

TABLE 25-1
Peripheral Intravenous Access Sites for Pediatric Patients*

Preferred Sites	Veins
Hand	Digital, metacarpal
Forearm	Supplementary cephalic, basilic, median antebrachial
Antecubital fossa	Median basilic, median cephalic, median cubital
Upper (arm (below axilla)	Basilic, cephalic
Foot (before walking age)	Greater saphenous, lesser saphenous
Scalp (before 18 mo)	Occipital, metopic, temporal
Lower leg (before walking age)	Greater saphenous, lesser saphenous

Secondary Sites†	Veins
Wrist	Superficial veins: infiltration in this area may result in pressure on the radial nerve
Abdomen	Superficial veins: rarely used, usually limited to neonates and chronically hospitalized patients; infiltration may result in damage to abdominal wall
Axilla	Axillary vein: usually limited to neonates; infiltration may cause pressure on structures in chest cavity
Knee	Popliteal vein: usually limited to neonates due to decreased mobility

*Sites listed in order of preference; consider individual characteristics

†Secondary sites should be considered only when preferred sites are not available.

(Figure 25-3) for greater flow rates, smaller gauge size (24 and 26), shorter length, nonkinking material, and devices made of Aquavene™, an elastomeric hydrogel that expands in gauge and length after 30 minutes in the vein, allowing a smaller catheter to be inserted and a longer dwell time than traditional catheters.[44] Small-gauge catheters such as the 26 and 24 for neonates and the 24 and 22 for children and adolescents are the choice when up to 2 weeks of IV therapy is prescribed. After this time, peripheral access sites diminish and use of a longer lasting or central device may be warranted.

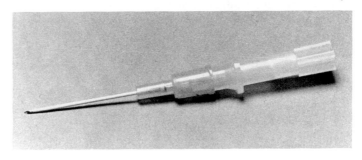

FIGURE 25-3 Small gauge thin-walled Teflon peripheral IV catheter, suitable for use with children. (Courtesy: Critikon, Inc., Tampa, FL)

INTRAVENOUS INSERTION TECHNIQUES

General IV insertion techniques will not be discussed in this chapter; however, some special techniques for achieving venous access in children will be highlighted.

To dilate veins in children, a smaller tourniquet may be necessary, and in neonates, a rubber band with a tape tab provides an easily removable tourniquet for scalp IVs (Figure 25-4).[14] In some cases, no tourniquet is used. Additional aids to vein location and dilatation may include warm soaks or transillumination.[36] Insertion of IVs in children requires stabilization of the extremity before venipuncture, so that movement of the child does not dislodge the newly inserted device and require subsequent sticks. A firm but gentle insertion technique is necessary for a successful venipuncture in a child because blood return in the flashback chamber may not appear as readily and the characteristic "pop" of entering a vein may not be felt. Choose the nondominant extremity first for IV access when possible; in unusual sites such as scalp and abdomen, the rule is to place the IV in the direction of venous flow or toward the heart.

Equipment and supplies are set up before venipuncture, usually in a treatment room if possible, thus preserving the child's room and bed as a "safe" place, where invasive procedures are not performed.[43] In an intensive care environment, supplies may be prepared away from the bedside so as not to cause undue anxiety before the actual venipuncture. In the home, supplies are usually set up in an area where lighting is maximized and a flat surface, such as a kitchen table, can be used as a work area.

Equipment for IV insertion includes the following:[6]

IV tubing with volume control device as warranted by age of child and type of infusion:

Volumetric pump

Microdrop calibrated chamber

Smallest container that will last for 24 hours

Stabilization equipment:

Armboard

Site protector

Short extension tubing with Luer lock connections

Tourniquet or rubber band

Antimicrobial solution for site cleansing

Adhesive tape

Sterile gauze or transparent dressing

Injection cap

1 to 3 mL of flush solution in a syringe

Gauze

Gloves

IV pole (if necessary)

IV device ranging from 25 gauge to 20 gauge depending on size of child and viscosity of infusate

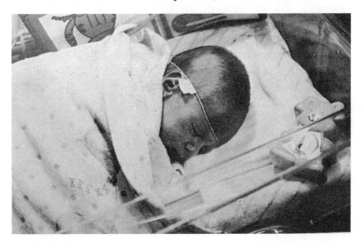

FIGURE 25-4 Rubberband used as a tourniquet on baby's scalp. (Courtesy: A. M. Frey)

The number of attempts at IV access should be no more than two to three, except in extreme emergency. Limiting venipuncture attempts decreases physical and emotional trauma to a child and can preserve venous integrity. Occasionally in children, threading of the IV catheter can be difficult. Threading of the catheter into the vein can be facilitated by making sure the catheter tip has entered the vein lumen after flashback of blood, by advancing the IV device slightly. Other measures include attaching a small connector tubing with flush solution, and flushing gently as the catheter is advanced. Sometimes, just waiting a few seconds until the child has calmed down can decrease incidence of venous spasm and facilitate catheter threading. As with any intricate skill, IV insertion in children requires patience and practice until the learning curve is diminished and skill level increases. Figures 25-5 through 25-8 demonstrate IV insertion in a 5-month-old

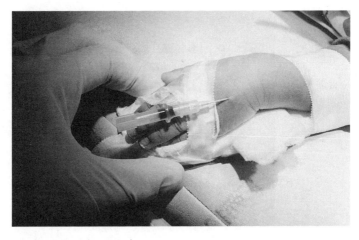

FIGURE 25-5 Blood enters the flashback chamber of the IV catheter, then the 24 gauge catheter is advanced slightly. (Courtesy: A. M. Frey)

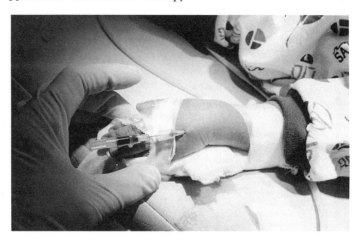

FIGURE 25-6 The catheter is advanced fully, stylet is pulled back, and tourniquet is removed. (Courtesy: A. M. Frey)

baby with meningitis who is receiving IV antibiotics intermittently through a heparin lock.

Once venous access has been obtained, the next strategy involves stabilization of the IV.

Stabilizing the Intravenous Line

Stabilization is essential, primarily in the younger child whose level of comprehension concerning the importance of not manipulating the IV site is minimal. All IVs placed in the head are taped in a U-shaped chevron pattern, and the extension tube is looped into a coil so that if the child pulls on the IV, the tension of the pull will affect the coil, not the IV site. A small, open-ended paper cup is placed on top of the site to act as a protective

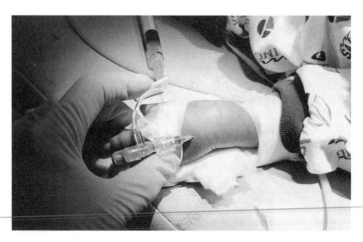

FIGURE 25-7 The stylet is removed and T connector is attached to hub of IV catheter. Catheter is flushed gently to assess patency. (Courtesy: A. M. Frey)

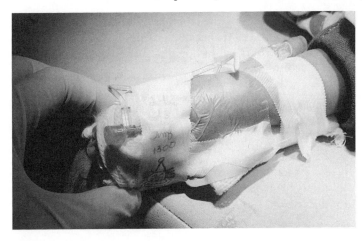

FIGURE 25-8 Clear sterile dressing is applied, the site is labeled, and the injection cap is attached to T connector. Fingertips and IV site remain visible. (Courtesy: A. M. Frey)

covering. Sites requiring stabilization include the hand and the arm, both of which generally require armboard support. The advantage of this type of stabilization is that it restricts the child's range of movement, thereby decreasing the risk of dislodgement of the IV needle. The foot also demands stabilization, primarily to use saphenous vein. Venous accessibility in the foot is not only more difficult, but it results in mobility restriction from the stabilizing legboards that are used to keep young children, especially under age 2, from manipulating the needle (Figure 25-9). An important aspect of IV access in the foot involves maintenance of normal joint configuration by placing padding under the foot, thus maintaining the natural bend at the ankle and avoiding foot drop or contracture injuries. Coverings such as stretch netting may keep little fingers away from the IV site, while providing easy visualization. The top "ribbed" portion of a sweatsock, slipped over

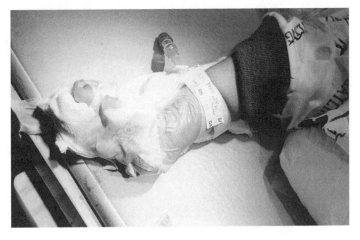

FIGURE 25-9 Foot IV site. Note that joint configuration is maintained and toes and IV site are visible. (Courtesy: A. M. Frey)

the IV, can serve the same function for home IV access. A roller bandage should not be used to cover an IV site because it is time-consuming to unravel and makes site assessments difficult. Surgical cutdown is less popular now that smaller, longer-term IV devices are available.

Surgical Cutdown

If routine vein accessibility is extremely difficult, a surgical cutdown performed by the surgical team may be indicated. The most common cutdown sites are the saphenous vein of the foot and the radial vein in the forearm. Because this procedure requires venous laceration or minor surgery, the site must be cleaned subsequently with antiseptic solution of povidone–iodine and povidone–iodine ointment at least biweekly to prevent local infection.

Emergency Intravenous Access

Obtaining successful IV access is essential to provide efficacious pediatric advanced life support. In many cases, during a "code" situation, peripheral veins have collapsed because of cardiac arrest and poor perfusion. Time for performance of a surgical cutdown can range from 2 to 40 minutes, with a median time of 8 minutes.[27] Intravenous access should be obtained within 5 minutes from the start of a resuscitation effort. After traditional routes have been attempted, often simultaneously, intraosseous (IO) access is a realistic goal. *Intraosseous infusion* is defined as infusion of blood, fluids, or drugs through a rigid needle directly into the bone marrow cavity.[34] From 1922, when first described by Drinker and colleagues,[13] through the 1940s to 1960s, this technique was widely used. As IV device technology improved, facilitating peripheral venous access, IO technique lost popularity. Since 1983, interest in IO therapy has increased because of a letter to the editor of *American Journal of Diseases in Children* that questioned the abandonment of this route.[52]

Intraosseous technique is based on the fact that fluid injected into the medullary cavity of the bone is quickly taken up by the extensive network of venous sinusoids, and drugs given by the IO route and the central venous route are equally effective, working faster than those administered by peripheral IV.[34] The best site for IO infusion in children up to 5 or 6 years old is the anterior medial aspect of the tibia, 1 to 3 cm below the tibial tuberosity, thus avoiding the growth plate at the end of the bone[27,34,40] (Figure 25-10).

Other sites include distal medial tibia, midanterior distal femur, iliac crest, humerus, and sternum in children less than 3 years of age, before which time, the sternum is too thin to support the IO needle.[40] Contraindications to IO access include site infections, fractures, burns, and bone disorders, such as osteogenesis imperfecta (brittle bone disease) and osteopetrosis (marble bone disease), where bones may fracture easily.[34,40]

Intraosseous access is indicated during emergency situations, such as respiratory or cardiac resuscitation efforts, when two attempts at peripheral IV access are unsuccessful.[34] A short rigid needle with a stylet is used to obtain IO access (Figure 25-11); alternately, a lumbar puncture needle may be used for infants although this needle can bend easily and is awkward to insert. Disposable bone marrow aspiration needles are now manufactured for IO access; 16, 18, or 20 is the recommended gauge size because a smaller lumen needle can become blocked with bone fragments or bend on insertion. After antimicrobial cleansing of the desired site, the IO needle is inserted perpendicular to the bone surface at a slight angle away from the epiphyseal plate. A screwing motion is

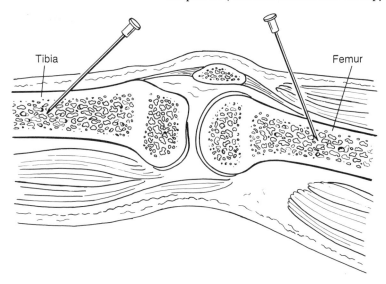

FIGURE 25-10   The anterior medial aspect of the tibia (lateral view) is the best site for intraosseous access in the child under 6 years of age.

used to insert the needle into the bone until decreased resistance is noted and the needle stands without support, usually at a depth of 1 cm in an infant or child. Further advancement may cause penetration of the opposite wall of the bone and result in extravasation of infusates. Some IO needles are now manufactured with a premarked shaft to indicate depth. After insertion, the stylet is removed and bone marrow content, similar to blood, is aspirated; this sample may be used for readings of $PaCO_2$ and pH, important parameters indicating success of resuscitative efforts.[34] A short connector tubing and flush solution, similar to that used with IV catheters, is connected to the hub of the IO needle and a split sterile gauze dressing and tape is placed to secure the site. If the

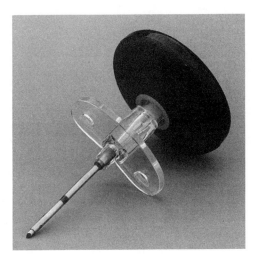

FIGURE 25-11   Intraosseous needle with Diekmann modification (two laterally opposed side ports, positioned near distal tip to ensure flow if tip is obstructed by bone fragment). (Courtesy: Cook Critical Care, Bloomington, IN)

child is awake, intradermal anesthesia before IO needle placement is advised. The site should be observed for infiltration of infusates into surrounding tissues; the same bone should not be used for repeated access if infiltration occurs.

Types of infusions given by the IO route are listed in Table 25-2. Infusates may be administered by gravity, manual pressure, or infusion pump.

Complications are relatively rare. Increased chance of osteomyelitis has been related to long-term use of the IO route, as well as infusion of hypertonic solutions. Other complications can include cellulitis, abscess, or local necrosis; fat embolism, although a possibility, has not been reported in children, probably because of the low fat content of bone marrow in children, especially under the age of 4.[34] Success rates with IO therapy have been reported to be as high as 97%.[46] However, further studies are needed, and replacement of the IO needle with IV access is recommended as soon as conventional IV access is feasible.

TABLE 25-2
Intraosseus Infusions

Fluids	Medications	Blood Products
5%, 10%, and 50% dextrose	Analgesics	Whole blood
Saline	Anesthetics	Packed red blood cells
Lactated Ringer's solution	Anticonvulsants	Plasma
Parenteral nutrition	Antisera	Albumin
	Antibiotics	Dextran
	Catecholamines	
	Miscellaneous Atropine	
	Calcium	
	Digitalis	
	Dopamine	
	Dobutamine	
	Epinephrine	
	Heparin	
	Insulin	
	Lidocaine	
	Levarterenol	
	Phenytoin	
	Sodium bicarbonate	
	Contrast media	

(From Glaesser, P. N., & Losek, J. D. [1986]. Emergency intraosseous infusions in children. *American Journal of Emergency Medicine, 4*, 35; Miccolo, M. A. [1990]. Intraosseous infusion. *Critical Care Nurse, 10*, 35–47; Mofenseon, H. C. [1988]. Guidelines for intraosseous infusions [Letter to the editor]. *Journal of Emergency Medicine, 6*, 145–146; Arbeiter, H. I., & Greengard, J. [1944]. Tibial bone marrow infusions in infancy. *Journal of Pediatrics, 25*, 1.)

Intermediate-Term Midline Intravenous Access

In recent years, use of IV devices that are placed peripherally, but are of longer length, and are left in place for a longer period of time, has become popular. As with most medical equipment, adult-sized versions of these devices are tested initially, and then research in children is commenced. The Standards of Practice of the Intravenous Nurses Society (INS) define central IV devices as those whose proximal tip is located in the subclavian, superior vena cava, or inferior vena cava.[26] Peripheral IV site changes should be done frequently to avoid infectious complications. However, in cases where intermediate-term IV therapy is desired and surgically placed central lines are not indicated, midline-located IV catheters have fulfilled a need. In children, these catheters have proven to be efficacious for treatment of such disorders as cystic fibrosis, osteomyelitis, Lyme disease, Crohn's disease, and a variety of other conditions that require several weeks of IV antibiotic, antifungal, or nutritional therapy, where peripheral IV access with short traditional catheters would be impractical.

A sample of such catheters currently available includes the Landmark™ catheter in 24 and 22 gauge, with a length of 3 to 6 inches. This catheter is made of Aquavene, the same material as the longer dwelling, short peripheral catheter that expands in size and length. The Landmark™ catheter is placed in the veins of the antecubital fossa, above or below the bend of the elbow, and threaded into the upper arm, where larger vein lumen and increased blood flow provide dilution of the infusate.[21] In addition, peripherally inserted central catheters (PICCs) have been inserted so that the tip is purposely placed in a vein in the upper arm.[55] Varying degrees of success have been reported with use of these devices and more research, particularly in the pediatric population, is certainly a mission for the IV nurse. Insertion and care of the Landmark™ catheter is covered in Chapter 12.

Central Intravenous Access

When longer term IV access is desired because of unavailability of peripheral sites or a need for long duration or lifelong therapy is identified, central venous access is indicated. Many types of devices exist for this purpose, including umbilical catheters, PICCs, surgically placed cuffed tunneled catheters, and totally implanted devices. Choice of device depends on the duration and type of therapy prescribed, patient and family input, and disease process. Although these devices are described in detail in earlier chapters, features unique to the pediatric population will be outlined.

Umbilical Catheterization

Most sites for neonatal IV therapy are similar to those for children discussed earlier in this chapter. However, a catheter unique to the neonatal population is the umbilical vessel catheter. Umbilical catheterization is common practice in many neonatal and intensive care units for treatment of acutely ill infants. This mode of therapy provides an easy route for IV administration. There are many undesirable risks such as thrombosis, embolism, vasospasm, vascular perforation, infection, and hemorrhage.[6] To prevent these complications, a specially designed umbilical catheter with the following features should be selected.

1. Flexibility
2. Relatively rigid walls for accurate pressure monitoring

3. A single end-hole to avoid clotting in the tip

4. Smoothness of the tip to prevent perforation of the vessel wall during catheter insertion

5. Radiopaqueness to radiographically visualize the location of the tip of the catheter

6. Small capacity so that only a small amount of blood need be withdrawn to clear the catheter for blood sampling

7. Size from 3.5 to 5 Fr. catheter

Arterial versus Venous Catheterization. Let us now examine the difference between arterial and venous umbilical catheterization. Within minutes of birth, the umbilical arteries normally constrict; delays in the process, however, occur in states of hypoxia and acidosis. The vast majority of infants are catheterized in the first day of life because catheterization is generally not possible past the fourth day of life.

The procedure for umbilical catheterization begins with the surgeon's preparation for asepsis, including handwashing, gloving, masking, and gowning. This step precedes the preparation of the umbilical stump with an iodine solution, followed by cleansing with alcohol, and subsequently draping of the sterile field and exposing the umbilical area. Dissection begins at the umbilical cord around 1.5 cm from the skin until the umbilical vessels are identified. Two thick-walled, pinpoint-sized arteries are easily distinguishable from a large, thin-walled vein. The heparinized catheter is passed through either the umbilical artery or vein, depending on the type of therapy desired.

Arterial catheterization accomplishes five goals: (1) blood sampling, (2) measurements of arterial pressures, (3) parenteral or antibiotic therapy in the vascularly compromised child, (4) exchange transfusions, and (5) arterial pH and blood gases. Venous umbilical catheterization accomplishes four goals, including (1) and (3) above as well as providing a means for a direct measurement of central venous pressure and a route for the infusion of TPN.[30]

Placements differ between the umbilical venous route and the arterial route. Ideally, the tip of the umbilical venous catheter should be positioned in the inferior vena cava near the right atrium in good position for central venous pressure and TPN administration. Comparatively, the umbilical arterial catheter is best positioned above the level of aortic bifurcation in good position for arterial measurements and exchange transfusions.

Once the catheter is placed correctly and position is confirmed radiographically, a suture may be placed superficially through the stump, tying it firmly to the catheter for anchorage.[29] The catheter is generally connected to a three-way stopcock for pressure monitoring, blood drawing, and fluid administration. When fluid administration is not necessary, the line may be heparinized. It is of the utmost importance to maintain patency of the indwelling catheter because blood clots can otherwise form. Flushing with heparin (1 U/mL IV fluid) should be done daily.

Increased thrombosis when administering fluids through an umbilical artery has been reported; therefore this mode of therapy should be used with caution. The nursing assessment for pending complications should include the following:

1. Examine buttocks to detect blanching caused by arterial spasms.

2. Closely monitor the umbilical line with Luer lock attachments to prevent disconnection of the tubing with resultant hemorrhage.

3. Closely monitor peripheral edema, unequal femoral pulses, and respiratory distress, which could indicate emboli formation.

4. Perform daily dressing changes with the application of povidone–iodine ointment to decrease the risk of sepsis.

If complications arise, report them immediately to the appropriate physician so immediate medical attention can be provided. Early intervention can reduce the risk of morbidity and mortality when using the umbilical access for IV therapy.

Because of the risk of complications and the short duration when using the umbilical vessel for IV therapy, many physicians now prefer to use an alternate peripheral site, such as the scalp or hand, or other central venous access.

Nontunneled Central Catheters

Nontunneled catheters include subclavian, jugular, and femoral catheters, as well as PICCs. These catheters are referred to as "nontunneled" to distinguish them from longer-dwelling cuffed Silastic catheters that are surgically tunneled under the skin. Nontunneled subclavian catheters usually have small lumens and a short length and may have from one to four lumens (Figure 25-12). These catheters are made of a stiffer material such as polyvinylchloride for easier insertion the short distance through the skin into the vein. In children, these catheters may be inserted nonsurgically, using a local anesthetic, in such sites as the internal or external jugular vein, the subclavian vein, or the femoral vein. If a child is very apprehensive, anxious, or uncooperative, a sedative such as chloral hydrate may be indicated before the procedure.

Catheter stiffness, high incidence of thrombus, and easy dislodgement limit use of these catheters to a relatively short period of time, ranging from a few days to up to 4 weeks.[53] Catheters may be changed over a wire if lumens become blocked or sepsis is suspected, although benefit of this practice is yet to be definitely proven and it remains controversial. In children, subclavian catheters are often used for IV access in critical situations, such as a multiple trauma patient brought to the emergency room or children in the pediatric intensive care unit, where several weeks of IV access and possible need for

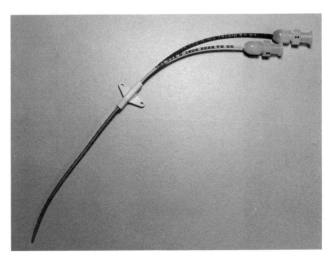

FIGURE 25-12 Subclavian double-lumen catheter. (Courtesy: A. M. Frey)

parenteral nutrition exists. Catheters placed in jugular and femoral locations can be occluded by anatomy, as babies tend to have a shortened neck and frequently adduct their legs, causing kinking in the catheter placed in the neck or groin. Femoral location is also the location of the diaper area and the dressing may become soiled frequently and exposed to infective organisms that are more prevalent in this location. Subclavian catheter insertion in neonates is technically difficult and can result in life-threatening complications such as pneumothorax, hydrothorax, hemothorax, and massive hemorrhage.[12] Fortunately, alternate choices for central venous access are available, and the peripherally inserted central catheter (PICC) is one of these choices for neonates to adults.

The PICCs were fairly common in the adult intensive care unit in the 1960s and have made a comeback in recent years.[53] Newer versions come in tiny sizes (27, 25, and 23 gauge) for neonates and infants to larger sizes (20, 18 and 16 gauge) for older children and adults. Double-lumen PICCs are also available, but large introducer and catheter size negates use of these in young children and those with tiny veins. Peripherally inserted central catheters are associated with fewer complications than surgically placed catheters[8] and insertion can be done without the risks of general anesthesia. Pediatric-sized PICCs are manufactured of Vialon (BD-Deseret) or softer Silastic-type material shown to have low incidence of irritation and thrombus formation, allowing PICCs to remain in place for months to years.[35] These catheters may be inserted in children in the hospital, outpatient, or home setting (Figure 25-13). In neonates, PICCs are inserted into the veins of the antecubital fossa, as well as axillary, saphenous, popliteal, and external jugular veins[8] (Figure 25-14). In older children who have reached walking age, the basilic and cephalic veins in the antecubital fossa, or slightly above or below this site, are ideal. Insertion of PICCs is covered in Chapter 14; the technique is similar in adults and children, although a child may be more anxious and less likely to be cooperative, and may need restraint and use of local anesthetic for easier insertion.

The complication rate with PICCs in children is minimal and includes clotting or occlusion as the most documented complication, particularly in neonates, where small

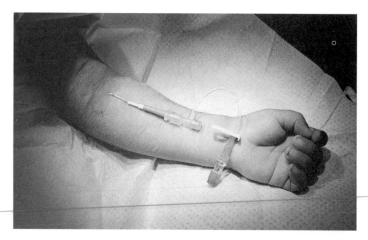

FIGURE 25-13   PICC in place without dressing, in left median cubital vein of a 3-year-old with repeat surgery for Hirshsprung's disease; after surgery, child was NPO on TPN. (Courtesy: A. M. Frey)

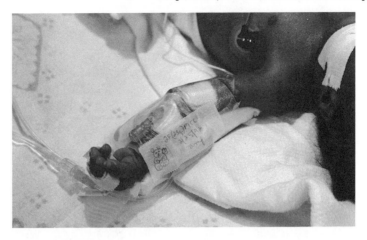

FIGURE 25-14 PICC in place, with dressing on site, in left basilic vein of neonate with hypoplastic ventricle. Patient is receiving prostaglandin infusion via the PICC. (Courtesy: A. M. Frey)

gauge size and low flow rates may lead to catheter blockage. This complication has led several researchers to recommend use of flow rates greater than 2 mL/hr, as well as addition of heparin (1 U/mL) to IV fluids.[8] Other complications include phlebitis, leaking, edema, erythema, and suspected or confirmed sepsis. Sepsis rates range from 0% to 11% in studies of infants.[16] In one study comparing peripherally and surgically placed central catheters in neonates, complication rate and dwell time were the same.[47] In addition to neonates, PICCs are also used for intermediate (2 weeks to several months) IV access in infants through adolescents for treatment of such conditions as cystic fibrosis, Crohn's disease, osteomyelitis, joint infections, brain abscesses, inflammatory bowel disease, pancreatitis, and any other condition requiring intermediate-term antibiotic, antifungal, or parenteral nutrition therapy, as well as therapies required by pediatric oncology patients.

Tunneled Central Venous Catheters
Tunneled catheters are most often chosen for long-term venous access, as are implanted ports, which will be discussed in the next section. In the early 1970s, Broviac developed the first tunneled catheter for patients who required long-term TPN.[5] Broviac catheters (Bard/Davol) have since become frequently used when long-term central IV access is needed, such as with children who have cancer. The Groshong catheter (Bard/Cath Tech), developed in the 1980s, is also tunneled, but is made of more thin-walled silicone than the Broviac.[57] Single- and double-lumen Broviacs and single- and double-lumen Groshongs are used in children; the triple-lumen Broviac tends to be somewhat large for pediatric use. Both catheters contain a Dacron polyester cuff that anchors the catheter in place subcutaneously several weeks after insertion[7] (Figure 25-15). Both catheters have a Luer-locking proximal hub(s) outside the patient; the Broviac has an open distal tip on the internal portion, whereas the distal tip of the Groshong is closed with a two-way slit valve. More detailed descriptions of tunneled catheters are provided in Chapter 15.

If no contraindications to general anesthesia exist, tunneled catheters are often inserted in the operating room. Local anesthesia and possibly a sedative medication may

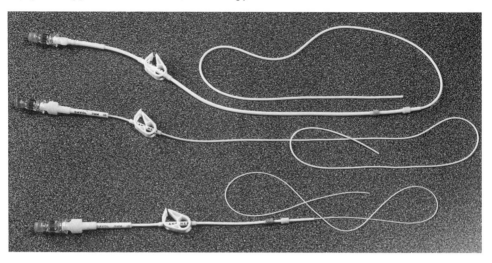

FIGURE 25-15 Neonatal- and pediatric-sized Broviac catheters with and without Dacron cuff and Vita-cuff. (Courtesy: Bard Access Systems, Cranston, RI)

be used in older children for catheter placement in the treatment room or at the bedside. Often, several procedures are coordinated with catheter insertion to avoid unnecessary trauma while the child is awake; for example, a newly diagnosed leukemia patient may have one visit to the operating room for Broviac insertion, bone marrow biopsy, and lumbar puncture.

In the larger child, the catheter is usually inserted percutaneously into the subclavian vein. In infants and neonates, because of the small size of the subclavian vein, this approach can be extremely dangerous. Therefore, in infants and children under age 5, the catheter is usually inserted through the facial vein or the external or internal jugular vein to the superior vena cava (Figure 25-16).

After proper placement is verified by chest x-ray, subcutaneous tunneling of the catheter is done—either up the parietal occipital area or down the chest wall to the fourth or fifth intercostal space, depending on the catheter type. This distal exit site from the original phlebotomy site provides a barrier from infection,[38] facilitates catheter maintenance, and provides the child with full-range neck mobility.

In some children, chest access sites are not available because of many previous central lines and vein thrombosis, or other surgery or complications. An alternate site for catheter placement is the femoral vein to the inferior vena cava, particularly in children under walking age. The proximal portion of the catheter is then tunneled under the skin of the abdomen or out onto the thigh.

Care of tunneled catheters is described in detail in previous chapters, and includes dressing changes, flushing to maintain patency, and prevention of infection and dislodgement. Care of tunneled catheters is continually researched, and procedures for children are based on manufacturers' guidelines, catheter volume, experience with adults, and ongoing and previously published research studies. Dressing materials range from use of no dressing in the well-healed nonimmunocompromised patient, to an adhesive bandage, gauze pad, or transparent dressing. Dressing changes are usually done using clean or sterile technique on a 2- to 3-times weekly schedule. Catheter patency is maintained with

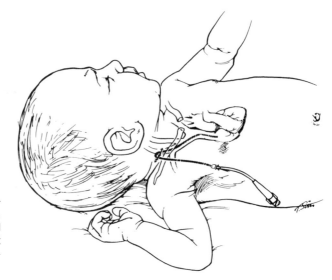

FIGURE 25-16 Example of pediatric infant-sized Broviac catheter. Note that the catheter is threaded into the external jugular to the right atrium and tunneled subcutaneously down the chest wall.

saline or heparinized saline in the strength of 10 to 100 U/mL, given from once or twice daily to once weekly. These protocols vary among institutions and are continuously reviewed based on research studies and the needs of the child.

The complications most frequently reported for tunneled catheters in children include infection, occlusion, and dislodgement, with the toddler age group exhibiting the highest complication level.[25] Broviac infection rates can range from 5% to 31.6% and are usually reported in terms of rate per 1000 catheter days to maintain consistency of data.[11] The most common organisms reported include *Staphylococcus aureus* and *Staphylococcus epidermidis*, as well as some gram-negative organisms, many of which are normal body flora.[10] Because of the high infection rate attributed to tunneled catheters, activities such as swimming and showering, where exposure to organisms can occur, may be prohibited, and alternate activities should be carefully planned for the child with a tunneled catheter in place. Occlusion may be corrected with urokinase (Abbokinase) or hydrochloric acid, depending on the cause of the occlusion.[24] Dislodgement may be avoided by carefully looping the external "tail" of the catheter under the dressing or to the chest; wearing of a T-shirt for all age groups with tunneled catheters is recommended. If breakage occurs, temporary repair may be done with a blunt-tip needle or IV catheter, so sterility and patency can be maintained until a more permanent splicing procedure can be accomplished.[53]

Implanted Ports

Venous access ports are implanted in the chest, upper abdomen, or in the forearm, with the catheter threaded into a central vein. Low profile pediatric ports have been available for several years and are made of stainless steel, titanium, or plastic, or a combination of those materials (Figure 25-17). Ports are a good choice for long-term venous access for the pediatric patient older than 3 years because before that age, lack of subcutaneous tissue may cause the port to erode through the skin. Because the port requires access at least monthly with a needle, this is an important consideration when advising patients and family about venous access devices. A port is ideal for the child who requires

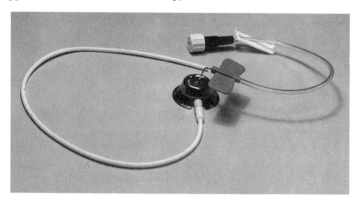

FIGURE 25-17 Low profile pediatric implanted port accessed with 22-gauge, 3/4 inch, 90° angle, noncoring needle. (Courtesy: A. M. Frey)

intermittent therapy, can tolerate the needle access, and does not like the inconvenience of an external catheter, such as oncology, short-bowel, or cystic fibrosis patients.[5]

Ports are accessed from the top or side, depending on the design, with a noncoring needle; a 22-gauge, 1/2-inch needle for a forearm port and a 22-gauge, 3/4- to 1-inch needle for a chest port are usually adequate for the viscosity and flow of pediatric infusions. Needles are changed every 7 to 10 days while the port is being used; dressings over the accessed port can be changed with the needle change or more frequently. When the port is not being used for infusion of medications, parenteral nutrition, transfusion therapy, or blood sample withdrawal, patency is maintained by flushing the port with heparinized saline, usually in the volume of 3 to 5 mL and the strength of 100 U/mL on a monthly basis.[23]

Complications reported with ports are similar to those identified for tunneled catheters, but the reported infection rate is lower (0%–9%) than with externalized catheters.[25] Although risk of port dislodgement is minimal, the noncoring needle may be dislodged and cause infiltration and possible tissue injury if vesicant drugs are being administered. Slight discomfort has been reported with needle access of the port, but this diminishes in time, and a high level of satisfaction has been reported with this device.[45] The port may be accessed by a hospital or home IV nurse, by the parents, or in some cases, by patients themselves, after return demonstration of correct technique. Of consideration in the cystic fibrosis population is use of the arm port versus the chest port, because chest physiotherapy, involving percussion of the chest, is a large part of the treatment plan for cystic fibrosis, and a chest port may obstruct therapy. Complete port description and care may be found in Chapter 15.

Of consideration to children and parents is catheter care, safety, cost, and body image. For instance, in toddlers, catheter dislodgement may easily occur; an infant may bite through the catheter during the teething period. A child who is extremely afraid of needles may not do well with an implanted port, which has to be accessed with a needle periodically. Conversely, an older child or adolescent may choose an implanted port over a tunneled catheter to avoid disturbance of body image. If the central device is to be used for continuous infusions or cycled daily therapies, such as TPN, a Broviac may be a better choice; if intermittent treatments are prescribed, a port might be the better device. Pediatric hospitals often employ clinical nurse specialists who can demonstrate pros and cons of each device, assist families in their choice of venous access, introduce children with similar devices, and help decrease anxiety about insertion and care of the device.

PEDIATRIC INTRAVENOUS THERAPIES

Primary indications for pediatric IV therapy include fluid balance, medication administration, cancer therapy, nutrition support, and transfusion therapy. Although these topics are covered fully in other chapters, features unique to the neonatal and pediatric patient are highlighted here.

Fluid Therapy

Fluid requirements during IV therapy are a concern. At what rate should IVs be administered to a child? Obviously, the answer to this question is determined by the child's stature and metabolic rate. The amount of fluid required for maintenance levels depends very much on insensible water loss from lungs, skin, urine, and stools and from metabolic expenditures from both internal or external stress levels.

Assessing Fluid Needs
Before deciphering fluid requirements, familiarization with the three different methods for assessing 24-hour maintenance fluids is crucial: namely, the meter squared, caloric, and weight methods. The methods listed below are according to the guidelines from Graef and Cone.[18]

1. The *meter squared* method has an arbitrary estimate of requirement of 1500 to 1800 mL fluid per square meter. The advantage of this method is its simplicity; its disadvantage is in the accessibility of a visual nomogram.

2. The *weight* method uses the child's weight in kilograms to estimate fluid needs. The advantage of this method also is its simplicity; the disadvantage is that it is less accurate in the patient who weighs more than 10 kg.[18]

3. The *caloric* method calculates that the usual expenditure of fluid is approximately 150 mL for every 100 calories metabolized. This method too is simple, but not totally accurate unless actual calorie requirements and energy intake are continuously assessed.

Maintenance fluid requirements for neonates and children differ in volume allowed in 24 hours, but fluid needs of both groups are calculated in milliliters per kilogram weight (Table 25-3).

The methods just discussed only address maintenance replacement according to insensible losses and do not address the additional metabolic expenditures that require further replacement therapy. For example, the most common cause of incremental fluid and caloric needs is temperature elevation. An increase in temperature elevation by 1°C increases the child's caloric needs by 12%. Conversely, a child who is hypothermic has a caloric decrease of 12% per degree Celsius, which decreases the fluid requirements.

Other conditions that affect incremental fluid requirements include gastrointestinal losses, small intestinal drainage, and ongoing diarrhea. The physician and the nurse should assess the entire metabolic situation before prescribing the amount and type of IV therapy a child needs. A precise intake and output record is the most valuable assessment

TABLE 25-3
Guide to Protein, Caloric, and Fluid Requirements per Day for the Pediatric Patient

Age	Protein/kg	Calories/kg
Premature	2.5 g	120–150
Term newborn	2.5 g	100–120
1–3 yr	1.5–2 g	70–100
4–6 yr	1.5 g	70–100
7–10 yr	1–1.5 g	70–100
11–14 yr	1 g	50–100
15–18 yr	1 g	50–70

Fluid Requirements by Weight

0–10 kg	100 mL/kg
11–20 kg	100 mL/kg—first 10 kg
	50 mL/kg—second 10 kg
21 kg and up	100 mL/kg—first 10 kg
	50 mL/kg—second 10 kg
	20 mL/kg—after 20 kg

(From Goldberg, M., & Tyrala, E. [1981]. *Parenteral nutrition guide* [3rd ed., p. 19]. Philadelphia: St. Christopher's Hospital for Children. Used with permission of the authors.)

tool for determining fluid requirements. When abnormal losses occur via the kidneys, it is wise to determine the extent of the loss and replace it rather than estimate according to the previously mentioned methods.[54] To ensure accuracy in judging fluid needs, most children receiving IV therapy are on strict intake and output, including diaper weighing.

How do fluid requirements differ in a neonate? Their fluid requirements are greater proportionately because of their higher percentage of total body water; therefore, infants are at greater jeopardy for both fluid overload and dehydration. Also, electrolytes must be followed closely by laboratory tests to determine whether the neonate is in a state of isotonic versus hypertonic dehydration. Actual water requirements vary between a newborn, a low-birth-weight infant, and a high-risk infant. The exact amounts of calories, water, and electrolytes required depend on the newborn's gestational age, body stores, and metabolic rates. The smaller and more immature the infant is, the greater is the total body water content. For example, the water content of a 28-week gestational age infant is 85% of total body weight, as compared to the term infant, whose water content is only 70%.[30] To arrive at specific fluid requirements, all these factors are accounted for, and a strict intake and output record is maintained.

Other factors that affect fluid requirements in the neonate include many therapeutic devices affecting metabolic rates. For example, radiant warmers and single-walled incubators may be effective in maintaining the infant's temperature, but this temperature elevation in turn increases the infant's insensible fluid losses. Phototherapy, though effectively used in the treatment of hyperbilirubinemia in the neonate, will increase insensible fluid losses and cause water requirements to be greater.[29] These various losses must be included when determining fluid replacement. If the child's fluid requirements are not met, a number of physiologic and metabolic states may occur, including evidence of weight loss in association with hyperosmolality, hypernatremia, and increased hematocrit, as well as evidence of metabolic acidosis, dehydration, and frequently, in infants, multiple apnea spells and increased bilirubin.

Conversely, administration of excess fluid, either IV or, occasionally, as a result of respiratory support systems, can be associated with edema, congestive heart failure, patent ductus arteriosus, and even bronchopulmonary dysplasia[32] in the neonate.

Accurate intake requires precision in IV administration. It is paramount that the flow of IV fluids be delivered at a constant rate. Even the smallest error can cause serious problems, especially in the compromised child. Rates in pediatrics generally vary from 5 to 80 mL/hr depending on the size of the child. Adolescent fluid requirements are similar to those for adults, ranging from 100 to 175 mL/hr. Intake and output is monitored hourly; fluids are delivered via gravity or by electronic infusion device for more accuracy through a peripheral or central IV device.

Intravenous Antibiotic and Medication Therapy

Multiple drug therapy is more the norm than the exception in today's high acuity pediatric patient. A recent survey by this writer noted that approximately 170 IV medications are administered to pediatric patients at St. Christopher's Hospital for Children in Philadelphia; approximately 60 or more of these medications are used for home IV therapy in children. A large portion of these drugs includes antibiotics, antivirals, and antifungals administered IV for such conditions as meningitis, osteomyelitis, Lyme disease, joint infections, prophylaxis before and after abdominal surgery, bacterial and fungal central line infections, systemic herpes, and sepsis.

Neonates are generally at greater risk of becoming septic, possibly caused by an acquired congenital disorder resulting in intestinal obstruction, immaturity in lung compliance resulting in respiratory distress syndrome, immaturity of the gastrointestinal tract resulting in necrotizing enterocolitis, and immaturity of the immune system. All these problems mandate antibiotic coverage by the IV route because of the neonate's immature gastrointestinal system and decreased tolerance to the systemic effect of the infection.

Pharmacokinetic parameters must be considered when administering IV medications to a child. These parameters include absorption, distribution, metabolism, and excretion, and each is affected by patient maturity and disease process.[37] Absorption of an IV drug depends on adequacy of the IV access and the length of delivery time; IV absorption is usually immediate. Distribution occurs when a drug, having entered the circulatory system, (it takes about 1 minute for blood to circulate through a child's body[58]), is distributed to the tissues. Most drugs are distributed via the extracellular fluid, others via binding with protein or fat molecules. Because the neonate has a higher level of total body water than the adult (80% versus 60%), water-soluble drugs, such as theophylline, have to be given at higher doses.[37] Neonates and malnourished children have decreased levels of plasma proteins, and drugs that bind to protein, such as nafcillin (Unipen), may be given in lower doses to these children. Some drugs may also compete with binding sites on the albumin molecule, displacing bilirubin from these sites in neonates, and increasing risk of hyperbilirubinemia. These drugs include salicylates, sulfonamides, phenytoin (Dilantin), furosemide (Lasix), and sodium benzoate.[19] Many commercially available medications and drug diluents contain sodium benzoate in the form of the preservative benzyl alcohol; this preservative has been linked to toxicity and death in premature infants, and care should be taken to stock only preservative-free diluents in the nursery and neonatal intensive care unit.[39] Because neonates have less subcutaneous fat, medications that are lipid soluble, such as diazepam (Valium), should be given in smaller doses. The liver plays a large part in drug metabolism. In the neonate with an immature hepatic system or the child with liver disease, decreased liver function may cause altered metabolism of such drugs as phenobarbital, phenytoin, and carbamazepine.[19] Many drugs are excreted via the renal system. Again, less efficient renal function caused by immaturity in the neonate or disease process in the older child, may result in decreased excretion of drugs, with longer half-life, and possibility of toxicity. In these patients, penicillins and aminoglycosides are given at greater dosage intervals (every 12 or 18 hours versus every 6 or 8 hours). In children with cystic fibrosis, where extrarenal clearance pathways eliminate drugs more quickly, IV aminoglycosides, such as tobramycin (Nebcin), must be given at two to three times the normal dose.[37]

Intravenous medications may be administered to children using a variety of methods, including manual IV push, volume-control set, syringe pump, or retrograde infusion. Sample minimal dilution guidelines are provided in Table 25-4. Each method is applicable to specific drugs and desired therapeutic outcome. Before and after IV administration of certain drugs, levels of medication in the blood are tested to determine the safe dosage range for therapeutic effectiveness. These levels are known as *trough level*, or the lowest drug level drawn just before giving a scheduled dose, and *peak level*, or the highest drug level, drawn 30 minutes after the drug and postflush have infused.[31] Monitoring of these levels and the clinical status of the patient and being aware of pharmacokinetic parameters will provide a good picture of the effects of IV medication administration in the child.

Dosages for pediatric patients are individualized and usually calculated in milligrams per kilogram for most IV drugs, milligrams per square meter for chemotherapy, and micrograms per kilogram for IV drugs used for resuscitation and advanced pharmacologic life support. A rule of thumb is that most drugs are packaged in single adult-sized doses, so a portion of a vial is usually needed for a child's dose. If more than two vials of a drug are needed for a single pediatric dose, calculations should be rechecked.

Of great concern to many practitioners is the correct administration of IV medications administered to a child during advanced life support. Some institutions use bedside charts, particularly in pediatric critical care areas, which list the individual doses of resuscitative drugs for the weight of that child. In addition, large, multidose charts listing doses of drugs and sizes of equipment used in a pediatric code may be posted in the emergency or treatment room areas. This information is extremely helpful to nursing and medical personnel who work with adult patients and are not readily familiar with these dosages from experience. Tables 25-5 and 25-6 list pediatric life support medications, dosages, and infusions.

Cancer Therapy

Because of research, discovery of new drug combinations, and aggressive therapy, the mortality rate for children with cancer has decreased greatly since the 1960s. Common cancers in children include leukemia, neuroblastoma, rhabdomyosarcoma, Wilms' tumor, retinoblastoma, lymphomas, Hodgkin's disease, and brain tumors. These cancers are treated with a team approach that includes physicians, clinical nurse specialists, staff nurses, social workers, child-life therapists, pharmacists, surgeons, and home IV and hospice nurses. Childhood cancer is treated with a combination of surgery, radiation,

TABLE 25-4
Minimum Dilutions and Maximum Flow Rates for Antibiotics

Drug	Minimum Diluent*	Concentration of Initial Dilution*	Final Maximum Concentration for IV Use†	Maximum Rate of Administration‡		
				mg/min	mL/min	mL/hr
Amikacin§		50 mg/mL; 250 mg/mL	2.5 mg/mL	17	6.8	408
Gentamicin		10 mg/mL; 40 mg/mL	1.6 mg/mL	3	2	120
Kanamycin		75 mg/2 mL; 500 mg/2 mL	5 mg/mL	17	3	180
Tobramycin		10 mg/mL; 40 mg/mL	1.6 mg/mL	4	2.5	150
Ampicillin	125 mg vial–1.2 mL	125 mg/mL	135 mg/mL	100	0.74	45
	250 mg vial–1.0 mL	250 mg/mL				
	500 mg vial–1.8 mL	250 mg/mL				
	1 g vial–3.5 mL	250 mg/mL				
Carbenicillin	1 g vial–2.0 mL	400 mg/mL	50 mg/mL	33	0.66	40
	5 g vial–9.5 mL	400 mg/mL				
Ticarcillin	1g vial–2.0 mL	400 mg/mL	50 mg/mL	33	0.66	40
	3 g vial–6.0 mL	400 mg/mL				
Cefamandole	1 g vial–3.0 mL		100 mg/mL	333	3.3	200
Clindamycin		150 mg/mL	6 mg/mL	30	5	300
Keflin	1 g vial–4.0 mL		100 mg/mL	333	3.3	200
Methicillin	1 g vial–1.5 mL	500 mg/mL	20 mg/mL	200	10	600
Nafcillin	500 g vial–1.7 mL	250 mg/mL	33 mg/mL	100	3	180
	1 g vial–3.4 mL	250 mg/mL				

*Based on manufacturer's suggestions as stated in package inserts.

†Based on usual adult dose and minimum volume of infusion recommended by manufacturer.

‡Based on usual adult dose, minimum volume of infusion, and minimum time of infusion recommended by manufacturer.

§Package insert for Amikacin states above values for infants.

(Prepared by and for Children's Medical Center, Dallas, February 1981.)

chemotherapy and biologic response modifiers. Children are usually randomized to be treated according to certain protocols, which are the subject of widespread, ongoing, multicenter research studies. Such aggressive therapy usually requires adequate long-term IV access because attempts to administer a vesicant drug by peripheral IV in an agitated child can result in extravasation injury to the child and occupational exposure to a toxic drug for the nurse. Tunneled catheters, implanted ports, and PICC lines are common access devices used in pediatric oncology patients. The function of various antineoplastic agents and administration guidelines are discussed in Chapter 24; dilution guidelines for pediatric chemotherapy are found in Table 25-7.

Parenteral Nutrition Therapy

Parenteral nutrition is discussed in Chapter 20. You will recall that the major breakthrough in parenteral feedings occurred in the late 1960s when Stanley J. Dudrick and his colleagues at the University of Pennsylvania reported their results with central venous

TABLE 25-5
Intravenous Drugs for Pediatric and Neonatal Resuscitation

Drug	Dose
Sodium Bicarbonate (8.4%)	1.0–2.0 mEq/kg
	1.0–2.0 mL/kg
Epinephrine (1:10,000)	0.1 mL/kg
	0.01 mg/kg
Atropine (0.4 mg/mL)	0.02 mg/kg
	Min dose = 0.15 mg
	Max dose = 2.0 mg
Naloxone (Narcan) (0.4 mg/mL)	0.1 mg/kg
	Min dose = 0.5 mg
	Max dose = 2.0 mg
Dextrose 10% via peripheral IV	5.0 mL/kg
Dextrose 25% via central IV	2.0 mL/kg

(Adapted from *Emergency pediatric and neonatal resuscitation reference*, courtesy of Robert Brown, RN, MSN, PNP, Nurse Manager, Emergency Department and Transport Team; and nursing staff of Pediatric/Neonatal Transport Team, St. Christopher's Hospital for Children, Philadelphia, 1991.)

hyperalimentation. The success of Dudrick's early experiments with subclavian catheters led to further success with human infants and adults who could not be fed adequately by the enteral route because of severe gastrointestinal disorders.

Dudrick devised a simple statement of criteria that differentiates patients who potentially can benefit from TPN therapy into categories. These categories include those

TABLE 25-6
Infusions

Medication	Preparation (add amounts calculated to D_5W to = 100 mL)	Dose	Range
Dopamine		1 mL/hr = 1 μg/kg/min	2.0–15.0 μg/kg/min
Dobutamine	(6 × kg) mg		2.0–15.0 μg/kg/min
Nitroprusside			0.5–5.0 μg/kg/min
Epinephrine	(0.6 × kg) mg	1 mL/hr = 0.1 μg/kg/min	0.1–1.0 μg/kg/min
Norepinephrine			
Lidocaine	(60 × kg) mg	1 mL/hr = 10 μg/kg/min	10.0–50.0 μg/kg/min
Isoproterenol	up to 20 kg: (0.6 × kg) mg	1 mL/hr = 0.1 μg/kg/min	0.1–1.0 μg/kg/min
	20–40 kg: (0.3 × kg) mg	1 mL/hr = 0.05 μg/kg/min	
	40 kg and up: (0.12 × kg) mg	1 mL/hr = 0.02 μg/kg/min	

(From *Emergency pediatric and neonatal resuscitation reference*, courtesy of Robert Brown, RN, MSN, PNP, Nurse Manager, Emergency Department and Transport Team; and nursing staff of Pediatric/Neonatal Transport Team, St. Christopher's Hospital for Children, Philadelphia, 1991.)

TABLE 25-7
Chemotherapy Dilution Guidelines for Pediatric Patients

Drug	Strength	Administration
Alkylating agents BCNU (Carmustine)	3.3 mg/mL (10% ethanol)	IV infusion slowly over 30–60 min, burning of vein if infused too rapidly
Cyclophosphamide (Cytoxan)	20 mg/mL	IV push or infusion
Dacarbazine (DTIC)	10 mg/mL	IV injection or infusion over 15–30 min
Mechlorethamine (Mustargen, nitrogen mustard)	1 mg/mL	IV push
Triethylene thiophosphoramide (Thiotepa)	15-mg vial (5 mg/0.6 mL)	IV push, intravesical in 30–60 mL of distilled water
Antibiotics Dactinomycin (actinomycin D, Cosmegen)	0.5 mg/mL	IV push infusion over 10–15 min
Doxorubicin (Adriamycin)	2 mg/mL	IV push or infusion over 3–15 min
Mithramycin (Mithracin)	0.5 mg/mL	IV push or infusion
Mitomycin (Mutamycin, mito-mycin C)	0.5 mg/mL	IV push or infusion
Streptozocin (Zanosar)	100 mg/mL	IV push or infusion
Antimetabolites Cytarabine (Cytosar-U, Ara-C)	20 mg/mL or 50 mg/mL	IV push or infusion, subcutaneous, intrathecal
Methotrexate (MTX, Mexate)	Injection prescribed amount 10 mL	IV push, IV infusion
Miscellaneous Cisplatin (Platinol)	1 mg/mL	IV push or infusion
Vinca alkaloids Vinblastine (Velban)	1 mg/mL	IV push, infusion in D_5W or NS
Vincristine (Oncovin)	1 mg/mL	IV push, infusion rapidly

Sparrow Hospital Division of Nursing Statement of Policy for Pediatric Chemotherapy Dilutions: A. Pediatric IV push chemotherapeutic drugs will be admixed to establish a minimum volume of 3 mL. B. The following guidelines will be used when admixing and administering IV pediatric chemotherapeutic drugs.

(From CRNIs role in pediatric chemotherapy administration. [1986]. *Journal of the National Intravenous Therapy Association, 9,* 467. Used with permission of J. B. Lippincott and Intravenous Nurses Society.)

patients who cannot eat, will not eat, or cannot eat enough.[50] Total parenteral nutrition should be used only in patients having inadequate gastrointestinal function, thereby disallowing feeding by the enteral route (especially because TPN costs are very high). Partial parenteral nutrition (PPN) can provide a supplemental source of nutrition for short periods of time in children who eat, but do not eat adequate amounts for growth. Total parenteral nutrition is becoming one of the most important therapeutic parameters in the successful management of certain pediatric diseases. The widespread use of TPN has sustained numerous children while their gastrointestinal tracts develop enough absorptive capacity to tolerate basal caloric requirements.

Pediatric patients receiving PPN and TPN usually fall into two major categories: those with either congenital or acquired anomalies of the gastrointestinal tract or those infants with intractable diarrhea syndromes. The gastrointestinal tract anomalies that generally require TPN include intestinal obstruction (obstruction in the intestinal lumen), gastroschisis (a congenital fissure in the wall of the abdomen that remains open), and necrotizing enterocolitis (necrosis of the small or large bowel caused by sepsis or hypoxia). The most dramatic treatment requires major resection of both small and large bowel and TPN may be needed for several weeks, sometimes months.[48] Other pediatric diseases that may require IV nutrition include cystic fibrosis, renal failure, congenital heart disease, cancer, and Crohn's disease. With the addition of TPN into their therapy regime, affected children can be expected to gain weight normally with only parenteral nutrients. In addition, TPN supplies enough calories to maintain the positive nitrogen balance required for normal growth and development. Criteria used to identify children for parenteral nutrition include greater than 5% weight loss, serum albumin level below 3 g/dL, growth ratio below fifth percentile when height and weight are plotted on growth charts, and total lymphocyte count less than 1000/mm³ (excluding granulocytopenic patients).[20]

Solutions are generally made by hospital or home IV agency pharmacy staff, and the admixture of solutions is done under a laminar air hood. The general constituents for TPN—amino acids, a dextrose calorie source, electrolytes, minerals, trace elements, and vitamins—provide amounts of nutrients sufficient to promote growth and maintain a positive nitrogen balance. Nitrogen balance is maintained through the amino acids intake; calories are obtained by glucose. Intravenous fat preparations are currently used to supply essential fatty acids. Electrolytes are usually added to the TPN solution in amounts established for IV maintenance requirements. Calcium, magnesium, phosphorus and other minerals are incompletely absorbed from the gastrointestinal tract. Therefore, the parenteral needs for minerals are significantly lower than oral needs, and the amounts in the TPN solution rarely exceed half the usual oral amounts. Trace elements may be needed and are now included in commercial solutions; vitamins are added according to children's recommended daily allowances. [*Note:* The yellow color of the TPN solution results from the addition of multivitamins. Because multivitamins limit the shelf life of TPN to 24 hours, home TPN patients are taught to add vitamins and other medication additives such as heparin and cimetidine (Tagamet)].

Pediatric requirements for IV nutrition follow general guidelines and are based on protein, calorie, and fluid needs per kilogram of body weight. See Table 25-3 for specific requirements for children of various ages.

Amino acids provide protein for growth. General pediatric recommendations for daily protein intake in the child are listed in Table 25-3. One gram of protein should deliver at least 30 calories.[49] Protein is administered in the strength of 10% amino acid solution in children and 6% amino acid solution in neonates. The less concentrated solution is used in neonates because it more closely approximates amino acid concentration of the healthy breast-fed infant.

Carbohydrate is infused in the form of dextrose, which provides energy for body tissues. If carbohydrate supply is inadequate, the body will break down protein or fat to provide metabolic needs. Dextrose provides the main calorie source; recommended daily amounts are 20 to 30 g/kg in children weighing less than 10 kg and 25 to 30 g/kg in children weighing more than 10 kg.[49] Because the dextrose in TPN is hydrated, it provides not 4, but 3.4 kcal/g. For example, 100 mL D5W contains 5 g dextrose, or 17 kcal; 100 mL D10W contains 10 g dextrose, or 34 kcal. The strength of dextrose that can be administered peripherally in a child is 10% to 12.5%.[49] Greater concentrations, given through a peripheral IV, can cause sclerosis, phlebitis, and extravasation injury if infiltration occurs. Although concentrated dextrose is needed to provide calories, the volume of fluid needed to dilute very concentrated dextrose is prohibitive to fluid balance in children, especially neonates. Higher concentrations of dextrose (up to 25%) in less volume of fluid may be delivered via central catheter.

The other source of non-protein calories is lipids, delivered as a fat emulsion. Originally, fat infusion was kept to a minimum, only 2% to 10% of daily calorie intake, because it was thought that higher fat intake resulted in pulmonary changes. This hyperlipemia is now thought to have been brought on by rapid infusion rate, not amount of intake, so a slower infusion rate over a longer period of time is now the rule, and fat intake now comprises 40% to 60% of total calories required daily.[49]

Fat emulsions come in strengths of of 10%, with 1.1 kcal/mL and 20%, with 2 kcal/mL. Both may be infused peripherally or centrally. Fats are essential for neurologic development in the infant; however, fatty acids may displace bilirubin from albumin, causing a rise in bilirubin level and an increased risk of kernicterus.[22] Accurate bilirubin levels should be drawn 4 hours after the fat emulsion has infused; if lipid infusion is continuous, the blood sample should be centrifuged before bilirubin assay.[22]

The second major area of responsibility for the nurse is in the delivery of TPN by a constant and proper infusion rate. The amount and rate of flow are governed by the optimal sugar utilization as determined by the renal threshold and the patient's specific requirements. If too little fluid is given, the sugar will be well below the threshold and the maximum caloric intake will not be reached. If too much solution is given, the renal threshold is exceeded and a sugar spill will be noted in the urine. The infusion rate should be checked frequently, at least every hour. Urine Tes-Tapes should be done after every void in neonates. A positive 2+ urine × 2 or a 3+ or 4+ urine requires immediate nursing intervention. If this occurs, the physician should be notified; a serum glucose may be ordered and the infusion rate may be adjusted or insulin may be added, depending on the individual needs of the patient. Electronic infusion devices serve as helpful aids in monitoring desired rates, especially in children. For this reason, TPN is always administered to the pediatric patient via an EID.

When a child is first started on TPN, the percentage of dextrose infused is gradually increased from 5% to a maximum of 20% to 25% via central line, according to the caloric needs and tolerance of the child (Table 25-8). Infusions may run over 24 hours for the very sick hospitalized child or may be gradually cycled down by 4-hour increments daily, maintaining the same volume infusion over less time. Cycling down to about 12 hours daily of TPN infusion allows far more freedom for the child, particularly the child on home TPN, who may infuse at night while asleep, and still follow a fairly normal lifestyle of school and activities. Portable infusion pumps, widely used in home IV therapy, also allow more freedom, do not require an IV pole, and can be placed in an unobtrusive carrying case. Weaning on and off the TPN solution used to be popular practice, allowing time for the pancreas to adjust to the change in glucose levels; this weaning process has been found to be unnecessary, except in special situations.

Depending on caloric expenditure based on stress levels, lipids may be provided prophylactically biweekly or daily to supplement caloric requirements. Administration of piggyback lipids through a nonfiltered system is common in hospital practice today. The lipids must be connected as close to the venous junction as possible.

As mentioned earlier, electrolytes, vitamins, minerals, and trace elements are provided in accordance with the child's daily requirements. Sample pediatric TPN solution mixtures are provided in Table 25-9.

TABLE 25-8
Administration Regimen for Central Alimentation Beyond First Year of Life

1. Initial (bottle #1)
   Glucose 10% to which electrolytes are added. If hyperglycemia does not develop within 24 hr, increase glucose to 15%.
2. Bottle #2
   Glucose 15% to which electrolytes are added. If all parameters are stable for 24 hr, add protein to the next bottle.
3. Bottle #3
   Glucose 15%. Protein in low concentration 1 g/kg/day. If all parameters are stable, increase protein, up to 2 g/kg/day if desired.
4. Bottle #4
   Glucose 20%. Protein may be increased to maximum requirements. If all parameters are stable and if necessary, sugar load may be increased to 20%.
5. Subsequent bottles of infusate
   Glucose maximum = 20%–25%.

(From Goldberg, M., & Tyrala, E. [1981]. *Parenteral nutrition guide* [3rd ed.]. St. Christopher's Hospital for Children, Philadelphia. Used with permission of the authors.)

TABLE 25-9
Routine TPN Stock Solution*

Solution	Starter Strength (mL)	Full Strength (mL)
Amino acid solution (8.5%)	100	165
D/W 50%	125	220
NaCl (2.5 mEq/mL)	5	5
MgSO$_4$ (4 mEq/mL)	2	2
Ca gluconate (0.45 mEq/mL)	9	13
KPO$_4$ (4.4 mEq/k/mL) 3 mmol P/mL)	1	1.5
KCl (2 mEq/mL)	3	2
MVI	2	2
H$_2$O	252	89
Total volume	500	500
kcal/mL	0.49	0.86
Glucose concentration	12.5%	22%
Protein concentration	1.7 g/100	2.8 g/100

* Trace elements added: ZnSO$_4$, CuSO$_4$, MnSO$_4$, CrCl$_2$, and Fe^{3+}. Weekly supplementation (IM injection): vitamin K, folate, and vitamin B$_{12}$.

(Prepared by and for Children's Medical Center, Dallas, July 1980.)

The third area of nursing responsibility is patient assessment. The nurse monitors the patient's physical status daily and screens, intervenes, and reports abnormal findings of temperature spikes, inappropriate glucose spills, chills, rashes, irritability, decreased level of consciousness, and so forth. Any observable abnormality is immediately reported to the physician. Serum levels of various chemistry and hematology tests are assessed daily for the first week and then decreased to a weekly schedule for the stable hospitalized or home TPN patient. See Figure 25-18, Total Parenteral Nutrition Flow Sheet, for a schedule for assessing these parameters.

The fourth major area of nursing intervention in a child receiving TPN is psychological support. Most TPN patients are infants who are acutely ill and deprived of maternal warmth and comfort. Even though a child on central TPN may be NPO, cuddling and holding the child should assist in meeting maternal needs. Also, allowing parents every opportunity to participate in their child's care is extremely important. First, the nurse should assess the family's level of comprehension about TPN and intervene by offering support in their areas of weakness and insecurities to decrease parental anxiety. As soon as the decision is made to place a child on TPN, it is best to use the preoperative teaching methodology of explaining purpose, procedures, and potential complications. Of course, all further questions can be handled on a daily basis. Permitting this open channel of communication not only supplies parents with the knowledge needed to become involved, but assists them in comprehending the purpose of TPN and why adherence to the protocol of TPN therapy is so important.

As with all therapies, disadvantages to TPN stem from potential complications. Every nurse must fully understand the possible complications of TPN therapy, including the symptoms of each specific complication. Complications are subdivided into three categories: catheter insertion, postinsertion, and metabolic complications.

Catheter Insertion Complications
1. Infection
2. Malposition
3. Perforation of structures (*ie*, artery, vein, lymph nodes, lung)

Postinsertion Complications
1. Infection
2. Thrombosis
3. Superior vena cava syndrome

Metabolic Complications

1. Hyperglycemia	4. Mineral disorder
2. Hypoglycemia	5. Hyperammonemia
3. Electrolyte imbalance	6. Hyperbilirubinemia

Most of the aforementioned complications can be treated or even prevented. Maintaining high-caliber aseptic techniques when handling the TPN line reduces the potential risk of sepsis. Certain metabolic complications are preventable through close nursing monitoring, although some predisposing metabolic abnormalities may require immediate medical intervention. With the incremental advances in technology and the formation

TPN FLOW SHEET

NAME _____

Age _____
Date starting TPN _____
Central/Peripheral _____

Day Starting TPN	BASELINE	1	2	3	4	5	6	7	8	9	10	11	12	13	14	15	16	17	18	19	20	21	22	23	24	25	26	27	28
DATE																													
Weight	•	•	•	•	•	•	•	•	•	•	•	•	•	•	•	•	•	•	•	•	•	•	•	•	•	•	•	•	•
*Length/H.C.	•	•						•							•							•							•
Protein/kg/24 hr	•	•	•	•	•	•	•	•	•	•	•	•	•	•	•	•	•	•	•	•	•	•	•	•	•	•	•	•	•
mL/kg/24 hr	•	•	•	•	•	•	•	•	•	•	•	•	•	•	•	•	•	•	•	•	•	•	•	•	•	•	•	•	•
Cal. kg/24 hr	•	•	•	•	•	•	•	•	•	•	•	•	•	•	•	•	•	•	•	•	•	•	•	•	•	•	•	•	•
Na/K	•	•	•	•	•		•	•			•			•	•			•				•							•
Co₂/Cl	•	•	•	•	•		•	•			•			•	•			•				•							•
BUN	•				•			•						•	•			•				•							•
Creatinine	•				•																								
Glu	•	•	•	•	•		•	•			•			•	•			•				•		•					•
Ca/Phos	•										•											•							•
TP/Alb	•																					•							•
Mg/Zn	•																					•							•
SGOT/SGPT	•							•														•							•
GGT	•							•						•								•							•
Bili T/D	•							•						•								•							•
Triglyceride	•							•						•				•				•							•
Cholesterol	•							•						•								•							•
HGB/MCV	•							•						•								•							•
Retic	•							•						•								•							
NUTRITIONAL ASSESSMENT	•														•														
Absolute Lymphocyte CT	•														•														
Transferrin	•																												
Skin Testing	•																												
Skin Folds	•																												
INFECTION																													
Culture sent & results	•																												
Chest X-ray (Central line only)	•						•							•								•							•

* Indicates study should be done
* Length-Weekly if 2 years - HC-Weekly if 1 year

544

TABLE 25-10
Blood Volumes at Various Ages

Premature infant	105 mL/kg
Term infant	80 mL/kg
3 months to adult	70–75 mL/kg

(From Luban, N., & Keating, L. [Eds.] [1983]. *Hemotherapy of the infant and premature* [pp. 5–65, 69–80, 95–124]. Arlington, VA: American Association of Blood Banks; Nathan, D., & Oski, F. [Eds.]. [1981]. *Hematology of infancy and childhood* [pp. 1491–1500]. Philadelphia: W. B. Saunders.)

of TPN teams, even the most prominent complication, sepsis, has decreased to acceptable rates. In the practice of TPN therapy, the catheter sepsis rate in children may rise as high as 10% because of the increased risks and general behaviors of children (*eg*, teething children have been known to bite the TPN catheter).

Pediatric Transfusion Therapy

Indications and techniques for transfusing blood and blood products to children are similar to those described for adults in Chapter 21. The major differences between adults and children include decrease in blood volume from neonate to adult, maturation of the immune system with regard to blood typing, blood counts through various stages of development, and requirements for transfusion therapy. Table 25-10 lists blood volumes for various ages. A transfusion procedure unique to the neonate is exchange transfusion, as described below.

The red blood cell of the infant is nucleated at birth and has a reduced half-life (23.3 days) in contrast to that of the adult (26–35 days).[33] Synthesis of fetal hemoglobin (HbF) declines rapidly after birth when adult hemoglobin (HbA) rises concomitantly. The higher affinity for oxygen of HbF facilitates transfer of oxygen from mother to fetus in utero, but persistence of HbF after birth may result in respiratory distress and tissue hypoxia in the neonate because of the inability of HbF to release oxygen to the tissues.[28] Manipulations of the infant, such as suctioning and IV starts, as well as crying, can increase peripheral leukocyte counts. Neutropenia, not neutrophilia, in the newborn, is a more common indicator of sepsis. Platelet counts do not differ greatly from neonate to adult, but neonates may easily develop thrombocytopenia from extrinsic sources.

The immune system of the neonate matures during infant stages of development. Circulating antibodies are derived from the mother during the last several prenatal weeks; therefore, premature infants have a less efficient humoral immunity. As a baby is exposed to outside antigens, antibody production begins, and for the first several days of life, mother's serum is used for compatibility testing. In infants older than 1 week and those previously transfused, compatibility testing is done on the blood of the baby. Group O red blood cells that are Rh negative or the same Rh as the infant are frequently used. In addition, red blood cells are tested for cytomegalovirus (CMV) and are only given to

◄ **FIGURE 25-18** Total Parenteral Nutrition Flow Sheet, St. Christopher's Hospital for Children, Philadelphia, PA. (From Goldberg, M., & Tyrala, E. [1981]. *Parenteral nutrition guide*, [3rd ed.], pp. 42–43. Used with permission of the authors.)

neonates if CMV negative. The freshest cells possible are used to avoid potassium load in young infants.

Specific indications for transfusion therapy are outlined extensively in Chapter 21. In general, indications for transfusion therapy in children include acute hemorrhage, anemia, abnormal component function or component deficiency, and removal of harmful substances, such as bilirubin, during exchange transfusion. Reduction in the blood volume of a child by 30% to 40% produces clinical evidence of shock. When 20% of blood volume is lost and may recur, transfusion is also indicated.[42] Central venous pressure is the best indicator for restoration of blood volume to normal; pulse rate is a less reliable guide, and 24 to 36 hours may pass before hemoglobin reflects true extent of blood loss. Reduced hemoglobin and hematocrit 3 to 6 hours after hemorrhage suggests loss of 20% to 25% of blood volume, whereas normal hemoglobin 6 hours after hemorrhage suggests that substantial blood loss has not occurred.[42] A red blood cell mass deficit occurs with chronic anemia, and transfusion with packed cells is not indicated until hemoglobin level drops below 6 g/dL.[42] Assessment of the patient's cardiopulmonary status and activity level, along with hemoglobin, should be considered before transfusion because an unstressed child can tolerate hemoglobin values of 3 to 6 g/dL without signs of heart failure. Also, because the most common form of anemia seen in children is iron deficiency anemia (which is rarely treated with transfusion), other treatments may be more indicated, including iron therapy, folic acid, or vitamin B_{12}.

Decreased production or altered function of platelets is usually caused by maternally induced disorder (ie, aspirin intake prenatally), congenital disorder, acquired disorder (ie, ITP), or chemotherapy-induced thrombocytopenia. Indications for transfusion of platelets, plasma, and plasma components are similar to those in adults, and Table 25-11 lists some parameters for blood component therapy in children.

Infusion of IV gamma globulin or IV IgG warrants specific mention because the use of this plasma derivative in children has grown substantially since the 1980s, when safe, effective IV preparations became licensed in the United States. Before that time, children with humoral immunodeficiencies were treated with intramuscular injections or infusions of plasma. The large volume of intramuscular IgG required adequate muscle mass, it was uncomfortable because injected volume was large, and IgG levels rose slowly and

TABLE 25-11
Blood Component Therapy for Pediatric Patients

Blood Product	Indication	Dosage/Rate
Red blood cells (packed)	Treatment of anemia without volume expansion	10 mL/kg, not to exceed 15 mL/kg at 2–5 mL/kg/hr
Platelets	To control bleeding associated with deficiency in platelet number or function	1 U (50–70 mL)/7–10 kg body weight
		Run over 30 min to maximum of 4 hr; IV push or drip
Fresh frozen plasma	To increase levels of clotting factors in children with demonstrated deficiency	Acute hemorrhage: 15–30 mL/kg as indicated
	Occasionally volume expansion in acute blood loss	Clotting deficiency: 10–15 mL/kg at 1–2 mL/min

(Adapted from *Transfusion therapy guidelines for nurses*. [1990]. National Blood Resource Education Program, Public Health Service, National Institutes of Health, U.S. Department of Health and Human Services.)

were only maintained for a short time before another injection was needed to help bolster infection-fighting capabilities. Larger doses of IgG can be given via the IV route, thus maintaining adequate serum levels with more convenient administration. Approved indications for IV IgG include deficiencies of the humoral immune system and ITP. Treatment of immunodeficiency requires monthly infusions of from 100 to 400 mg/kg for life; acute ITP is treated with 400 mg/kg up to 1 g/kg until platelet rise is noted.[51] In children, a viral infection often precludes onset of ITP, and 80% to 90% of children exhibit spontaneous remission in 6 to 12 months. Platelet count in ITP lowers because antibody-coated platelets are destroyed by splenic phagocytes, and IV IgG is prescribed to elevate platelet counts so that potentially fatal episodes of hemorrhage can be avoided. Palliation of other childhood disease entities, such as neonatal sepsis, cystic fibrosis, and bacterial infection in human immunodeficiency-positive children, is the topic of ongoing research, largely because of the ability of gamma globulin to be administered by the IV route in the neonate to the adolescent.

Blood and blood products in children may be administered via 27-, 26-, or 24-gauge peripheral IV in neonates and via 24- or 22-gauge in older children. An infusion pump, capable of infusing blood, is recommended for transfusion therapy in children; in neonates, blood may be prefiltered by the blood bank, and then infused from a syringe on a syringe pump. Pediatricians request blood and blood products in mL/kg increments, instead of units, because a single unit of packed red blood cells may equal the entire blood volume of several infants. In children, volume and fluid balance considerations negate the simultaneous infusion of saline, particularly in neonates; instead, the peripheral or central IV device must be flushed with 1–3 mL of saline before and after the transfusion. Rate of blood transfusion may be very slow or even staggered with boluses of dextrose in neonates. Five percent to 10% of red cell volume should be infused slowly over the first 15 minutes, then the rate increased to an hourly IV rate tolerated by the child.[28]

Specific physical assessment areas indicative of hematologic function in children include color changes in skin, lips, conjunctiva, mucous membranes, and nails, such as blue for cyanosis, pale for anemia, or yellow for jaundice. Look at fingernails and toenails for clubbing, skin for petechiae, and mucous membranes for bleeding. Blood oozing from old venipuncture sites is often a precursor to onset of disseminated intravascular coagulation (DIC). When a tourniquet is placed on an extremity, evidence of petechiae distal to the tourniquet may be indicative of ITP or other platelet disorders.

In addition to physical assessment, history should include previous exposure to toxins (which may be a cause of aplastic anemia), and any previous transfusions, including the reason, and patient reaction. Psychological support of the family is indicated, in addition to education about transfusion therapy and alternatives, if available. Agency policy is necessary regarding refusal of transfusion by a parent or guardian, and state laws differ on this topic; in most cases, a waiver must be signed if transfusion is refused.

In an exchange transfusion, most or all of the infant's blood is replaced with compatible red blood cells and plasma from one or several donors. In the early 1950s, exchange transfusion was first used for management of HDN; with the introduction of anti-D immune globulin (Rhogam) in the 1960s, the number of infants with this disease greatly declined. Indications for exchange transfusion include hemolytic disease of the newborn, caused by Rh or ABO incompatibility, DIC, sepsis, respiratory distress syndrome, and polycythemia, or "thick blood syndrome," where some of the infant's blood is removed and replaced with plasma. The most common indication for exchange is

HDN. Two causes of HDN include Rh incompatibility, where the second Rh + baby of an Rh − mother is affected when anti-D antibodies in the mother, developed in response to the first pregnancy, cross the placenta and destroy the red blood cells of the second baby. At birth, the infant will be anemic and exhibit increased levels of unconjugated (indirect) bilirubin. Deposition of excess bilirubin in the brain can cause kernicterus, a type of encephalopathy. Exchange transfusion is considered when bilirubin levels increase more than 1 mg/dL each hour, or reach 15 to 16 mg/dL in the neonate and 20 mg/dL in the full-term infant.[22] Although hemolytic disease from ABO incompatibility is more common, it is usually mild enough to be treated with phototherapy or a single blood transfusion, until the infant's liver matures enough to clear bilirubin out of the blood. ABO incompatibility occurs most frequently when a type O mother carries an A or B fetus.[42] In ABO incompatibility, the direct Coombs' test may be only weakly positive, whereas, with Rh incompatibility, the Coombs' is strongly positive. In contrast to Rh disease, ABO HDN may occur in the first infant.

Red blood cells alone, or in conjunction with fresh frozen plasma, may be used for exchange transfusion. To treat Rh HDN, type O, Rh blood crossmatched with the mother is used; for ABO HDN, use Rh compatible, type O blood.

A double-volume or two-volume exchange is usually performed where exchange transfusion is equal to twice the patient's blood volume. This replaces about 85% of the newborn's blood and lowers the bilirubin level in blood by about 50%, but does not have any effect on extravascular bilirubin. Albumin may be administered before the exchange to bind bilirubin, allowing a greater amount to be removed during the procedure. Ideally, two vascular access sites are used to allow simultaneous withdrawal and infusion, including sites such as the umbilical vessels and peripheral or central veins. If only one access is available, the push–pull method is used. Calcium and dextrose levels are closely monitored during the exchange because blood preservatives may cause levels to decrease. Complications can include those related to the catheter, discussed earlier in the chapter, as well as those related to transfusion therapy.

SUMMARY OF PEDIATRIC CARE

As outlined in INS Standards of Practice, an IV nursing team is an integral part of nursing care for the pediatric patient. Because children vary from neonate to adolescent in physiologic as well as developmental level, special consideration and increased time may be necessary to provide efficacious IV therapy. Consultation to staff nurses regarding safe drug administration and transfusion therapy to children is an integral part of the pediatric IV team function. Assisting families with choice of venous access, providing skilled insertion of that device, as well as follow-up care and teaching have become integral roles for IV nurses. Both IV teams and nutrition support teams have demonstrated lower complication rates and increased quality of care.

In conclusion, specific principles in caring for pediatric patients receiving IV therapy have been discussed, as well as the fluid and nutritional requirements and diseases that necessitate pediatric IV therapy. By familiarizing nurses with this current information, it is hoped that their understanding of the complexities involved in caring for a child receiving IV therapy will be deepened.

REFERENCES

1. Arbeiter, H. I., & Greengard, J. (1944). Tibial bone marrow infusions in infancy. *Journal of Pediatrics*, *25*, 1.
2. Batton, D. G., Maisels, J., & Applebaum, P. (1982). Use of peripheral intravenous cannulas in premature infants: A controlled study. *Pediatrics*, *70*, 488.
3. Blake, F. G., Wright, F. H., & Wachter, E. H. (1970). *Nursing care of children* (p. 11). Philadelphia: J. B. Lippincott.
4. Berner-Howry, L. B., McGillis-Bindler, R., & Tso, Y. (1981). *Pediatric medications* (pp. 3–28). Philadelphia: J. B. Lippincott.
5. Broviac, J. W., Cole, J. J., & Schribner, B. H. (1973). A silicone rubber atrial catheter for prolonged parenteral alimentation. *Surgery, Gynecology and Obstetrics*, *136*, 602.
6. Bryant, B. G. (1990). Drug, fluid, and blood products administered through the umbilical artery catheter: Complication experiences from one NICU. *Neonatal Network*, *9*, 27–46.
7. Camp-Sorrell, D. (1990). Advanced central venous access, selection, catheters, devices, and nursing management. *Journal of Intravenous Nursing*, *13*, 361–370.
8. Chathas, M. K. (1986). Percutaneous central venous catheters in neonates. *Journal of Obstetric, Gynecologic, and Neonatal Nursing*, *15*, 324–331.
9. Clarke, T. A., & Reddy, P. G. (1979). Intravenous infusion technique in the newborn. *Clinical Pediatrics*, *18*, 550–554.
10. Corey, B. E. (1989). Major complications of central lines in neonates. *Neonatal Network*, *7*, 17–28.
11. Decker, M. D., & Edwards, K. M. (1988). Central venous catheter infections. *Pediatric Clinics of North America*, *35*, 579–612.
12. Dolcourt, J. L., & Bose, C. L. (1982). Percutaneous insertion of Silastic central venous catheter in neonates. *Pediatrics*, *70*, 484.
13. Drinker, C. K., Drinker, K. R., & Lund, C. C. (1922). The circulation in the mammalian bone marrow. *American Journal of Physiology*, *62*, 1–92.
14. Fay, M. J. (1983). The special challenges of pediatric IVs. *Dimensions of Critical Care Nursing*, *2*, 24.
15. Frey, A. M. (1991). The immune system. Part II. Intravenous administration of immune globulin. *Journal of Intravenous Nursing*, *14*, 397–405.
16. Geidell-Oellrich, R., Murph, M. R., Goldberg, L. A., & Aggarwal, R. (1991). The percutaneous central venous catheter for small or ill infants. *American Journal of Maternal Child Nursing*, *16*, 92–96.
17. Glaesser, P. N., & Losek, J. D. (1986). Emergency intraosseous infusions in children. *American Journal of Emergency Medicine*, *4*, 35.
18. Graef, J., & Cone, T. (1977). *Manual of pediatric therapeutics*. Boston: Little, Brown.
19. Guyon, G. (1989) Pharmacokinetic considerations in neonatal drug therapy. *Neonatal Network*, *7*, 9–12.
20. Haas-Beckert, B. (1987). Removing the mysteries of parenteral nutrition, *Pediatric Nursing*, *13*, 37–41.
21. Hadaway, L. (1990). A midline alternative to central and peripheral venous access. *Caring*, *9*, 45–50.
22. Hahler-D'Angelo, J., & Welsh, N. P. (Eds.). (1988). Pediatric drug and IV therapy. In *Medication administration and IV therapy handbook* (pp. 305–307). Springhouse, PA: Springhouse Corp.
23. Harris, L. C., Rushton, C. H., & Hale, S. J. (1987). Implantable infusion devices in the pediatric patient: A viable alternative. *Journal of Pediatric Nursing*, *2*, 174–183.
24. Holcombe, B., Forloines-Lynn, S., & Garmhausen, L. W. (1992). Restoring patency of long-term central venous access devices. *Journal of Intravenous Nursing*, *15*, 36–41.
25. Ingram, J., Weitzman, S., Greenberg, M. L., Partin, P., & Filler, R. (1991). Complications of indwelling venous access lines in the pediatric hematology patient: A prospective comparison of external venous catheters and subcutaneous ports. *American Journal of Pediatric Hematology/Oncology*, *13*, 130–136.
26. *Revised intravenous nursing standards of practice*. (1990). *Journal of Intravenous Nursing*, (Suppl.), S47.
27. Kanter, R. K., Zimmerman, J. J., Straus, R. H., & Stoeckel, K. (1986). Pediatric emergency intravenous access: Evaluation of a protocol. *American Journal of Diseases of Children*, *140*, 133.
28. Kasprisin, C. A. (1985). Transfusion therapy for the pediatric patient. In R. Rutman & W. Miller (Eds.). *Transfusion therapy* (pp. 179–185). Rockville, MD: Aspen Systems Corp.
29. Kitterman, J., Phibbs, R., & Tooley, W. (1970). Catheterization of umbilical vessels in newborn infants. *Pediatric Clinics of North America*, *17*, 895–896.
30. Klaus, M. H., & Fanaroff, A. (1979). *Care of the high risk neonate* (2nd ed.). London: W. B. Saunders.
31. Korth-Bradley, J. M. (1991). A pharmacokinetic primer for intravenous nurses. *Journal of Intravenous Nursing*, *14*, 124.
32. Levitt, E. (1980). Neonatal IV therapy. *Journal of the National Intravenous Therapy Association*, *3*, 169.

33. Luban, N., & Keating, L. (Eds.). (1983). *Hemotherapy of the infant and premature* (pp. 5–65, 69–80, 95–124). Arlington, VA: American Association of Blood Banks.

34. Manley, L., Haley, K., & Dick, M. (1988). Intraosseous infusion: Rapid vascular access for critically ill or injured infants and children. *Journal of Emergency Nursing, 14,* 63.

35. Markels, S. (1990). Impact on patient care: 2652 PIC catheter days in the alternative setting. *Journal of Intravenous Nursing, 13,* 347.

36. Mattson, D., & O'Connor, M. (1986). Transilluminator assistance in neonatal venipuncture. *Neonatal Network, 4,* 43.

37. Matyskiela-Frey, A. M. (1985). Pediatric dosage calculations. *Journal of the National Intravenous Therapy Association, 8,* 373–379.

38. Meyenfeldt, M., Stapert, J., DeJong, P., Soeters, P. B., Wesdorp, R. I., & Greep, J. M. (1980). TPN catheter sepsis: Lack of effect of subcutaneous tunneling of PVC catheters on sepsis rate. *Journal of Parenteral and Enteral Nutrition, 4,* 514–517.

39. Meyer, H. M. (May 28, 1982). *Letter to Hospital Pharmacists.* Rockville, MD: U.S. Department of Health and Human Services, Federal Drug Administration.

40. Miccolo, M. A. (1990). Intraosseous infusion. *Critical Care Nurse, 10,* 35–47.

41. Mofenseon, H. C. (1988). Guidelines for intraosseous infusions (Letter to the editor). *Journal of Emergency Medicine, 6,* 145–146.

42. Nathan, D., & Oski, F. (Eds.). (1981). *Hematology of infancy and childhood* (pp. 1491–1500). Philadelphia: W. B. Saunders.

43. Piercy, S. (1981). Children on long term IV therapy. *Nursing 81, 11,* 66–69.

44. Plesko, L. (1989). Streamlined catheterization. *Neonatal Intensive Care, 2,* 36, 38.

45. Poole, M. A., Ross, M. N., Haase, G. M., & Odom, L. F. (1991). Right atrial catheters in pediatric oncology: A patient/parent questionnaire study. *American Journal of Pediatric Hematology/Oncology, 13,* 152–155.

46. Rosetti, V., Thompson, B., Miller, J., Mateer, J. R., & Aprahamian, C. (1985). Intraosseous infusion: An alternative route of pediatric intravenous access. *Annals of Emergency Medicine, 14,* 885–888.

47. Shulman, R. J., Pokorny, W. J., Martin, C. G., Pettit, R., Baldaia, L., & Roney, D. (1986). Comparison of percutaneous and surgical placement of central venous catheters in neonates. *Journal of Pediatric Surgery, 21,* 348–350.

48. Teitell, B. C. (1978). *The role of the pediatric TPN nurse with pediatric oncology patients.* Paper presented at ASPENS Third Clinical Congress.

49. Testerman, J. E. (1989). Current trends in pediatric total parenteral nutrition. *Journal of Intravenous Nursing, 12,* 152–162.

50. Third National Cancer Survey. Nutritional Cancer Institute. (1977). *CA—A Cancer Journal for Clinicians* (p. 27). American Cancer Society.

51. *Transfusion therapy guidelines for nurses.* (1990). National Blood Resource Education Program, Public Health Service, National Institutes of Health, U.S. Department of Health and Human Services.

52. Turkel, H. (1983). Intraosseous infusions (Letter to the editor). *American Journal of Diseases of Children, 137* 706.

53. Viall, C. D. (1990). Your complete guide to central venous catheters, *Nursing 90, 20,* 34.

54. Watson, E. H., & Lowery, G. H. (1958). *Growth and development of children.* Chicago: Year Book Medical Publishers.

55. Weeks-Lozano, H. (1991). Clinical evaluation of Per-Q-Cath for both pediatric and adult home infusion therapy. *Journal of Intravenous Nursing, 14,* 249–256.

56. Weibley, T. T., & Fraze, D. E. (1985). Intravenous Teflon catheter cannulation in the premature infant. *Neonatal Network, 3,* 29–33.

57. Wickham, R. S. (1990). Advances in venous access devices and nursing management strategies. *Nursing Clinics of North America, 25,* 345–364.

58. Zenk, K. E. (1986) Administering IV antibiotics to children. *Nursing 86, 16,* 50–52.

REVIEW QUESTIONS

1. When starting an IV in a toddler, the best approach would be:
   a. "Let's go and start your IV now."
   b. "You were bad, so we're going to give you a needle."
   c. "Where do you want your IV?"
   d. "Can we start your IV now?"

2. The scalp would be an ideal site for IV access in which of the following children?
   a. a neonate with gastroschesis
   b. a 2-month-old with hydrocephalus
   c. a 20-month-old with leukemia
   d. a 16-month-old in respiratory arrest

3. The IV catheter gauge ideal for most pediatric patients is which of the following?
   a. 16
   b. 18
   c. 20
   d. 24

4. The ideal place to start an IV in a child is:
   a. at the bedside
   b. in the treatment room
   c. in the mother's lap
   d. in the home of the patient

5. After two attempts at IV access during resuscitative efforts, the following site should be used:
   a. intraosseous
   b. intrathecal
   c. intra-arterial
   d. intracardiac

6. An IV site unique to the neonatal population is the:
   a. scalp
   b. foot
   c. abdomen
   d. umbilicus

7. For long-term intermittent access in an adolescent, the central access device of choice would be the:
   a. Broviac catheter
   b. Hickman catheter
   c. subclavian catheter
   d. implanted port

8. The best method for calculating fluid therapy for a child is:
   a. caloric method
   b. weight method
   c. age method
   d. meter squared method

9. Criteria for infusion of TPN include:
   a. low serum albumin
   b. high lymphocyte count
   c. growth ratio below 50th percentile
   d. low protein-to-fat ratio

10. The purpose of neonatal exchange transfusion is to:
   a. elevate neutrophil count
   b. prevent congestive heart failure
   c. lower bilirubin level
   d. change blood type

CHAPTER 26

Home Infusion Therapy

GROWTH OF HOME CARE

The growth of home infusion therapy and alternative site treatment has opened countless opportunities for IV nurses nationwide. This growth is the product of social, economic, and political forces that have shaped our overall system for delivering health care.

Nationally, home care is a growing enterprise. The United States Commerce Department calls it one of the fastest growing sectors of the medical market.

CONTRIBUTING FACTORS

Present growth is attributed to an expanding aging population, advances in technology, and changes in reimbursement policies. As the over-65 population increases from less than 12% of the total population to 21% by the year 2030, this group will see rapid growth. By the year 2020, baby boomers will reach age 85 and older and could number 9 million. Medical technology has allowed many procedures and treatments that once were confined to the hospital to be provided safely and effectively in the home. Changes in federal policy in the early 1980s eliminated limits on the number of home nursing visits that could be provided, liberalized the requirement for prior hospitalization, and allowed proprietary home health agencies to become Medicare-certified in states without home health licensure laws. Pressure from private payors and managed care companies has contributed to the growth of home infusion care.

HOME INFUSION PROGRAMS

Home infusion programs may function under the auspices of any number of parent organizations. State and county health departments are the most commonly used example of governmental agencies providing home health care services. Visiting nurse associations have always been providers of extensive Medicare services to clients in need. Proprietary agencies provide services on a fee-for-service basis to private individuals. Until 1981, such companies were precluded from participation in the Medicare program. Agencies under the controlling authority of local hospitals or conducted as joint ventures are generally hospital-based programs.

Sharon M. Weinstein: PLUMER'S PRINCIPLES & PRACTICE OF INTRAVENOUS THERAPY, FIFTH EDITION, © 1993 J. B. Lippincott Company

NURSING SUPPORT

Nursing support begins at the time of hospitalization with the key words "discharge planning." Never before has this been truer, as patients move from the security of the inpatient environment to assume responsibility for self-care in the comfort of their places of residence.

The *home care coordinator* is involved in identification of appropriate candidates for home infusion therapies. The inpatient teaching program is consistent with the type of therapy ordered and includes line management, dressing changes, flushing, hookup and disconnect, handling of equipment, aseptic technique, emergency interventions, recognition of signs and symptoms of possible complications, handling of inventory, and pump management. Specific teaching packets should be provided. Patients are not medical professionals, a teaching plan specific to the patient's individualized needs is essential. Language barriers often inhibit otherwise successful teaching programs. Every effort should be made to address the patient in language he or she best understands. Figures 26-1 through 26-3 provide examples of IV teaching in various languages. Final coordination with the supplier is made before discharge to ensure safe, timely arrival of pump, solutions, and related equipment.

The *home infusion nurse* is responsible for the care of the patient in the person's

¿Cómo está? Soy la enfermera encargada de administrarle el suero intravenoso.

▲ **HELLO, I AM YOUR I.V. NURSE. (FEMALE)**

Como esta? Soy el enfermero encargado de administrarle el suero intravenoso.

▲ **HELLO, I AM YOUR I.V. NURSE. (MALE)**

Vengo a revisarle la aguja del suero intravenoso.

▲ **I AM HERE TO CHECK YOUR I.V.**

Voy a aplicarle el suero intravenoso.

▲ **I AM HERE TO START YOUR I.V.**

Le cambiaremos la aguja intravenoso de lugar cada (2) - (3) dias.

▲ **WE CHANGE THE I.V. SITE EVERY (2) - (3) DAYS.**

Le duele en donde tiene inyectada la aguja intravenosa?   Si   No

▲ **DO YOU HAVE PAIN AT YOUR I.V. SITE?**   **YES**   **NO**

Tengo que cambiarle el lugar de la aguja intravenosa debido a que:

▲ **I NEED TO CHANGE YOUR I.V. TODAY BECAUSE OF:**

(a) le duele,	(b) tiene inflamacion,	(c) tiene la piel roja,	(d) es un procedimiento de rutina.
▲ **(A) PAIN**	**(B) SWELLING**	**(C) REDNESS**	**(D) ROUTINE**

Si le duele o si se le inflama el lugar donde tiene la aguja del suero intravenoso, hagaselo saber a la enfermera.

▲ **IF PAIN OR SWELLING BEGINS, TELL YOUR NURSE.**

SPANISH

FIGURE 26-1 Language for IV patient teaching: Spanish. (Courtesy: Jaclyn Tropp, CRNI)

Guten Tag/ Abend, ich bin die Krankenschwester zuständig für die Infusion.
▲ **HELLO, I AM YOUR I.V. NURSE. (FEMALE)**

Guten Tag/ Abend, ich bin der Krankenpfleger zuständig für die Infusion.
▲ **HELLO, I AM YOUR I.V. NURSE. (MALE)**

Ich muss Ihre Infusion kontrollieren.
▲ **I AM HERE TO CHECK YOUR I.V.**

Ich muss Ihen eine Infusion geben.
▲ **I AM HERE TO START YOUR I.V.**

Wir wechseln die Infusionsstelle alle (2) - (3) Tage.
▲ **WE CHANGE THE I.V. SITE EVERY (2) - (3) DAYS.**

Haben Sie Schmerzen an der Infusionsstelle?   Ja   Nein
▲ **DO YOU HAVE PAIN AT YOUR I.V. SITE?**   **YES**   **NO**

Ich muss heute Ihre Infusionsstelle wechseln, wegen:
▲ **I NEED TO   CHANGE YOUR I.V. TODAY BECAUSE OF:**

(a) Schmerzen   (b) Schwellung   (c) Rötung   (d) Routinemässig
▲ **(A) PAIN**   **(B) SWELLING**   **(C) REDNESS**   **(D) ROUTINE**

Wenn Schmerzen auftreten oder Rotung beginnt, teilen Sie das bitte der Krankenschwester mit.
▲ **IF PAIN OR SWELLING BEGINS, TELL YOUR NURSE.**

GERMAN

FIGURE 26-2   Language for IV patient teaching: German. (Courtesy: Jaclyn Tropp, CRNI)

place of residence. If not affiliated with the hospital itself, skill levels of home infusion nurses should be qualified and documented. Care delivered by a credentialed IV nurse is preferred.

POLICIES AND PROCEDURES

Policies and procedures for the provision of home infusion services must be consistent with published Standards of Practice. Guidelines are provided by two accrediting bodies: the Joint Commission on Accreditation of Healthcare Organizations (JCAHO), and the Community Health Accreditation Program (CHAP) of the National League for Nursing (NLN).

Procedures must be comprehensive and address all infusion therapies provided as well as the governing body and management of the organization. Reviewers from both the accrediting bodies and the Medicare program (if a Medicare-certified agency) may inspect agency documents without prior notification. The home infusion therapy program must be found consistent with the organization's philosophy and purpose. A qualified professional must be responsible for the direction, coordination, and general

Come va? Io sono la sua infermiera.

▲ **HELLO, I AM YOUR I.V. NURSE. (FEMALE)**

Come va? Io sono il suo infermiere.

▲ **HELLO, I AM YOUR I.V. NURSE. (MALE)**

Sono qui per controllare la sua flebo.

▲ **I AM HERE TO CHECK YOUR I.V.**

Sono qui per metterle la flebo.

▲ **I AM HERE TO START YOUR I.V.**

Noi cambiamo di posto la flebo ogni (due) - (tre) giorni.

▲ **WE CHANGE THE I.V. SITE EVERY (2) - (3) DAYS.**

Li fa male dove sta la flebo?	Si	No
▲ **DO YOU HAVE PAIN AT YOUR I.V. SITE?**	**YES**	**NO**

Devo cambiarle la flebo oggi a causa di:

▲ **I NEED TO   CHANGE YOUR I.V. TODAY BECAUSE OF:**

(a) dolore,	(b) gonfiore,	(c) rossore,	(d) giro giornaliero.
▲ **(A) PAIN**	**(B) SWELLING**	**(C) REDNESS**	**(D) ROUTINE**

Se le fa male, o se comincia a gonfiaresi, lo dica all'infermiera.

▲ **IF PAIN OR SWELLING BEGINS, TELL YOUR NURSE.**

ITALIAN

FIGURE 26-3 Language for IV patient teaching: Italian. (Courtesy: Jaclyn Tropp, CRNI)

supervision of all professional services. Infusion nursing care must be provided by a registered professional nurse; must be in accordance with the client's plan of treatment; and must include comprehensive health and psychosocial evaluation, monitoring of the client's condition, teaching and training activities in the self-administration of medications given IV, subcutaneously, or intraspinally, and provide for the overall well-being of the client. Necessary drugs, biologicals, equipment, and supplies may be provided directly by the organization or by arrangement. Services must be coordinated with a designated case manager for each client who is responsible for ensuring that the following activities occur:

1. Initial assessment of the individual, family, and home environment
2. Development of a plan of care
3. Appropriate referral and follow-up
4. Coordination of services
5. Implementation of the plan of care
6. Ongoing evaluation
7. Plan for termination of care

STAFF DEVELOPMENT

Infusion therapy case managers are selected for their expertise and experience. The ability to provide intensive care services to patients in their places of residence is essential. The job description and evaluation process for this nursing professional must encompass the need for further development and education to remain abreast of the latest technologies, equipment, and infusion therapy procedures. Nurses providing home infusion therapy should work with mentors who can enable them to grow personally and professionally within their chosen fields.

AVAILABLE RESOURCES

The resources of professional societies and the role that such organizations play in staff development cannot be overlooked. These societies provide the collegiality and professional camaraderie that enable nurses to grow in this rapidly changing field. Intravenous nursing professionals should be encouraged to participate in such organizations on national and local levels. They should be encouraged to publish case studies about their success stories in home infusion care and to share their knowledge and expertise with others.

HOME INFUSION THERAPIES

The majority of IV procedures provided in the hospital can likewise be provided in the home. Home infusion therapies are diverse and encompass many modalities for patient care, including antibiotics, nutritional support, hydration, pain management, antiemetics, antineoplastics, blood and component therapy, venous sampling, and IV drugs such as cardiovascular agents, growth hormones, and colony-stimulating factors.

Antibiotics

Antibiotic therapy is an established procedure in the confines of one's home. Newer technology and the development of more potent β-lactam antibiotics have facilitated the growth of this treatment modality. To qualify for service, the patient should be medically stable, the infection should be one that can be treated on an outpatient basis, the patient

---

Available Resources to Assist in the Development of a Home Infusion Program

American Association of Blood Banks (AABB)
American Society of Hospital Pharmacists (ASHP)
American Society for Parenteral and Enteral Nutrition (ASPEN)
Community Health Accreditation Program (CHAP)
Intravenous Nurses Society (INS)
Joint Commission on Accreditation of Healthcare Organizations (JCAHO)
National Association for Home Care (NAHC)
Oncology Nursing Society (ONS)

should be compliant, and reliable venous access should be available. As with any drug, the first dose should be administered in a monitored clinical setting.

Nutritional Support

The advent of home parenteral nutrition (HPN) in the 1960s enabled physicians to support intestinally handicapped patients for indefinite time periods. Technical barriers to HPN have diminished over time. Advanced products, catheters, and technologies have enabled us to provide advanced nutritional support to patients with appropriate diagnoses. If the patient is receiving care under the Medicare program, the test of permanence must be met, and the patient must be in need of HPN for 90 days or more.

Usually administered as a cyclic infusion in the home setting, the patient receives a full day's requirement of fluid, glucose, lipid, and other nutrients over a shorter 10- to 12-hour period. (See Chapter 20.)

Hydration

The ability to maintain fluid balance in the patient in the place of residence is the goal of home hydration therapy. Hydration may also be given to augment the HPN program by providing supplemental potassium or insulin, or be implemented to prehydrate the patient in need of a cardiac fluid challenge or antineoplastic agent. Long-term administration of multiple electrolyte solutions is also possible.

Pain Management

Continuous or intermittent self-administration of IV analgesics in the home allows those in need to remain with their families with a degree of comfort not previously available. Again, manufacturers have kept pace with demands for more sophisticated equipment to ensure safe administration of these drugs in an unmonitored environment. Pain medications may be administered by a patient-controlled analgesia (PCA) or portable pump, through IV, intrathecal, epidural, subcutaneous, or other routes of administration. (See Chapter 23.)

Applicable Diagnoses for Home Total Parenteral Nutrition

Kwashiorkor
Nutritional marasmus
Other severe protein–calorie malnutrition
Malnutrition
Unspecified vitamin deficiency or other nutritional deficiency
Disorders for amino acid transport and metabolism
Intestinal disaccharidase deficiences/malabsorption
Disorders of lipid metabolism

Disorders of fluid, electrolyte, and acid–base balance
Cystic fibrosis
Disorders involving the immune mechanism
Anorexia nervosa
Nutritional and metabolic cardiomyopathy
Obstruction of duodenum
Regional enteritis
Idiopathic proctocolitis
Chronic liver disease and cirrhosis
Postsurgical nonabsorption
Cancer cachexia

Antiemetics

Antiemetic protocols aimed at intermittent infusion have facilitated the care of the patient in need of antineoplastic therapies and ensured patient comfort to a new level of care. A diversity of protocols provide antiemetic infusions as a single-agent treatment or combined with HPN therapies.

Antineoplastics

Chemotherapeutic agents are administered to patients in their homes by various IV systems. Nonvesicant chemotherapeutic agents are often given through peripheral cannulas, either short- or intermediate-term products. Vesicant and nonvesicant agents are being administered by centrally placed catheters, implanted catheters, and implanted pumps. (See Chapter 24.)

Blood and Component Therapy

Transfusions of blood and blood components are now performed on home patients. Compatible blood is taken to the home and transfused under the direction of a professional nurse. Policies and procedures for this type of service entail development of methods of securing the component, billing for service, remaining with the patient for the duration of the transfusion, emergency measures, transport of the blood/blood product, and follow-up. As with all therapies, the same level of care provided to patients in the inpatient setting is provided to patients in their residences. (See Chapter 21.)

Venous Sampling

Venous sampling for all types of laboratory testing is available in home infusion programs. Peak and trough levels, chemistry panels for the HPN patient, white blood cell counts for the oncology patient, and a diversity of other tests may be performed. Venous samples may be drawn through peripheral venipuncture, existing line, or central line sampling. As with all home procedures, care must be taken to ensure the safe handling and disposal of medical waste.

Intravenous Drug Administration

Intravenous drug administration is a rapidly growing area of home infusion therapy. Intravenous drugs administered in the home care setting include cardiovascular drugs, antihypertensive agents, heparin, interferon, colony-stimulating factors, chelation therapy (deferoxamine), growth hormone, gamma globulin, and others. Again, first dosing should occur in a clinically monitored environment. Emergency drugs should be readily available, and protocols for their use should be established in written policies and procedures.

CANDIDATES FOR HOME INFUSION THERAPY

The criteria used for patient selection play a key role in the success or failure of a home infusion therapy program. Patients are deemed appropriate based on an evaluation of certain parameters, including physical factors such as diagnosis and medical stability, venous access, drug therapy, laboratory profile, support system, educability, visual acuity, manual dexterity, and financial resources or limitations to treatment. Once the referral to home care has been made, the referral checklist or similar document should be initiated (Figure 26-4).

Diagnosis

The home infusion therapy ordered must be consistent with the patient's diagnosis and ability to be treated in an alternative care setting. Common diagnoses for antibiotic therapy include osteomyelitis, otitis media, sinusitis, cryptococcal meningitis, pneumonia, subacute bacterial endocarditis, primary bacteremia, cellulitis, urinary tract infection, pyelonephritis, septic arthritis, histoplasmosis, peritonitis, toxic shock syndrome, Lyme disease, rickettsial infection, acquired immunodeficiency syndrome (AIDS)-related opportunistic infections, and others.

All types of cancer patients are appropriate candidates for home infusion of antineoplastic agents, especially combination protocols. Many third-party payors restrict reimbursement for antineoplastic agents to the alternative care setting and have set limits on inpatient treatments. Even if treatment is initiated on an inpatient basis, the protocol that was started or the investigational treatment may be continued in the home care setting. Related infusion therapies for the oncology patient might include nutritional support, IV pain management, antiemetics, leucovorin rescue regimens, and intraperitoneal protocols.

Medical Stability

Medical stability is essential if patients are to perform all required procedures themselves. If a patient is not medically stable but has medical approval for home care, a family member may assume full responsibility for performing all techniques. A backup person may be needed, depending on the individual home situation. Policies and procedures outlining medical stability must be developed and approved by the home care provider's medical board. Such a policy might indicate that the patient must be afebrile for the 24-hour period before discharge, or if febrile, the patient must be on antibiotics that have been started as an inpatient. The patient should have a comprehensive assessment before leaving the hospital (Figure 26-5).

Vascular Access

Vascular access appropriate to the planned course of treatment is essential if the home infusion program is to be a success. Home nutritional support is best given through an acceptable central venous access route. When IV nurses are involved in product selection, the patient's clinical needs will be met. Use of a dual-lumen port or tunneled line is helpful and should be encouraged. Measures must be in place to deal with the potential for cannula occlusion, and appropriate drugs such as urokinase should be readily available. Teaching protocols for line management will vary with the type of access involved. Teaching plans must be patient specific and address all areas of maintenance and self-care (Figure 26-6).

Drug Therapy

Often the type of drug therapy ordered will determine the appropriateness of a candidate for the home infusion program. Most drugs given in the inpatient setting are also acceptable in a home infusion program. Dobutamine, for example, requires frequent

(*text continues on page 565*)

Home Infusion Referral Checklist

Home Care Provider:

[ ] _____

[ ] _____

INFORMATION TO:	DATE/INITIAL

INFORMATION TO:

A. DISCHARGE PLANNER INFORMED _____

B. IV TEAM INFORMED _____

C. HOME AGENCY INFORMED: _____

Name of agency _____

Address _____

Phone # _____ FAX # _____

Local contact _____

D. LOCAL PHYSICIAN IDENTIFIED (if applicable) _____

Name _____

Address _____

Phone # _____ FAX # _____

TYPE OF REFERRAL:

A. Parenteral nutrition _____

B. Enteral nutrition _____

C. IV antibiotics _____

D. Pain management _____

E. Nupogen _____

F. Chemotherapy _____

G. Catheter care _____

H. Other _____ _____

TEACHING COMPLETED:

A. HOME INFUSION _____ _____

B. SUBCLAVIAN/CATHETER CARE _____

[ ] Port   Type _____

[ ] Hickman/Groshong   [ ] Subclavian   [ ] Other _____

Lumens _____

SUPPLIES NEEDED FROM HOSPITAL UPON DISCHARGE:

_____

_____

_____

_____

DELIVERY DATE _____   START OF INFUSION _____

DATE OF REFERRAL FROM PHYSICIAN _____   DATE OF DISCHARGE _____

SIGNATURE/INITIAL _____ ____   TITLE _____

_____ ____   _____

_____ ____   _____

FIGURE 26-4 Home Infusion Referral Checklist.

CLINICAL HOMECARE LTD.
70 NEW DUTCH LANE, FAIRFIELD, NJ 07004
(201) 227-0222   1-800-955-9922

INITIAL PATIENT ASSESSMENT
(page one)

DATE: ___ — ___ — ___

PATIENT DATA

PATIENT NAME	SIGNIFICANT OTHER/CAREGIVER

ADDRESS

PHONE

BIOGRAPHICAL DATA

M.D.	MARITAL STATUS	DEPENDENTS	S.S. #	CLINICIAN
ADDRESS	OCCUPATION			
PHONE	D.O.B.	AGE		R.N.

HISTORY

CURRENT DIAGNOSIS

ALLERGIES

CURRENT THERAPY	GOALS/ANTICIPATED DURATION OF THERAPY

CHIEF COMPLAINTS

HISTORY/PERTINENT MEDICAL/SURGICAL DATA

REVIEW OF SYSTEMS/NURSING DIAGNOSIS

VITAL SIGNS: _____ PULSE: _____ BP: _____ RESP: _____

WEIGHT: _____   HEIGHT: _____

COMMENTS:

HEAD/NECK: ☐ WNL   ☐ MASSES   COMMENTS/DIAGNOSIS
☐ PAIN   ☐ TENDERNESS
☐ WOUNDS ☐ DRAINAGE ☐ SWELLING

GI: ☐ WNL   ☐ NAUSEA   ☐ VOMITING   COMMENTS/DIAGNOSIS
☐ ANOREXIA ☐ BLEEDING ☐ PAIN ☐ ASCITES
ABN
☐ CONSTIPATION ☐ DIARRHEA ☐ BOWEL ☐ MASSES
SOUNDS
☐ DISTENTION ☐ HERNIA ☐ OSTOMY

NEURO: ☐ WNL   ☐ HEADACHE   COMMENTS/DIAGNOSIS
☐ TREMORS ☐ VERTIGO ☐ ATAXIA ☐ APRAXIA
☐ APHASIA   ☐ PARESIS   ☐ SYNCOPE
☐ SEISURES
☐ EPISODES OF UNCONSCIOUSNESS

RESPIRATORY: ☐ WNL   ☐ TRACH   TRACH CARE:
☐ DYSPNEA   ☐ SOB   ☐ ORTHOPNEA
☐ CYANOSIS ☐ ABN LUNG SOUNDS ☐ COUGH   COMMENTS/DIAGNOSIS
☐ SPUTUM   ☐ COLOR   ☐ PAIN
IPPB
☐ O2 AT_____ L MIN/VIA _____☐ USED

G-U: ☐ WNL ☐ FREQUENCY   COMMENTS/DIAGNOSIS
☐ URGENCY ☐ PAIN ☐ BURNING ☐ OSTOMY
EXTERNAL
☐ RETENTION ☐ INCONTINENCE ☐ CATH
INDWELLING   CATH
☐ CATH   ☐ CHANGED   SIZE_____
☐ CATH IRRIGATION ☐ ABN APPEAR. OF URINE

MUSCULO-SKELETAL: ☐ WNL   COMMENTS/DIAGNOSIS
☐ RIGIDITY   ☐ STIFFNESS   ☐ ROM LOSS
☐ JOINT   ☐ SWELLING   ☐ PAIN

NUTRITION: ☐ WNL   ☐ SPECIAL DIET   COMMENTS/DIAGNOSIS
☐ DIET NOT UNDERSTOOD ☐ DIET NOT FOLLOWED
☐ INADEQUATE NURTRITION
☐ INADEQUATE FLUID INTAKE
☐ CHEWING PROBLEM ☐ WEIGHT LOSS

CARDIOVASCULAR: COMMENTS/DIAGNOSIS
☐ WNL ☐ EDEMA
☐ PALPITATIONS ☐ FAINTING ☐ CYANOSIS
☐ NECK VEIN DISTENTION   ☐ CHEST PAIN
POOR
HEART SOUNDS: ☐ QUALITY ☐ IRREGULAR
☐ PERIPHERAL PULSES: ☐ PRESENT ☐ ABSENT
☐ PACEMAKER   RATE_____
☐ MURMUR ☐ GALLOP
☐ **VASCULAR ACCESS**

ENDOCRINE: ☐ WNL   ☐ SWEATING   COMMENTS/DIAGNOSIS
☐ BLURRED VISION   ☐ POLYURIA
☐ POLYDIPSIA   ☐ INSULIN REACTION
☐ URINE S/A

SKIN: ☐ WNL ☐ RASH ☐ JAUNDICE   WOUND CARE:
☐ PRURTIUS   ☐ POOR SKIN CARE
☐ POOR SKIN TURGOR ☐ BRUISES ☐ DECUBITUS   COMMENTS/DIAGNOSIS
WOUND LOCATION _____
MEASUREMENTS _____
STAGE _____

FIGURE 26-5   Initial patient assessment form. (Courtesy: Clinical Homecare Ltd., Fairfield, NJ).

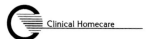 Clinical Homecare

INITIAL PATIENT ASSESSEMENT
(page two)

PATIENT NAME	DATE	PERSON COMPLETING FORM	CLINCIAN

MEDICATION PROFILE

CURRENT MEDICATIONS _____

PAST MEDICATIONS _____
ALLERGIES _____

PATHOLOGICAL COMPLICATIONS: ☐ GI ☐ RENAL ☐ HEPATIC ☐ NEUROLOGICAL ☐ DERMATOLOGICAL ☐ OTHER _____ NAME OF PERSON ADMINISTERING MEDICATIONS _____

UNDERSTANDS MEDICATION AND DOSAGE SCHEDULES ☐ YES ☐ NO   COMPLIANCE WITH MEDICATION REGIMEN: ☐ YES   ☐ NO

NURSING DIAGNOSIS	COMMENTS

PSYCHOSOCIAL ASSESSMENT

☐ SOCIAL SUPPORT SYSTEMS ADEQUATE ☐ POOR/UNSAFE PSYCHOSOCIAL CLIMATE   ☐ NEED FOR ANCILLARY SERVICES: TYPE: _____

CAREGIVER: ☐ AVAILABLE   ☐ LIVES IN RESIDENCE   ☐ AVAILABLE AT ALL TIMES IN CASE OF EMERGENCY/EQUIPMENT MALFUNCTION

☐ FAMILY INVOLVED AT LEVEL POSSIBLE _____

NURSING DIAGNOSIS	COMMENTS

FUNCTIONAL LIMITATIONS/SAFETY FACTORS ASSESSMENT

FUNCTIONAL STATUS/SAFETY FACTORS: ☐ APPROPRIATE FOR HOME CARE ☐ OTHER _____
☐ PHYSICAL IMPAIRMENTS: ☐ MENTAL STATUS ☐ HEARING ☐ EYESIGHT ☐ SPEAKING ☐ DEXTERITY ☐ AMBULATIONS ☐ OTHER _____

NURSING DIAGNOSIS	COMMENTS

ENVIRONMENTAL/SAFETY FACTORS ASSESSMENT

ENVIRONMENT: ☐ SAFE/APPROPRIATE/ADEQUATE FOR PRESCRIBED THERAPY ☐ OTHER _____
ADEQUATE: ☐ ROOM FOR SAFE MOBILIZATION & EQUIP. ☐ STORAGE SPACE ☐ ELECTRICAL/OUTLETS ☐ REFRIG/APPLIANCES ☐ PHONE ☐ CLEAN WORKING AREA

NURSING DIAGNOSIS	COMMENTS

COGNITIVE/TECHNICAL SKILLS ASSESSMENT (Rate on scale of 1 to 10, 10=Above Average, 5=Average, 1=Below Average)

_____ ABILITY TO UNDERSTAND INSTRUCTIONS/PROCEDURES   _____ ABILITY TO PERFORM TECHNICAL PROCEDURES WITH APPROPRIATE TECHNIQUE
_____ ABILITY TO COMMUNICATE EFFECTIVELY AND APPROPRIATELY   _____ OVERALL COGNITIVE/TECHNICAL SKILLS

NURSING DIAGNOSIS	COMMENTS

THERAPY

THERAPY (PRESCRIPTIONS, DRUGS, EQUIPMENT, SUPPLIES ORDERED)

NURSING IMPRESSIONS/RECOMMENDATIONS

PLAN

FIGURE 26-5 (Continued)

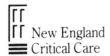

New England Critical Care

PATIENT TEACHING CHECKLIST/ CERTIFICATION OF INSTRUCTION

PATIENT NAME: _____

CAREGIVER: _____

TYPE OF THERAPY: _____

DATE: _____

CONTENT (Check all that apply) (Fill in blanks as indicated)	THEORY/SKILL REVIEWED (INITIAL/DATE)	RETURN DEMONSTRATION COMPLETED (INITIAL/DATE)	SUMMARY/COMMENTS RE: PATIENT/CAREGIVER'S SUCCESS WITH TEACHING
1. Reason for Therapy_____			
2. **Drug/Solution**_____			
☐ Dose _____			
☐ Schedule _____			
☐ Label Accuracy _____			
☐ Storage _____			
☐ Container Integrity _____			
☐ Side Effects _____			
3. Aseptic Technique _____			
☐ Handwashing _____			
☐ Prepping Caps/Connections _____			
☐ Tubing/Cap/Needle Changes _____			
4. Access Device Maintenance _____			
Type/Name: _____			
☐ Device/Site Inspection _____			
☐ Site Care/Dsg. Changes _____			
☐ Catheter Clamping _____			
☐ Maintaining Patency _____			
☐ Saline Flushing _____			
☐ Heparin Locking _____			
☐ Fdg. Tube Declogging _____			
☐ Self Insertion of Device _____			
5. Drug Preparation _____			
☐ Premixed Containers _____			
☐ Compounding ☐ Recipe _____			
☐ 3:1 Lipid Transfer _____			
6. Method of Administration _____			
☐ Gravity _____			
☐ **Pump (Name):** _____			
☐ Continuous ☐ Intermittent _____			
☐ Cycle/Taper: _____			
7. Administration Technique _____			
☐ Pump Rate/Calibration _____			
☐ Priming Tubing ☐ Filter _____			
☐ Filling Syringe _____			
☐ Loading Pump _____			
☐ Access Device Hookup/Disconnect _____			
☐ Head Elevation _____			
8. Potential Complications _____			
☐ Pump Alarms/Troubleshooting _____			
☐ Phlebitis/Infiltration _____			
☐ Clotting/Dislodgement _____			
☐ Infection ☐ Air Embolus _____			
☐ Breakage/Cracking _____			
☐ Electrolyte Imbalance _____			
☐ Fluid Balance _____			
☐ Glucose Intolerance _____			
☐ Aspiration _____			
☐ N/V/D/Cramping _____			
☐ Other: _____			

FIGURE 26-6 Patient teaching checklist. (Reprinted with permission from Oncology Nursing Press. Coker, M., & Lampert, A. [1990]. *Oncology Nursing Forum, 17*[6], 923–925.)

CONTENT (Check all that apply) (Fill in blanks as indicated)	THEORY/SKILL REVIEWED (INITIAL/DATE)	RETURN DEMONSTRATION COMPLETED (INITIAL/DATE)	SUMMARY/COMMENTS RE: PATIENT/CAREGIVER'S SUCCESS WITH TEACHING
9. Self Monitoring: _____ ☐ Weight ☐ Temperature _____ ☐ I & O ☐ Urine S & A _____ ☐ Fingersticks _____ ☐ Other: _____			
10. Supply Handling/Disposal _____ ☐ Disposal of Sharps _____ ☐ Disposal of Supplies _____ ☐ Cleaning Pump _____ ☐ Changing Batteries _____ ☐ Blood/Fluid Precautions _____ ☐ Chemo/Spill Precautions _____			
11. ☐ Electrical Safety _____			
12. Contact Information Given to Patient Re: _____ ☐ Inventory Checks _____ ☐ Deliveries _____ ☐ Nursing _____ ☐ Reimbursement _____ ☐ Service Complaints _____			
13. Written instructions/phone numbers given to patient ☐ Yes ☐ No If No/Why: _____			

NURSE'S INITIAL	SIGNATURE	NURSE'S INITIAL	SIGNATURE

CERTIFICATION OF INSTRUCTION

I agree that I have been instructed as described above and understand that the above functions will be performed in the home, outside a hospital or medically supervised environment.

_____
PATIENT/LEGAL GUARDIAN SIGNATURE   DATE

_____
CAREGIVER'S SIGNATURE (IF NOT PATIENT)   DATE

_____ RN
WITNESS (NECC NURSE)   DATE

FIGURE 26-6   (Continued)

electrocardiographic monitoring; this may easily be accomplished in a full-service home care program.

Laboratory Profile

Procedures must be in place for routine laboratory work-ups and transmission of reports of such studies to the ordering physician. Changes in laboratory values, including panic values, should be reported immediately and adjustments made in the treatment plan consistent with the patient's clinical condition. Laboratory testing for the HPN patient might include twice-weekly chemistry profiles, transferrin levels, and application of an anergy panel (Multitest) 2 days before resuming antineoplastic therapy. The patient receiving antibiotic or antifungal agents might require routine peak and trough levels, blood cultures, and white blood cell counts.

Support System

The patient's life-style is an important consideration. If removed from a controlled hospital environment, will the patient be responsible for avoiding potentially dangerous situations? Does the patient live alone or with a family member who can provide the emotional support needed for a successful course of treatment? The home setting should be evaluated for safety, availability of clean and dry storage for supplies or refrigeration for drugs and supplies, and sufficient space to permit privacy while performing procedures. Safe ambulation, adequacy of outlets, convertors, and battery power for ambulatory drug delivery systems are all important factors to be considered. Emotional stability and individual level of motivation with a desire to be involved in self-care are essential to the success of treatment.

Educability

Principles of adult learning must be considered when assessing appropriateness for home infusion therapy. The patient should be capable of learning and performing all procedures. Ideally, with the educational process initiated at the time of admission and early identification of potential home infusion candidates, the teaching process will be enhanced and learning levels will be high. Illiteracy may be overcome by audio or audiovisual training programs.

Visual Acuity

Visual acuity is required for maintaining sterility and avoiding potential touch contamination of supplies. Magnifying or reading glasses may be required.

Manual Dexterity

Manual dexterity is needed to manipulate supplies and equipment used in the infusion without touch contamination. Manipulation of supplies, Luer connections, junction-securement devices, and Huber needles may present a problem to the patient with arthritis or another degenerative disorder.

Financial Resources

Before acceptance, a patient's insurance benefits are assessed for homecare coverage. Although many patients have outstanding health care benefits for inpatient care, the benefits for home infusion therapy may be limited or nonexistent. Reimbursement for home care services is covered in depth at the close of this chapter.

PLAN OF TREATMENT

The physician, as gatekeeper, writes the plan of treatment for the patient in need of home infusion therapy. The individualized plan, in addition to routine infusion orders, should also define functional limitations, goals of treatment, and duration of treatment; for some modalities, a letter of medical necessity is required.

SELECTING A HOME INFUSION PROVIDER

Discharge planners, home care coordinators, and social workers are involved in the process of selecting a home infusion provider. If the hospital offers its own service or a preferred provider arrangement exists, this process is facilitated. Otherwise, the selection may be an ordeal unless specific criteria have been developed and parameters are followed.

Training

The home infusion provider should be involved in the training process; continuity of care from hospital to home is enhanced when the relationships are developed early and when the patient and family members feel a high degree of confidence in the professional responsible for training and support services. The inpatient training program should be started as early as possible. Training should be individualized and consistent with the patient's needs and the type of therapy or modalities ordered. Training includes line management, dressing changes, infusion techniques, flushing, handling of equipment, sterility, recognition of signs and symptoms of possible complications, handling of inventory, and pump management. Teaching packets and visuals should be provided whenever possible. A teaching plan for the patient should be developed, reviewed, and signed and a copy should become a part of the patient's clinical record. A second copy should accompany the patient to the place of residence. Teaching level and return demonstrations should be validated, as seen in Figure 26-7.

Support

Before discharge, the patient should safely demonstrate the ability to perform all required procedures to comply with the regimen. The patient must have the necessary knowledge for the prevention, recognition, and appropriate action required for any potential complication. The home infusion provider should review the patient's Bill of Rights, Responsibilities for Participation in the Home Infusion Program, and the Assignment of Benefits documents. Final coordination is made before discharge. The nurse should visit the patient on the day of discharge. Supplies should be checked, inventoried, and stored in an appropriate designated area. Support should be provided to the patient and family

Clinical Homecare

Corporate Headquarters: 70 New Dutch Lane, Fairfield, New Jersey 07004

PATIENT TRAINING RECORD

INITIAL ☐   REVIEW ☐

INSTRUCTED/DEMONSTRATION			COMMENTS
	Instructed	**Demonstrated**	
Storage	☐	☐	
Handwashing	☐	☐	
Preparation of equipment	☐	☐	
Sterile technique	☐	☐	
Aseptic technique	☐	☐	
Adding needle	☐	☐	
Basic nutrients	☐	☐	
Insertion of tubing spike	☐	☐	
Priming tubings	☐	☐	
Use of pump	☐	☐	
Connect catheter to tubing	☐	☐	
IV therapy completion	☐	☐	
Initiation of infusion cap	☐	☐	
Cleansing port	☐	☐	
Flushing catheter	☐	☐	
Heparinization	☐	☐	
Drip rate setting	☐	☐	
Care and observation of entrance site	☐	☐	
Care and observation of exit site	☐	☐	
Dressing Change	☐	☐	
Daily observation	☐	☐	
Temperature taking	☐	☐	
Possible catheter related problems	☐	☐	
Symptoms and signs of complications w/use of IV	☐	☐	
Emergency procedures &	☐	☐	
Disposal of Medical Waste	☐	☐	
Emergency CHC phone #	☐	☐	

RN SIGNATURE _____   DATE

PATIENT SIGNATURE _____   DATE

PLEASE PRINT NAME

FORM #205•192

FIGURE 26-7 Patient training record. (Courtesy: Clinical Homecare Ltd., Fairfield, NJ)

during initial procedures and throughout the duration of treatment. The documentation process should be reviewed with the patient and procedures established for daily monitoring and ongoing support. A monthly report and report of case conferences should be sent to the physician; the hospital may also request copies of these forms. Open lines of communication will enable the infusion provider to meet the patient's current and ongoing needs for care and will ensure a high degree of confidence on the part of the referral source.

Service

The home care program chosen must be a full-service program, one that is able to meet the patient's total needs for nursing, supplies, delivery, inventory, and storage. Such needs should be considered expectations and should be consistent with the highest standards of accrediting organizations. The service must be available on a 24-hour basis, with response time limited to 30 minutes or less.

EQUIPMENT NEEDS

Equipment needs in the home infusion program will vary with the type of therapy ordered and the need for electronic infusion instrumentation. When a single modality, such as antibiotic therapy, has been ordered, the supply needs are simple. More complex regimens, such as HPN, require additional supplies and equipment. Typical supply needs for starting and continuing the patient on various therapies are found in Figures 26-8 and 26-9. Various electronic instruments are available for infusion purposes in the alternative care setting. Backup support should be available on a 24-hour basis in the event of pump or product failure.

COMPLIANCE

Positive outcomes should be the treatment goal—restoring the patient to a functional capacity and enabling the patient and family to return to a functional level consistent with the stage of disease and its process are essential. Outcome measurements, based on those developed by JCAHO and CHAP, enhance the level of care provided and ensure excellence. Ongoing monitoring of the patient's status is needed; compliance with the protocol is evaluated and documented. The compliant patient administers the drugs and treatments as ordered; follows aseptic practice; reports signs and symptoms of complications; monitors and records weights, temperature, urine glucose determinations, and other parameters; and delights in the ability to provide self-care.

PATIENT'S ROLE IN HOME CARE

The patient is responsible for specific aspects of this care, including compliance, monitoring, line management, operation of electronic infusion equipment, and other duties. The patient, before acceptance into a home infusion program, is responsible for knowing patient rights and responsibilities (Figure 26-10). In addition to signing a copy of these responsibilities and acknowledging receipt of that information, the patient is also asked to sign an agreement and consent for services (Figure 26-11). In this way, the patient is

---

PATIENT STARTUP
• PAIN MANAGEMENT
• CADD 5800

BAGS: Drug Cassette _____ Amt. _____ Other _____ Amt. _____

PUMP: Type - CADD PCA SERIAL #

Special Delivery Instructions:

      On all portacath patients, send Solopak heparin and Solopak saline - 5cc

      On all subclavian catheter patients, send Solopak heparin and Solopak - 3cc

---

QTY./EA.   DESCRIPTION   CODE #

ROUTE OF ADMINISTRATION: [ ] PORT   [ ] SUBCLAV.   [ ] INTRATHECAL   [ ] EPIDURAL

QTY./EA.	DESCRIPTION
SAB	CADD 5800 extension
1 BX (I)	ALCOHOL PREPS
1 BX (I)	**POVIDONE PREPS**
2-3	DRESSING KIT
1 (I)	SHARPS CONTAINER
1 (I)	MAIL CONTAINER FOR RETURN OF SHARPS
1 ROLL (I)	1" HYTAPE
1 ROLL (I)	TRANSPORE TAPE
14	HEP FLUSH 100U/ML
14	SALINE FLUSH
1 EA. (I)	HIBICLENS
1 EA. (I)	PATIENT MANUAL
1 EA. (I)	CLAMP
6 EA.	CLICK LOCK
6 EA.	CLICK LOCK CAPS
TYPE OF ACCESS:	NEEDLE-SPECIFIC _____

INITIAL SHIPMENT ONLY; MONITOR UTILIZATION PRIOR TO FURTHER SHIPMENT OF THESE PRODUCTS

FIGURE 26-8 Supply list for patient start-up on CADD 5800 for pain management.

made aware of the terms of the agreement and consent for service, release of medical information, and financial responsibility for the services provided. This form may also include an Assignment of Benefits, guaranteeing payment to the provider.

INFECTIOUS WASTE MANAGEMENT

Within the home care program, provisions must be made for handling infectious patient waste. The Environmental Protection Agency (EPA), a federal regulatory board, has developed many advisories regarding infectious waste. With passage of the Medical

(*text continues on page 574*)

PATIENT STARTUP
• TPN
• STATIONARY AVI PUMP

BAGS: Drug Cassette _____ Amt. _____ Other _____ Amt. _____

PUMP: Type - AVI #

Special Delivery Instructions:

On all portacath patients, send Solopak heparin and Solopak saline - 5cc

On all subclavian catheter patients, send Solopak heparin and Solopak - 3cc

QTY./EA.	DESCRIPTION	CODE #

ROUTE OF ADMINISTRATION: [   ] PORT   [   ] SUBCLAV.   [   ] INTRATHECAL   [   ] EPIDURAL

QTY./EA.	DESCRIPTION
SAB	AVI
1 BX (I)	ALCOHOL PREPS
1 BX (I)	**POVIDONE PREPS**
2-3	DRESSING KIT
	MASKS (2 per dressing kit)
1 (I)	SHARPS CONTAINER
1 (I)	MAIL CONTAINER FOR RETURN OF SHARPS
1 ROLL (I)	1" HYTAPE
1 ROLL (I)	TRANSPORE TAPE
14	HEP FLUSH 100U/ML
14	SALINE FLUSH
12 EA. (I)	22 GA. 1" NEEDLE
10 EA. (I)	10CC SYRINGE
4 EA. (I)	22 3/4 PORTA (STANDARD BORE)
1 EA. (I)	HIBICLENS
1 EA. (I)	CLINISTIX
1 EA. (I)	THERMOMETER
1 EA. (I)	PATIENT MANUAL
1 EA. (I)	CLAMP
12 EA.	CLICK LOCK
12 EA.	CLICK LOCK CAPS
1 EA.	3 PRONG OUTFIT ADAPTER
	1.2 MICRON FILTER
1 EA. (I)	I.V. POLE
2 EA.	VENOSET
1 EA.	LITER 5% D/W OR 0.45NS PER ORDER

INITIAL SHIPMENT ONLY; MONITOR UTILIZATION PRIOR TO FURTHER SHIPMENT OF THESE PRODUCTS

FIGURE 26-9 Supply list for patient start-up on stationary AVI pump for TPN.

Clinical Homecare

Corporate Headquarters: 70 New Dutch Lane, Fairfield, New Jersey 07004

PATIENT RESPONSIBILITY

As a patient with Clinical Homecare you have the responsibility to:

1. Provide to the best of your knowledge accurate and complete information about present complaints, past illnesses, past and current treatments and other matters that would affect your treatment plan, and the ability to benefit from services.

2. Report unexpected changes in your condition.

3. Make it known whether you clearly comprehend the treatment plan, services offered, and what is expected of you.

4. Follow the plan of care including instructions given by care providers to implement this plan.

5. Agree to a schedule of services, and if unwilling or unable to comply with this schedule notify Clinical Homecare or your nurse.

6. Accept responsibility for your actions if you refuse treatment or do not comply with staff instructions.

7. Be respectful and considerate of the individual rights of the home care staff.

8. Provide as soon as possible a copy of any advanced directives if applicable, to be included in your medical record.

I understand the above Patient Responsiblities.

X _____   _____   _____
        SIGNATURE   PRINT NAME   DATE

FIGURE 26-10 Form to demonstrate patient's understanding of own responsibility for IV home care. (Courtesy: Clinical Homecare Ltd., Fairfield, NJ)

Clinical Homecare

Corporate Headquarters: 70 New Dutch Lane, Fairfield, New Jersey 07004

AGREEMENT AND CONSENT FOR SERVICES   Page 1 of 2

Patient Name: _____

Terms of Agreement and Consent for Infusion Services: I understand that by signing this agreement, I authorize provision of products and services to me by Clinical Homecare Corporation (CHC). I also understand that I am to remain under the medical care of my attending physician throughout the course of my treatment. My attending physician has explained the risks and benefits of home infusion therapy to me, and has informed me of my rights and responsibilities in the care process, and I fully understand them.

I understand that if I request additional home health services, other than home infusion therapy, CHC may refer me to another provider which is not owned or operated by CHC. In those cases, I will not hold CHC responsible or liable for those services provided by another vendor, and will not hold CHC liable for furnishing me with the names of other home health care providers.

Medical Information Authorization: I authorize my hospital, or physician, or medical agency to provide CHC with any and all records concerning my medical history, services rendered, or treatment received.

Release of Medical Information: I authorize CHC to furnish to my insurance carrier(s) or its agents, any medical information pertaining to my medical history, services rendered, or treatment provided needed to process claims. I also release CHC from responsibility or liability that may arise from the release or reproduction of such information or documents.

Financial Information: I understand that I am financially responsible for all products and services provided by CHC that are not reimbursed by my insurance carrier(s). In the event that my insurance carrier does not accept "assignment of benefits," I understand that correspondence and payments may be sent directly to me. I agree that when such payments are received, I can pay for CHC products and services by either personal check, or by directly endorsing the insurance payment by writing "pay to the order of Clinical Homecare Corp." and my signature.

_____   _____
Signature (Patient or *Guarantor)   Date

_____   _____
Witness   Date

Patient Name: _____

Address: _____

Assignment of Benefits: I authorize direct payment to Clinical Homecare Corp. of any insurance benefits otherwise payable to me for products or services provided. I also authorize my insurance carrier(s) to furnish Clinical Homecare Corp. with any and all information concerning my insurance benefits and status claims submitted by Clinical Homecare Corp.

_____   _____
Signature   Date

_____   _____
Witness   Date

FIGURE 26-11 Form for agreement and consent for infusion services. (Courtesy: Clinical Homecare Ltd., Fairfield, NJ)

Clinical Homecare

Corporate Headquarters: 70 New Dutch Lane, Fairfield, New Jersey 07004

Acceptance of Equipment:

I understand that the equipment listed below, which I have received, is the property of CHC and is being rented to me. I agree to use the equipment in accordance with the instructions provided by the nurse and manufacturer's operating manual. I also agree to return the equipment to CHC in working order and in good condition allowing for reasonable wear and tear within 10 days of the completion of my therapy.

I understand that CHC is not a manufacturer of the equipment and makes no representation or warranties expressed or implied with respect to the merchantability or fitness for a particular purpose of any equipment or supplies otherwise.

I understand that I am responsible for proper wiring of the premises where the equipment is used, for ensuring that the electrical outlets utilized are in good working condition, and for ensuring that the equipment when utilized is properly grounded in accordance with the manufacturer's operating instruction.

In no event shall CHC be liable for special, consequential, or incidental damages, either direct or contingent.

DESCRIPTION/MODEL NAME AND NUMBER   SERIAL NUMBER

_____   _____

_____   _____

Signature (Patient or Guarantor)   Date

_____   _____

Witness   Date

_____

The undersigned certifies that he/she has read the above and received a copy. The undersigned also certifies that he/she is the patient, or is duly authorized by the patient as their general agent to execute the above and accept its terms.

_____   _____

Signature (Patient or Guarantor)   Date

_____   _____

Witness   Date

* If guarantor, state here relationship to patient and reason why patient is unable to sign:

_____

MEDICAL SUPPLIES ARE NOT RETURNABLE FOR CREDIT OR EXCHANGE

FIGURE 26-11   (Continued)

Waste Tracking Act of 1988, Congress mandated to the EPA the investigation and development, if needed, of guidelines for handling home-generated medical waste. The home care provider should establish policies and procedures for handling such waste, particularly when patients reside in more remote, less accessible areas of the country. Prepackaged kits are available from a number of manufacturers and include sharps disposal systems as well as the more sophisticated ChemBLOC Spill Kit (Figure 26-12).

REIMBURSEMENT

Reimbursement for home infusion therapies is somewhat complex and depends on the nature of the business itself. For example, a Medicare-certified home health agency may bill for supplies associated with a Medicare Part A visit; the same agency may not bill under Part A for HPN.

Claims Documents

Claims forms generally encompass the universal billing form number 82 (UB–82) or Health Care Financing Administration (HCFA–1500 for Medicare B claims). The carrier may accept patient identifying information on the HCFA–1500 if accompanied with a UB–82 listing itemized charges. Some payors provide their own billing forms. Most payors require an itemized invoice listing all drugs or nutritional solutions and supplies delivered to the patient in the calendar month billed. A Statement of Medical Necessity is also required along with the physician's prescription for therapy. Pain management prescriptions may require triplicate prescriptions, consistent with the state pharmacy laws in the state in which the product is being mixed. The Assignment of Benefits, as previously discussed, is required to authorize the insurer to pay directly the provider for the product and service.

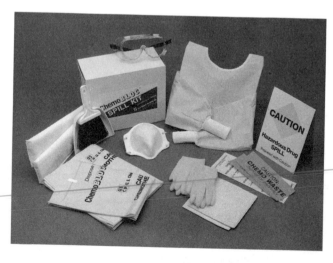

FIGURE 26-12 Home health care kit for final disposal in ChemoBLOC container. (Courtesy of U.S. Clinical Products, Dallas, TX)

TABLE 26-1
Home Intravenous Infusion Coverage

Payor	Antibiotic	Chemo	Hydration	Pain	HPN
Medicare A	—	Yes	—	No	—
Medicare B	No	Yes	No	Yes	No
Medicaid	—	Yes	—	Yes	Yes
PEN	No	No	No	No	Yes
HMO/PPO	Yes	Yes	Yes	Yes	Yes
Commercial	Yes	Yes	Yes	Yes	Yes
CHAMPUS	Yes	Yes	Yes	Yes	Yes

CHAMPUS, Civilian Health and Medical Programs for Uniformed Services; HPN, home parenteral nutrition; HMO, health maintenance organization; PPO, preferred provider organization; PEN, parenteral/enteral nutrition program.

Patient Copayment

Even on a reasonable charge basis, home infusion services are costly, and the patient may be required to pay a copayment. Medicare Part B will cover 80% of applicable allowable for the type of therapy provided; the remaining 20% is the responsibility of the patient. Commercial insurers routinely require 20% copayments on the part of the patient.

Third-Party Payors

Third-party payors for home infusion therapies include Medicare, Medicaid, commercial insurance, health maintenance organizations (HMOs), preferred provider organizations (PPOs), and managed care companies. The HMOs, PPOs, and managed care payors make determinations on a case-by-case basis and generally do not go "out of contract." An overview of various payment plans for therapies may be found in Table 26-1.

BIBLIOGRAPHY

Baldwin, D. (1992). Management of IV hazardous materials and hazardous wastes in the work environment. *Journal of Intravenous Nursing, 15*(2), 50.

Beason, R., Bourguignon, J., Fowler, D., & Gardner, C. (1992). Evaluation of a needle-free intravenous access system. *Journal of Intravenous Nursing, 15*(1), 11–13.

Malloy, J. A. (1990). Home care accreditation through Joint Commission on Accreditation of Healthcare Organizations. *Journal of Intravenous Nursing, 13*(3), 185–187.

Moeser, L. C. (1991). Anaphylaxis: A preventable complication of home infusion therapy. *Journal of Intravenous Nursing, 14*(2), 114.

Sheehan, K., & Gildea, J. (1985). Home antibiotic therapy: A less than ideal candidate. *Journal of the National Intravenous Therapy Association, 8*(3), 157.

Studebaker R. (1985). Home health agencies: Functions and reimbursement. *Journal of the National Intravenous Therapy Association, 8*(1), 43.

Terry, J. (1983). Home care utilizing Silastic catheters. *Journal of the National Intravenous Therapy Association, 6*(5), 348.

Weinstein, S. (1987). Regulatory concerns: Home care. *Journal of the National Intravenous Therapy Association, 10*(3), 175–184.

Weinstein, S. (1984). Intravenous therapy within the scope of home health services. *Journal of the National Intravenous Therapy Association, 7*(1), 39.

REVIEW QUESTIONS

1. The growth of home care is attributed to which of the following factors?
   a. aging population
   b. technology
   c. reimbursement
   d. baby boomers

2. Governmental agencies providing home care services include:
   a. state health departments
   b. county health departments
   c. university health clinics
   d. public clinics

3. Policies and procedures for the provision of home infusion services must be consistent with:
   a. published Standards of Practice
   b. JCAHO guidelines
   c. CHAP criteria
   d. ASHP standards

4. A case manager is responsible for which of the following activities?
   a. initial assessment
   b. development of a care plan
   c. appropriate referral and follow-up
   d. ongoing evaluation

5. Home infusion therapies may include:
   a. antibiotics
   b. parenteral nutrition
   c. hydration
   d. antiemetics

6. The first dose of an antibiotic drug should be given:
   a. in the home
   b. in a monitored environment
   c. by the patient
   d. by a professional

7. Patients are deemed appropriate candidates for home infusion therapy after assessment of:
   a. venous access
   b. drug therapy
   c. laboratory profile
   d. educability

8. Common diagnoses for antibiotic therapy include:
   a. Lyme disease
   b. osteomyelitis
   c. otitis media
   d. bronchitis

9. The plan of treatment in a home care program is written by the:
   a. pharmacist
   b. nurse
   c. physician
   d. branch manager

10. Claims documents include which of the following?
    a. UB–82
    b. HCFA–1500
    c. Part B billing form
    d. Part A billing form

Glossary

ABO System—a basic heredity blood group system; it denotes a patient's blood group

Adjuvant chemotherapy—the use of drugs in addition to surgery and/or radiation therapy administered to eradicate metastatic disease

Agglutination—clumping of red blood cells when incompatible bloods are mixed

Agglutinin—an antibody causing agglutination with its corresponding antigen

Alkylating agents—agents that kill cells by cross-linking DNA strands (*ie*, disturbing the normal structure) in the DNA molecule.

Alopecia—the loss of hair from the body and/or the scalp

Analogue—a compound that resembles another in structure, *eg*, fluorouracil is an analogue of uracil

Anorexia—absence or loss of appetite for food

Antibody—a substance present in the plasma that incites immunity; is capable of reacting with the specific antigen that caused its production

Anti–free-flow administration set—stops when removed from the electronic infusion device, yet allows gravity flow when the user takes action

Antigen—an immunizing agent capable of inducing the body to form antibodies

Antimetabolites—anticancer drugs that substitute for or block the use of an essential metabolite

Antimicrobial—an agent that destroys or prevents development of microorganisms

Antimicrobial ointment—a semisolid preparation used to prevent the pathogenic action of microbes

Antineoplastic agent—a medication or treatment for cancer

Antitumor antibiotics—anticancer drugs that interfere with cellular production of DNA and/or RNA

Arterial pressure monitoring—monitoring of arterial pressure through an indwelling arterial catheter connected to an electronic monitor

Arteriovenous (AV) fistula—the surgical anastomosis of an artery and vein

Arteriovenous (AV) grafts—the insertion of a synthetic device connecting a vein and an artery

Aseptic technique—mechanisms employed to reduce potential contamination

Assay determination—decision based upon an analysis and/or examination

Auscultation—process of listening for sounds in the body

Autologous—products or components of the same individual

Bacteria—a microorganism that may potentiate a diseased state

Blood grouping—the testing of red blood cells to determine antigens present and absent

Body surface area—surface area of the body determined through use of a nomogram; important when calculating dosages

Bone marrow—the inner spongy tissue of a bone where red blood cells, white blood cells, and platelets are formed

Cancer—the general name for more than 100 diseases in which abnormal cells grow out of control; a malignant tumor

Cannula—a hollow tube made of plastic or metal; used for accessing the vascular system

Catheter—a hollow tube made of plastic used for accessing the vascular system

Cell kill—the number of cancer cells killed at a given dose by an antineoplastic drug

Chemical incompatibility—a change in the molecular structure or pharmacologic properties of a substance, which may or may not be visually observed

Chemotherapy—the treatment of cancer patients with chemical agents designed to kill cancer cells

Cognitive—behaviors that place primary emphasis on the mental or intellectual processes

Cold agglutinin–a red blood cell agglutinin that acts at relatively low temperature; part of a disease process caused by a transient infectious disease; may be idiopathic

Color coding–system developed by manufacturers that identifies products/medications by the use of a color system. These color code systems are not standardized and may vary with manufacturer.

Compartment syndrome–compression of circulation evidenced by impaired pulses, compromised circulation, and pain

Compatibility–capable of being mixed and administered without undergoing undesirable chemical and/or physical changes or loss of therapeutic action

Compatibility test–all tests performed on donors and recipients to determine compatibility of blood; also known as the cross-match

Complement–a group of proteins in normal blood serum and plasma that in combination with antibodies causes the destruction of particular antigens

Contamination–introduction of pathogens or infectious material from one source to another

Corrective action–a defined plan to eliminate deficiencies

Cross contamination–movement of pathogens from one source to another

Curative–therapy that is either healing or corrective

Cutdown–surgical procedure for exposure and cannulation of a vein

Delayed reaction–adverse effect occurring after 48 hours and up to 180 days post-transfusion

Delivery system–a product(s) that allows for the administration of medication. These systems can be integral or have component parts. Delivery systems encompass all products used, from the solution container down to the cannula.

Disinfectant–an agent that eliminates all microorganisms except spores, generally used on inanimate objects

Distal–furthest from the heart; furthest from point of attachment; below previous site of cannulation

Distention–increase in size due to pressure within

Document–a record written or printed that contains original, official, or legal information

Documentation–a recording in written or printed form containing original, official, or legal information

Dome–a plastic component used in hemodynamic monitoring

Dose-limiting toxicity–the degree of toxicity that dictates the maximum amount of drug that safely can be administered

Electronic infusion device–an electronic instrument that is used to regulate the flow rate of the prescribed therapy. These are often referred to as EID.

Embolus–a blood clot or other foreign substance that is carried in the blood stream. It has the potential to impede and/or obstruct circulation.

Epidemiology–the division of medical science concerned with defining and explaining the interrelationships of the host, agent, and environment in causing disease

Epidural–located on or over the dura mater

Epithelialized–the growth of epithelial cells over a wound or over and around a catheter site

Erythema–redness of the skin

Extravasation–inadvertent administration of vesicant solution/medication into surrounding tissue

Filter–a porous device used to prevent the passage of undesired substances

Free-flow–nonregulated, inadvertent administration of fluid

Fungi–vegetable cellular organisms that subsist on organic matter

Gram negative bacteria–organism remaining unstained by the Gram's method; such as Klebsiella, *Escherichia coli, Pseudomonas, Serratia,* etc., associated with infusate contamination and arterial catheters

Gram positive bacteria–organism holding the dye after being stained by the Gram's method; such as *Staphylococcus epidermidis, Staphylococcus aureus,* etc., associated with venous catheter contamination

Hematocrit–an expression of the volume of red cells per unit of circulating blood

Hemodynamic pressure monitoring–the measurement of pulmonary artery pressure, arterial pressure, cardiac output, etc., via an electronic monitor

Hemoglobin–the iron-containing pigment of red blood cells functioning primarily in the transport of oxygen from the lungs to the tissues of the body

Hemolysis–rupture of the red cell membrane causing the release of hemoglobin

Hemorrhage–abnormal discharge of blood, either external or internal

Hemostasis–cessation of the flow of blood through a port or vessel

HLA system–human leukocyte antigens; a complex array of genes that are involved in immune regulation and cell differentiation

Hypercalcemia–serum calcium concentrations above normal levels

Hypertonic–solution more concentrated than that with which it is compared; a fluid having a concentration greater than the normal tonicity of plasma

Hyperuricemia–uric acid blood concentrations above normal levels

Hypotonic–solution less concentrated than that with which it is compared; a fluid having a concentration less than the normal tonicity of plasma

IgA–immunoglobulin A; a class of immunoglobulins in body secretions

IgG–immunoglobulin G; a class of immunoglobulins or circulating antibodies in the blood that frequently cause sensitization

IgM–immunoglobulin M; a class of immunoglobulins or circulating antibodies in the blood that are capable of binding complement

Immediate reaction–adverse effect occurring immediately or up to 48 hours post-transfusion

Immunocompromised–decrease resistance to disease

Immunoglobulin–a protein with antibody activity

Immunohematology–the study of blood and blood reactions

Implanted port/pump–vascular access device placed totally beneath the skin surface by surgical procedure

Incident–an unusual occurrence that requires documentation and action because of potential or implied consequences

Incompatible–incapable of being mixed or used simultaneously without undergoing chemical or physical changes or producing undesirable effects

Infection–invasion of the body by living microorganisms

Infiltration–the inadvertent administration of non-vesicant solution/medication into surrounding tissues

Infusate–parenteral solution administered into the vascular system

Integumentary–cutaneous; dermal

Intermittent intravenous therapy–administered at prescribed intervals with periods of infusion cessation

Intraosseous–within the cavity of a bone that is filled with marrow

Intrathecal–inside the spinal cord

Intrinsic contamination–contamination during product manufacture

Isolation–the separation of potentially infectious persons and/or materials

Isotonic–solution having the same concentration as that with which it is compared, *ie*, plasma

Laminar flow hood–a contained work area in which the air flow within a confined area moves with uniform velocity along parallel flow lines with a minimum of eddies

Latex injection port–a resealable rubber cap designed to accommodate needles for administration of solutions into the vascular system

Leukopenia–total number of leukocytes in the circulating blood less than normal, the lower limit of which generally is regarded as $5000/\mu/L$

Lumen–the interior space of a tubular structure, such as a blood vessel or cannula

Lymphedema–swelling of an extremity caused by obstruction of the lymphatic vessel(s)

Malignancy–uncontrolled growth and dissemination of a neoplasm

Medical act–procedure performed by a licensed physician

Metastasis–the spread of cancer to sites distant from the site of origin

Microabrasion–break in skin integrity which may predispose the patient to infection

Microaggregate–microscopic collection of particles such as platelets, leukocytes and fibrin, that occurs in stored blood

Microaggregate blood filter–filter that removes potentially harmful microaggregates and reduces non-hemolytic febrile reactions

Microorganisms–extremely minute living matter which can only be seen with the aid of a microscope

Monoclonal antibody–antibodies produced by a clone of cells derived from a single cell in large quantities for use against a specific antigen

Morbidity–number of infected persons or cases of infection in relation to a specific population

Mortality—ratio of number of deaths in a population to number of individuals in that population

Multiple-dose vial—medication bottle designed to be entered more than one time that is hermetically sealed with a rubber stopper

Nadir—the lowest level to which a blood count drops in response to an antineoplastic agent

Needle—a slender, pointed, hollow metal device

Neoplasm—a new growth or tumor, either benign or malignant

Nitrosoureas—anticancer drugs that produce metabolites that attack DNA in a manner analogous to alkylating agents

Non-permeable—ability to maintain integrity

Non-vesicant—intravenous medications, including but not limited to medications administered for cancer, which generally do not cause damage or sloughing of tissue

Obturator—instrument used to occlude a hollow cannula

Occluded—a cannula blockage due to precipitation and/or clot formation

Oncology—the study of tumors

Osmolarity—number of solutes contained in solution measured in milliosmoles per liter

Outcome—the interpretation of documented results

Palliative—treatment that may be provided for comfort and/or temporary relief of symptoms and does not cure

Palpable cord—a vein that is rigid and hard to the touch

Palpation—examination by touch

Parenteral—denoting any route other than the alimentary canal, such as intravenous

Parenteral nutrition—nutrients that are administered intravenously; comprised of carbohydrates, proteins, and/or fats, and additives such as electrolytes, vitamins, and trace elements

Paresthesia—abnormal spontaneous sensations (*eg,* burning, prickling, tingling, or tickling without physical stimulus)

Particulate matter—relating to or composed of fine particles

Pathogens—disease-producing microorganisms

Percutaneous puncture—puncture performed through the skin

Peripheral—pertains to veins of the extremities, scalp, and external jugular

Peripheral neuropathy—dysfunction of postganglion nerves, ranging from paresthesia to paralysis

Phlebitis—inflammation of a vein; may be accompanied by pain, erythema, edema, streak formation, and/or palpable cord. Rated by a standard scale (see phlebitis topic). A possible precursor to sepsis

Phlebotomy—withdrawal of blood from a vein

Physical incompatibility—an undesirable change that is visually observed

Plant alkyloids—anticancer drugs derived from plants, such as the periwinkle (vincristine and vinblastine)

Positive pressure—maintaining a constant, even force within a lumen to prevent reflux of blood; achieved while injecting by clamping or withdrawing needle from cannula

Post-infusion phlebitis—inflammation of a vein occurring after cannula removal

Pounds per square inch (psi)—a measurement of pressure, psi equals 50 mm Hg or 68 cm H_2O

Preservative-free—contains no added substance capable of inhibiting bacterial contamination

Process—actual performance and observation of performance based on compliance with policies, procedures, and professional standards

Product integrity—intact, uncompromised product; condition suitable for intended use

Proximal—nearest to the heart; closest to point of attachment; above previous site of cannulation

Pruritis—itching

Psychomotor—behaviors that place primary emphasis on the various degrees of physical skills and dexterity as they relate to the thought process

Purulent—containing or producing pus

Push—direct injection of a medication into a vein or access device

Quality assurance—an ongoing, systematic process for monitoring, evaluating, and problem solving

Radiopaque—ability to be detected by radiographic examination

Rh system—a blood group system denoting the presence or absence of D (Rh) red cell antigen

Risk management—process that centers on identification, analysis, treatment, and evaluation of real and potential hazards

Roller bandage—a roll of gauze or other material used for protecting an injured part, for immobilizing a limb, for keeping dressings in place, etc.

Sclerotic–fibrous thickening of the wall of the vein resulting in decreased lumen size. On palpation, usually feels hard to the touch

Semi-quantitative culture technique–a laboratory protocol used for isolating and identifying microorganisms

Sensitization–the initial exposure of an individual to a specific antigen that results in an immune response

Sepsis–the presence of infectious microorganisms or their toxins in the blood stream

Single-use vial–medication bottle intended for one-time use that is hermetically sealed with a rubber stopper

Skin-cannula junction–point at which the cannula enters the skin

Statistics–the science of collecting, classifying, and interpreting information based on the numbers of things

Stomatitis–sores on the inside of the mouth

Structure–describes the elements on which the program is based. These elements include resources such as federal and state laws, professional standards, position descriptions, patient rights, policies and procedures, documentation forms, quality controls, corrective action programs, etc.

Stylet–a rigid metal object within a catheter designed to facilitate insertion

Surfactant–material whose properties reduce the surface tension of fluid

Surveillance–the active, systematic, ongoing observation of the occurrence and distribution of disease within a population and of the events or conditions that increase or decrease the risk of such disease occurrence

Tamper-proof–inability to alter

Thrombocytopenia–decreased thrombocytes or platelets

Thrombolytic agent–a pharmacologic agent capable of dissolving blood clots

Thrombophlebitis–inflammation of the vein with clot formation

Thrombosis–formation of a blood clot within a blood vessel

Trace elements–minute amounts of essential elements present in the body

Transfusion reaction–any adverse effect to the transfusion of whole blood or its components or derivatives

Transparent semipermeable membrane (TSM)–a sterile dressing that allows visualization, is water resistant, and is air permeable

Trendelenburg–a position used to increase venous distention in which the head is lower than the feet

Tunneled catheter–a central catheter designed to have a portion lie within a subcutaneous passage before exiting the body

Valsalva maneuver–the process of making a forceful attempt at expiration with the mouth, nostrils, and glottis closed

Vascular access–means of approaching or entering the vascular system

Venipuncture–puncture of a vein for any purpose

Vesicant–intravenous medication that causes blisters and tissue injury when it escapes into the surrounding tissue(s)

Volumetric–relating to measurement of or by volume

Answers to Questions

Chapter 1 ————————————————

No questions for Chapter 1

Chapter 2 ————————————————

1. B
2. D
3. D
4. D
5. C

Chapter 3 ————————————————

1. D
2. D
3. A
4. A
5. B

Chapter 4 ————————————————

1. A
2. D
3. B
4. B
5. A

Chapter 5 ————————————————

1. D
2. C
3. C
4. A
5. B,C
6. D
7. D
8. D
9. D
10. A

Chapter 6 ————————————————

1. C
2. A
3. A
4. D
5. B
6. B,D
7. A,B,C,D
8. A,B,C,D
9. B
10. A,B,C,D

Chapter 7 ————————————————

1. A,B
2. A,C
3. A
4. A,B,C,D
5. A
6. B
7. A,B,D
8. A
9. A,B
10. D

Chapter 8 ————————————————

1. A
2. B
3. A,B,C,D
4. B
5. C
6. A
7. B
8. A,B,C
9. A,B,C,D
10. A,B,C

Chapter 9

1. A,C
2. D
3. A,B,D
4. A
5. A,B
6. A,B
7. A,B,C
8. A
9. B
10. C

Chapter 10

1. D
2. A
3. B
4. D
5. C
6. B
7. A
8. D
9. C
10. A

Chapter 11

1. A
2. B
3. A
4. C
5. C
6. B
7. D
8. B
9. A
10. C

Chapter 12

1. C
2. B
3. C
4. C
5. D
6. A
7. C
8. B
9. A
10. D

Chapter 13

1. B
2. B
3. A,B,C,D
4. A
5. C
6. D
7. B
8. D
9. A,B,D
10. A,B,C,D

Chapter 14

1. A
2. B
3. A
4. B
5. C
6. D
7. B,C
8. D
9. C
10. C

Chapter 15

1. C
2. A,B,C
3. A
4. A
5. A
6. D
7. A
8. B
9. C
10. D

Chapter 16

1. B
2. D
3. A
4. A,B,D
5. A,C
6. A,B
7. A,B,C
8. A
9. A,B,C
10. A

Chapter 17

1. A,B,C
2. C
3. D
4. A,B,C
5. A
6. A
7. C
8. B
9. C
10. A

Chapter 18

1. A,B,C
2. B
3. A,C
4. B
5. A
6. A,C
7. B
8. A
9. A
10. A

Chapter 19

1. A
2. B
3. C
4. A,B,C
5. A
6. A
7. B
8. A
9. A,B,C,D
10. A

Chapter 20

1. C
2. C
3. D
4. B
5. A
6. D
7. B
8. B
9. B
10. B

Chapter 21

1. A
2. C
3. A
4. D
5. B
6. C
7. A
8. C
9. C
10. A

Chapter 22

1. B
2. B
3. C
4. A,B
5. A,B,C
6. A,B,D
7. A,B,C,D
8. D
9. A,B,D
10. D

Chapter 23

1. A,B,C,D
2. A
3. A,B
4. A,D
5. A,B
6. A,B,C,D
7. C,D
8. C
9. A
10. A,B,C,D

Chapter 24

1. D
2. A,B,C,D
3. A
4. B
5. D
6. A
7. A,B,C,D
8. D
9. D
10. B

Chapter 25 _____

1. A
2. A
3. D
4. B
5. A
6. D
7. D
8. A
9. A
10. C

Chapter 26 _____

1. A,B,C
2. A,B
3. A,B,C,D
4. A,B,C,D
5. A,B,C,D
6. B,D
7. A,B,C,D
8. A,B,C
9. C
10. A,B

Standards of Practice: Nutrition Support Nurse

American Society for Parenteral and Enteral Nutrition (A.S.P.E.N.)

INTRODUCTION

A.S.P.E.N. is a professional society whose members are health care professionals—physicians, nurses, dietitians, pharmacists, and nutritionists—who are dedicated to optimum nutritional support of patients in health care settings and at home.

The diversity of A.S.P.E.N.'s professional membership reflects the basic importance of good nutrition to optimal health and the multidisciplinary team approach to sound nutritional support.

These Standards have been developed, reviewed, and approved by the following A.S.P.E.N. groups: Standards Committee, Nurses' Committee, Executive Committee, and Board of Directors.

These Standards of Practice for Nutrition Support Nursing should be used in conjunction with the following A.S.P.E.N. publications:

Definitions of Terms Used in A.S.P.E.N. Guidelines and Standards

Standards for Nutrition Support, Hospitalized Patients

Standards for Nutrition Support, Home Patients

Standards of Practice, Nutrition Support Dietitian

Standards of Practice, Nutrition Support Pharmacist

A.S.P.E.N. has developed these standards to promote the health and welfare of those patients in need of enteral and parenteral nutrition. The standards represent a consensus of A.S.P.E.N.'s members as to that minimal level of practice necessary to assure safe and effective enteral and parenteral nutrition care. A.S.P.E.N. disclaims any liability to any health care provider, patient, or other persons affected by these standards.

SCOPE OF PRACTICE

Role. Nutrition Support Nursing is the care of individuals with potential or known nutritional alterations. Nurses who engage in specialized nutrition support use specific expertise to enhance the maintenance and/or restoration of an individual's nutritional health. Physiological, metabolic, and behavioral principles, as well as technological advances, are considered when interventions that use the nursing process are planned. The nursing process includes ongoing assessment and planning of care, the provision of care, and an evaluation of the individual's response to the care delivered.

The Nutrition Support Nurse may function as a member of a multidisciplinary nutrition support service, team, or committee that coordinates the provision of specialized nutrition support in the hospital, home, or other settings. Because the care delivered by other health care professionals interfaces with Nutrition Support Nursing, common practice areas are approached from a collegial point of view.

Nutrition Support Nursing encompasses all nursing activities that promote optimal nutritional health. Nursing interventions are based upon scientific principles. These interventions are revised when changes occur in the individual's situation and/or when research data can be translated into new or different clinical practice. The scope of practice includes but is not limited to: direct patient care; consultation with nurses and other health professionals in a variety of clinical settings; education of patients, students, colleagues, and the public; participation in research; and administrative functions.

Goals.   Nutrition Support Nursing uses nursing expertise to optimize the maintenance or restoration of an individual's nutritional health. Identification of measurable outcomes requires data collection and frequent assessment. The Nutrition Support Nurse participates in the development and review of standards of care for nutrition support for the institution or provider. The following outcomes are specific to the individual who requires nutrition support nursing care:

- The individual demonstrates the anticipated responses to nutrition support interventions.
- The individual/family demonstrates a knowledge of nutritional requirements and self-care measures to meet these requirements.
- The individual experiences no preventable complications resulting from nutritional support interventions or related nursing care.
- The individual/family uses nutrition support methods that maintain or improve nutritional status.

CHAPTER I. ASSESSMENT

The Nutrition Support Nurse, in collaboration with other members of the health care team, assesses the individual who is or may become malnourished for adequacy of nutritional status.

Required Characteristics

1.1. The Nutrition Support Nurse shares in the responsibility of assuring that an appropriate nutritional assessment has been performed. This assessment may include the following parameters:
    1.1.1. Current weight
    1.1.2. History of weight changes (rapidity of changes, presence of edema or ascites)
    1.1.3. Height (plus head circumference in infants)
    1.1.4. Age
    1.1.5. Sex
    1.1.6. Clinical signs of malnutrition
    1.1.7. Laboratory evidence of malnutrition
    1.1.8. Nutrient intake prior to admission, including type and amount of supplements
    1.1.9. Food intolerance and allergies

1.1.10. Mechanical or physiological changes that affect (a) ingestion, digestion, absorption, or metabolism or (b) nutrient needs, *eg*, infancy, adolescence, or pregnancy

1.1.11. Psychological changes that affect nutrient intake

1.1.12. Acute and/or chronic diseases or conditions

1.1.13. Medications/substances with potential for drug/drug, drug/nutrient, or nutrient/nutrient interactions

1.1.14. Social, cultural, and religious factors that affect food preferences, ability to purchase and prepare food, and food intake patterns

1.1.15. Activity level

1.1.16. Periodic reassessment of any of the above

CHAPTER II: THERAPEUTIC PLAN

The Nutrition Support Nurse, in collaboration with other health care professionals and the individual/family, participates in the development of a therapeutic plan of care for the individual.

Required Characteristics

1.1. There is documentation of a nursing plan, policy, and/or procedure/protocol for nutritional care which is compatible with the multidisciplinary therapeutic plan of care.

1.2. There is documentation that the individual/family has been informed of and/or participated in developing the nursing plan of care.

1.3. The nursing plan of care considers goals of therapy, discharge planning, and individual/family education needs.

CHAPTER III: IMPLEMENTATION

Nursing interventions in collaboration with other health care professionals ensure that the individual receives the prescribed feeding formulation in a safe, accurate, and cost-effective manner, using an appropriate delivery system and access device.

Required Characteristics

1.1. The Nutrition Support Nurse participates in the development and review of procedures/protocols and policies related to the administration of feeding formulations and to the management of access devices.

1.2. The Nutrition Support Nurse participates in quality assurance activities related to the administration of feeding formulations and to the management of access devices.

1.3. The Nutrition Support Nurse participates in educational activities, for nursing staff and other members of the health care team, that are related to the administration of feeding formulations and the management of access devices.

1.4. Nursing interventions for the individual/family are appropriate to prevent or manage any side effects or complications related to (a) the feeding formulation or its administration, and/or (b) the access device.

1.5. The Nutrition Support Nurse participates in selection and monitoring of delivery systems appropriate for the administration of feeding formulations.

CHAPTER IV: PATIENT MONITORING

The Nutrition Support Nurse, in collaboration with other members of the health care team, monitors and evaluates the individual's response to nutrition support therapy.

Required Characteristics

1.1. The medical record includes documentation of the Nutrition Support Nurse's evaluation of the individual's responses to nursing interventions and overall progression with regard to the plan of care.

CHAPTER V: PROMOTION OF SELF-CARE

The Nutrition Support Nurse, in collaboration with other health care professionals, assists the individual/family to maintain a level of independent care that is both safe and appropriate.

Required Characteristics

1.1. There is documentation that the Nutrition Support Nurse provided and evaluated interventions to assist the individual/family toward maximum self-care.

1.2. There is documentation that the individual/family participated in the development of short- and long-term goals and in decisions about related resources needed after discharge from acute care.

1.3. There is documentation that the individual/family has acquired the necessary self-care skills.

CHAPTER VI: RESEARCH AND EDUCATION

The Nutrition Support Nurse has acquired current knowledge in the area of nutrition support and participates in continuing education.

Required Characteristics

1.1. The Nutrition Support Nurse participates in educational offerings.

1.2. The Nutrition Support Nurse incorporates current and appropriate research findings into clinical practice.

(Reprinted with permission of A.S.P.E.N.)

Standards of Practice: Standards for Home Nutrition Support

American Society for Parenteral and Enteral Nutrition (A.S.P.E.N.)

INTRODUCTION

A.S.P.E.N. is a professional society whose members are health care professionals—physicians, nurses, dietitians, pharmacists, and nutritionists—dedicated to optimum nutrition support of patients during hospitalization and rehabilitation.

A.S.P.E.N.'s diverse professional membership emphasizes the basic importance of good nutrition to good medical practice and the multidisciplinary team approach to sound nutrition.

These Standards have been developed, reviewed, and approved by the following A.S.P.E.N. groups: Standards Committee, Executive Committee, and Board of Directors.

The following terms were defined during the revision of the home nutrition support standards and are used in these standards.

1. Home nutrition therapy—the provision of nutrients and any necessary adjunctive therapeutic agents to patients by administration into the intestine or stomach or by intravenous infusion for the purpose of improving or maintaining a patient's nutrition status in the home environment.

2. Referring physician—the physician who develops and retains the ultimate authority for the patient's treatment plan.

3. Physician/nutrition support team—physician or nutrition support team under the guidance of a physician.

4. Treatment plan—orders established and signed by the referring physician for the care of the home patient (*ie*, the medical orders including: nutrients, medications, activity orders, access site orders, etc).

5. Care plan—a plan of professional clinical activities developed by the home nutrition therapy provider to implement the treatment plan.

6. Home nutrition therapy provider—the organizations providing the nutrients, medications, supplies, equipment, and professional clinical services to a home nutrition therapy patient in accordance with these standards.

7. Feeding formulation—a ready-to-administer mixture of nutrients.

These Standards of Practice for Home Nutrition Support should be used in conjunction with the following A.S.P.E.N. publications:

Definitions of Terms Used in A.S.P.E.N. Guidelines and Standards

Standards for Nutrition Support, Hospitalized Patients

Standards of Practice, Nutrition Support Dietitian

Standards of Practice, Nutrition Support Pharmacist

Standards of Practice, Nutrition Support Nursing

Standards of Practice, Nutrition Support Physician

A.S.P.E.N. has developed these standards to promote the health and welfare of those patients in need of enteral and parenteral nutrition. The standards represent a consensus of A.S.P.E.N.'s members as to that minimal level of practice necessary to assure safe and effective enteral and parenteral nutrition care. A.S.P.E.N. disclaims any liability to any health care provider, patient, or other persons affected by these standards.

ORGANIZATION STANDARDS

Standard 1.   The referring physician/nutrition support team (NST) responsible for home nutrition support shall be clearly identified and their roles defined.

1. The physician who has expertise in home parenteral and enteral nutrition support is primarily responsible for the patient's nutrition care. The physician acts in concert with a registered nurse, a dietitian, and a registered pharmacist. Each of these health care professionals shall have appropriate education, specialized training, and experience in home parenteral and enteral nutrition.

2. Home nutrition support services shall be initiated, modified, supervised, evaluated, and coordinated by the physician/NST.

Standard 2.   The physician/NST caring for home parenteral and enteral nutrition patients shall be guided by written policies and procedures specifically designed to address the needs of the home patient or the patient in transition to home care.

1. There shall be written policies and procedures concerning the scope and provision of home parenteral and enteral nutrition services.

2. These written policies and procedures shall be developed by the physician/NST in conjunction with other professionals, as appropriate.

3. These policies and procedures shall be reviewed at least every 3 years and revised as appropriate to reflect optimal standards of care.

4. Written policies and procedures shall include but not be limited to:
   4.1 The roles, responsibilities, and 24-hour availability of care from the physician/NST and home nutrition therapy provider.
   4.2 Defined criteria for patient eligibility and selection, which might include: medical suitability; rehabilitative potential; social and economic factors; and educational, psychological, and emotional factors pertinent to the patient and others who are significantly involved in this care.
   4.3 A mechanism for referral to a knowledgeable and experienced home nutrition therapy provider for acquisition and delivery of enteral or intravenous nutrients, equipment, and supplies, with consideration for patient's freedom of choice.
   4.4 Education of patient/caregiver.
   4.5 A mechanism for patient monitoring (*eg*, frequency of follow-up contact, laboratory studies, response to nutrition therapy, and physical examination).

4.6 A mechanism for referral to consultative medical services and services of other professionals (eg, psychologists and social workers) and nonprofessionals (eg, patient support groups), as appropriate.

4.7 Reimbursement mechanisms for payment for services, equipment, and supplies.

4.8 Preparation, storage of, and techniques for administering a feeding formulation in the home.

4.8.1 Feeding schedules.

4.8.2 Care of feeding tubes and equipment for patients receiving enteral formulas.

4.8.3 Care of catheters and tubing for patients receiving intravenous nutrition.

4.8.4 Care and maintenance of electronic infusion devices.

4.8.5 Care and maintenance of feeding formulations.

4.9 Prevention, management, and timely response to complications in the home, and emergency consultation with professional staff.

4.10 A mechanism for timely communication and collaboration among the physician/NST, home nutrition therapy provider, patient, caregiver, and other health care professionals involved.

4.11 A mechanism for quality assurance, which shall include but not be limited to mortality, hospital readmission, and complications.

Standard 3.   Home parenteral and enteral nutrition services shall be documented.

1. Medical records shall be maintained for every patient receiving home parenteral and enteral nutrition and shall include but not be limited to:

1.1 Designation of a physician with expertise in parenteral and enteral nutrition having primary responsibility for patient's home nutrition care.

1.2 All pertinent patient diagnoses and prognoses, including long- and short-term treatment objectives.

1.3 A nutrition assessment and medical evaluations, with follow-up as appropriate.

1.4 Scope and results of initial and ongoing education of patient/caregiver.

1.5 Treatment plan shall include orders established and signed by the referring physician for care of the patient (which include medical orders for nutrients, medications, activity level, access-site care).

1.6 A care plan including consideration of functional limitations of the patient, activities permitted, psychosocial needs, suitability of home environment for provision of home nutrition services, and name(s) of other individual(s) who will assist in care of the patient if required.

1.7 A current medication profile including prescription and nonprescription drugs, home remedies, and known allergies or sensitivities.

1.8 Signed and dated progress notes for each contact between the patient and physician/NST or home nutrition therapy provider (*eg*, home visit, clinic visit, telephone contact, and rehospitalization). Progress notes shall report response to nutrition therapy including but not limited to results of serial monitoring, complications, and revisions in the therapeutic regimen.

1.9 Signed and dated progress notes for each contact between the home nutrition therapy provider and the physician/NST including but not limited to results of serial monitoring, complications, and revision in the therapeutic regimen.

1.10 A summary statement at termination of nutrition therapy including but not limited to the reason for terminating treatment, complications, patient outcome, and followup.

Standard 4. The home parenteral and enteral nutrition treatment and care plan shall be reviewed, evaluated, and updated regularly by the physician/NST to determine overall appropriateness, effectiveness, and safety.

1. Evaluation of patient's need for and response to home parenteral and enteral nutrition shall be the responsibility of the physician/NST.

2. This review and evaluation shall be performed and documented periodically as dictated by patient's medical and nutrition status.

3. The treatment and care plan shall be revised based on the review, and changes shall be communicated and implemented.

PATIENT SELECTION STANDARD

Standard 5. Indications and contraindications for home parenteral and enteral nutrition are as follows:

1. The patient shall be carefully evaluated prior to selection for home parenteral and enteral nutrition.

   1.1 A patient who is a candidate for home enteral nutrition should be unable to meet nutrient requirements by voluntary oral intake. A patient who is a candidate for home parenteral nutrition should be unable to meet nutrient requirements via the gastrointestinal tract safely and adequately.

   1.2 The patient's home environment should be such that the physician, in consultation with the appropriate social worker or other health professional, concludes that home therapy is more appropriate than long-term institutional care.

   1.3 The treatment and care plan should be designed to achieve the home parenteral or enteral nutrition objectives.

   1.4 The patient's home environment should be appropriate for the safe use of home parenteral or enteral nutrition support.

   1.5 The patient/caregiver should be willing and able to perform home parenteral or enteral nutrition support procedures.

   1.6 The patient/caregiver should be knowledgeable about therapeutic expectations, risks, benefits, and responsibilities (financial and other) of home parenteral or enteral nutrition and should agree to participate.

2. The patient/caregiver should understand the rationale, risks, benefits, and therapeutic options regarding nutrition support.

3. The patient and/or family should understand the cost of equally suitable nutrition support approaches and alternatives, insurance coverage, and financial responsibilities.

4. An evaluation of the nutrient needs of the patient shall be performed prior to the initiation of home parenteral or enteral nutrition support.

4.1 Nutrition requirements shall take into account the patient's disease state, nutrition status, activity level, and growth requirements.

4.2 The anticipated duration and route of nutrient administration shall be determined.

4.3 The goals for home parenteral or enteral nutrition support shall be established in consideration of the immediate and long-term needs of the patient.

TREATMENT PLAN STANDARDS

Standard 6. The home parenteral and enteral nutrition treatment plan shall be determined and documented prior to the initiation of treatment and on an ongoing basis.

1. Elements of the treatment plan should include but are not limited to:
   1.1 Nutrition goals.
   1.2 Prescribed nutrients (type and dose of calories, protein, fluid volume, vitamins, minerals, trace elements, and electrolytes).
   1.3 Infusion times and rates.
   1.4 On-and-off tapering schedule.
   1.5 Specialized techniques of preparation and administration in the home setting.
   1.6 Care of access device, equipment, solutions, and formulas.
   1.7 Prescriptions for home parenteral or enteral solutions, medications, items, etc.
   1.8 Clinical monitoring (see Standard 13).
   1.9 Laboratory monitoring (see Standard 13).
   1.10 When appropriate, methods for transition from parenteral to enteral or oral nutrition and from enteral to oral nutrition.

2. Short-term goals should be developed and may include resolution of disease progression, wound healing, progression to enteral support, and oral nutrition.

3. Long-term goals should be developed and may include maintenance of normal nutrition and rehabilitation to physical and social independence.

4. Objectives should be developed prior to the initiation of nutrition support and on an ongoing basis as needed dependent on medical and nutrition evaluations.

Standard 7. The route(s) selected to provide home parenteral or enteral nutrition support shall be appropriate to meet assessed nutrient requirements and achieve treatment plan goals and objectives.

1. The safest, most cost-effective route that meets the patient's needs and preferences should be used.

2. The physician/NST should recognize that as the patient's therapy progresses, the optimal feeding mode may change and may, at times, include a combination of oral, enteral and parenteral feedings.

3. Use of the enteral route is preferred for patients who have a functioning and accessible gastrointestinal tract that can be safely used.

Standard 8. The selected home parenteral or enteral formula shall be appropriate for the disease process and compatible with other medications, therapy, and access route, and shall meet nutrient needs.

1. The formulation selection and modification should be directed by the physician/NST.

2. The patient should be given a copy of the prescriptions for the feeding formulation and other medications.

IMPLEMENTATION STANDARD

Standard 9.   The access device and infusion method shall be appropriate for home use.

1. Selection of the access device should be based on safety and efficacy, and consideration should be given to patient preference.

2. The placement of parenteral and enteral devices should be performed or supervised by a physician proficient in such placement.
   2.1 Parenteral access
       2.6.1 Central venous lines or implanted ports should be placed by a physician.
       2.6.2 Peripherally inserted central catheter (PICC) lines should be placed by a physician or a nurse (where allowed by state nursing licensure boards).
   2.2 Enteral access
       2.2.1 Nasogastric tubes should be placed by a health care professional or patient/caregiver who has been properly trained and is proficient in such placement.
       2.2.2 Nasoduodenal or nasojejunal tubes must be placed by a physician or a health care professional designated by the physician.
       2.2.3 Percutaneous enterostomy (gastrostomy or jejunostomy) tubes must be placed by a physician or under the guidance of a physician; subsequent replacement may be done by a health care professional or patient/caregiver proficient in such placement, as designated by the physician.

3. Policies and procedures shall be established to address access to implanted ports and central venous lines, and reintroduction of each type of feeding tube.

4. The nutrient infusion method or electronic infusion device selected should be suitable for home use.
   4.1 Selection should be based on safety and cost-effectiveness.
   4.2 Consideration should be given to patient preference, volume to be infused, type of regimen (cyclic, continuous, or intermittent), and activity level of the patient.

Standard 10.   The patient/caregiver shall receive education and demonstrate competence in the preparation and administration of home parenteral and enteral nutrition support.

1. The patient/caregiver receiving home parenteral nutrition should be instructed in:
   1.1 Proper storage of formulated and admixed parenteral feeding formulations.
   1.2 Inspection of home parenteral nutrition containers and contents.
   1.3 Aseptic technique required for the admixture procedure and administration via access device.

    1.4 Compatibility and stability of nutrition and coadministered solutions under refrigeration or at room temperature.

    1.5 Infusion method.

    1.6 Use of parenteral infusion equipment.

    1.7 Proper disposal of used containers, tubing, and needles.

    1.8 Drug–nutrient and nutrient–nutrient interactions.

    1.9 Medication information and administration.

2. The patient/caregiver receiving home enteral nutrition should be instructed in:

    2.1 Proper storage for ready-to-feed or formula that requires mixing.

    2.2 Inspection of enteral products for contents and expiration date.

    2.3 Clean technique for preparation of formula, administration, and reuse of supplies and equipment.

    2.4 Stability of formula at room temperature.

    2.5 Infusion method.

    2.6 Use of enteral feeding equipment.

    2.7 Timing, method of administration, and compatibility of any medications via enteral access.

    2.8 Drug–nutrient and nutrient–nutrient interactions.

    2.9 Medication information and administration.

    2.10 Product hang time.

3. Educational material tailored to the patient and the therapy is provided to the patient/caregiver for use at home.

4. Patient/caregiver education should include periodic reassessment and retraining as needed.

Standard 11.   The patient/caregiver shall receive education and demonstrate competence in access route care.

1. The patient/caregiver receiving parenteral infusions should be trained in:

    1.1 Aseptic techniques to access and maintain the access device.

    1.2 Connecting and disconnecting the intravenous tubing to the catheter.

    1.3 Post-infusion flushing to prevent catheter occlusion.

2. The patient/caregiver receiving enteral feedings should be trained in:

    2.1 Clean techniques for handling the tube.

    2.2 Maintaining the access site.

    2.3 Flushing the tube to maintain patency.

Standard 12.   The patient/caregiver shall receive education and demonstrate competence in the recognition and appropriate response to complications.

1. Patient/caregiver should be able to recognize and respond to indications of potential metabolic complications.

2. Patient/caregiver should be able to recognize mechanical and procedural problems that include but are not limited to:

    2.1 Catheter or tube occlusion, leakage, breakage, or dislodgement.

    2.2 Equipment malfunction or breakage.

    2.3 Infusate contamination or precipitate or inhomogeneity.

3. Patient/caregiver should be able to recognize and report any signs/symptoms of a localized or systemic infectious process.

4. Patient/caregiver should know when and whom to contact when complications occur.

PATIENT MONITORING STANDARD

Standard 13. The patient shall be monitored for therapeutic efficacy, adverse effects, and clinical changes that may influence specialized nutrition support.

1. Protocols should be developed for periodic review of the patient's clinical and biochemical status.
2. Routine monitoring should include:
   2.1 Continued need to therapy.
   2.2 Nutrient intake.
   2.3 Review of current medications.
   2.4 Signs of intolerance to therapy.
   2.5 Weight changes.
   2.6 Biochemical, hematologic, and other pertinent data including clinical signs of nutrient deficiencies and excesses.
   2.7 Adjustment to therapy.
   2.8 Changes in lifestyle.
   2.9 Psychosocial problems.
   2.10 Changes in the home environment.
3. Assessment of the patient's major organ functions should be made periodically.
4. Psychosocial aspects of the patient/caregiver should be reassessed periodically.

TERMINATION OF THERAPY STANDARD

Standard 14.   Prior to discontinuation of parenteral or enteral nutrition support one of the following criteria shall be applicable:

1. Parenteral nutrition should not be discontinued until nutrient requirements can be met by enteral or oral nutrition.
2. Enteral nutrition should not be discontinued until nutrient requirements can be met by oral nutrition.
3. Parenteral or enteral nutrition support should be discontinued whenever the patient's medical condition, especially complications, so indicates.
4. Parenteral or enteral nutrition support should be terminated when the physician and patient judge that the patient no longer benefits from the therapy. The decision to discontinue support must be made according to accepted community standards of medical care and in compliance with applicable law.

(Reprinted with permission of A.S.P.E.N.)

Index

Page numbers followed by *f* indicate figures; page numbers followed by *t* indicate tabular material.